# Reconstructive
# Plastic Surgical Nursing

*Observation* tells us the fact, **reflection** the meaning of the fact . . . *observation* tells us how the patient is, **reflection** tells us what is to be done.

*The trained power of attending to one's own senses, so that these should tell the nurse how the patient is, is the* sine qua non *of being a nurse at all.*

*Florence Nightingale 1882*

# Reconstructive Plastic Surgical Nursing

Clinical Management and Wound Care

**Jill E. Storch** RN, RM, BEd, MEd St, MRCNA

*Research Associate (Nursing) to Professor GI Taylor AO*
*Reconstructive Plastic Surgery Research Unit*
*University of Melbourne*
*Australia*

**&**

**Jan Rice** RN, Plas Surg Cert.

*Manager, Education and Clinical Services*
*Wound Foundation of Australia*
*Department of Pharmacy Practice*
*Victorian College of Pharmacy/Monash University*
*Melbourne, Australia*

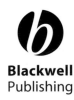

**Blackwell**
Publishing

Editorial offices:
Blackwell Publishing Ltd, 9600 Garsington Road, Oxford OX4 2DQ, UK
    Tel: +44 (0)1865 776868
Blackwell Publishing Inc., 350 Main Street, Malden, MA 02148-5020, USA
    Tel: +1 781 388 8250
Blackwell Publishing Asia Pty Ltd, 550 Swanston Street, Carlton, Victoria 3053, Australia
    Tel: +61 (0)3 8359 1011

First published 2005 by Blackwell Publishing Ltd

Library of Congress Cataloging-in-Publication Data
Storch, Jill E.
    Reconstructive plastic surgical nursing : clinical management & wound care / Jill E. Storch and Jan Rice.
        p. ; cm.
    Includes bibliographical references and index.
    ISBN-13: 978-1-4051-0165-3 (pbk. : alk. paper)
    ISBN-10: 1-4051-0165-2 (pbk. : alk. paper)
    1. Surgical nursing.  2. Surgery, Plastic.  3. Wounds and injuries–Nursing.
    [DNLM: 1. Perioperative Nursing–methods.  2. Reconstructive Surgical Procedures.  3. Surgery, Plastic–methods.
4. Wounds and Injuries–nursing. WY 161 S884r 2005]  I. Rice, Jan, R.N.  II. Title.
RD99.S89  2005
617.9'520231 – dc22
                                                                                            2004029531

ISBN-13: 978-14051-0165-3
ISBN-10: 1-4051-0165-2

A catalogue record for this title is available from the British Library

Set in 9 on 11 pt palatino
by SNP Best-set Typesetter Ltd., Hong Kong
Printed and bound in India
by Replika Press Pvt, Ltd

The publisher's policy is to use permanent paper from mills that operate a sustainable forestry policy, and which has been manufactured from pulp processed using acid-free and elementary chlorine-free practices. Furthermore, the publisher ensures that the text paper and cover board used have met acceptable environmental accreditation standards.

For further information on Blackwell Publishing, visit our website:
www.blackwellnursing.com

# Contents

Contents

Contents

# Foreword

Pioneered by Sir Harold Gillies in the UK, modern plastic surgery evolved during the two Great Wars to restore to society the mutilated unfortunates of these two conflicts. Gillies established concepts and principles of plastic surgery that were rapidly taken up by clinicians across the Western World leading to the establishment of many dedicated plastic surgery centres.

Sir Benjamin Kenneth Rank (Benny, or BKR to his associates) trained under Gillies and established plastic surgery in Australia, first at the Heidelberg Repatriation Hospital, then at the Royal Melbourne Hospital and finally at Preston and Northcote Community Hospital (PANCH) in Melbourne, Australia, where he negotiated the development of a specialist 60 bed premises named the Victorian Plastic Surgery Unit (VPSU). This unit became Australia's major plastic surgery teaching unit for both medical and nursing graduates and launched the careers of many committed clinicians.

BKR surrounded himself with a dedicated team of nurses in the theatre and in the two wards. The nursing authors of this book, Jill Storch and Jan Rice, established a long relationship of more than three decades with the VPSU and have combined their extensive experience to provide this 'first' in the plastic surgery nursing literature.

Jill and Jan's introduction to the evolution of modern plastic surgery was both unique and timely. The 'anatomical renaissance' was about to happen as microsurgery transformed distant tissue transfer from a multistage protracted scenario of uncomfortable tube pedicle operations – confined usually to the young – to a one stage transplant. However, these highly complex microsurgical procedures, which involved suturing of the blood vessels of the transplant to those at the recipient site, were not without their problems. These operations were at first protracted (often extending for more than 12 hours) and when they went wrong they really went wrong – the whole transplant was lost! Never before did *'so much depend on so few'* – the nightingales in the theatre and in the ward.

Jill Storch was in charge of the operating theatres (ORs) when the world first free skin flap was performed at PANCH by a couple of modern surgical pioneers, 'volunteer' scrub nurses and a long suffering and loyal anaesthetic team. Nearly every microsurgical transplant that followed was a *'first'*, whether bone, nerve, muscle or tendon. The waters were unchartered, the learning wave was steep and we were often dumped. So much depended on the dedication of Jill and her staff in the operating theatre, the organisational skills of the unit managers, and proficiency of the nursing staff in the plastic surgery wards, to prevent the flap from floundering.

Initially, at the VPSU, Jill Murphy, an experienced Australian (UK trained plastic surgery nurse) set up an accredited specialist six months plastic surgery nurse training course. When 'Murph' moved up the professional ladder, Jill Storch took over this role for more than eight years, establishing the course at university level allowing students to move from graduate diploma to clinical doctorate level within the specialty of plastic surgery nursing. Her colleague, Jan Rice, became an expert in wound management and set up a clinical and educational service at a major university teaching centre that continues to this day providing on-site and distance learning programmes.

This book, therefore, is unique. Written by these two nurse clinicians (who often assumed the role of 'surgeons') and based on their vast national and international experience over more than 30 years at an important time in the history of plastic surgery. It is intended for the training of nurses and covers the patient's pathway through their preoperative, operative and postoperative care. It covers a wide range of plastic surgical procedures and wound types that will confront both the trainee and the trained nurse.

Practice concepts are based on the important foundations of anatomy, physiology and pathology commencing at the cellular level. The format is easy to read, the style clear and concise, the illustrations are liberal, with summary boxes and figures as useful *aide mémoires* to bring the text to life, and the references, cross-references and internet sources are helpful.

This book is a valuable guide for both the nurse and the doctor. The authors are to be commended on this labour of love and their dedication. It is a privilege to know Jill and Jan, to have worked and learnt from them, and to have been asked to write this Foreword.

**G. Ian Taylor** AO
*Director*
*The Jack Brockhoff Reconstructive Plastic Surgery*
*Research Unit of the Royal Melbourne Hospital and*
*University of Melbourne*
*Melbourne, Australia*

# Preface

The preservation and maintenance of the functional integrity of the skin is fundamental for the basic survival of the human organism. The history of reconstructive plastic surgery and its associated nursing care is historically founded on the management of patients with simple and complex wounds regardless of their congenital, traumatic or disease based aetiology.

Although a large number of professional surgical nurses are charged with providing technical and general nursing care, much of what physiologically occurs at the microcirculatory and the cellular level within a wound, is little understood or appreciated. If professional nurses are to make a difference to patient outcomes, in addition to traditional care, this scientific knowledge is essential to holistic patient management.

Taking an evidence-based scientific approach to clinical nursing is challenging, as much of what can be classified as 'nursing practice' or 'patient care' has not been identified or researched in depth at the clinical level. The challenge is to be able to state the 'point of difference' the nurse's presence makes to the care of the patient at all stages of management.

**Section I** outlines a basic nursing framework through which patient care may be approached.

**Sections II–VI** have endeavoured to discuss patient care by integrating functional anatomy, contemporary reconstructive plastic surgical research, and nursing research, in an effort to assist the nurse practitioner in understanding 'the why?' in addition to 'the what?' of their clinical actions.

For the plastic surgery nursing expert there is perhaps little described in this book that is new. For the beginner practitioner, and those many nurses working in integrated surgical units, this book endeavours to convey a framework through which nurses charged with caring for patients treated under the clinical umbrella of reconstructive plastic surgery, may gain a greater understanding of their daily practice, and contribute to 'best practice' clinical and patient outcomes.

The authors of this book have had a long and enduring professional passion for reconstructive surgery nursing practice. It is hoped that the information contained within will assist those who are also involved in this clinically demanding area of patient care.

# Applying this Book to Clinical Practice

The authors of this book had four principal objectives in the presentation of this book:

1. The first was to present the concept of 'caring' through a simple practice framework that could be applied to address complex nursing care within reconstructive plastic surgery nursing. To this end, Chapter 2 outlines practice principles on how to approach the complexities of plastic surgery nursing and patient/client care. These principles are applied wherever possible throughout Sections II–VI. To gain optimal advantage from this book an examination of Chapter 2 is strongly advised prior to advancing to Sections II–VI.

2. The second was to address wound management as it is applied within plastic surgery. Section II discusses this subject in detail, including the functional anatomy of the skin, wound assessment, dressing products and practical wound management in a broad range of settings.

3. The third was to provide an outline of the perioperative episode and its influence on patient care in the postoperative period. Section III discusses the principal issues required for safe patient outcomes for both adults and children.

4. The fourth was to combine the first three objectives to provide a pathway through which nursing care of common reconstructive plastic surgical procedures could be addressed. By using a range of means throughout this book, including clinical photos, diagrams, tables, and review boxes which refer the reader to relevant sections elsewhere in the book, we hope we have, in some way, achieved this goal.

Author notes:

- The recently published *Blueprints – Plastic Surgery* (2005, Blackwell Publishing), by Jesse A. Taylor, is highly recommended as a pocketbook for easy orientation to common plastic surgical procedures.
- For US readers, in May 2005 the American Nurses Association released *Plastic Surgery Nursing: Scope and Standards of Practice*, available online at http://wwwnursingworld.org/.
- Subsequent new information, including companion Blackwell Publishing publications and writer contacts to support this book, will be available online at http://www.plasticsurgerynursing.info.

# Abbreviations Used in This Book

| | |
|---|---|
| ABCD | Asymmetry – border – colour – diameter |
| ABPI | Ankle brachial pressure index |
| ADL | Activities of daily living |
| AJCC | American Joint Committee on Cancer |
| ASA | American Society of Anaesthesiologists |
| ASPSN | American Society of Plastic Surgical Nurses |
| AVIS | Arterio-venous impulse systems |
| AWBM | Acute wound bed management |
| BCC | Basal cell carcinoma |
| BHS | Beta haemolytic streptococcus |
| BOTOX® | botulinum toxin type A |
| BP | Blood pressure |
| CFC | Chlorofluorocarbon |
| CFU | Colony forming units |
| CVP | Central venous pressure |
| CWBM | Chronic wound bed management |
| DVT | Deep vein thrombosis |
| ECG | Electrocardiogram |
| EWMA | European Wound Management Association |
| FTSG | Full thickness skin graft |
| HRT | Hormone replacement therapy |
| ICF | Intracranial fluid |
| ICN | International Council of Nurses |
| ICU | Intensive care unit |
| IM | Intramuscular |
| IV | Intravenous |
| LMW | Low molecular weight heparin |
| MASH | Mobile army service hospitals |
| MIDS | Modular internal distraction system |
| MLD | Manual lymphatic drainage |
| MM | Malignant melanoma |
| MRI | Magnetic resonance imaging |
| MRSA | Methicillin resistant *Staphylococcus aureus* |
| MSH | Melanin stimulating hormone |
| mtDNA | Mitochondrial DNA |
| MWH | Moist wound healing |
| NANDA | North American Nursing Diagnosis Association |
| NICU | Neonatal intensive care unit |
| nm | nanometres, used to measure the wavelength of light |
| NP | Negative pressure |
| NS | Normal saline |
| NSAID | Non-steroidal anti-inflammatory drug |
| NUK® | a brand of teat useful in the feeding of babies with cleft lip or cleft palate |
| PACU | Post anaesthesia care unit |
| PCA | Patient controlled analgesia |
| PE | Pulmonary embolism |
| PEG | Percutaneous endoscopic gastrostomy |
| PEM | Protein-energy malnutrition |
| PONV | Post-operative nausea and vomiting |
| POP | Plaster of Paris |
| psi | pounds per square inch – a measure of pressure |
| PTSD | Post-traumatic stress disorder |
| PWBM | Palliative wound bed management |
| RACE | Rest – alignment – compression – elevation |
| RCN | Royal College of Nursing (UK) |
| RCT | Randomised controlled trial |
| RICE | Rest – immobilisation – comfort – elevation |
| RR | Recovery room |
| SCC | Squamous cell carcinoma |
| SCD | Sequential compression devices |
| SMAS | Superficial musculoaponeurotic system |
| STSG | Split thickness skin grafts |
| TCA | Trichloroacetic acid |
| TED | Thrombo-embolitic device/deterrent |
| TENS | Transcutaneous electrical nerve stimulation |
| TMJ | Temporomandibular joint |
| TRAM | Transverse rectus abdominis muscle |

**TSA(N)PT** Topical sub-atmospheric (negative) pressure therapy, called negative pressure therapy throughout this book
**UAL** Ultrasonic assisted liposuction
**VAC** Vacuum assisted closure
**VQ** ventilation-perfusion scan (lung scan to check for pulmonary embolism)

**WBA** Wound bed assessment
**WBM** Wound bed maintenance/management
**WBP** Wound bed preparation
**WBR** Wound bed repair
**WHO** World Health Organization

# Section I
## Reconstructive Plastic Surgery Nursing Practice – Foundation and Practice Framework

# Chapter 1

# Reconstructive Plastic Surgery Nursing Practice

## Origins and definitions

The origin of the science, art and practice of reconstructive plastic surgery is based on the care of wounds, regardless of aetiology, and the restoration of the accepted normal functional ability and aesthetic form of conditions following the presentation of congenital malformations, trauma or disease.

The original term 'plastic surgery' is derived from the Greek words *plastikos* or *plassein*, meaning 'to mould', and *chirurgia*, the Latin word for surgery[1,2]. Its formal use was first noted in a medical lexicon in the early 19th Century when a German surgeon, Von Graefe, used it in a monograph describing how he had remoulded a nose by reconstructing the patient's skin to restore both function and aesthetics[1,2].

Although the term 'to mould' in contemporary terminology implies more of a concern with an artificial or contrived design, within surgery it is related to restoring particular form and function by redefining and/or replacing the missing tissue mould/s or form/s.

Early records, (the writings of Susrutra, India, circa 600–800 BC), demonstrate that particular shapes of the nose and ear lobes commanded respect thought to reflect the status of the tribe or individual[1,2]. Amputation of these body parts was a common punishment, used to ostracise criminals – and even respected citizens of conquered cities – to denote their fall from power. In some cultures, the practice of nasal amputation for adultery was seen as the ultimate way to make the perpetrator unattractive. This also marked out the individual within society. Those who led their countries' armies in search of increasing land and influence often suffered from nasal amputations as a result of sword and knife fights. Duels between opposing men were common practice to settle disagreements over money, personal family integrity, or the female sex. All these conflicts resulted in various forms of facial trauma.

Subsequently, influential and wealthy victims of this injury sought physicians who attempted to use the patient's normal skin tissue for the restoration of the physical and aesthetic form of the nose, rather than using metal covers or wooden prostheses. Personal aesthetics were important, with ear reconstruction a particularly popular reconstructive procedure.

It was recorded by the famous physician of the age, Celsus, that in Roman times, defects were closed by the use of advancement flaps – another form of skin movement. The search continued, with many attempts being made to reconstruct the nose using skin designed as a connected, tubed skin flap (referred to as a pedicle) from the forehead, or from the upper forearm to the nose[1,2]. These pedicles were disconnected when healing was deemed to have taken place or to have failed. Even greater heights of research into these concepts were achieved when the European work was translated into the English language during the 19th Century. The rationale for determining success or failure of skin flaps would not be fully understood until the flow of blood in the body was recognised in the 1930s to be a closed circulatory process.

Although there were great advances in the middle of the 20th Century, few individuals have contributed to the early written history of reconstructive plastic surgery more than Gaspare Tagliacozzi (1549–1599)[1,2] (Figure 1.1).

In 1597, Tagliacozzi wrote:

*'We restore, repair, and make whole those parts . . . which nature has given but which fortune has taken away, not so much that they delight the eye but that they may buoy up the spirit and help the mind of the afflicted.'*[1,2]

His exquisite detailed writings on a philosophy of practice, surgical principles, and the methods and importance of splinting and immobilisation, have become cornerstones for the modern practice of plastic surgery[1,2]. This was in the historical period of

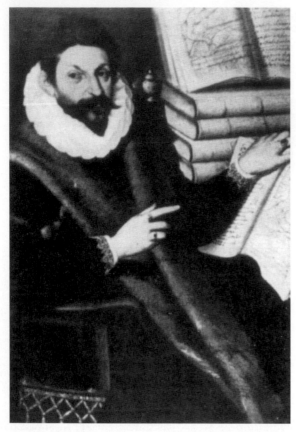

Figure 1.1 Gaspare Tagliacozzi (1549–1599). Reprinted from: Wood-Smith D. & Porowski P.C., 1967, with permission from Elsevier.

the Renaissance with major conflicts emerging between science and religion. The Church, which was dominant at this period, condemned Tagliacozzi's writings, stating that by attempting to reconstruct the nose, he was interfering with the work of God. Shortly after his death, his remains were exhumed from their initial resting place and reburied in unconsecrated (unblessed) ground[2]. It was not until 1958 that Pope Pius XII stated that aesthetic surgery was theologically valued as it restored to perfection God's greatest creation – Man[2].

## The legacy of the early reconstructive plastic surgical masters

The personal and community sense of what is believed to be 'normal' largely drives the individ-

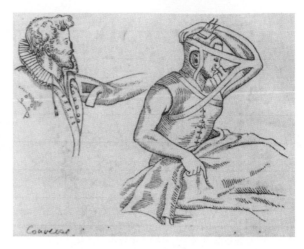

Figure 1.2 Gaspare Tagliacozzi – drawing of defect of the nose repair by tube pedicle taken from the left arm – (1549–1599). With permission: Wood-Smith D. & Porowski P.C., 1967, Elsevier.

ual's need for functional and aesthetic independence in a society that places so much value on so-called 'physical perfection' and independent function[1–6]. Reconstructive surgery has its history and origins in repair techniques designed to restore the normal function and appearance of the human body, regardless of its aetiology.

The ongoing development of modern techniques is based on the inherited principles of the early masters and modern applied clinical research. This is enhanced by continuing attention to detail by modern physicians, nurses and allied health personnel.

Figures 1.2–1.8 provide a profile of the movement in the pictorial history from Gaspare Tagliacozzi (1549–1599) to the present time.

Since the 1960s there has been a revolution in macrovascular and microvascular circulatory research, with the latter leading to a major upsurge in the specialty area of microvascular surgery. This important area of research began a significant change in the thinking and practice of reconstructive flap, replant, and transplant surgery.

Many early physicians contributed to reconstructive plastic surgery with the invention of surgical instruments (i.e. skin graft knives) and techniques that assist in making reconstructive surgery an art as well as a science. Registered nurses working in operating rooms will be familiar with specialised

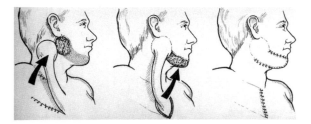

**Figure 1.3** Transfer of tubed skin to repair jaw defect – pre microsurgical free flap era (early to mid 20th Century). Reprinted from: McGregor I.A. & McGregor A., 1995, with permission from Elsevier.

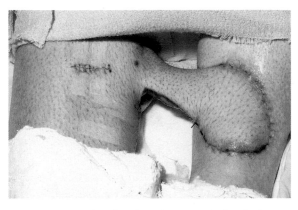

**Figure 1.5** Cross leg flap (1978) – a surgical technique developed in the early part of the 20th Century. Skin flap raised from back of the leg and placed on anterior surface to cover compound fracture of the tibia – donor site skin grafted – flap disconnected from donor area at about 3–4 weeks.

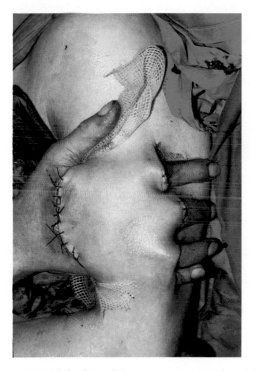

**Figure 1.4** Mobile skin of the upper arm raised and degloved palm of the hand inserted temporarily to aid survival of vital structures until decisions were made as to the reconstructive technique – pre microsurgical free flap era (late 1960s).

instruments that bear the name of renowned researchers and practitioners developed over centuries.

## Establishing specialist surgical treatment units

History records that during the Roman wars, the Roman army set up strategically placed camps along the routes as they marched towards their battle objectives. These camps enabled those who had the potential to survive to be physically carried and treated, one to two days' walk from the battlefield. These way-stations often became small towns through the development of self-managing infrastructures. They also subsequently served as a source of healed troops available for the front if required, and for messages to be quickly sent to the headquarters of the region, and returned to the front line generals. This allowed an unobstructed pathway to Rome from wherever the armies were fighting, and the return of orders or battle plans. The remains of many of these villages and towns can be seen in certain areas of, for example, the European and English countryside.

The next important phase was during the 19th Century (Napoleonic wars) with the introduction of the concept of horse-drawn ambulances set up to return surviving soldiers to the front as soon as

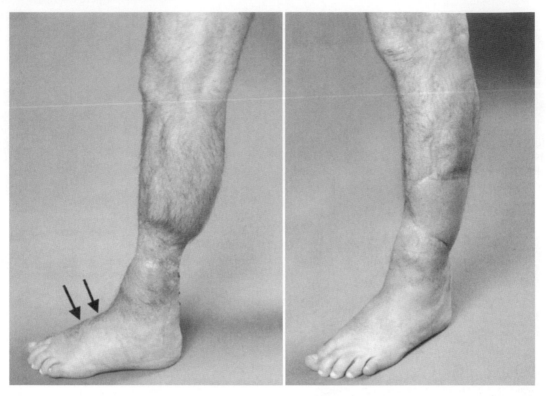

**Figure 1.6** Microsurgical free flap reconstruction reorientating lymphatic channels to correct post traumatic lymphoedema. With permission: Professor G.I. Taylor, Reconstructive Plastic Surgery Research Unit, University of Melbourne, Australia.

possible after primary retrieval care. This was undertaken at army medical camps that were close to the battle. This model was aimed at replacing the short- and medium-term high mortality rate of the ferocious battles, by reinforcing the numbers of soldiers with the 'patched up' injured.

Although it may be considered that the original reason for the establishment and goals for the origins of 'ambulances' through horse-drawn mobile transport was largely inhumane, the process had an extremely long-term and positive outcome. With continuing upgrading of the retrieval processes, this allowed those soldiers and support staff who may have died on the battlefield (i.e. from bleeding, or systemic infection developing from minor injuries), to return to intermediary and larger hospitals. Improved hospital organisation and the development of interdisciplinary healthcare teams, with the primary goal of the individual's physiological and psychological recovery, changed the basis of the original motive for ambulance development.

The introduction of retrieval helicopters (MedEvac) by the American medical corps during the Korean and Vietnam wars to Mobile Army Service Hospitals (MASH), clearly established the important and fundamental 20th and 21st Century principles for fast patient retrieval, resuscitation and stabilisation where recovery from injury, or life-threatening medical conditions, was possible, rather than the expected death[11].

## Key events and discoveries

Several important events and discoveries are responsible for the practice of modern reconstructive plastic surgery and a parallel need for expert nursing care:

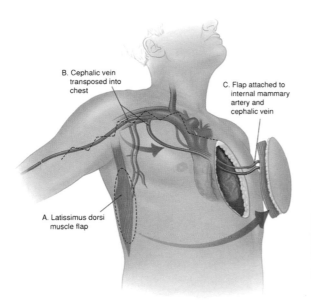

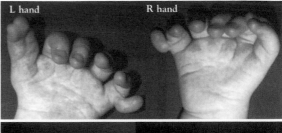

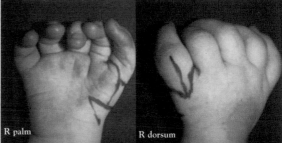

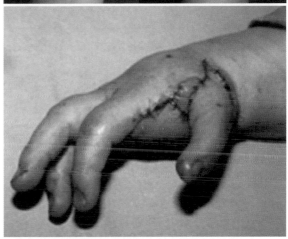

**Figure 1.7** Complex microsurgery used to reconstruct the chest wall following cardiac by-pass surgery with wound complications (post infection and failed local flaps). With permission: Professor G.I. Taylor.

**Figure 1.8** Re-orientation of anatomical structure and form in a child with congenital malformations of both hands, using advanced microsurgical techniques. With permission: Professor G.I. Taylor.

**World War I:** During WWI the large number of mutilated bodies and casualties flowing from, for example, the Battle of the Somme, and many other tragic battles, saw the overflow of military medical hospitals in the field and in the home countries. It became clear to some surgeons that there was a need for specialist surgical units to deal with specific injuries based on a multidisciplinary approach.

One such unit was at a specialist hospital in Sidcup, Kent, in the United Kingdom, set up for the treatment of those individuals, particularly pilots, with facial injuries including fractures and burns. From this emerged a team of eminent army surgeons and dentists from the British Commonwealth countries, the United Kingdom, and United States of America, led by the distinguished English surgeon Sir Harold Gillies. Gillies had a specific interest in reconstructive surgery of the face, and non-healing burn wounds. Professor T.P. Kilner from the UK, and Sir Archibald McIndoe from New Zealand, a cousin of Gillies who had studied in America, also joined the team.

Leading English plastic surgeons demanded of government healthcare institutions that nurses interested in this emerging specialist area be allocated to these newly dedicated units to assist the surgical teams, where they could be educated in the specific care needs of this promising and demanding specialty[3].

These and other US surgeons also became formidable figures in the development of new surgical instruments, and for the foundation of the modern

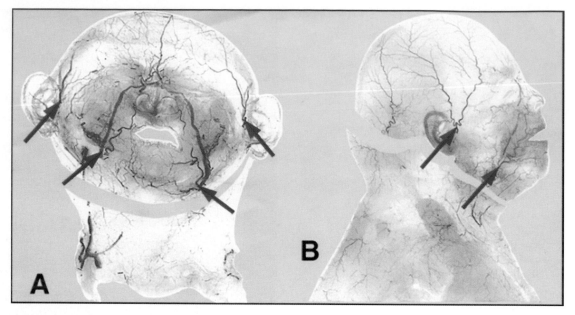

**Figure 1.9** The future – potential total face and scalp transplant based on current microcirculatory research. With permission: Professor G.I. Taylor.

concepts and principles now used for many successful reconstructive techniques. This changed surgery from a salvage concept to a reconstructive and recovery concept. Box 1.1 outlines the general founding principles that arose from the development of this group approach[1-3].

---

**Box 1.1** Development of the modern founding principles for successful reconstructive plastic surgery.

- The value of organisation (trained specialists, case segregation and centralisation of facilities)
- The value of teamwork (co-ordinating the skills required to achieved the required results – control of anaesthetic gases delivered by endotracheal intubation, surgeons, dentists, nurses, allied health, psychosocial assistance)
- The ability to learn from trial and error (using empirical methods, procedures of proven value could be selected to meet the individual patient's needs).

---

**Anaesthesia:** The discovery of safe anaesthetic gases with pain-controlling actions, combined with the development by Magill to provide anaesthesia by inserting a tube via the mouth, or nose, into the trachea allowed open access to the face, for surgical reconstruction[1-3]. Individuals with congenital malformations and disease would also be the beneficiaries of these developing anaesthetic skills that exponentially increased the range of surgical procedures available to the general public.

**Tracheostomy:** The value of tracheostomy, in selected patients, for long-term airway management, became apparent as it allowed repeated surgical exposure of the face for secondary and tertiary reconstructive surgery.

Other modern scientific discoveries and approaches include:

- The introduction of antibiotics
- Improved understanding of resuscitation methods
- Innovative and creative reconstructive practices
- Support for the recognition of the psychosocial implication of body image

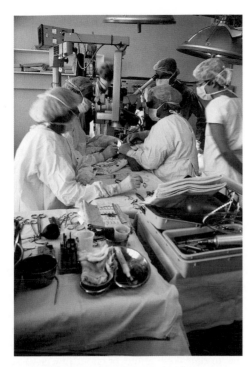

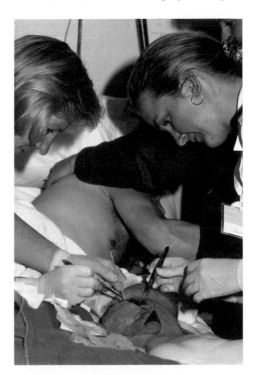

**Figure 1.10** Modern major microscopic reconstructive surgery team in the operating room – Victorian Plastic Surgery Unit, Melbourne, Australia (2003).

**Figure 1.11** Specialist nurse clinicians working as a team applying split skin grafts to a complex wound – Victorian Plastic Surgery Unit, Melbourne, Australia.

- The development of modern prosthetic camouflage techniques
- The initiative of a whole team approach

### *Important outcomes for victims of war*

Military and civilian victims and patients who may not have been able to function or engage with the world because of mutilating facial or hand injuries caused by bombs, burns, gunshot or mine explosions, were top priority. This allowed many soldiers and civilians to return to a reasonably acceptable life in the community[1-3].

Although mortality rates continued to be high, increasing survival rates significantly posed new challenges for creative resuscitation methods, surgical reconstruction, nursing care and rehabilitation – largely unavailable in earlier times.

Thus with the forming of these practice principles, historical events, anaesthetic techniques, discovery of antibiotics, new drugs, the increased application

of scientific thinking, the collective modern age of plastic surgery came about and reconstructive plastic surgery began to be recognised as an entity in its own right. As stated, this was substantially related to the massive and destructive world wars of 1914–1918 and 1939–1945[1-3].

With increasing advances in the science of microbiology, hygiene practices, antibiotics, anaesthesia, and analgesia, the demand for surgery amplified the need for reconstructive methods of all parts of the body following birth defects, trauma or disease.

## Modern application of founding principles

The early setting down of the concepts and principles of the specialty had far-reaching influences throughout the world, particularly the USA, and this saw an explosion of research, and progress in thinking and practice, much of which remains the cornerstone of modern operating and patient care practice today.

### Trauma

Clinical research was also increasingly signifying that time between injury, resuscitation and stabilisation was 'the golden hour'. The vastly improved techniques of anaesthesia, pain management, timely rescue and retrieval surgery, and infection control would become dominant.

Increased understanding of the pathophysiology of injury, infection and the need for expert wound management saw the major upgrading of acute medical episodes, trauma retrieval and burns management practices in civilian societies. This also opened up increasing opportunities for nurse clinicians to engage in specialist nursing practices. Expert nurses became strongly established in emergency rooms, operating theatres, critical care and team-based postoperative surgical units, expert wound care, and rehabilitation programmes[7].

### Advances in microsurgery

The introduction of the operating microscope, with fine suture material increased the medical and surgical capability to repair severed nerves and restore macro- and microscopic blood flow. For contemporary reconstructive surgery and its associated wound management, research into the immune system, microcirculation of the skin, and these technical advances provided the facility to repair nerve continuity, providing some potential for restoration of sensory protection to important body regions. Advances were also made in limb salvage and, in suitable patients, replant surgery (Figure 1.7)[2–7].

### Development of a multidisciplinary approach – congenital malformations, trauma and disease

Modern plastic surgery can provide sophisticated and complex methods for restoration of the integrity of the skin and bone with multifaceted surgical reconstructive flap procedures, frequently undertaken in association with other surgical specialty areas, such as neurosurgery, orthopaedics, otolaryngology, maxillofacial, dental and ophthalmic surgery[2,4–6,8]. Major trauma of the face, or upper and lower limbs, head and neck cancer, or loss of a breast from cancer, require substantial and creative skills to restore or re-create adequate functional and desired aesthetic attributes.

In addition, a range of procedures are undertaken to improve function and enhance appearance for presenting congenital malformations such as breast anomalies, defects of the hands and feet, craniofacial malformations and soft tissue conditions such as haemangioma. Burns that may contribute to distorting and functionally debilitating scar contractures in the whole body of the growing child, or adults, often require multiple and ongoing surgical procedures to increase mobility and restore function and aesthetic form.

### Aesthetic surgery – primary and as adjuncts to reconstructive surgery

The practice of reconstructive plastic surgery cannot be separated by the desire to achieve an optimal aesthetic outcome. Strictly aesthetic surgical procedures may be undertaken alone or as adjuncts to reconstructive undertakings.

Skin resurfacing using chemical peels, dermabrasion or laser therapy and major surgical interventions such as rhinoplasty, facelift, liposuction for body contouring and removal of large areas of adipose tissue and skin, represent a large portion of the procedures that can be undertaken to assist the client to sustain or regain a more youthful appearance[2,4–6,8]. It is often overlooked that many of these procedures also contribute to attaining an acceptable aesthetic surgical outcome following major reconstructive flap surgery for trauma and disease, as secondary or tertiary procedures.

### Recent advances in reconstruction concepts

**Tissue expansion:** one of the most recent noteworthy advances in reconstructive surgery has been the development and use of tissue expansion. Normal skin adjacent to injured tissues is expanded significantly, enhancing the use of the patient's own skin and allowing for continuity of normal tissue surfaces.

**Synthetic prosthesis:** when the available normal skin is insufficient or inappropriate for the desired function and/or form, the use of modern synthetic materials for synthetic prosthetics (i.e. titanium osseo-integration techniques to artificially replace, for example, a nose or an ear, (see Chapter 25)) is of such high quality that these can also be considered in the 'reconstructive' equation[4-6].

**Electronics:** although most patients will elect to have restorative surgery that uses their own skin, the increasing development of electronics and computerised 'spare parts' is an option to preserve other parts of the body (i.e. upper and lower limbs) from further scarring, or to speed up the process by foregoing some of the steps required in multistaged procedures[2,4-6].

**Other advances** in contemporary knowledge and research that are pushing the frontiers of plastic surgery even further include[2,4-6]:

- Micro blood flow to the skin
- Understanding of the structure and function of the nervous system
- Gene therapy
- Projected application of human stem cell research
- Control of immune responses to foreign proteins.

## The evolution of specialist reconstructive plastic surgery nursing practice

The place of nurses as carers can be traced back through the history of the religious orders, and particularly through the extraordinary works of the more recent history by Edith Cavell (1865–1915) during the Crimean War, and the writings of, for example, Florence Nightingale.

As outlined above, during World War II in the UK, previously held ideas of the importance of a team approach started to gain momentum and finally became a reality with the survival of many soldiers with major burns and facial injuries. This created an urgent push for the development of reconstructive surgery teams to be set up with surgeons, anaesthetists, dentists, nurses, prosthetists and rehabilitation therapists working within a dedicated specialist unit[3].

The main purpose of these multiskilled reconstructive plastic surgery teams was to focus on primary, secondary and tertiary reconstruction of large numbers of injuries to the face and upper and lower limbs from gunshot and aircraft crash injuries, and extensive and debilitating burns – an early feature of aircraft crashes. The team objectives were to enable the injured person to return to the community as functionally, aesthetically and psychosocially prepared as possible. This significantly expanded traditional wound care but also required new nursing skills in the management of skin grafts, complex skin flaps and tube pedicles[2,3,10-13].

This concept of teams and quality training quickly spread to America and countries within the British Commonwealth, increasing the number of prominent surgeons desiring to support reconstructive plastic surgery as a separate discipline within the overall discipline of surgery[2].

In a parallel move, surgeons in the USA instigated education and training programmes in public hospitals, defence forces and private hospital settings[1,2]. Specific requirements for nurses to participate as surgical assistants, acute care patient providers, astute observers of change in neurovascular wound status, wound care specialists, and to be technically skilled in burns and specific dressing management, became standard. This universal need assisted in educating experienced and specialist nurses to emerge as experts with a fundamental and strategic place in patient care[2,11].

The latter period of the 20th Century saw many profound changes in applied scientific and medical research, technology, methods of healthcare delivery and the emergence of short-stay patient care[8]. For some of those registered nurses drawn to the care of patients within the discipline of reconstructive and aesthetic plastic surgery, positive opportunities have arisen to extend the professional nursing role outside the traditional hospital environment[8].

Change has provided an expanded range of career options in specialist operating theatres, surgeons' assistants, science-based wound care practice, and private nurse practitioners with expansion of skills into community care, education and research. The increasing numbers of free-standing plastic surgery centres and surgeons' rooms/offices have also enabled the specialist nurse to be a primary member of the team[9-11].

It is often suggested that what separates reconstructive plastic surgery and its nursing care from other surgical and nursing disciplines is the constant high level of attention to detail at every point of patient care, and the importance of an overall team approach[3,9,10].

Early texts demonstrate the complexity of nursing care from a different perspective than is seen today (i.e. the common use of migratory tube pedicles)[10,11] (Figure 1.3).

Modern surgical techniques may be more sophisticated, but the complexity of patient care remains. A sound knowledge of anatomy, pathophysiology, wound healing, wound observations, the neurovascular system, expert clinical assessment, and critical analytical skills, are essential.

Regardless of the surgical approach to the expanding range of sophisticated treatment combinations, the ability to meet the challenges and scope of reconstructive plastic surgery nursing requires registered nurses who are highly educated, critical thinkers, competent practitioners in all areas of general nursing, including specialist wound care, and patient education. Added to this is a high level of knowledge and understanding of the underlying pathophysiology of congenital malformations, disease, injury, and the fundamental importance of psychosocial effects of illness and disability. In that sense, the registered nurse who is an expert in whole patient care, in addition to this specialist area, will continue to be a primary asset to optimal patient outcomes[8–11].

## Professional educational programmes

**USA:** The American Society of Plastic Surgical Nurses (ASPSN), based in the USA, is the leading professional plastic surgical nursing organisation in the world. It has developed practice standards that focus principally on national USA Standards of Professional Performance, and Standards of Care as measurable practice outcomes[9–11]. These are applied through the nursing process, and the ethical and legal right of the patient to engage in the decision making process. ASPSN has strengthened its commitment to excellence in clinical and patient outcomes by providing postgraduate nursing education and certification standards that underpin the professional place of plastic surgical nurses in specialist patient care[9–11].

**Australia:** A similar organisation has been established in Australia, based in Melbourne, and although it has a significant number of members, it lacks the strength of the numbers within the ASPSN. Nonetheless, its commitment to education, through regular meetings and educational formats, has added

to the knowledge base of many professional nurses working within the specialty in hospital and office-based establishments.

The Australian Catholic University, a national university, conducts accredited postgraduate education in plastic surgery and wound management for nurses from graduate diploma to PhD level at their Melbourne campus.

Many short comprehensive courses are also conducted by the Victorian Plastic Surgery Unit at the St Vincent and Mercy Hospital campus, and the Wound Foundation of Australia, sited at the Parkville campus of Monash University, incorporates the wound management of flaps and skin grafts in face-to-face, and national and international wound management distance education programmes. See recommended websites at the end of this chapter.

**UK:** In the UK, similar groups have emerged to address professional and clinical issues and these work closely with the dominant plastic surgical and multidisciplinary groups. These include the British Association of Plastic Surgery Nurses (BAPSN) and the British Association of Head and Neck Oncology Nurses.

## References

(1) Converse J.M. *Reconstructive plastic surgery – principles and procedures in correction, reconstruction and transplantation, Vol. 1.* London: W.B. Saunders, 1964.
(2) McCarthy J.G. (ed.). *Plastic surgery volumes 1–8.* London: W.B Saunders, Harcourt Brace, 1990.
(3) Rank Sir B.K. *The story of plastic surgery 1868–1968.* Reprinted from the Centenary Issue of The Practitioner Symposium: Retrospect and Prospect 1868–1968. July, 1968, 201:114–121.
(4) Aston S.J., Beasley R. & Thorne C.N.M. *Grabb and Smith's plastic surgery,* 5th edn. New York: Lippincott & Raven Publishers, 1997.
(5) Ausher B.M., Erikson E. & Wilkins E.G. *Plastic surgery: indications, operations and outcomes.* St Louis: Mosby, 2000.
(6) Ruberg R.L. & Smith D.J. *Plastic surgery – a core curriculum.* St Louis: Mosby, 1994.
(7) Howell E., Wildra L. & Hill M.G. *Comprehensive trauma nursing – theory and practice.* Illinois: Foresman and Company, 1988.
(8) Fortunato N. & McCullough S. *Plastic and reconstructive surgery. Mosby's Perioperative Nursing Series.* St Louis: Mosby, 1998.

(9) Hackett P. Standards of clinical nursing practice for plastic surgical nursing. *Plastic Surgical Nursing*, 1997 (spring); **17**(1):23–32.

(10) Jenkins M. *Plastic surgery nursing*. London: Macmillian, 1964.

(11) Wood-Smith D. & Porowski P.C. (eds). *The nursing care of the plastic surgery patient*. St Louis: Mosby, 1967.

(12) American Society of Plastic Surgical Nurses. *Introduction to standards of clinical practice*, 1997. http://www.aspsn.org/about/standards/introduction/html

(13) Goodman T. *Core curriculum for plastic and reconstructive surgical nursing*. Pitman, N.J.: American Society of Plastic Surgical Nurses Inc., 1996.

## Recommended websites

**History of plastic surgery**
http://www.plastic-surgeon.org/pshistry.htm
http://www.emedicine.com/plastic/topic433.htm

**History of professional nursing practice**
http://www.aahn.org/
http://www.library.vcu.edu/tml/bibs/nsghis.html
http://195.12.26.123/social/nursing_intro.htm
http://www.lib.flinders.edu.au/resources/sub/healthsci/a-zlist/history.html
http://www.plasticsurgery.com.au/history/index.shtml

**Nursing pioneers**
http://www.edithcavell.org.uk/
http://www.florence-nightingale.co.uk/

**Professional organisations**
http://www.aspn.org (USA)
http://www.changingfaces.co.uk/whoswho.html (UK)
http://www.theblackhole.co.uk/ (UK)

# A Clinical Practice Framework for Modern Reconstructive Plastic Surgical Nursing

## Reconstructive plastic surgery nursing roles and responsibilities

Reconstructive plastic surgeons essentially define their professional care role within three general practice approaches, as shown in Box 2.1[1–4].

---

**Box 2.1** Practice approaches utilised by reconstructive plastic surgeons.

| | |
|---|---|
| **Preservation** | of life – of the whole patient, or body part |
| **Correction or restoration** | of physical function – of the whole patient, or body part |
| **Restoration or improvement** | of physical appearance – of the whole patient, or body part. |

---

Whilst it may be said that the goals of the disciplines of medicine[1–4] and nursing appear to be somewhat the same, there are emerging major distinctions between the focus and level of specific practices, risk management, professional responsibility and accountability by clinical nurses for each individual patient[5–36].

Nursing has been universally described within the holistic attributes of the complex concept of 'caring'[5–11]. This text will seek to adopt the principles of 'caring' through the accepted ethical and legal responsibilities of the professional nurse clinician, whose responsibilities are the safekeeping of patients following reconstructive plastic surgery, reflected within the concept and applied principles of the triad of safety, comfort and independence (Figure 2.1).

---

**Box 2.2** Professional practice pathway for reconstructive plastic surgery nursing.

| | |
|---|---|
| **Safety** | provide a whole, safe and secure physiological and psychological environment for the patient |
| **Comfort** | relieve and manage patient pain and discomfort |
| **Independence** | plan and help restore the individual patient's ability for independent self-care or facilitate assisted self-care. |

---

## Developing a reconstructive surgery nursing practice pathway

### Utilising 'caring' as a practice concept

'Caring' within an ethical framework has been the primary focus and platform on which nursing has been built and the concept has been researched extensively by many prominent nursing theorists[5–11] to develop a complete framework that defines nursing as a discrete discipline with its own areas of legal responsibility and accountability. Despite descriptions of various nursing models that reflect the concept of 'caring' for nursing practice having been suggested in the literature – and sometimes applied in practice – a consensus on a straightforward universal model is yet to emerge to meet the needs of the extensive and expanding range of nursing interventions and responsibilities.

Contemporary nursing practice is not only focused on the physiological needs of the human organism but is also deeply conscious of the psycho-

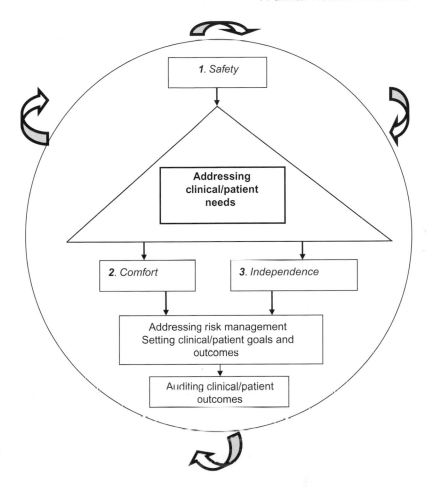

**Figure 2.1** Triad of clinical nursing management.

social issues that arise prior to, during and after illness[20–28]. The desire for integration of the two principal aspects of the physiological and psychosocial needs constitute the present notion of 'caring' as understood by professional nurses[1–28].

Although medical officers largely determine the direction of overall management for patient outcomes[2], some specific distinctions between the professional roles of all team members – for example, medical, nurses and allied health – need to be made to reflect the practice and legal requirements of all licensed practitioners.

In modern community care the essential needs for clean air, clean water and clean food can be translated into clinical physiological outcomes for patient and wound management. For example, evaluating the essential provision of oxygen for cellular function, fluids for circulatory integrity, and dietary needs for

nutritional integrity. In addition to this is the essential need to address psychosocial issues that have the capacity to alter optimal medical and nursing outcomes.

Professional nurses are familiar with practice standards that assist and guide the development of clinical practice pathways, or practice algorithms. These can provide patient management directions to follow in order that medical and nursing outcomes can be met with minimal disruption to the patient[20–23]. They may also afford the means to address the avoidance of adverse outcomes and a method of measuring quality patient care through outcome standards.

Orthodox or ritualistic formulas do not always meet all practice needs but they can frequently provide an opportunity to develop a critical way of thinking within the particular contexts of care. This helps to ensure the nursing process has been applied, best practice has been employed, and legal and ethical standards have been addressed and met.

Figure 2.1 outlines a triad for clinical nursing management. This demonstrates a model for an approach, which should be seen as dynamic; that is, the patient is at the centre of the total circular and repeatable approach. Figure 2.2 outlines a practice pathway for reconstructive plastic surgery nursing.

## Nursing morbidity, co-morbidity, nursing risk management, evidence-based practice, setting clinical nursing goals and healthcare outcomes

The following section of this chapter will introduce and discuss supporting principles and their application through introducing the concepts and clinical

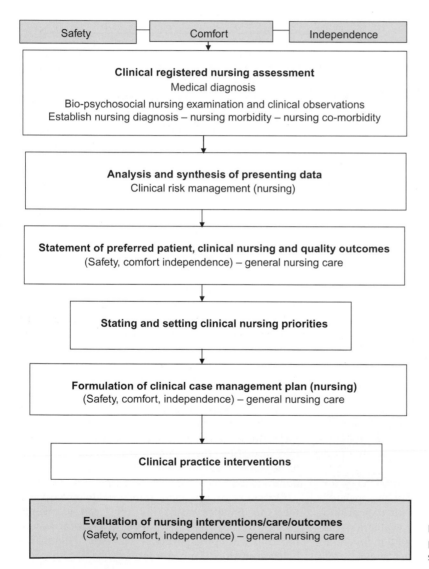

**Figure 2.2** A clinical practice pathway for reconstructive plastic surgery nursing.

principles of nursing co-morbidity, nursing risk management, and by addressing procedural practices and clinical nursing outcomes.

Box 2.3 outlines the practice principles that underpin reconstructive plastic surgery nursing based on Figures 2.1 and 2.2.

---

**Box 2.3** Practice principles for reconstructive plastic surgery nursing.

- Advanced scientific knowledge that encompasses applied anatomy, pathophysiology, and proficiency in applied technical and nursing care skills
- Patient assessment that addresses the aetiology and mechanism of injury of the presenting condition, pathophysiology, and the patient's psychosocial needs
- Applied clinical nursing decisions based on the nursing care process (assessment/nursing diagnosis), clinical risk management, setting goals and outcomes that address clinical and patient needs
- Science-based, or expert experiential wound assessment and overall management skills of wounds at all stages of repair, maintenance and/or palliative needs
- Advanced clinical neurovascular observation, analytic and reporting skills[14]
- A high level of focus on setting achievable clinical and patient stated goals and accomplishing the best overall outcome through the application of critical thinking skills.

---

## Establishing a basic terminology to address clinical nursing practice

---

**Box 2.4** Terminology.

Mortality, in medical terms, means loss of life (i.e. death) as an outcome. This may be accidental, unexpected, deliberate, or a natural but expected event.

Medical co-morbidity means the physiological factors or issues that arise as a result of an illness or primary medical disease, for example:

- Facial fractures leading to respiratory deficits and pneumonia
- Diabetes mellitus leading to vascular ulcers.

Nursing morbidity and nursing co-morbidity may be similarly applied to both of the above, for example:

---

- Altered mobility
- Patient self-care and independence deficits
- Skin breakdown
- Difficulties with hygiene
- Nutritional deficits
- The identification of psychosocial impact of altered normality
- Patient education to prevent primary, or secondary, adverse events.

---

## Nursing morbidity and nursing co-morbidity

In many nursing textbooks, expressions such as 'nursing issues'[16–28] are frequently used, but this terminology implies 'medical' issues reflecting the patient's medical condition, rather than defining nursing morbidity and co-morbidity. Many areas of the recent journal research literature and e-journals refer to these as 'nurse sensitive' interventions.

Although the terms 'nursing morbidity' or 'nursing co-morbidity' are not described in the nursing literature, it is becoming increasingly apparent that with the deliberate separation of the professional nursing role, this may fast become legally necessary[11–16].

## Identifying core clinical issues

The emerging and wider development of independent practice nurses with legal rights to patient assessment, prescribing particular drugs and nursing treatments will see further expansion of the identification of the nursing role.

Although nursing theorists and practitioners are moving towards defining and describing specific terminology for the role of practice nurses, certain terms in general healthcare remain universal, for example: patient mortality, patient morbidity and co-morbidity. Applying this terminology within the nursing care role and responsibilities could be seen to be in line with the professional nursing adoption of other universal healthcare terms, for example: (nursing) assessment, diagnosis, risk management, and clinical outcomes. The specific defining and clinical application of these universal terms within nursing care may provide the potential to express both the collaborative and the independent practice boundaries of the medical, nursing and allied health-care roles.

As an example, a seriously ill patient with limited cognitive and physical abilities related to medical morbidity (primary adverse episode: brain attack), will also present with nursing morbidity (at primary risk for adverse events, i.e. mobility issues). The combination of these factors may lead to nursing co-morbidity (i.e. the development of pressure ulcers) and prevention may be suggested to be a legal nursing responsibility.

Where there is a failure to utilise an objective risk assessment tool, reflecting medical morbidity and nursing morbidity, a breakdown in the provision of prevention measures and development of, for example, a pressure ulcer, it may become a specific nursing issue (nursing co-morbidity, secondary adverse events). That is, it may be suggested within a legal interpretation that minimisation or prevention of pressure ulcers, by the available evidence-based care, is a nursing responsibility, regardless of the status or level of medical co-morbidity of the patient.

This issue, and others in which nurses are expected to initiate a primary and ongoing patient assessment process (i.e. multidisciplinary responsibility for patients with an inability to self-care/manage, nutritional deficits), must be more clearly stated, and structurally and formally organised to avoid these adverse events.

Thus nursing co-morbidity (secondary adverse events) may be said to be the emergence of those issues of safety, comfort and altered independence that may arise as the result of medical or nursing morbidity, or secondary issues that arise from patient care designated as specific nursing actions. Additional examples may be the application of evidence-based provision of therapeutic oxygen, optimal pain management, skin care, wound assessment, wound dressing management, and the initiation of palliative wound bed care[20–28].

The use of universal terms can allow for the development of a much clearer understanding of the medical and nursing role for a reduction of the existing ambiguities. Identifying the issues that constitute nursing morbidity and co-morbidity can assist the important areas of nursing risk management processes and clinical practice. This understanding can also underpin addressing clinical nursing risk management, nursing outcomes, clinical benchmark-ing and the continuing educational needs of professional nurses[11–19].

## Applying evidence-based practice and expert experience

### Background

Best practice, acceptable clinical performance, and outcome standards developed by healthcare professionals, essentially reflect the available evidence-based research, accepted expert experience, the context of care required, and large areas of untested rituals[11–28].

It is important to recognise the significance of human illness within its context and culture, and that not all nursing assessment and proposed interventions can possibly be scientifically proven. Many decisions are based on judgement rather than known facts. This is referred to as 'independent discretionary judgement' and relies on the relevant knowledge, multiple exposure to a range of simple and complex experiences, and the ability to undertake critical thinking that takes in the context of the presenting situation and preferred patient outcomes.

The medical condition, nursing implications, contextual and cultural environment including empathy, compassion and the differences and significance of the patient's individual interpretation of their illness that impinge on the proposed patient care plan, should always be a significant feature in the nurse's decision making. This contextual and cultural focus should not be easily discarded from the rich heritage of professional nursing practice without evidence of its lack of efficacy, or meaning for the individual patient. In addition, any attempt to discard/limit the scope or timeframes of therapeutic nursing practices that reflect a sensitive response to known or unexpected human needs should not be accepted unless there is objective evidence of the lack of the value for such actions, e.g. listening to the patient.

Professional nursing requires increasing practical clinical research, adoption of risk management, evidence-based practices or accepted specialised/expert experience, and continuing education that can deliver preferred clinical and patient outcomes to underpin a committed sense of ethical and accountable practices[16–38].

Wide areas of plastic surgery nursing interventions can be scientifically supported by what is referred to as 'applied research' that is based on known physiology, scientific and medical texts.[20–28] But substantial areas of practice protocols and clinical outcomes, particularly those related to patient observations or specialised wound care, continue to be based on the individual patient, expert experience, or are in response to doctor's orders. The undertaking of valid objective clinical nursing research to drive specific nursing actions is limited.

Projects in the USA that have looked at nursing outcomes reflecting North American Nursing Diagnosis Association (NANDA) designations have highlighted the lack of objective-based practice research available to address a large range of independent actions/responsibilities assigned to nurses.

The value of using practice standards based on evidence-based practices, expert experiences, and risk management practices, is that many potential problems or complications can then be minimised or avoided, reducing mortality and morbidity, and protecting precious healthcare resources with a public demonstration of healthcare governance.

International and national Cochrane evidence-based reviews for best practice medical guidelines have proved extremely useful, but have also clearly demonstrated the scarcity of well-designed experimental, clinical or epidemiological studies to strongly recommend specific practices for totally safe implementation in nursing.

In examining the evidence for the effectiveness of healthcare interventions, it is important to consider the quality of that evidence. There are several different formats for describing strength of evidence and two are outlined in Boxes 2.5 and 2.6.

See recommended websites at the end of this chapter.

---

**Box 2.5** Types of evidence.

- Systematic review of evidence from randomised controlled trials (RCTs)
- Results from one or more high quality RCTs
- Results from non-randomised trials
- Results from non-experimental studies (descriptive, case series, etc.)
- Expert opinion

---

**Box 2.6** Strength of evidence.

| | |
|---|---|
| Level I | For a randomised controlled trial, the lower limit of the confidence interval, expressed as a range, for a measure of effect is still above a meaningful benefit in healthcare terms |
| Level II | For a randomised controlled trial, the lower limit of the confidence interval, expressed as a range, for a measure of effect is less than a meaningful beneficial effect in healthcare terms; but the point estimate of effect still shows effectiveness of the intervention |
| Level III | Measures of effectiveness are taken from non-randomised studies of groups of people where a control group has run concurrently with the group receiving the intervention being assessed |
| Level IV | Measures of effectiveness are taken from non-randomised studies of groups of people where intervention effects are compared with previous or historical information |
| Level V | Evidence is from single case studies |

---

## Risk management within clinical nursing practice

---

**Box 2.7** Common definitions of the term 'risk'.

| | |
|---|---|
| Acceptable risk | actual or potential compromising factors that can be stabilised |
| Unacceptable risk | actual or potential compromising factors that cannot be stabilised |
| Calculated risk | risk taken with all factors considered and addressed where possible |
| Uncalculated risk | failure to assess or comprehend the risks that may lead to adverse consequences |
| Minimal or diminished risk | little or no identified risk |
| Risk aversion | avoidance of taking a risk |
| Risk assessment | identification of actual and/or potential factors that may incur any form of risk, acceptable or unacceptable |
| Risk management | strategies to prevent or minimise injury or adverse events occurring |

*Continued*

| | |
|---|---|
| **Medical risk** | proposed or initiated medical treatments that will, or has the potential to, place the patient in danger of injury, adverse event or death |
| **Nursing risk** | conditions emerging from existing or arising systemic conditions, psychosocial disturbances, difficulties in mobility, unresolved pain or nutritional deficits that may predispose to risks in patient safety, comfort or independence. |

## Clinical governance

Clinical governance is a framework that helps clinicians (including nurses) to continuously improve quality and safeguard standards of care. It aims to integrate all the activities that impact patient care into one strategy.

This involves improving the quality of information for patient care, promoting collaboration, team working, and partnerships, as well as reducing variations in practice, and implementing evidence-based practice. Some recommended websites providing guidelines for application of clinical governance in clinical nursing practice follow the references for this chapter.

## *Developing strategies for risk management in general nursing practice*

Risk management is focused on the evaluation of a situation and the objective strategies that are applied so that the margin for error is eliminated or minimised[29–40]. This does not infer that the application of objective risk taking is to be avoided. For example, many areas of clinical research are based on controlling risk factors within the guidelines of the project, which allow the research to be halted when adverse events arise (i.e. drug trials).

The application and practice of risk management has been adopted in almost every area of human activity, including healthcare, government and business, with the aim of minimising or preventing harm or injury, managing cost effectiveness and reducing the level of patient, client, or staff dissatisfaction and potential for litigation. In healthcare it is linked to prevention of adverse events, clinical and patient outcomes, and is an important basis for determining overall quality management outcomes.

For professional nurses, the identification and management of risk that is nursing based is a dynamic and proactive process that seeks to prevent or minimise any known or unknown factors that can impact on, or alter, the preferred progress or outcome of a 'nurse sensitive' intervention[29-38]. It is a course of action for optimising opportunities, and minimising or excluding risks that may lead to adverse events which have the potential to cause patient death, disability, personal financial loss and/or legal action or long-term psychological dysfunction.

## Risk management in reconstructive plastic surgery nursing

For plastic surgery nurses, the sheer diversity of age groups, conditions and requests of patients who are referred for plastic surgery, can produce significant clinical risks and psychosocial care challenges[1–4].

Patients who are grieving, angry and non-compliant, psychologically disturbed, dissatisfied with their care/outcomes and resent the attitudes of the carers, can present nurses with additional tests of their clinical skills in problem identification and professional management. Advanced skills in nursing assessment paralleling medical assessment, and the application of objective processes that address actual or potential complicating factors, give a leading edge in prevention of adverse events[1–4,17–28].

Despite what is expected of recently graduated professional nurses, it takes many years of postgraduate education and experience to practise critical thinking at a high level (extrapolation)[27]. On that basis, it is extremely important to provide aspiring experts an educational and practice framework of care that addresses specific pathways of patient care. This can allow for growing knowledge and experience to develop a professional who is able to practise with independent discretionary judgement, confidence, and remain with a sense of compassion and caring.

Whilst there is significant argument in the literature regarding prescriptive learning, there are rules and formulas required in science, legal precedence, and ethical responsibilities that provide the basis for objective critical thinking, superior decision making, and planning for the avoidance of adverse events for which there are major consequences/outcomes for the patient and the professional nurse.

## Developing and auditing core nursing healthcare goals, outcomes and benchmarks

| Box 2.8 Example definitions of clinical outcomes. | |
|---|---|
| Clinical outcomes | mortality (death), morbidity (disability), uneventful (returning to normal health) |
| Functional outcomes | exit level of patient/client independence (mobility) and self-care, need for assistance (disability) |
| Quality outcomes | the quality of the care provided by all professional groups and the level of patient approval of outcome relating to quality of life on exit (excellent, discomfort, dissatisfaction, unacceptable) |
| Economic outcomes | the cost of attaining or not meeting the preferred clinical and quality outcomes within a defined timeframe |
| Aesthetic outcomes | the cosmetic result of the surgery, including the consequences of adverse events or abnormal healing, related to patient physiological responses |
| Healthcare benchmarks | the highest outcome standard set according to the accepted scientific research, which is expected to provide an outcome based on the applications of accepted best practice[22]. |

### Healthcare outcomes

Although the quality of overall patient outcomes related to medical interventions has long been a principal focus[2], an increasing number of discussion papers have emerged regarding the specific roles of professional nurses and allied healthcare groups, in the whole range of patient care encounters[12–19]. Within the domain of healthcare, the following

terms: patient outcome, clinical outcome, medical outcome and quality outcome, are essentially defined as the end results of decisions made and the prescribed treatments or interventions. These are paralleled with overall patient management achieved within a cost structure framework, measured against set benchmarks.

### Setting clinical benchmarks

Evidence-based practice and accepted expert practice can assist in setting clinical benchmarks, which are balanced against professional standards. These benchmarks can reflect the stated expected outcomes that are set by groups of practice experts. The actual outcomes are then measured against what is desired or expected by the community and this is the basis of quality improvement processes.

The measurements applied should take into consideration important variables that can influence 'bottom-line' financial results, such as the level of expertise and technology available, use of risk management strategies, patient compliance, psychosocial factors (context and cultural issues) related to the patient, time factors, financial influences and restraints.

Whilst many professional health carers view the imposition of measurement on patient care as an unmerited interference between the patient and the professional healthcare provider, others believe that responsibility and accountability for the quality and outcome of public and private investment money justifies the means used to provide practice and financial transparency.

### Purpose of setting benchmarks for nursing outcomes

The move to models of short stay in a range of healthcare centres has seen radical changes in the approach to all facets of patient care, including the scrutiny of cost effectiveness by nursing practices. Some American institutions are undertaking major projects aimed at designing research models for the evaluation of 'nurse sensitive' outcomes and benchmarks. That is, the outcomes and stated benchmarks that reflect areas of designated nursing responsibility.

The utilisation of the North American Nursing Diagnosis Association (NANDA) framework is seen in the USA as an appropriate reference marker to establish benchmarks and outcomes. This presents a major difficulty outside the USA, as there is little or no universal agreement on what the professional nursing role may specifically constitute.

Obtaining a worldwide agreement on specific nursing outcomes and benchmarks, in differing contexts of care, presents a major professional hurdle. Although this may delay or prevent any real advancement in the immediate future, the process is important to voice generic outcome areas that are currently considered and evidenced as being nurse sensitive.

Substantial debate continues as to the efficacy of systems that may have the potential to confine nursing practice to a set of numbers, particularly in the area of care that requires a high focus on empathy, compassion and psychosocial issues. Added to this is the fear that professional staffing and funding will be directed to an increasingly narrow scope of patient care that is accepted only on an objective and measurable basis, i.e. short stay patients with minimal morbidity.

Conversely, it is argued that unless nursing clearly defines and confirms the parameters of its practice environment and potentials by evidence, or expert experience that makes a difference, its functional responsibilities may increasingly be at the dictates of others who would set the educational and the experiential standards necessary for professional nurse registration. The establishment of nurse sensitive benchmarks and outcomes can help to establish evidence of the essential role of this area of professional care.

For a substantial number of plastic surgical patients, the development of new surgical techniques, low invasive procedures, proactive preoperative assessment, modern generation dressings, wound management and drainage system care, pain management, home care, and excellence in discharge planning, has resulted in day, or 24-hour, surgery.

Short stays are now experienced by approximately 80% of patients, and have substantially increased the intensity of the demands placed on nursing and allied health staff. This has required a reprioritising and redefining of many areas of nursing responsibility, education, and processes for the delivery of clinical nursing management[1-4]. Nowhere is this more so than in discharge planning, patient education, and complexity of care for the patient in the community.

Professional benchmarking of those activities designated as 'nursing sensitive' is providing an oppor-

tunity to advance nursing research and develop evidence-based approaches into how and why much of nursing management is undertaken and understood. With the current dynamic state of the application and evaluation of research practices to many medical conditions not previously treated, constant and ongoing monitoring of practices and setting of staged clinical and patient outcomes are now required.

## Setting preferred clinical and patient goals and outcomes

With the development of overall patient healthcare outcomes, clinicians are challenged to set standards for their own practices, in order that the preferred clinical, and patient outcome/s may be met. Essentially, these outcomes can only be met by setting interim goals within the educational, clinical and financial resources available to clinicians, and with the co-operation of the patient.

Fundamental to the process of setting outcomes is the individual goals set to meet these outcomes. They must be practically achievable within the resources available, and within the patient's capacity to accomplish treatment modalities, and suggested discharge programmes.

Setting unrealistic goals and outcomes is preparing for failure, patient disappointment, anger, and the potential for legal redress.

Boxes 2.9 and 2.10 outline a suggested framework for setting patient outcomes under the headings of patient safety, comfort and independence.

---

**Box 2.9** Patient safety.

**Safe physiological parameters:** the patient's need for safe physiological parameters are assessed and applied within stated timeframes (as appropriate) with self-care, or assisted management to achieve the stability of:

- The respiratory system
- The cardiovascular system
- Renal and fluid balance
- Neurological status
- Nutritional need
- Hygiene and skin care status
- Wound management and prevention of infection
- Psychosocial status.

**Clinical nursing risk management** is applied for minimisation or prevention of adverse events in relation to:

- Wound management – secondary injury
- Pain management – unresolved pain or discomfort
- Nutritional deficits
- Altered mobility
- Development of deep vein thrombosis (DVT) – pulmonary embolus (PE)
- Development of pressure ulcers
- Patient falls
- Medication errors.

**Preferred needs for patient safety** are assessed to provide the appropriate level of required:

- Patient dependence
- Patient interdependent (co-dependent) care
- Patient independent care.

**Education and information:** the patient is provided with an appropriate level of ongoing education and information in relation to prescribed/recommended care that provides a high level of confidence in the quality of safety provided.

---

### Box 2.10 Patient comfort.

**Specific processes** are proposed to provide a pain/discomfort-free environment within a pre-emptive and an allocated timeframe, including:

- Objective-based assessment (i.e. numerical scales) of individual patient needs, and the patient's individual statements of need
- Use of applied pharmacology
- Use of adjunct (including alternative practices) comfort measures, as appropriate, to reinforce pharmacological comfort measures.

**Pain/discomfort** is objectively assessed in order that:

- All treatments undertaken, including wound care, are pain and discomfort-free
- Optimal levels of mobility can be experienced
- An optimal level of independent patient decision-making and self-care can be demonstrated and experienced.

**Empathy**, reassurance and positive reinforcement are put into practice within a range of objective and adjunctive measures, to provide patient comfort

**Patient satisfaction**: the patient is able to express satisfaction with the level of comfort experienced and treated through the use of objective assessment methods (i.e. numerical scales)

## Auditing of preferred clinical and nursing outcomes

Boxes 2.11 and 2.12 outline suggested examples of how set outcomes may be audited.

---

### Box 2.11 Patient independence.

**Patient needs** for the most advantageous levels of mobility and self-care are assessed to effectively support the patient needs at the levels of:

- Dependent – total care required
- Interdependent (co-dependent) – requires assistance
- Independent – can manage all care.

**Support:** the patient is supported according to an objective-based assessed level in order that there is:

- Provision for nursing measures based on the assessed levels of individual independent needs
- A protective framework to secure the patient from adverse events related to altered mobility
- Ongoing education and open lines of communication for the patient to express any psychosocial needs related to altered independence
- Regular advice to patient or primary carers of the independence and psychosocial needs of the patient, with appropriate measures put into place to provide optimal clinical and patient outcomes.

---

### Box 2.12 Audit of patient safety.

There was:

- An identification of existing medical and nursing morbid and co-morbid factors
- An identification of those primary physiological and psychological factors that have the potential to compromise patient safety
- Utilisation of specific risk management approaches and the utilisation of outcome planning for prevention or minimisation of physiological and psychological adverse events whilst in care and on discharge
- Patient acknowledgment, acceptance and permission sought to institute specific processes proposed to provide a safe environment
- Patient education instituted to initiate and support safe practices
- Objective patient satisfaction sought, in relation to the quality of nursing care experienced, during all levels of inpatient, discharge and rehabilitation care.

**Box 2.13** Audit of patient comfort.

There was:

- An identification and application of optimal and proactive/pre-emptive methods of pain management specific to the individual patient's needs
- An objective evaluation of pain management processes utilised, and altered as appropriate to patient needs
- Provision of personal pain management education
- A process to seek patient acknowledgment and acceptance of specific processes proposed and used to provide a pain-free environment in care and on discharge
- An objective process, that sought expressions of patient satisfaction for a quality of nursing care experienced, and alterations to care made as necessary during the whole inpatient, discharge and rehabilitation care period.

**Box 2.14** Audit of patient independence.

There was:

- Identification of physical mobility including self-care entry and exit level:
  - Dependent – total care required
  - Interdependent (co-dependent) – requires assistance
  - Independent – can manage all care
- Utilisation of risk management to ensure prevention of injury related to any altered mobility that may compromise, or adversely alter, the preferred level of independence
- Information provided to primary carers or significant other/s as appropriate
- Patient or primary carer support provided with education at all levels of self-care deficits experienced
- Ongoing communication seen as an essential process for informing and obtaining consensus on recommended care
- Provision of physiological and psychological adjuncts, education and support necessary to improve the level of mobility and self-care as required
- An objective process that sought expressions of patient or primary carer satisfaction for quality of nursing care, experienced in whilst in care, on discharge, and during the rehabilitation phase.

## General ethical and legal issues for nurses

### The importance of addressing unmet patient expectations

The individual's motives for seeking, for example, purely aesthetic surgery, may be presented to the surgeon in a variety of ways. Collaboration between surgeon and nurse in the assessment process to identify underlying actual problems or potential problems is extremely important. Professional involvement in this area of plastic surgery requires an understanding of the basic psychological profiling of personality types. This allows clinicians to recognise individuals who have unrealistic expectations and/or major psychiatric disturbances.

Some patients will initially appear satisfied and then, in the early or later postoperative phase, express varying levels of dissatisfaction with the surgical outcome or overall treatment. For selected individuals, psychiatric assessments and counselling may provide a strong basis for a mutual understanding of what is and is not possible.

Professional nurses working in this area of the specialty must recognise their limitations and be able to decline roles that they may not be educationally or experientially prepared for, such as advanced psychological counselling, patient education, or solicited or unsolicited surgical advice to the patient[15–21]. Financial compensation may be sought if the patient believes he or she has been inappropriately counselled regarding treatment regimes, and the expected aesthetic outcomes are not realised. It is also very important to set up conflict/aggression training/management and risk management protocols, that provide safety and exit strategies for staff to 'escape' from angry, dissatisfied or potentially violent patients or clients[13,14,22].

### Responsibility and accountability in clinical practice

The development of nursing as a professional discipline has seen a parallel rise in the extent of ethical responsibility and legal liability, and the associated accountability assigned to nurses[23]. Specific patient care roles ascribed to the professional nurse vary from one country to another, but in Western culture, areas of emerging litigation are, as much as anything else, defining the professional role of nurses. Many actions may be considered unethical but not illegal (e.g. the manner in which the patient is spoken to). Essentially, unethical behaviour is that which is against the standards that the profession sets for its members, and brings the profession into disrepute, as opposed to illegal actions (e.g. assault on a patient) which constitutes a breach of the law.

The International Council of Nurses (ICN), representing the professional nursing bodies of most countries around the world, has developed and published generic ethical standards and guidelines for its members, outlining universal and specific standards of care that address nursing education, nursing practices and patient care. Standards of care in nursing are essentially a reflection of the common law principles that govern the behaviour of the community of particular countries[11-15].

Most cases of healthcare litigation fall into the category of contributory negligence: inappropriate actions by registered clinicians that are believed to have contributed to patient injury, major dissatisfaction or death. For nurses, medication errors, inadequate knowledge and inappropriate application of evidence-based wound care, withholding of adequate prescribed pain management, and the development of pressure ulcers, have seen increases in litigation where patients believe that professional care has not reflected expected or defined practice standards, or been at the level of expectation, and where injury may have, or has, resulted[20-38].

## Patient consent and emerging areas of litigation against nurses

The issues that surround the principles of what constitutes 'informed consent' are central to common law, and the matter of informed consent is at the core of the planning of any proposed invasive procedure, or (for particular groups) blood transfusion.

In common law within healthcare practice, the performance of a medical or nursing intervention without any consent constitutes 'battery', and the performance of a procedure without informed consent is considered 'negligence'. Within this, it is accepted that patients have a right to autonomy, to expect that no harm will result, and that professionals have a duty of care to ensure that these rights are respected and maintained.

For nurses undertaking an increasingly independent role in designing patient interventions and patient education, and accepting an advocacy role in a patient's care, there is an exponential rise in legal accountability for accepted responsibility and applied practices[39-44].

In plastic surgery, most cases of litigation that come to court are reported to be the result of a perceived, or real, lack of initial and ongoing communication. Misunderstandings between doctor and patient, or doctor, patient and nursing clinician(s), are also high on the list.

Some patients undergoing, for example, aesthetic surgery, skin peels or laser treatments may have unrealistic expectations that cannot be met. The patient's eagerness and need to have the procedure undertaken, see the wound(s) healed, and to return to work or the community, often places unreasonable pressure and unrealistic time constraints on all concerned. This is the time when mistakes or adverse events often occur.

In other instances, assessment processes may be complicated by inadequate acknowledgement of known or perceived patient psychological concerns or underlying psychiatric problems. Working in association with psychotherapists or clinical psychologists who have an interest in, and understanding of, the issues regarding body image, can be useful in determining clinical and legal risks, and the appropriateness of the requested procedure(s).

Following surgical procedures, any initial or continuing refusal by medical or nursing clinicians to acknowledge that the patient truly believes that there is a problem, or was not appropriately informed of potential complications, is often the beginning of a chain of events that leads to expensive and lengthy court proceedings.

In some cases, if both patient and clinician are to be protected from litigation, it is mandatory to:

- Re-assess the proposed procedure (more than one interview with the patient)
- Discuss any anticipated adverse clinical outcomes (e.g. scar outcomes)
- Use professional and empathic communication skills combined with written documentation of all clinical conversations and patient responses.

All preoperative preparation should include plainly written patient information sheets about the planned surgery and proposed postoperative care, including timeframes.

The documentation of principal responsibilities and the increasing use of the terms 'nurse sensitive outcomes' and 'clinical nursing indicators' are important advances in the evolving recognition of therapeutic nursing undertakings and provide an additional and objective protective layer against the occurrence of adverse events. Risk management in reconstructive plastic surgery nursing can be applied to any surgical or nursing setting including office-based settings.

Specific guidelines can be set up to provide pathways for addressing episodes of potential general and specific risks that may occur because of the nature of the practice. For example, poor patient selection may lead to poor outcomes. A perceived, or real, postsurgical or nursing adverse event may lead to the potential for medical, nursing or office staff to be injured by abusive or dissatisfied patients. This has become a significant issue of our times and the extent of abuse or retribution sought in such cases should not be underestimated.

It must also be recognised that few things are completely risk-free but management goals are to reduce the risk to as low a threshold as possible. Risk management should not be seen as a panacea to rid healthcare of all the actual and potential problems that arise for patients or staff. Its judicious use can be an important adjunct to proper physical and psychological assessment processes and an important recognition of potentially complicating factors that have the potential to cause injury or adverse events. Adverse event reporting, with ongoing auditing of clinical and quality outcomes, provides opportunities to alter practices where necessary and avoid the potential for litigation.

### When adverse events do occur

Legal liability, in almost every aspect of life, is one of the most controversial issues in modern Western society. It must be remembered that many cases of litigation arise more than one year after the event (often more than seven), making it difficult for witnesses to recall a full or even a vague memory of an event that appeared, at the time, not to be adverse.

For nurses, when adverse events do occur, or there is doubt in the patient's or clinician's mind, accurate identification of the principal issues, precise times, individuals present, conversations held, and detailed documentation of the actions taken to correct the problem are essential.

The primary, and ongoing, use of risk management assessment documentation can provide clear evidence of the nurse's intention to protect the patient in those areas designated as nursing responsibility and accountability. If critical or adverse incidents do occur, defensive statements (for example: *'there were not enough staff on that day'*, *'I didn't have the time'*, *'the doctor ordered me to do it'*, or *'I didn't understand'*) are no longer accepted within the litigation process.

With the professionalism of nursing come expectations of knowledge, understanding the consequences of an action or inaction, accountability, patient advocacy, and the questioning of medical or hospital management orders that may have the potential to initiate an adverse outcome. In many instances, legal concerns arise from the belief that 'treatment not documented is a treatment not done'[30,39–44]. This places some doubt in the process of documenting 'only in/by exception'.

## The importance of documenting nursing interventions

Ongoing professional communication with basic descriptions, in language that is understood by the patient (e.g. is an interpreter required?), and engaging with the patient to ensure that permission is given prior to undertaking interventions, wherever possible, and regardless how small, are essential.

All care should be documented in circumstances where the risk of any injury is even remotely possible, or has occurred. For example, where the patient has some degree of existing physical or psychological disability that may alter his or her ability to fulfil any additional activities, or co-operate fully.

The importance of the basic professional responsibility to document risk management, clinical pathways, case management, clinical observations and clinical responses, and reporting adverse changes in the patient's condition, cannot be over-emphasised. The few minutes needed to maintain such records could make the difference between a well-informed team producing a positive patient and clinical outcome, and the disappointed patient with an uninformed attitude leading to legal problems, substantial financial compensation, and significant question marks over the nurse's competence[42].

In modern legal culture, expert nurse witnesses are now being utilised by prosecuting and defence lawyers to support particular lines of advocacy and interpretation of nursing documentation that defends or denies an offence(s) committed by the nurse or nurses. Such is the increasing status of some advanced nurse practitioners as expert witnesses, that their place in assisting lawyers and the courts to objectively understand the nurse's role, required responsibility and accountability in patient care, is becoming standard practice[30,39-44].

# References

(1) Aston S.J., Beasley R. & Thorne C.N.M. *Grabb and Smith's plastic surgery*, 5th edn. New York: Lippincott & Raven, 1997.

(2) Ausher B.M., Erikson E. & Wilkins E.G. *Plastic surgery: indications, operations and outcomes*. St Louis: Mosby, 2000.

(3) McCarthy J.G. (ed.). *Plastic surgery*, volumes 1–8. W.B Saunders, Harcourt Brace, 1990.

(4) Ruberg R.L. & Smith D.J. *Plastic surgery – a core curriculum*. St Louis: Mosby, 1994.

(5) Watson J. Introduction: an ethic of caring and nursing. In: *The ethic of care and the ethic of cure. Synthesis in chronicity*. (ed. Watson J.) New York: National League of Nursing Publication, 1979.

(6) Benner P. *From novice to expert: excellence and power in clinical practice*. Menlo Park: Addison-Wesley, 1984.

(7) Benner P. & Wrubel J. *The primacy of caring. Stress and coping in health and illness*. Menlo Park: Addison-Wesley, 1992.

(8) Leininger M.M. *Care: the essence of nursing and health*. Detroit: Wayne State University Press, 1984.

(9) Kyle T.V. The concept of caring: a review of the literature. *Journal of Advanced Nursing*, 1995; 21(4):506–5.

(10) Pegram A. How do nurses perceive care? *Journal of Clinical Nursing*, 1992; 1(1):48–9.

(11) Walsh M. *Nursing frontiers: accountability and boundaries of care*. Oxford: Butterworth-Heinemann, 2000.

(12) Hackett P. Standards of clinical nursing practice for plastic surgical nursing. *Plastic Surgical Nursing*, 1997 (spring); 17(1):23–32.

(13) United Kingdom Central Council for Nursing, Midwifery and Health Visiting. *Standards for records and record keeping*. London: UKCC, 1993.

(14) American Nurses Association. *Standards for clinical nursing practice*, 2nd edn. Washington DC: ANA, 1998.

(15) Australian Nursing Federation. *Standards of nursing practice*. http://www.anf.org.au

(16) Lang N.M. Discipline-based approaches to evidence-based practice: a view from nursing. *Joint Commission Journal on Quality Improvement*, 1999 (October); 25(10):539–44.

(17) Patten J.A. A case study in evidence-based wound management. *British Journal of Nursing*, 2000 (June); 9(12): (suppl) S38–40, S42, S44 passim.

(18) Glanville I., Schirm V. & Wineman N.M. Using evidence-based practice for managing in advanced practice nursing. *Journal of Nursing Care Quality*, 2000 (October); 15(1):1–11.

(19) Navito D.G. Advanced practice: guidelines for evidence-based clinical practice. *Nursing Outlook*, 2000; 48:58–59.

(20) McCance K.L. & Huether S.E. *Pathophysiology: the biologic basis for disease in adults and children*, 3rd edn. St Louis: Mosby, 1998.

(21) Smeltzer S.C. & Bare B.G. (eds). *Brunner and Suddarth's textbook of medical-surgical nursing*, 9th edn. Philadelphia: Lippincott, 2000.

(22) Black J., Hokason Hawks J. & Keene A.M. *Medical-surgical nursing* 6th edn. *Clinical management for positive outcomes* – single volume. Philadelphia: W.B. Saunders, 2001.

(23) Mallett J. & Dougherty L. (eds). *The Royal Marsden Hospital manual of clinical nursing procedures*, 5th edn. Oxford, UK: Blackwell Science, 2000.

(24) Fortunato N. & McCullough S. *Plastic and reconstructive surgery: Mosby's Perioperative Nursing Series*. St Louis: Mosby, 1998.

(25) Anderson L. The Plastic Surgical Nurse: Nurse Specialist for the 1990s. *Nursing Clinics of North America*, 1994; 29(4):817–25.

(26) Corbett R. Colours of the spectrum: plastic surgery and reconstructive nursing. *Nursing Spectrum* (Washington, D.C., USA), 1995 (Aug 21) 5(17):16.

(27) Castledine G. & McGee P. (eds) *Advanced and specialist nursing practice*. Oxford, UK: Blackwell Science, 1998.

(28) *Best practice: evidence-based practice information sheets for health professionals*. 2004. Distributed by Blackwell Publishing. http://www.joannabriggs.edu.au

(29) Bernstein P. *Against the gods: the remarkable story of risk*. New York: John Wiley & Sons Inc., 1998.

(30) Sharp C.C. *Nursing malpractice: liability and risk management*. Auburn House Publishing, 1999.

(31) Aufseer-Weiss M.R. & Ondeck D.A. *Medication use and risk management: hospital meets home*. Concurrent Review Nurse Health Services, New York: Cigna Healthcare, 2001.

(32) Autar R. Nursing assessment of clients at risk of deep vein thrombosis: DVT: the Autar DVT scale. *Journal of Advanced Nursing*, 1996; 23:763–70.

(33) Bergstrom N., Braden B., Kemp M., Champagne M. & Ruby E. Predicting pressure ulcer risk: a multisite study of the predictive validity of the Braden scale. *Nursing Research*, 1998 (September/October); 47(5):261–66.

(34) Black R.E. Priority setting in case management based on need and risk. *Journal of Case Management (United States of America)*, 1995 (autumn); 4(3):79–84.

(35) Calfee B. Clinical insights for office practice management: risk management. *Orthopaedic Nursing*, 1998 (Jan/Feb); **17**(1):25–6.

(36) Harris A. Risk management in practice: how are we managing? *Clinial Performance in Quality Healthcare (UK)*, 2000; **8**(3):142–9.

(37) Harris M.R. Reducing risk of complex response: an invisible outcome. *Nursing Administration Quarterly*, 1997 (summer); **21**(4):25–31.

(38) Jones C. Risk assessment and clinical risk management. *British Journal of Psychiatry*, 1997 (September); **177**:290.

(39) McIlwain J.C. Clinical risk management: principles of consent and patient information. *Clinical Otolaryngology*, 1999 (August); **24**(4):255–61.

(40) Tingle J. Clinical guidelines: legal, clinical risk management issues. *British Journal of Nursing*, 1997 (June 12–25); **11**(6):639–41.

(41) Guido G.W. Advanced nursing practice: legal concerns. *AACN Clinical Issues*, 1995 (Feb); **6**(1):99–104.

(42) Hadfield-Law L. Take action to protect yourself. *Journal of Wound Care*, 2001; **10**(1):501–3.

(43) Power S. Legal and accountability issues. *Nursing Times*, 2000 (Apr 13–19); **96**(15):45–8.

(44) Trott M.C. Legal issues for nurse managers. *Nursing Management*, 1998 (June); **29**(6):38–41.

## Recommended websites

**History and application of the Cochrane Review for evidence-based practice**
http://www.cochrane.org
http://www.cochrane.org/consumers/sysrev.htm

**Clinical governance – nursing**
http://www.rcn.org.uk/publications/pdf/ClinicalGovernance2003.pdf
http://bmj.bmjjournals.com/cgi/content/full/321/7263/737

# Chapter 3

# Body Image Issues and Reconstructive Plastic Surgery

## Body image

In basic terms, 'body image' is the subjective impression, or real belief or awareness, that one has of one's own or another's physical appearance, and how a person believes they are perceived. The importance of body image disturbances have been recognised and accepted within a specific entity of nursing diagnosis, in the USA, by the Seventh National Conference on the Classification of Nursing Diagnosis[1-16].

Reconstructive plastic surgery nursing body image disturbances may be best understood through the areas outlined in Box 3.1.

### Box 3.1 Principal causes of body image disturbances.

- Presence, effects and outcomes of congenital malformations:
  - Major functional disturbances
  - Aesthetic disfiguration
  - Major body (psychiatric) image disturbances – dysfunctional insight into/of self, or/of others
- Adverse physical outcomes of injury or disease:
  - Major functional disturbances
  - Aesthetic disfiguration
- Other – congenital gender disorders – genetic and/or hormonal aberrations
- Identity conditions secondary to adverse medical events – poor/mediocre surgical outcomes
- Cultural beliefs and customs – loss of body parts associated with loss of position, power or body image within the 'tribe' or societal group
- Desire to feel 'normal' or to meet the perceived or real community styles of the time
- Desire to delay or overcome the ageing process
- Congenital conditions.

These are predominately classified under craniofacial syndromes with distorted bony and soft tissue of the face and other body parts[1-4]. This is discussed more fully in Section V.

## Gender identity disorders – physiological/psychological

Birth observed congenital malformation (e.g. hermaphrodite) is a chromosomal abnormality where both testicular and ovarian tissue exist in the same person.

Some visual differences may initially be evident, and this is usually the primary clue to the syndrome, but will require confirmation by genetic blood tests. The decisions that the parents and paediatric medical team (including geneticists) make regarding the appropriate gender the child will be assigned, must be based on physiological and psychosocial, short and long-term planning.

### In the adolescent and adult

Uncertainty regarding gender identity or ambiguity within the concept of body image is a poorly understood and highly complex medical condition, which requires multidisciplinary team management, understanding and empathy.

Addressing the individual's desire for trans-sexual or gender reassignment procedures should be undertaken in centres where there is a team-based infrastructure for the entire range and extent of the often multiple surgical procedures required, including geneticists, endocrinologists and specialists in supportive psychosocial management.

The facilities must be available throughout the entire multifaceted process – from request for the procedure to post-discharge care. Adverse events such as surgical complications, or psychological (i.e. unhappiness with the procedural outcome) must be expertly managed to avoid unfavourable outcomes. Such is the complexity of this condition that some patients may request a reversal of the entire surgical process. See recommended websites at the end of this chapter.

## Major body image disturbances – non-congenital

These are principally known as body dysmorphic syndrome or maladaptive personality traits[1-4,13,14]. They may emerge where patients develop inappropriate perceptions and unrealistic expectations of their body, themselves generally, and of others.

These disturbances may be physically, psychologically, perceptually, culturally or spiritually based. Negative feelings and fear of isolation and rejection, can pre-empt various stages of depression, anxiety, loss of self esteem, and decreasing levels of interaction with the immediate family and/or the community. Severe psychological disturbances may lead to intermittent or continuing degrees of self-harm, potentially leading to accidental death or suicide[1-16].

Each individual will have varying degrees of sensitivity for their own personal needs. For patients with purely ambiguous requirements and unrealistic expectations, psychiatric/psychological assessment may be necessary to ascertain the basis of their pathology[1-16]. This may assist in ascertaining objectivity of motives which then allows the surgeon, without prejudice, to reconsider undertaking any operation that is not conceived out of practical and balanced motives for change.

## Specific medical conditions associated with body image

An additional condition known as body image agnosia is described where the patient has a marked inability to visualise or have a sense of body parts. This is commonly the result of stroke or brain damage due to an accident. As research continues on the brain and its response to genetic, physiological and environmental conditions, our behavioural responses/activities become more evident. The brain and its function remain a source of wonder and constant research.

## General development and attitudes to body image

The image we have of our bodies is a principal key and powerful component of our individual/unique identity, and our place in the immediate and wider environment. It is different in each individual and may be an expression of, or allied to one's personal level of, self esteem. It is a conscious and unconscious act of self perception, self belief, and self awareness. It is linked to group and community attitudes and is largely responsible for how we identify ourselves, those who surround us, and our intrinsic place in society. The sense of body image can have a positive or dominating negative effect on our behaviour, and what we personally see as physically and psychologically essential in our day-to-day existence[1-15].

Development of body image is suggested to be evolutionary, beginning at six months of age in both males and females in all societies and cultures[3]. It continues throughout life and may be individually or collectively expressed, sought and experienced to varying degrees, through experienced behavioural patterns, and engagement with alternative cultural or political groups.

The acceptance, abhorrence or denial of one physical form or another is documented through the centuries and has largely been demonstrated through art or sculpture and in more recent history, photography and television. In modern societies, peer and media pressure to conform to a particular view or fashion is enormous. The need to be considered 'normal' can be overwhelming for those who do not feel 'normal' and particularly those wishing to be part of a group who represent a youthful image, attractiveness, power and/or success.

Cultural attitudes to congenital malformation or loss of body parts can be psychologically devastating and impose major restrictions on the relative place of the individual in that particular community (e.g. isolation from the family group, inability to marry or being seen as mentally abnormal). Alternatively, in some cultures, individuals born with congenital malformations are seen as closer to God than others – much blessed and cared for.

Frequently, many outward physical differences (e.g. Down's syndrome, craniofacial malformations) may be improperly associated with varying degrees of intellectual ability.

For human beings to function normally within society, it is important that they should not be wrongly or inappropriately judged by their apparent or perceived, physical difference. Most individuals can expect to have a positive quality of life if it is possible to combine special educational requirements with reconstructive surgery, growth and intellectual testing and development programmes with positive ongoing family and community support.

## The concept of beauty

The concept of beauty is stated to have few or no universal criteria and varies from one culture to another and, in Western-style communities, from one century to another. It is both a male and female phenomenon[1].

Humans have always been aware of, and concerned with, appearance. In some societies, the presence or absence of some external appendages were judged to be the mark of God, or conversely, as the mark of the Devil or an evil sign. In addition, many individuals' long-felt fear and revulsion at seeing those who are malformed, who appear significantly different from the tribal norm, or who are severely injured, made parallels with madness and/or badness. This feeling is deeply centred within the conscious and subconscious of most cultures and tribal groups with predominant ruling groups forming general parameters to determine what constitutes an acceptable or normal appearance. Deviations from these parameters can have societal, psychological and lifestyle repercussions for those who do not appear to conform to norms.

Since the 1970s, 'attractiveness' has also emerged as an intrinsic part of a normal and accepted body image and sense of identity for males. An explosion in the wide range of stylish male clothes, jewellery, hairstyles, requests for aesthetic surgery, fitness, and diet, has contributed to the provision of an increasing range of individual options[1,14,15].

The exploitation of the concept of youth and particular interpretations of what constitutes beauty or individuality, with a marketing focus on cosmetics, surgery, clothes, adornments, cars and lifestyles, can all contribute to projecting a particular image or set of images. These images are orchestrated to promote sales of products and a particular sense of identifying with so-called fashionable groups of the day. The scale of marketing of image, style, wealth, and certain forms of exhibitionism in modern society is unprecedented. The use of plastic surgery is viewed by many as an accepted extension of other forms of restyling and redefining oneself[1].

The principal goal of patients who seek purely aesthetic surgery is to create an altered or completely different profile, or to restore youthful looks to enhance a sense of positive body image and feeling of personal wellbeing. For many individual patients, even slight physical changes (e.g. slight nasal alteration) provided by surgery may also bring about positive lifestyle changes. For others, body image distortions may emerge in overall general terms and then develop in more discrete ways, focusing on the minutiae of areas such as ageing spots or slight weight gain.

## Reconstructive plastic surgery and body image

Reconstructive surgery for congenital malformations, trauma, disease processes and body image disturbance, including procedures to address the ageing process, may be life-changing for those who suffer from functional and aesthetic problems that give them a sense of profound physical difference and social isolation[1-16]. The restoration of normal anatomical and aesthetic form to assist individuals in addressing their personal sense of normal function and body image is one of the basic precepts on which reconstructive plastic surgery is based.

Reconstructive plastic surgery is unique in that patients and surgeons rarely separate the reconstructive procedures designed, and undertaken, from the expectation that procedures will also include optimal aesthetic outcomes.

For many patients, proactive recognition of the need for immediate and ongoing social support services can provide an environment of safety, allowing rehabilitation to proceed with minimal disruption or distress.

Issues of perceived or real inadequate communication between the patient and clinicians, a major lack of understanding of loss of body image, the patient's need for independence, refusal of the clinicians to listen or to accept that a problem may exist, are stated as the principal reasons patients express dissatisfaction with management, and turn to litigation. Substantial clinical skills of observation, empathy, listening, communication, and providing comfort in the face of injury, a malignant disease causing major life disruption or potential loss of life, can alert the nurse to the need for professional counselling for actual or potential psychological disturbances.

## Combining reconstructive and aesthetic surgery – meeting patient expectations

Much of contemporary reconstructive plastic surgery for congenital malformations, disease and following major trauma, aims, where possible, to minimise the physical defects, psychological effects and the need for additional or multiple restorative and aesthetic procedures. This requires planning complex procedures and using the patient's own tissue to reconstruct the missing bone and/or tissue wherever the defect, perceived or otherwise.

In particular areas of reconstructive plastic surgery for major trauma or significant disease, surgeons will often focus initially on lifesaving (i.e. survival) and repair (i.e. preserving function) procedures. Addressing total aesthetic/cosmetic patient needs (i.e. appearance) may not be appropriate at the time of primary surgical intervention and these issues may need to be addressed, through additional procedures, at a later date.

The rationale for the need of staged procedures may not be completely understood by the patient or significant others, who may register shock at the initial sight of the patient's appearance. Patient education and reinforcement of the stages planned must be discussed more than once to ensure at least some basic understanding of the associated risks.

The 'one stage' surgical procedure is a goal that is pursued wherever possible; secondary procedures are used to 'tidy up' minimal functional or aesthetic aberrations, or recurring problems[1–5]. Many patients desire excision, restorative/functional and aesthetic surgery to occur simultaneously. Expectations can be high and unrealistic and patients must be educated about the limitations of surgery for some procedures. Objective patient selection criteria are critical, and should reflect practice standards. For example, for patients with breast cancer who experience grief, fear, a loss of body image, identity, and a sense of decreased sexuality immediate reconstruction following mastectomy may be appropriate. Where this is an option, it can provide an early framework through which coping with the perception and fear of death and psychosocial issues is made easier for them. Where immediate reconstruction is not appropriate, the proposed immediate and ongoing treatment regime must be thoroughly explained and provided in writing to the patient and significant others. It is essential to provide empathy and patient education, and ensure that the patient understands the issues and rationale for proposed staged care plans.

## General nursing management issues

First of all, a comprehensive assessment and understanding of the aetiology, nature of the malformation, injury or illness is fundamental. Secondly, it is critical to identify the actual and clinical potential adverse physical and psychosocial events and consequences for the patient. This may require the recognition of the specific needs of particular cultural or ethnic groups with specific issues relating to body image, self image, loss of body parts, and loss of independence. This can provide a foundation for recognising nursing morbid and co-morbid factors (see Chapter 2) and planning and achieving clinical nursing outcomes that allow for an approach that reflects excellence in total patient care.

An expanded view of the patient's health and quality of life needs can be achieved by a review of the patient's need for assistance in undertaking independent functions including hygiene, nutrition, wound dressings, and rehabilitation with the collaboration of allied health professionals.

## Specialist psychosocial nursing assessment needs for reconstructive surgery patients

### Individuality

Each patient is unique, and initial and ongoing holistic assessment processes require this to be taken into consideration. For example, patients who have experienced a debilitating hand injury or major burns may be left with a range of major psychological body image disturbances, depending on the degree and causation of the experience.

Severe injury or disease that results in the loss of the patient's ability to return to their preferred occupation, loss of income and relative place in society, can severely affect body image and self-confidence. This may result in a range of psychosocial issues and dysfunctional behaviour with major depressive and potential suicidal thoughts or actions.

### Cultural issues

A patient's poor command or understanding of the English language, or a clinician's inadequate understanding of different cultural norms, can lead to poor communication, misunderstandings, frustration, anger and non-compliance. The use of specialist medical interpreters (other than family members) where possible, and ensuring that messages are conveyed accurately, can create an environment of trust, reducing fear, anger and misunderstandings of primary or additional proposed reconstructive procedures.

### Post-traumatic stress disorder

The emergence of early, or delayed, post-traumatic stress disorder (PTSD), can also be a feature of major, long-term unexpected critical incidents for individuals or groups. Many distressing events may profoundly affect an individual's ability to distance themselves from, or come to terms with, critical incidents where, for example, they may have experienced unpredicted near-death events personally, or witnessed unforeseen severe injury or death of family, friends or workmates.

Undertaking primary clinical physiological and psychological assessments, data analysis, providing information and education, requires professional education and certified skills commensurate with the task. Nurses not trained in clinical psychology should not attempt to counsel patients in this critical area of care.

Empathy, listening for clues to how the patient feels, initial support, and timely communication to the surgeon of the patient's remarks, attitude and feelings, are essential. These primary patient responses are particularly important when clinical observations denote significant physiological and/or psychological disturbances, unexpected and unusual anxiety, anger and non-compliant behaviour.

### Clinical responses

It is important for early identification of any actual or potential psychosocial problems to be made, as clinical treatment may necessitate proactive urgent referrals to a consultant in psychiatry or psychology, for assessment and potential therapeutic drug treatment, including counselling.

Nurses should diligently avoid engaging in any clinical actions for which they have no education or experience as, in the final analysis, nurses will be, and are being, held responsible for particular adverse outcomes that pertain to assigned nursing responsibilities.

## Avoiding litigation – principles

For the patient, the quality of what is finally externally visible is essentially the ultimate and critical measure of their expectations[1-6], quality of surgical and nursing care, and perception of attention to detail at all levels.

The need to assist individuals to appear 'normal', at least externally, requires a continuing search for creative methods of reconstruction that support the patient in a psychological sense of wellbeing and an acceptable quality of life. This quest is intrinsic within the origins of reconstructive plastic surgery.

In the final analysis, it is almost impossible to separate the protective, functional, aesthetic/cosmetic and psychosocial needs of any patient undergoing reconstructive or aesthetic surgery; consequently, the overall term 'plastic surgery' is again being used in some countries to describe the full extent and complexity of the specialty[2,4-6]. Unfortunately, because of an overemphasis on the cosmetic or aesthetic side of plastic surgery, the reconstructive aspects are often displaced within the total concept of the specialty.

An excellent principle is to obtain a clear sense of the consequences or risk of any proposed intervention that is potentially injurious to the patient. Clear, informed and professional ethically based practices, communication and documentation skills are fundamental to addressing contemporary nursing practice.

Evidence-based or expert experience should be used as the basis for designing nursing protocols and risk management strategies, and outlining achievable outcomes.

The patient's informed consent for any interventions must be obtained. That is, the advantages, disadvantages, potential complications, preferred outcomes, preferred timeframes, and outlines of pathway for care must be provided both orally and in unambiguous documented formats wherever possible[3,11,12,15].

Patients/clients, legislators, and the legal profession expect that optimal protection for the patient from potential adverse events is the primary consideration by all professional carers, particularly where the potential for injury is raised beyond the normal thresholds. This is the principle of, 'first, do no harm'.

This book will primarily devote its focus on a proposed model for applied clinical nursing that includes clinical nursing risk management through the setting of goals and outcomes, pre- and postoperative patient needs, relating wound care to specific areas following reconstructive surgical procedures, and selected areas of aesthetic body enhancement.

## References

(1) Alam M. & Dover J.S. On beauty: evolution, psychosocial considerations, and surgical enhancement. *Archives of Dermatology*, 2001; June (137):795–807.

(2) Aston S.J., Beasley R. & Thorne C.N.M. *Grabb and Smith's plastic surgery*, 5th edn. New York: Lippincott & Raven Publishers, 1997.

(3) Ausher B.M., Erikson E. & Wilkins E.G. *Plastic surgery: indications, operations and outcomes*. St Louis: Mosby, 2000.

(4) McCarthy J.G. (ed.) *Plastic surgery*, volumes 1–8. Philadelphia: W.B Saunders, Harcourt Brace, 1990.

(5) Fortunato N. & McCullough S. *Plastic and reconstructive surgery. Mosby's Perioperative Nursing Series*. St Louis: Mosby, 1998.

(6) Anderson R.C. & Maksud D.P. Psychological adjustments to reconstructive surgery: plastic surgical nursing. *Nursing Clinics of North America*, 1994 (Dec); **20**(4):712–24.

(7) Borah G., Rankin M. & Wey P. Psychological complications in 281 plastic surgery practices. *Plastic Reconstructive Surgery*, 1999 (Oct); **19**(2):74–6, 106.

(8) Partridge J. The psychological effects of facial disfigurement. *Journal of Wound Healing*, 1993 (May); **2**(3):168–72.

(9) Clarke A. & Cooper C. Psychosocial rehabilitation after disfiguring injury or disease: investigating the needs of specialist nurses. *Journal of Advanced Nursing*, 2001; **34**(1):18–26.

(10) Grossbart T.A. & Sarwer D.B. Cosmetic surgery: surgical tools – psychosocial goals. *Seminars in Cutaneous Medical Surgery*, (USA), 1999 (Jun); **18**(2):101–11.

(11) Gorney M. & Martello J. Patient selection criteria. *Clinics in Plastic Surgery*, 1999 (Jan); **26**(1):37–40.

(12) Moser S. Social service collaboration: meeting the patient's psychosocial needs. *Plastic Surgical Nursing* (USA) 1993 (summer); **13**(2):84–5, 119.

(13) Sarwer D.B. The 'obsessive' cosmetic surgery patient: a consideration of body image dissatisfaction and body dysmorphic disorder. *Plastic Surgical Nursing*, 1997 (winter); **17**(4):193–7.

(14) Pertschuk M.J., Sarwer D.B., Wadden T.A. & Whitaker L.A. Body image dissatisfaction in male cosmetic surgery patients. *Aesthetic Plastic Surgery*, 1998 (Jan–Feb); **22**(1):20–4.

(15) Spencer K.W. Selection and preoperative preparation of plastic surgery patients. *Nursing Clinics of North America*, 1994 (Dec); **29**(4):697–710.

(16) Goodman T. *Core curriculum for plastic and reconstructive surgical nurses*, 2nd edn. Pitman N.J.: American Society of Plastic Surgical Nurses Inc., 1996. http://www.aspn.org

## Recommended websites

**Gender reassignment**

http://www.hmso.gov.uk/si/si1999/19991102.htm (Sex discrimination Act UK – 1999)

http://encyclopedia.thefreedictionary.com/Gender%20reassignment%20therapy (male to female)

http://www.plasticsurgery.co.nz/grs-main.asp (male to female)

# Section II
Wound Management – Reconstructive Plastic Surgical Nursing

# Introduction to Wound Management within Reconstructive Plastic Surgery Nursing Practice

1. Primary clinical management definitions
2. Introduction to wound management within reconstructive plastic surgery nursing practice

## 1. PRIMARY CLINICAL MANAGEMENT DEFINITIONS

### Acute care

Acute care is defined as the medical and/or nursing plan of care provided to a patient requiring treatment for a sudden episode of illness which may, or may not, be life-threatening. This may result from accident, trauma, disease, or following surgery[1-9].

### Chronic care

Chronic care has its roots in the ancient Greek word *chronos*, meaning 'time' and implying 'long lasting'. Chronic wound management is based on this definition[2-12].

Because healthcare in the Western world is focused mainly toward acute medical or surgical care, and to preventing or curing disease, chronic care is suggested to be an unfamiliar term to many. This is according to *Chronic Care in America: A 21st Century Challenge*, a report published by The Robert Wood Johnson Foundation in the USA (http://www.rjwf.org). The term 'chronic care' refers to a continuum of care required over a prolonged period for people who have lost, or never acquired, functional abilities.

Dorothy Rice, part of the team at the Institute for Health and Aging at the University of California, San Francisco, who wrote the report, emphasised that chronic care refers to fragmented services that the chronically ill need. Chronic care can include medical care, rehabilitative care, and personal assistance for

conditions that last for years. Chronic conditions are often in the incurable category and it is reasonable that a defined plan of care, paralleled to palliative care, is considered. The goal of care in these circumstances, is often one of optimal maintenance, and the support of the independent means, which the client has achieved, or is capable of achieving and maintaining.

In modern societies, the term 'chronic care' is often used interchangeably with long-term care in reference to nursing homes, and home care agencies. Newer terminology for nursing homes, such as 'aged care facilities' or 'supported residential facilities' more clearly define the range of care available to those who require support or total care.

For many clients, the expression 'nursing home' can be a negative one implying that they are ill, infirmed, disabled or dying and totally lacking any independence, so requiring 'nursing' care when in some cases the opposite may be the case. In addition, many clinicians state that the term often has demeaning connotations for those professional nurses caring for the aged, who are actively encouraging clients towards interdependence (co-dependence) and independence with a high level of self maintenance for as long as possible.

### Palliative care

*'Palliative care is an approach that aims to improve the quality of life of patients, and their families, facing the problem associated with life threatening illness, through the prevention and relief of suffering by means of early identification and impeccable assessment and treatment*

*of pain and other problems, physical, psychosocial and spiritual.'*

World Health Organization (http://www.who.int/cancer/palliative/definition/en/)

Palliative wound care is based on this definition[3,4,7].

---

**Box 4.1** Palliative care aims.

Palliative care aims to:

- Provide relief from pain and other distressing symptoms
- Affirm life
- Regard dying as a normal process
- Neither hasten nor postpone death
- Integrate the psychological and spiritual aspects of patient care
- Offer a support system to help patients live as actively as possible until death
- Offer a support system to help the family cope during the patient's illness and in their bereavement
- Use a team approach to address the needs of patients and their families, including bereavement counselling, if indicated
- Enhance quality of life, which may also positively influence the course of illness
- Be applicable early in the course of illness, in conjunction with other therapies that are intended to prolong life, such as chemotherapy or radiation therapy
- Include those investigations needed to better understand and manage distressing clinical complications.

---

## Palliative care for children

Palliative care for children represents a special, albeit closely related, field to adult palliative care. A representation of WHO's definition of palliative care that is appropriate for children and their families is detailed in Box 4.2 (these definitions may also be applied to paediatric chronic disorders, including wound care). http://www.who.int/cancer/palliative/definition/en/

---

**Box 4.2** WHO definition for children – outline.

- Palliative care for children is the active total care of the child's body, mind and spirit, and also involves giving support to the family.
- It begins when illness is diagnosed, and continues regardless of whether or not a child receives treatment directed at the disease.
- Health providers must evaluate and alleviate a child's physical, psychological, and social distress.
- Effective palliative care requires a broad multidisciplinary approach that includes the family and makes use of available community resources it can be successfully implemented even if resources are limited.
- It can be provided in tertiary care facilities, in community health centres and even in children's homes.

---

## 2. INTRODUCTION TO WOUND MANAGEMENT WITHIN RECONSTRUCTIVE PLASTIC SURGERY NURSING PRACTICE

### Addressing wounds across a spectrum of care

---

**Box 4.3** Utilising wound management practice terminology.

- **Acute** wound bed management (AWBM)
- **Chronic** wound bed management (CWBM)
- **Palliative** wound bed management (malignancy) (PWBM-M)
- **Palliative** wound bed management (non-malignant) (PWBM-NM)

---

### Background – wound care practices

Wound management clinicians and educators require basic clinical pathophysiological indicators of what constitutes the changing formula of a wound from acute to chronic, and chronic to palliative (within or outside the cancer wound framework). There appear to be some differences of opinion as to when a wound moves from one present classification

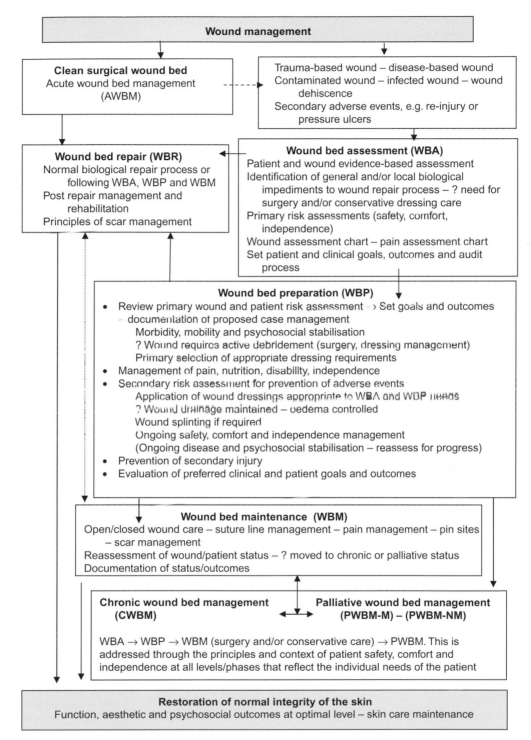

**Figure 4.1** A clinical practice pathway for wound management in reconstructive plastic surgery nursing.

**Box 4.4** Wound management pathway terminology.

| | |
|---|---|
| **Moist wound healing (MWH)** | the pathophysiological concepts and principles on which current evidence-based wound management is approached and practised[2–11] |
| **Wound bed assessment (WBA)** | the pathophysiological, evidence-based assessment of a wound and its bed at all stages of repair or failure to repair |
| **Wound bed preparation (WBP)** | instituting balance into the physiological and psychosocial processes, preparation of an actual or potential wound (surgical, non-healing chronic or palliative wounds), for the purpose of initiating/restoring the repair process or long-term patient safety, comfort and independence |
| **Wound bed maintenance (WBM)** | maintenance of the optimal pathway (physiological, psychosocial) to repair (surgical, non-healing chronic or palliative wounds) for the purpose of initiating/restoring the repair process or long-term patient safety, comfort and independence |
| **Wound bed repair (WBR)** | the integration of the physiological and psychosocial processes that facilitate wound repair/healing (surgical, non-healing chronic or palliative wounds) for the purpose of initiating/restoring the repair process or long-term patient safety, comfort and independence |
| **Palliative wound bed maintenance (PWBM)** | the whole care of the patient and wounds that recur as a result of cancer or specific disease processes that are of a long-term chronic non-healing nature (ulcerated, cavity, dehisced wounds) and may not or do not respond to the traditional surgical, non-surgical wound management practices, or alternative medical practices. This category could also include, for example, stomas and chronic fistulas. |

to another, when it is required to be based on a scientific criterion.

The terminology (see Box 4.3) suggests a pathway for wound care by defining specific management processes that need to be identified and scientifically addressed.

Steps in normal tissue repair are not arbitrary but rather overlapping, with the body's life support systems working uncompromisingly to sustain the positive changes in a forward movement (repair/survival).

Unwarranted changes in the direction of wound treatments that cannot be scientifically justified, are a source of disrupted care, potential secondary injury, pain, patient anxiety, and an increasing loss of confidence by the patient in the wound care process. This may finally end in a failure of the originally set clinical outcomes, and a source of grief and anger, by the patient.

The question then becomes whether the patient and wound care remains in the acute phase, or has moved into a chronic wound phase, due to a failure to understand the exact and inexact scientific basis of wound repair. In some units this change may be suggested to be after 21 days, the preferred healing timeframe of the epidermal resurfacing, including the formation of initial tissue strength in the dermis, within a clean surgical wound. This phase of movement may be referred to as acute-on-chronic period, in that contamination is present, healing is inhibited, and progress appears to be stagnant or in decline. The inability to initiate and complete the healing process within an objective timeframe that provides a highly protective state to the organism, may then see the wound fall into the chronic or palliative category unless reassessment and alternatives are sought to restore the positive progress of cellular and tissue repair.

## Discussion

Based on Boxes 4.3 and 4.4, a practice pathway was developed (Figure 4.1) as an educational tool for postgraduate students to identify particular regions of the wound healing process, and to enable clinicians to address wound care through an overall framework.

The current evidence-based data that are available regarding wound healing are essentially based on the known principles of physiology, microbiology, animal studies, cadaver and *in vivo* studies of the blood supply to the skin. Included within these are the outcomes of clinical observations, various clinical trials reviewing dressing products, and expert experience[1-25]. Basic principles and approaches to wound care have been established, based on both scientific and experiential data and this has significantly improved the healing outcomes of acute wounds, long-standing chronic wounds, and the management of cancer-based wounds.

Regardless of the progress made so far, it seems self evident that if there is to be a science-based wound management discipline, further studies are required that can provide a universal agreement on a lexicon, classification, and scientifically defined borders of what biologically constitutes an acute, chronic or palliative wound.

The ongoing scientific research, and works being undertaken on wound repair that focus on cellular functions, vascular disease, diabetes mellitus, leg ulceration diagnosis and treatment modalities, are examples of attempts to better define the complex pathophysiology that surrounds tissue repair.

Currently, there is a great deal of fragmentation in wound care delivery, and the overall costs to the community are gaining momentum. The development of patient care structures, reflecting evidence-based practices and case management delivering wound repair outcomes acceptable to governments, will likely be the projects that have a greater capacity for funding.

## General principles required for a wound to heal

In contemporary plastic surgical wound care, the recognition of a holistic approach has been significant in improving wound repair and/or quality of life outcomes in acute, chronic and palliative care-based wounds[3,4,7]. As in all medical and nursing care, the approaches taken reflect both the exact sciences (empirical, research-based) and the inexact sciences (social sciences).

The complexity of caring for individual patients and their wounds is more often based on good experiential judgement rather than fact. Nonetheless, independent discretionary judgement can be a combination of insights drawn from a range of many repeated constructive and non-constructive experiences and the current evidence-based research available.

The following principles (Boxes 4.5 & 4.6) for excellence in wound management within reconstructive plastic surgery are based on the existing and

---

**Box 4.5** Principles of wound management within reconstructive plastic surgery nursing – building a basic knowledge base.

- Acceptance of the requirement of a combined scientific and caring model (based on, for example, safety, comfort, independence) and approach to holistic patient care
- The developed concepts and principles of the model (Figure 4.1) aim to support the importance for developing a multidisciplinary team approach with the skills required to provide the total range of care for patients presenting within the practice of reconstructive plastic surgery[5]
- Acquiring a broad knowledge base of congenital malformations, trauma (mechanisms of injury), disease processes, and their effects on the tissue repair process
- Acquiring the knowledge and understanding of the process for undertaking a wound assessment based on the pathophysiology of injury and wound repair within the individual patient's needs.

---

**Box 4.6** Principles of wound management within reconstructive plastic surgery nursing: applying the knowledge base.

- Acceptance of the significance of an optimal blood flow to the wound and its surroundings
- The results of continuing research into the blood flow to the skin have significantly assisted in the acceleration in surgically restoring the integrity of the skin in injured zones (e.g. skin flaps) and limb salvage (e.g. microsurgery and replant surgery) procedures[21,22]
- Following tissue injury/trauma/disease, the recognition that until revascularisation within a clean wound has been established and stabilised, immobility is a decisive factor primarily for the first 48–72 hours and is fundamentally essential in re-establishing a local circulatory system for cellular recovery
- Immobility avoids shear, friction and movement within the injured tissues that would interrupt the development of neovascularisation and the re-anastomotic process[5,21,22]
- Applying the knowledge that clean, closed surgical wounds with each of the tissue layers interfaced, free from dead space, fluid/moisture in excess of normal

*Continued*

levels, or tissue tension, and with an internal moist warm environment, will have a high potential to heal, free from adverse events

- The scientific amount of moisture required remains unknown, but it is accepted that an environment of specific moisture and cellular warmth is essential, as it is observed in normal tissues within body zones[15–17]
- The increased understanding of the significant effects of critical contamination and infection within the injured area, and on the host
- This requires 'rebalancing' the wound bed/host bacteria levels significantly in favour of the host[11,12]
- The damaging effects of oedema on cellular function are becoming more scientifically understood and some wound treatment modalities (particularly chronic wounds) are increasingly being focused towards reduction of oedema before, or in concert, by addressing the overall needs of the wound to facilitate the repair process[2,13]
- The recognition that there is a significant relationship between unresolved acute pain, chronic pain, painful wound dressing changes, and the failure of wounds to repair[2–4,7,18,20]
- The acceptance of the role that normothermia contributes to normal cellular function and an optimal wound repair process[23]
- The acceptance and application of the research-based scientific concepts and principles of moist wound healing (MWH) as the foundation on which current normal biological tissue healing treatment modalities are based[14–16]
- This may be achieved by WBA, WBP and WBM that facilitate wound closure, including skin grafts, skin flaps, or modern wound dressings which imitate the protective cover normally afforded by the normal epidermis[17]
- Application of the concept of wound bed preparation (WBP) with practice principles as essential if the optimal environment for wound repair is to occur[17]
- Acceptance of the introduction of a range of evidence-based treatment modalities to address oedema, wound exudates, contaminated, and infected wound sites, in selected patients[24,25]. These include:
  - Electrical stimulation
  - Ultrasonic treatments
  - Special compression bandaging techniques
  - Negative pressure therapy.

accepted knowledge and practices currently adopted in order for optimal wound outcomes to occur[1–25]. These are not in order of priority as each is of equal importance, and based on the range of references provided at the end of the chapter, and the accepted clinical wisdom of the experts of the day.

## References

(1) Wysocki A.B. Skin anatomy, physiology, and pathophysiology. *Nursing Clinics of North America*, 1999 (Dec); **34**(4):777–97.
(2) Peacock E.E. Jr. *Wound Repair*, 3rd edn. Philadelphia: W.B. Saunders Company, 1984.
(3) Dealey C. *The care of wounds*, 2nd edn. Oxford, UK: Blackwell Science, 1999.
(4) Bryant R.A. (ed.) *Acute and chronic wounds: nursing management*. St Louis: Mosby Year Book, 1992.
(5) Robinson J.B. & Friedman R.M. Wound healing and closure. *Selected Readings in Plastic Surgery*, 8(1):1999–2000.
(6) Lazarus G.S., Cooper D.M., Knighton D.R., Margolis D.J., Pecoraro R.E., Rodeheaver G. & Robson M.C. Definitions and guidelines for assessment of wounds and evaluation of healing. *Archives of Dermatology*, 1994 (Apr); **130**(4):489–93.
(7) Carville K. *Wound care – manual*. Western Australia: Silver Chain Nursing Association, 1993, Revised edition 1995.
(8) Moy L.S. Management of acute wounds. *Dermatologic Clinics*, 1993 (Oct 11); **4**:759–66.
(9) Dubay D.A. & Franz M.G. Acute wound healing: the biology of acute wound failure. *Surgical Clinics of North America*, 2003 (Jun); **83**(3):463–81.
(10) Bates-Jensen B.M. Chronic wound assessment. *Nursing Clinics of North America*, 1999 (Dec); **34**(4): 799–845.
(11) Robson M.C. Wound infection: a failure of wound healing caused by an imbalance of bacteria. *Surgical Clinics of North America*, 1997 (June); **77**(3):637–50.
(12) Bowler P.G., Duerden B.I. & Armstrong D.G. Wound microbiology and associated approaches to wound management. *Clinical Microbiology Reviews*, 2001 (April); 244–269.
(13) Guyton A.C. & Hall J.E. *Textbook of medical physiology*, 9th edn. London: W.B. Saunders, 1996.
(14) Winter G.D. Formation of the scab and the rate of epithelialisation of superficial wounds in the skin of the domestic pig. *Nature*, 1962; **193**:293.
(15) Winter G.D. Epidermal regeneration studied in the domestic pig. In: Hunt T.K. & Dunphy J.E. (eds) *Fundamentals of Wound Management*. New York: Appleton-Century-Crofts, 1979.
(16) Bolton L.L., Monte K. & Pirone L.A. Moisture and healing: beyond the jargon. *Ostomy/Wound Management*, 2000 (Jan) **46**(1A Suppl):51S–62S quiz 63S–63S.
(17) Vowden K. & Vowden P. Wound bed preparation. http://www.worldwidewounds.com

(18) Moffatt, C. *Pain and trauma at wound dressing changes*: Position Document, 2002. http://www.worldwide wounds.com/News/News.html

(19) Mallett J. & Dougherty L. (eds).*The Royal Marsden Hospital Manual of Clinical Nursing Procedures*, 5th edn. Oxford, UK: Blackwell Science, 2000.

(20) Taylor G.I., Palmer J.H. & McManamny D. The vascular territories of the body (angiosomes) and their clinical implications. In: McCarthy J.G. *Plastic surgery: volume 1, general principles*. Philadelphia: W.B. Saunders, 1990.

(21) Taylor G.I., Gianoutsos M.P. & Morris S.F. The neurovascular territories of the body: an anatomic study and clinical implications. *Plastic Reconstructive Surgery*, 1994; **94**:1–5.

(22) Kurz A., Sessler D. & Lenhardt R. Perioperative normothermia to reduce the incidence of surgical wound infection and shorten hospitalisation. *New England Journal of Medicine*, 1996 (May); **9**(334):1209–15.

(23) Morykwas M., Argenta L.C., Shelton-Brown E. & McGuirt W. Vacuum-assisted closure: a new method for wound control and treatment: animal studies and basic foundation. *Annals of Plastic Surgery*, 1997; **38**:553–562.

(24) Argenta L.C. & Morykwas M. Vacuum-assisted closure: a new method for wound control and treatment: clinical experience. *Annals of Plastic Surgery*, 1997; **38**:563–577.

# Chapter 5

# The Functional Anatomy of the Skin and its Appendages

## Background

In order to understand the process of wound healing and ageing, nurse clinicians must have an excellent working knowledge and understanding of the anatomy and functions of living cells, and the physiology of how cells may be destroyed, and are suggested to die naturally.

The human body is made up of approximately 75 trillion cells, which constitute the building blocks of all body organs[1]. Figure 5.1 shows the basic structure of the cell.

The term 'cell' originates from the Latin word *cella*, or storeroom – a place for storing the elements that reproduce and sustain life. Two basic types of cells exist, **eukaryocytes**, or cells of living tissue, and **prokaryocytes**, cells of lower forms of life that have no true nucleus – such as bacteria or viruses.

All living cells contain a true central **nucleus**, with the exception of **erythrocytes**, or mature red blood cells (RBCs) which have a life span of approximately 45 days and are replaced by new, nucleated RBCs. **Leucocytes**, or white blood cells (WBCs), are multinucleated, reflecting their multifunctional purposes[1].

All living tissue cells consist of the same basic architecture (Figure 5.1), although some cells are, for example, flat, round or rectangular, according to the functional structure of the tissue they form part of. Living cells have a true nucleus, **cytoplasm**, and **organelles**, surrounded by a cytoplasmic membrane. These organelles all have specific structures and functions, and their activities are driven by the nucleus at the centre of the cell, powered by the **mitochondria**. Within the nucleus is the **nucleolus** containing the RNA and chromatin granules containing protein, and DNA that develops into chromosomes, which are the determinants of hereditary characteristics[1].

The **nucleus** is the central controlling body within a living cell. It is usually spherical, enclosed and protected by a membrane, and contains the genetic codes for sustaining all life systems of the organism. As such, it is responsible for responding to cell injury and directing growth and reproduction. Although not able to function independently, the mitochondria (the powerhouse of the cell that converts food to energy) contains its own DNA molecule, which is separate from the main DNA, or **genome**, of our cells[2–4]. The lifecycle of the mitochondria has been demonstrated to significantly influence the ageing process (i.e. self programmed to die), and ability of the cells to be replaced as required[2] (see Chapter 6).

Cells are suspended in a specialised gel-like substance that assembles them in a precise and orderly framework, preventing disorder and collision with each other during normal movement. Chaotic cellular movement and collisions result in injury to the outer protective membrane that protects the cell as a whole. This actually, or potentially, places the cells at risk by disrupting their essential functions, which may result in their demise[5–7]. Because of their basic fragility, cells within tissues, although packed with precision and order, also require a backup system for their protection. This is provided by negative or positive atmospheric pressures within the tissues to ensure constancy of order for optimal function[5]. The loss of one or both of these two fundamental physiological factors is a primary pathological cause of major wound disturbances and repair processes.

### Cells and tissues

Cells form tissues, and complex tissues form the human anatomical structures[1,5–12]. The skin is composed of compound cellular structures that emanate from multiple germ layers, and its total structure and function is an exquisite example of this complexity. Because of its multiple and complex protective functions, the skin, including its blood supply, is the largest organ of the body and can technically be described as one of the most important single organs of the body[1].

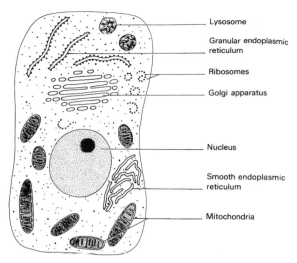

Figure 5.1 A typical cell and its most important components (*Blackwell's Dictionary of Nursing*, 1994).

Labels:
- Lysosome
- Granular endoplasmic reticulum
- Ribosomes
- Golgi apparatus
- Nucleus
- Smooth endoplasmic reticulum
- Mitochondria

---

**Box 5.1** Principal functions of the epidermis/skin.

- A waterproof wrapping for the entire body
- A protective lining for the internal digestive system
- The first line of defence against bacteria and other organisms
- A cooling system via sweat
- A sense organ that gives us information about pain, temperature, pressure and pleasure.

---

## The skin as a defensive and protective structure

### The epidermis

Skin tissue is the first line of the body's defence against external forces and bacterial invasion and its total design reflects these protective functions (Figure 5.2). It is the largest organ of the body, covering the entire body both outside (approximately 1.5–2 m²), and inside, lining it with squamous epithelium tissue. Thus the skin of the outer body is continuous with the mucous membrane of the oral, digestive, respiratory and urogenital systems[1,5–12].

The skin consists of two principal layers, the **epidermis** (or outer layer), and the **dermis** (or inner layer), which are separated by an extremely important structure called the **basement membrane**[1,5–12].

The epidermis consists of squamous epithelium (epidermal cells) tissue and consists of **labile** cells (unstable, as opposed to stable, or permanent, such as, nerve cells). Because of constant usage of this special tissue externally and internally, the architecture of these labile cells enables them, under normal wear and tear, to be readily and constantly replaced.

The presence of the dermis, with tissue consisting of more stable cells, is fundamental in the process of wound/skin repair. It is primarily composed of connective tissue (tissues that connect anatomical body structures, providing strength and resilience). As the deeper layer of the skin proper, it anchors the skin to the hypodermis, or fatty layer, and these are then attached to the underlying connective tissues linking together the anatomical structures of the body providing strength and bonding[1,5–12].

The dermis contains the microvascular structures through which the circulatory system nourishes and removes waste products from the epidermis, which has no discrete circulatory structure of its own. This microvascular structure connects back into the venous and lymphatic macro system, returning the blood flow to the heart, maintaining the normal architectural circulatory structure and movement.

### The appendages within the skin

As an extension of the surface epidermis, the appendages of the skin (the hair follicles and cutaneous sweat and sebaceous glands that project into the dermis) provide moisture and oil to the skin, keeping it soft and supple. In non-full thickness wounds, they contain epidermal cells with a blood supply that assists the labile cells replicating and resurfacing partial thickness wounds.

Full thickness wounds (e.g. full thickness burns) lose their appendages. In the presence of the epidermal/skin appendages, the epidermis has a highly sophisticated and complex process of constant resurfacing following normal wear and tear. Under normal circumstances, following injury to the epidermis and partial thickness of the dermis, the dermis (as a connecting tissue) also provides contracting forces in parallel with the resurfacing epidermal process.

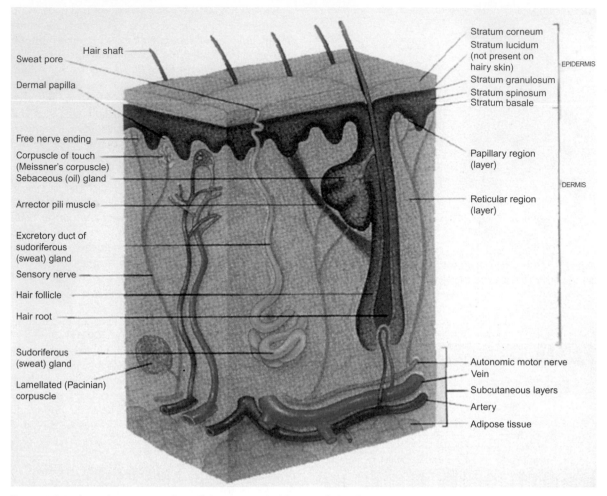

**Figure 5.2** Universal representation of the anatomical layers of the skin.

Trauma or disease that destroys the nucleus and/or mitochondria of the squamous epidermal and dermal connective tissue cells also renders the skin's cells inactive. Zones of tissue injury will have a range and mixture of living and dead cells. This is called a **wound**[5–12].

## The micro blood flow to the skin

One of the most significant results of modern vascular research within reconstructive plastic surgery has been the identification of the interconnections between the vascular territories (also referred to as **angiosomes** (Figures 5.3, 5.4 & 5.5). Blood flows to the skin through a circulatory system in a three-dimensional pattern (Figure 5.6), allowing all levels of the skin tissue to receive its primary needs according to its particular function (fixed or mobile)[13,14]. Angiosomes supply blood to specific body regions that contain both fixed and mobile skin (Figures 5.7 & 5.8)[13,14].

The identification and mapping of these territories has enabled major advances in the wound repair and

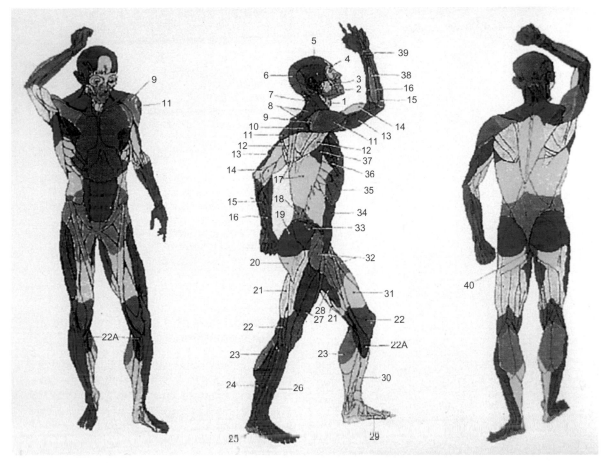

**Figure 5.3** Diagrammatic representation of the distribution of the arterial blood supply to the skin of the body, referred to as vascular territories or angiosomes. With permission: Professor G.I. Taylor.

the microvascular transfer of large areas of vascularised skin, and other tissues, including bone, to specifically match the areas required to be reconstructed. These studies are also the origin on which the concept and principles of 'tissue expansion' are based.

Muscle and skin tissue flaps based on the vascular territories can be moved locally with their blood supply remaining connected, or disconnected and reconnected, to similar size vessels at a distant site to repair structural and functional defects. This is of extreme importance in small or large zones of lost skin, particularly fixed skin areas,

and areas that protect significant underlying tissues such as damaged muscle, macrocirculations and nerves.

For optimal wound repair, it is the efficiency of the overall macro- and microcirculatory architecture, pressure and flow at each anatomical tissue level, emerging at the level of the skin, that is fundamentally important for the restoration of the effectiveness of the important functions of the skin. Regardless of the cause, disturbance or loss of a continuous and effective circulatory micro blood flow is one of most common reasons for failure of a wound to heal, and flaps to fail[6-13].

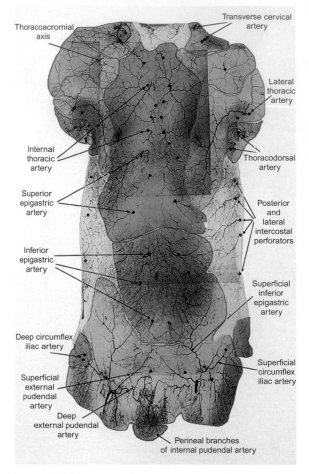

Thoracoacromial axis

Transverse cervical artery

Lateral thoracic artery

Internal thoracic artery

Thoracodorsal artery

Superior epigastric artery

Posterior and lateral intercostal perforators

Inferior epigastric artery

Superficial inferior epigastric artery

Deep circumflex iliac artery

Superficial circumflex iliac artery

Superficial external pudendal artery

Deep external pudendal artery

Perineal branches of internal pudendal artery

**Figure 5.4** Diagrammatic representation of the sources of the blood supply to the soft tissues and skin of the torso. With permission: Professor G.I. Taylor.

**Box 5.2** Principal functions of normal uninterrupted circulatory blood flow.

- Transports oxygen and nutrients to the cells and removes cytotoxic substances from the tissues at each tissue level
- Regulates pH through buffer systems ensuring cellular integrity
- Regulates body temperature
- Controls water movement in the intracellular and extracellular spaces
- Protects the organism by initiating the clotting system to prevent blood loss
- Initiates white blood cellular mechanisms to prevent and fight infection
- Aids in the synthesis of vitamin D, where adequate sunlight is available[1,14,15].

## The importance of a barrier against the external environment

Skin is indispensable in the maintenance of life, forming a protective barrier between the external environment and the internal organs[1]. Sweat and oil glands in the skin have very important protective functions that rely on the efficiency of the blood supply at the dermal level.

At the level of the epidermis, under normal conditions the skin has a pH of 4.4–5.5 (normal physiological blood pH is about 7.35–7.4) maintained by the sebum that exudes from glands in the skin and this provides the external body with a highly protective acidic cloak, or mantle[5-9,14,15]. This is the first line of defence against the potential invasion of opportunistic bacteria and foreign particulate matter, and penetration of environmental factors (for example, some chemicals and insect bites).

The outer cell membrane layer (the **cytoplasmic membrane**) envelops the whole cellular structure and contains multiple micro perforations. It is the 'sentry' for the inner cell contents. It is extremely selective and protective in respect of what is allowed to enter the inner contents of the cell, and the time-frame over which this may occur. Any products wishing to enter the inner cells' compartment for cellular and physiological energy to be produced, or drugs to be absorbed, must be water or fat soluble. As cells in different organs of the body are responsi-

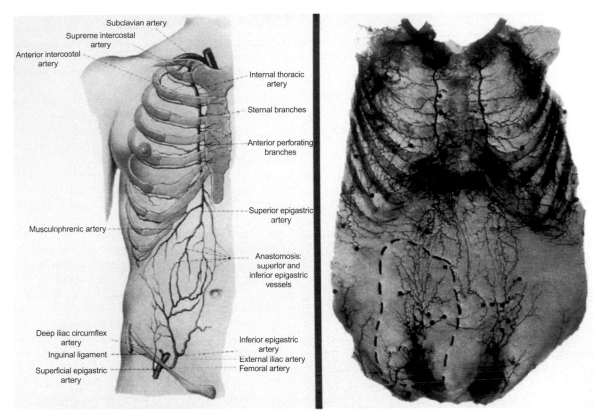

**Figure 5.5** Modern diagrammatic representation of the distribution and source of the blood supply to the transverse rectus abdominis muscle (TRAM) and skin of the abdomen, with clinical application to TRAM flap design for breast reconstruction. With permission: Professor G.I. Taylor.

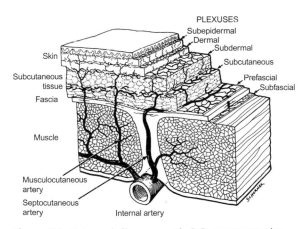

**Figure 5.6** Universal diagrammatic 3-D representation of the blood supply to the skin, from primary source vessel to skin (note the distribution of septocutaneous and musculocutaneous vessels). With permission: Professor G.I. Taylor.

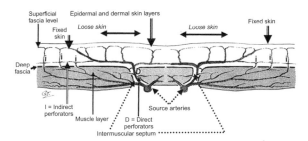

**Figure 5.7** Diagrammatic representation of the blood supply to the skin, indicating distribution of general blood flow into fixed and mobile skin, reflecting Figure 5.6. With permission: Professor G.I. Taylor.

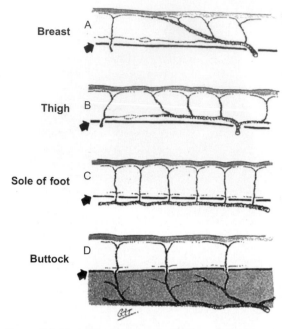

**Figure 5.8** Diagrammatic representation of the blood supply to the skin, indicating source of blood flow into the fixed and mobile skin of differing body regions. With permission: Professor G.I. Taylor.

ble for different functions, the outer cell membrane must select what is to be accepted as important, or repelled as a foreign invader.

Various lipids (fats) are synthesised in the cells of the **stratum corneum**. This is the outer cellular layer of the epidermis. The continuing presence of these lipids creates a near impermeable barrier to almost all water soluble toxins and other substances, such as excess water that comes into contact with the skin. Thus the stratum corneum provides an effective barrier against excess absorption in normal uninjured skin and, conversely, also intelligently controls water loss from the inside of the epidermis to the external environment.

Despite this, some hazardous environmental toxins are absorbed into the cells because they are highly fat soluble or water soluble, but may also be selectively repelled by the level of water or fat within the epidermis. It is the constant high level bombardment of toxic materials or particulate matter that can ultimately destroy the protective pH mantle by entering the cells and causing, for example, malignant tumours of the skin or mucous membrane[6].

## Resident skin organisms

The organisms *Streptococcus viridins* (Gram-negative) and *Staphylococcus epidermis* (Gram-positive) are resident bacteria and normally present on the skin in colonies of $10^3$ per gram of tissue[6]. Increase in the colonisation numbers increases the potential for wound infection such as MRSA (methicillin-resistant *Staphylococcus aureas*). MRSA is sometimes called 'golden Staph' because of the golden pigment seen in a microscopic view of the bacteria. This organism causes a particularly troublesome wound infection and is encountered in many hospital units due to its resistance to all but one or two extremely expensive antibiotics[14,15].

The presence of highly acidic sebum[6] and the maintenance of this biological level are important to reduce the potential for the development of infection. Injury to the skin, or dilution of this acidic mantle, increases the risk of bacterial entry. If the integrity of the basement membrane that connects the dermis and epidermis is broken, this further increases the risk, as this membrane acts as a secondary sentinel barrier to certain opportunistic neoplastic forces, and protects against bacterial invasion.

The basement membrane is sensitive to cell size and some molecules can penetrate this barrier (particularly those less than 40 kD) allowing opportunistic bacteria entry into the dermis, for example, MRSA which is 25 kD[6].

Finally, skin provides the underlying tissues with a cushioning protection from minor or moderate injury, substantially reducing potential injury to the deeper underlying tissues[6-12].

## Body temperature regulation

Thermoregulation of the human organism is an essential primary survival function. In normal conditions, internal body temperature is maintained constantly at approximately 36.8°–37°C (98.6°F), mainly through metabolic cellular functions creating body heat, and reflected ambient environmental temperatures.

In adults, under normal circumstances, the physiological balance between metabolic heat production and cellular needs is maintained exactly, principally related to the surface temperature of the skin. This is a function of the rate and volume of a warm arterial blood flow, controlled primarily by the sympathetic nervous system, which determines blood flow activity according to physiological needs, and the ambient environmental temperature[1].

Children are very sensitive to ambient temperature alterations, as their hypothalamus is immature, and they therefore require a high metabolic rate to cope within the parameters of normal activity and the distribution of water volume to body surface area. This is an extremely important physiological factor in the surgical and nursing management of children and adults undergoing major reconstructive surgery, particularly flaps and replant surgery[14,15].

---

**Box 5.3** The role of skin in body temperature regulation.

- Proper temperature regulation is vital to maintaining metabolic reactions
- Active cells, such as those of the heart and skeletal muscle, produce heat
- Heat may be lost to the local environmental surroundings from the skin
- The body responds to excessive heat by dilation of dermal blood vessels and sweating
- The body responds to excessive cooling by constricting dermal blood vessels, inactivating sweat glands, and causing shivering
- Sweating (except that which is a reflex response to emotional stress) can also assist in the control and regulation of body temperature but does not occur until core temperature exceeds 37°C, regardless of skin temperature
- As many cellular functions are undertaken within a relatively fine heat ratio, core temperature must be preserved as an essential priority for all body cells in order to function at an optimal level, particularly in relation to circulatory flow[6,14,15].

---

## Discussion

As stated, tissue cells must stay within the narrow range of acceptable core temperature values in order to undertake the functions that are responsible for maintenance of life. Modern research into the effects of body temperature on cellular function, particularly related to how specific temperature ratios influence the maintenance of the cellular pH, is providing a much clearer picture of the need to maintain core temperature for tissue repair. This is particularly important during, and after surgery, post injury, and in providing part of the rationale for ensuring a wound environment that requires tissue warmth for cell repair and replication[6,14,15].

For patients undergoing surgery, monitoring and regulation of core temperature in the intra-operative and postoperative phases, by mechanical and environmental means to maintain normal core thermoregulation (**normothermia**), is now seen to be as important as the monitoring and regulation of circulatory and respiratory functions[14,15] (see Chapter 15).

Nurse clinicians have a very dominant role in clinical monitoring, observations, clinical responses, and educating other clinicians regarding the need to maintain normothermia in all patients at risk, particularly children, the elderly, the injured and the critically ill.

## Water balance

The germinal or basal cell layer of the epidermis (the innermost layer closest to the dermis) holds 40% of the water in the epidermis[6,14,15]. Loss of water and electrolytes from the body, and maintenance of moisture levels in the skin and connective tissues, is principally controlled by the stratum corneum, or outermost layer of the epidermis. The stratum corneum is not completely impermeable to fluid, as it allows the loss of small amounts of fluid into the environment. This is called insensible loss, or perspiration, and can amount to approximately 600 ml daily in an adult under normal circumstances, and a significantly larger quantity under emotional or physical stress, or during acute illness[14,15].

Postoperatively, following extensive soft tissue injury, burns and major reconstructive surgery, this fluid loss must be considered in determining an accurate fluid balance. For example, the loss of a litre of water a day, as a minimum, is significant for a patient who has lost or is losing substantial amounts via ongoing low level haemorrhage, open wounds, drainage systems and dressings[14,15].

Major damage to the skin, multiple injury and burns are suggested as classic examples of situations where fluids and electrolytes are also lost proportionally to the extent and distribution of the injury, by interstitial (third space) fluid shifts[6,14,15]. There is a stated '**golden hour**' following injury where patients with substantial partial and full thickness burns can suffer (i.e. major hypovolaemia) with, for example, irreversible renal failure and potential death if disturbances in fluid balance are not recognised and immediately corrected. Overcorrection causes the reverse shift (hypervolaemia) which places the patient at serious risk and commonly results in renal and cardiorespiratory disturbances[6,14,15].

In wound care, immersion of the unstable epidermal tissue of limbs (e.g. chronic venous ulceration) in water for longer than 10–15 minutes can result in the skin absorbing up to three to four times their normal weight, causing pain, cellular damage, and patient distress. Monitoring of immersion time is important, and should be appropriate to the amount of moisture required for hygiene, removal of dressings, or the easy removal of collected flaking skin (dead cells)[6].

## Sensation

**Meissner's** and **Pacinian** corpuscles are located only in the palms of the hand and soles of the feet and are responsible for tactile and pressure responses. Within the dermis, unmyelinated nerve endings respond to temperature, pain, or injury such as insect bites[1].

Sensory receptors in the skin provide constant monitoring of the surrounding environmental conditions. Diverse nerve endings are principally concerned with touch, temperature and pressure. They are more concentrated in some areas than others, for example, more in the fingertips, fewer in the skin of the back.

Loss of peripheral sensory function in the feet (e.g. peripheral neuropathy in diabetes mellitus) can result in significant tissue injury following burns, or minimal pressure over long time periods[6,14,15].

Unlike the vascular system, which is distributed through a circulatory pattern with a collateral supportive system, the nervous system is more like a tree with branches, unconnected and somewhat inadequately supported within its own architecture when injury occurs[1]. When primary or secondary level nerves are cut (e.g. trauma) or destroyed by disease (e.g. disease of the facial nerve) there appears to be no collateral or backup system to replace their entire function, even in the long term[1].

Reconstructive surgery has had some encouraging results, but these have been minimal unless innervated tissue flaps are used. In the case of facial nerve palsy, cross facial nerve reconstruction, face lift procedures, and the use of tendons to create facial slings for assisting both function and aesthetics have pro-

vided some acceptable aesthetic results, but restoration of motor nerve function has been somewhat disappointing in most cases. Thus the importance of preserving the existing functioning motor and sensory nerves becomes extremely imperative.

## Synthesis of vitamin D

Ultraviolet light (sunlight) absorbed by the skin is believed to assist in the synthesis of vitamin D, which is essential for production of calcium for bone healing and for preventing osteoporosis and bone fragility[6]. The level of exposure required is the subject of research as it has been suggested that people who have little or no sun exposure are more at risk in the medium to long term for osteoporosis. This is particularly of interest for those who are institutionalised for long periods.

Although much is known about the benefits of many vitamins, research is ongoing to ascertain their scientific value for a range of healthcare issues, particularly in the area of their protection against disease, medical indications, dosages, and contraindications to use in certain medical circumstances. Because the body only absorbs what is immediately required and most vitamins are not stored for long periods in the body, the unsubstantiated benefits or, conversely, the actual and potential medical problems when vitamins are taken at high dosages on a daily basis, are of concern to many researchers and clinicians.

## Skin mobility – independence and wound repair

*'Skin is composed of layers. The deepest layer, binding skin to superficial skeletal muscle, is a bed of loose areolar tissue called the* tela subcutanea. *In animals other than man, a layer of skeletal muscle, the* panniculus carnosus *overlies areolar tissue (a type of connective tissue having little tensile strength). In man, however, superficial striated muscle is vestigial (of a primitive nature), and the platysma is the only remaining reminder of a useful adjunct to skin mobility'.*[4]

### *Functional anatomy*

Personal independence is largely dependent on the human's anatomical and physiological ability to be mobile. This mobility is supported by an extensive range of joint, deep and superficial tissue movements, strength of the connective tissues, and flexibility of the skin in certain regions of the body.

The skin, or outer cover, of most non-human small or medium-sized animals and quadrupeds, is predominantly mobile with a specialised connective tissue layer separating it from the underlying substrate tissue. This provides a necessary and extraordinary flexibility for the underlying muscle. The accommodating macro source blood vessels, and the micro blood vessels of the skin, allow those with this structural advantage to respond when speed is required for survival, hunting, or escape from the predators (flight or fight). Fundamental to this dynamic flexibility of the skin is the ability of the vascular structure to stretch and contract in response to functional needs without causing cellular, vascular or nerve trauma, or spasm[6,13].

Humans do not need the same degree of mobility for hunting, speed and survival as other animals, which can be observed in the looseness of the skin of, for example, the cat. As humans function in an upright position, there is a requirement for strategically placed fixed skin zones to combat or reverse the effects of normal gravitation pull[6]. To some degree, and in some regions, this is reversed with ageing and biological tissue changes in the skin. There are also some medical and congenital conditions that can affect normal collagen structural development and maintenance, for example, scleroderma.

Although human skin is stated to be of the intermediate type (i.e. neither entirely fixed, nor entirely mobile)[13], for ease of understanding it is usually stated to be fixed, or mobile (loose). The degree of skin movement is matched with a circulatory vascular pattern to parallel the functional requirements (Figure 5.8)[6,13]. When observed as a whole it can be seen that the human skin is a complex mix of both mobile and fixed tissues and these differences can be within centimetres of each other in, for example, the breast, abdomen and sternum.

## The importance of understanding skin mobility for wound repair

The degree of mobility of the human skin has an important influence on decisions that are made regarding options for surgical wound closure[6,13]. This mobility of the skin raises important issues that must be considered in respect of wound repair following trauma or surgery:

- In wound management of the injured skin, the degree of the skin's mobility in all anatomical zones (Figures 5.6–5.8) essentially dictates its primary ability to repair (contract and resurface with strength and resilience), protecting the underlying tissues[13]
- In wound repair, the temporary immobility (i.e. splinting) of the injured and surrounding zones is fundamental to prevent shear and friction on the repairing cells and tissues
- In reconstructive plastic surgery, the mobility of the skin essentially defines the procedure that is selected to repair the defect. Areas of loose or intermediate skin will usually allow the skin to be closed with minimal tension. Major loss of tissue may require the application of skin grafts, muscle flaps with skin grafts, or the movement of more mobile skin to less mobile skin zones, such as in the use of skin flaps[6,7,13] (see Section IV). For face lifting or rhytidoplasty, tightening the platysma forms an important basis of maintaining firmness of the facial/neck skin when the excess skin is removed and wrinkles are thus smoothed out[7]

Three principal biological effects are responsible for these varying levels of mobility or flexibility and these are kept in mind when assessing options for wound closure/management[6,13] (Box 5.4).

---

**Box 5.4** Importance of identifying fixed and mobile skin for wound repair treatment and outcomes.

- The movement (flexibility) and parallel circulatory responses needed to meet the functional dynamics of particular body areas
- The requirement for skin to be relatively fixed (e.g. over bone) at certain anatomical body points to reverse the effects of normal gravitational pull when in the upright position
- The positive (e.g. fixed tissue regions) and negative atmospheric forces (e.g. in mobile tissue regions) observed within particular body tissue zone/spaces[5].

## Sub-atmospheric (negative) pressure in the tissues

The integrity of homeostasis in the human body is initiated and maintained by a surfeit of visible and invisible functioning activities. The presence and maintenance of positive and negative pressure within the body tissues fall into this category[5].

When the skin is totally intact, and the total circulatory system is functioning effectively, there are said to be physiologically regulated negative and positive forces within certain tissue regions that assist in maintaining optimal interstitial fluid balance, or equilibrium, and organ function. This results in uninterrupted cellular stability and thus tissue compactness[5].

At the level of the skin, atmospheric pressure is normally accepted to be zero, and in most of the body's natural cavities in the body where there is free fluid in dynamic equilibrium with the surrounding interstitial fluid, sub-atmospheric or negative pressures have been recorded[5].

Although it has long been acknowledged by physiologists that negative and positive pressures exist in the body tissues, a recent research report has confirmed a state of normal physiological negative and positive fluid pressures within all body spaces and tissues, including the skin[5].

Within loosely bound and mobile tissues (e.g. the skin), a sub-atmospheric pressure forms a vacuum or suction effect providing additional cellular stability when movement or stress is exerted. This allows the skin to fulfil one of its functions by providing a sliding movement across other tissues without the effects of stress, tear, shear and friction, seen where the skin is fixed to its substrate fascial layer[6].

Sub-atmospheric (negative) pressures appear to be largely, but not only, derived from the intermittent pulse-like action of the extensive, expansive and complex arrangement of the lymphatic system, with some assistance from an active venous system through the actions of the muscles[5]. The actions of muscles adjacent to the lymphatics also provide support, squeezing them and pushing fluid upwards in a manner similar to providing the pumping action of the normal venous system. Injury to the local and surrounding tissues, particularly muscle, and a loss of skin integrity, may temporarily and/or permanently alter the reliability of this process[5].

It has been further established that in fixed skin, or tightly encased tissues or organs (e.g. the kidney, the brain), there is a range of positive pressure exerted from +6 to +13 mm Hg. These positive pressures provide fixed positioning and stabilising mechanisms for the major body organs against the normal trauma of body movement[5]. Conversely, this fixed positioning means that these organs are easily damaged when localised trauma does occur.

Box 5.5 provides examples of body areas with acknowledged negative pressures. Fixed tissue zones are suggested to be in positive pressure[5]. Box 5.6 outlines the suggested rationales for negative pressures within the tissues.

---

**Box 5.5** Examples of recorded sub-atmospheric (negative) pressures in the body.

| | |
|---|---|
| Intrapleural space | −8 mm Hg |
| Epidural space | −4 mm Hg to −6 mm Hg |
| Joint synovial spaces | −4 mm Hg to −6 mm Hg |
| Mobile/loose tissue | the average negative pressure is suggested to be in the range of −3 to −6 mm Hg[5]. |

---

**Box 5.6** Suggested physiological purpose of negative pressure (NP) in selected body tissues.

- NP assists in the stabilisation and controlled movement of the interstitial gel in which the body's cells are suspended
- NP assists in the timely removal of interstitial fluid that is excess to needs in mobile or loose tissue regions of the body, significantly reducing the development of oedema in normal tissue
- NP helps to eliminate or reduce potential dead space that is capable of allowing the accumulation of fluid, for example, oedema, in the interstitial spaces, which would affect the controlled stability and movement of cells. The assembly of cells in normal close and ordered proximity to the capillaries allows for the essential and optimal exchange of gases and nutrients, and assists in the orderly removal of fluid back into the general circulation
- NP provides a contamination-free physiological environment by the removal of cytotoxic wastes, allowing a milieu that is conducive to the initiation of tissue and vascular growth factors, which are required for the development of granulation tissue, collagen formation for dermal contraction, and epidermal resurfacing.

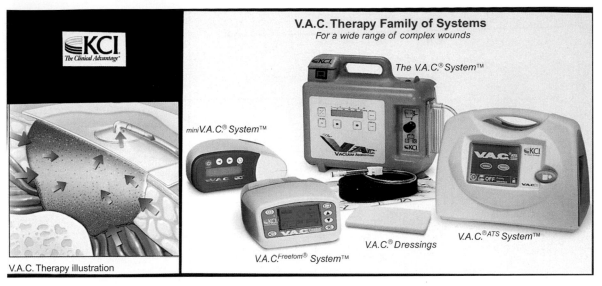

**Figure 5.9** Example of the range of vacuum assisted closure systems (VAC Systems®) available. With permission: KCI Medical Ltd., 2004.

## The Way Vacuum Assisted Closure Works

The MiniV.A.C.™ (Vacuum Assisted Closure) device assists in wound closure by applying localised negative pressure to draw the edges of the wound to the centre.

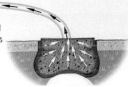

**Figure 5.10** Adapted example of application to dead space wound zone. With permission: KCI Medical Ltd., 2004.

See recommended websites at the end of this chapter for additional information on functional anatomy of the skin.

## Application to wound repair

This knowledge has important implications in the process of wound repair where oedema is not resolv-ing according to physiological expectations. Open or closed tissues may require scientifically designed compression bandaging (on the upper or lower limbs), or the application of negative pressure by a mechanical modality to force the excess fluid to the surface where there is dysfunction of the venous and/or lymphatic system (e.g. the KCI VAC®System[16-20], Figures 5.9–5.12).

The timely restoration of internal negative pressure within mobile skin tissues through ensuring the integrity of the vascular circulation in and surrounding the wound, eliminating dead space in the wound and sealing the wound from the environment, also appears to be a integral component for dermal contraction and epidermal resurfacing, by reducing wound tension and restoring normal cellular function[16-20].

Box 5.7 outlines emerging knowledge assisting in the understanding of the pathophysiological nature of the complexity of wound repair.

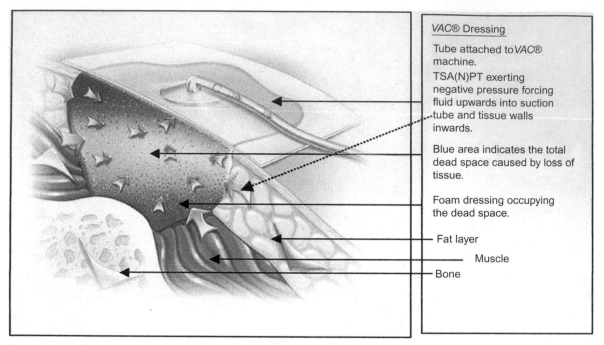

**VAC® Dressing**

Tube attached to *VAC®* machine.

TSA(N)PT exerting negative pressure forcing fluid upwards into suction tube and tissue walls inwards.

Blue area indicates the total dead space caused by loss of tissue.

Foam dressing occupying the dead space.

Fat layer

Muscle

Bone

**Figure 5.11** Adapted example of application to dead space wound zone. With permission: KCI Medical Ltd., 2004.

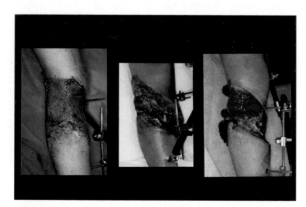

**Figure 5.12** Compound wound of the lower limb – VAC System® primarily applied following initial debridement – maintained for 48 hours followed by application of meshed split skin graft to attain early closure and protect underlying tissues and bone prior to major reconstructive free flap surgery (wound bed preparation). With permission: KCI Medical Ltd., 2004.

**Box 5.7** Current important research areas for wound repair.

- The structure, physiological control and distribution of the microcirculatory flow of blood to the skin[21]
- Surgical techniques that mechanically redirect blood flow to injured zones (collateral circulation)[21]
- The place and function of specific growth factors in normal tissues and complex wounds[22–29]
- Vascular pathology and the presence of stem cells for replacement of vascular structures[22–29]
- Hormonal control (nitric oxide) of blood flow in the skin[5]
- The complex functions of collagen and hyaluronic acid[5].

## References

(1) Williams P.L. & Warwick R. *Gray's anatomy*, 36th edn. Edinburgh, London, Melbourne, New York: Churchill Livingstone, 1980.

(2) Larsson N-G. Mice against Methusela. *Nature*, 2004 (May 27):417–23. http://info.ki.se/article_en.html?ID=1399

(3) Brierly E.J., Johnson M.A., James O.F. & Turnbull B.M. Mitochondrial involvement in the ageing process. Facts and controversies. *Molecular and Cellular Biochemistry*, 1997 (Sep); 174(1–2):325–8.

(4) Muller-Hocker J. Mitochondria and ageing. *Brain Pathology*, 1992 (Apr); 2(2):149–58.

(5) Guyton A.C. & Hall J.E. *Textbook of medical physiology*, 9th edn. Phil: W.B. Saunders, 1996.

(6) Peacock E.E. Jr. *Wound repair*, 3rd edn. Philadelphia: W.B. Saunders, 1984.

(7) Ausher B.M., Erikson E. & Wilkins E.G. *Plastic surgery: indications, operations and outcomes*. St Louis: Mosby, 2000.

(8) Bryant R.A. (ed.). *Acute and chronic wounds: nursing management*. St Louis: Mosby Year Book, 1992.

(9) Dealey C. *The care of wounds*, 2nd edn. Oxford, UK: Blackwell Science, 1999.

(10) Kerstein M.D. The scientific basis of healing. *Advances in Wound Care*, 1997; 10(3):30–36.

(11) Silver I.A. The physiology of wound healing. *Journal of Wound Care*, 1994 (Mar); 3(7):106–109.

(12) Robinson J.B & Friedman R.M. Wound healing and closure. *Selected Readings in Plastic Surgery*, 1999; 8(1).

(13) Taylor G.I., Palmer J.H. & McManamny D. The vascular territories of the body (angiosomes) and their clinical implications. In: McCarthy, J.G. *Plastic surgery: volume 1, general principles*. Philadelphia: W.B. Saunders, 1990, pp. 329–78.

(14) McCance K.L. & Huether S.E. *Pathophysiology: the biologic basis for disease in adults and children*, 3rd edn. St Louis: Mosby, 1998.

(15) Smeltzer S.C. & Bare B.G. *Brunner and Suddarth's textbook of medical-surgical nursing*, 9th edn. Philadelphia: Lippincott, Williams and Wilkins, 2000.

(16) Argenta L.C. & Morykwas M.J. Vacuum-assisted closure: a new method for wound control and treatment: clinical experience. *Annals of Plastic Surgery*, 1997; 38:563–77.

(17) Morykwas M.J., Argenta L.C., Shelton-Brown E.I. & McGuirt W. Vacuum-assisted closure: a new method for wound control and treatment: animal studies and basic foundation. *Annals of Plastic Surgery*, 1997; 38(6):553–62.

(18) Mullner T., Mrkonjic L., Kwasny O. & Vecsei V. The use of negative pressure to promote the healing of tissue defects: a clinical trial using the vacuum sealing technique. *British Journal of Plastic Surgery*, 1997; 50(3):194–9.

(19) Banwell P., Withey S. & Holten I. The use of negative pressure to promote healing. *British Journal of Plastic Surgery*, 1998; 51(1):79.

(20) Thomas S. *An introduction to vacuum assisted closure*. 2001. Available on website: http://www.worldwidewounds.com/2001/may/Thomas/Vacuum-Assisted-Closure.html

(21) Taylor G.I. & Dhar S. *Collateral circulation and the circulatory delay phenomena: Research report of current clinical investigations*. The Jack Brockhoff Reconstructive Surgery Research Unit at The Royal Melbourne Hospital and University of Melbourne, Australia, 2001.

(22) Risau W. Mechanisms of angiogenesis. *Nature*, 1997 (April); 386(17):671–4.

(23) Gavaghan M. Vascular haemodynamics. *AORN Journal*, 1998; 68(2):212–26.

(24) Henry T.D. Can we really grow new blood vessels? *Lancet*, 1998 (June 20); 351(9119):1826–7.

(25) Gill D. Angiogenic modulation. *Journal of Wound Care*, 1998 (September); 7(8):411–14.

(26) Schaper W. & Buschmann I. Collateral circulation and diabetes. (Editorial) *Circulation*, 1999 (May 4); 99(17):2224–6.

(27) Buschmann I. & Schaper W. The pathophysiology of the collateral circulation (arteriogenesis). *Journal of Pathology*, 2000; 190:338–42.

(28) Carmeliet P. Mechanisms of angiogenesis and arteriogenesis. *Nature Medicine*, 2000; 6(3):389–95.

(29) Germain L., Remy-Zolghadri M. & Augur F. Tissue engineering of the vascular system: from capillaries to larger blood vessels. *Medical and Biological Engineering and Computing*, (England), 2000 (Mar); 38(2):232–40.

## Recommended websites

**Functional anatomy of the skin**

http://www.meddean.luc.edu/lumen/MedEd/medicine/dermatology/melton/skinlsn/sknlsn.htm (excellent)

http://www.umm.edu/dermatology-info/anatomy.htm

http://www.telemedicine.org/anatomy/anatomy.htm

http://lm.ucdavis.edu/slide_sets/cha/101/Skin/title.html

# Physiology of the Ageing of the Skin Incorporating an Overview of Common Skin Lesions

## 1. PHYSIOLOGY OF AGEING SKIN

### Background

As previously outlined at the beginning of Chapter 5, the living cell, its structure and function, must be clearly comprehended if the ageing process and wound repair are to be clearly understood.

For every cell, there is a time to live and a time to die. Cell death is called **apoptosis**.

There are two ways in which cells die:

- They are killed by injurious agents – toxins, injury, disease
- They are induced to commit suicide – genetically programmed to die (the ageing process)[1–6].

The ageing process has recently been demonstrated to be related to the DNA in the mitochondria. For example, mitochondrial DNA (mtDNA) is replicated by an enzyme called mtDNA polymerase. This enzyme is capable of replication with a very high degree of precision because it has the capacity to proofread its work and, therefore, correct any errors made. On some occasions, errors do occur and this is referred to as a mutation. Mutations can potentially lead to tumours, particularly malignant tumours[4–6].

In a landmark Swedish study using mice[1], the scientists used genetic engineering and removed the proofreading ability of mtDNA. They then compared these mice with normal mice. Mutations were 3–5 times higher in the genetically engineered mice, with all the signs of ageing occurring more quickly, and the life span of these mice was significantly shorter[1].

In day-to-day living, as the skin wears and tears, it is fundamental for human survival that there is a high level of capacity to repair and replace labile and stable tissues by precise cellular function. To make these repairs, all cells need to multiply to replace injured or dead cells in parallel with the mtDNA. Accumulating mutations in the mitochondria slowly but significantly reduce the ability of cells to maintain this repair process. Ageing of the body's skin and organ tissues is the result, and finally, the basis of death[1–3].

Important long-term complex research studies are also being undertaken to further determine the relationship between the decline in efficacy of the mtDNA to replicate in the repair of tissues and the production of tumours[4–6]. All of these studies have their basis in the potential to genetically engineer out the suggested cellular 'imperfections' or mutations that occur, to prolong life and to prevent cancer in the body's organs.

### Pathophysiology, elastin, collagen and the ageing process

The process of normal physiological ageing of the body is observed at cellular level to commence at about the age of 20 years for both men and women[7–11]. Within the skin, the rate of synthesis of dermal fibroblasts begins a slow but constant decline. Ageing skin gradually thins, and slowly becomes more vulnerable to UVA, UVB, and UVC rays, injury, gravitational sagging, and loss of functions that are observed in youthful skin.

The process of ageing must also be thought of within the concept of what the cells of the tissues are undergoing, in relation to normal expected cellular changes, and abnormal cellular changes caused by exposure, polluting factors, drugs, disease, smoking, etc.

## Elastin and collagen

**Elastin** is the non-collagenous protein designed to give the tissues flexibility, and consists of the yellow elastic tissue fibres than can be microscopically observed in the skin.

**Collagen** is the most abundant protein in the body. It consists of bundles of white, glistening non-elastic fibres and is designed to provide strength and structure in the connective tissues. There are at least 13 recognised types of collagen (with only a few described) and different anatomical structures are made up of specific ratios. For example, rigid structures such as tendon and bone are made up of Type 1. Human skin, being more mobile or elastic, is 80% Type I and 20% Type III. The aorta is principally made up of Type III – arteries are 80% Type III and 20% Type I – the opposite ratio to skin but again reflecting the function of the part[7–12].

Types IV and VII are found in the basement membrane at the epidermal and dermal junction. This is essential for structural and anchoring support of the epidermis to the dermis, and finally to the underlying connective tissues[7–12]. Collagen also provides the scaffolding for elastin, which provides flexibility in certain structures, e.g. the skin.

The combination of collagen and elastin provides strength, resilience, and flexibility to allow the maximum mobility and physical protection over the human lifespan. This can be significantly improved by an optimal diet and regular exercise.

Many skin care products are targeted at the collagen and elastin that are responsible for contraction and flexibility of the facial skin[4–6].

The basic processes of ageing outwardly seen in the skin are a range of complex ongoing micro alterations that occur within the skin's overall structural changes, and these can be observed microscopically in the cells of the yellow elastin fibres, and the collagen fibres at the level of the basement membrane.

Further micro changes in skin that appear over the years are cellular changes that result in a gradual thinning at epidermal/dermal junction (basement membrane) and changes in the strength and resilience of the rete anchoring capacity (i.e. the

rete ridges flatten out)[7–11]. This increases the vulnerability to injury that is principally related to shear and friction, which is significant in the formation of pressure ulcers in the elderly, and the chronically ill patient.

Loss of the body's subcutaneous tissue results in loss of elastin, collagen, and fat. This results in thinned and flattened tissue layers, exhibited by wrinkling and sagging, which is further aggravated by gravity.

Collagen turnover and replacement slows and the biological 'memory' capacity of elastin fibres lessen with age. The average changes are generally quite slow when the skin is cared for, and protected from the elements, but can be hastened by a range of factors such as smoking, inadequate daily skin care, and excessive exposure to the sun, cold and the general elements.

For example, in a 20-year-old white male, the skin of the forearm is approximately 1.1 mm thick, while at 70 years it can be expected to be 0.8 mm thick. In comparable females the thickness will decrease from 0.8 mm to 0.75 mm.

The rete pegs of the basement membrane that anchor the epidermis to the dermis also continue to flatten out, significantly reducing thickness and strength, and depleting the skin's antibacterial protective functions. All of this contributes to thinner, flaccid skin and although this reduction in the dermal thickness may not appear to be great, it is noteworthy as it means simple trauma can significantly damage the skin by causing full thickness injury (i.e. skin tears, burns), and healing is considerably slower.

Macro external changes that occur are dryness, wrinkling, changes in pigmentation, and increased susceptibility to solar damage.

## Additional changes in the skin

Vascular changes in the skin, in particular the capillary loops, become smaller in number and size, contribute to alterations in wound healing in the ageing skin and further increase the susceptibility to primary and secondary injury.

Hormonal changes contribute to the decline in sebaceous gland function, promoting dryness of the skin, increasing the need to artificially replace the declining oil supply. With changes in hair growth, sensory perception and thermoregulation, all these factors combine to contribute to the overall vulnerability of the skin that comes with the ageing process.

### Photo-ageing of the skin – effects of UVA radiation on the skin

Most modern texts divide the skin into six main types, reflecting the response to ultraviolet A, B and C (UVA, UVB and UVC) rays, ranging from Type 1 (skin always burns and never tans) to Type 6 (skin always tans and never burns). The level of melanin content in the epidermis of the skin is an important agent in partially protecting the dermis, as the sun's rays on the skin stimulate the melanin stimulating hormone (MSH) centre in the brain, and feed back to the melanin cells to engage in protective cellular mechanisms.

One of the most discussed subjects in the pathophysiology of ageing skin is the initiation and control of destructive oxygen free radicals that are stated to have the capacity for the destruction of cell DNA – see recommended websites (the effects of solar radiation) at the end of this chapter.

Within the dermis are photon-absorbing chemicals, referred to as **chromophores**. The chromophores are capable of moving to an unstable, high energy state and the excess energy created is absorbed by nearby structures and oxygen molecules. The molecules become unstable and, because they are not paired, proceed to destroy other cells and vulnerable tissue. Carrots are among the many basic foods containing elements thought to be excellent scavengers of free radicals, but eaten in excess they cause the skin to take on orange/yellow colour. Because the theory and function of free radicals is not completely understood, the use of commercial antioxidants should be under the supervision of physicians, dieticians or pharmacists.

### Wrinkles

Face and neck wrinkles are the bane of many men and women. Although not fully understood, it is suggested that wrinkles, particularly those on the face and neck, are essentially caused by constant and repetitive mechanical forces (e.g. frowning) and downward gravity forces. These constant forces add to the normal reduction of the collagen matrix and the elastin recoil/contracting forces (elastic 'memory' within the elastin cells) that occurs with age.

This change stimulates the local fibroblasts, resulting in thickening of the connective tissue (fascia) that is attached to the face and neck muscles. This thickening forms lines of tension corresponding to the contracting forces attempting to repair the subtle cellular damage. Heavy cigarette smoking (which alters blood flow and thus slows the repair of damaged cells) and constant exposure to the sun (which dries the skin) also contribute significantly to the degree and extent of the developing wrinkles.

### Retention of physical strength

Although the skin may lose its capacity to recoil and remain firm to varying degrees, a good diet, minimal exposure to heat and cold, skin care and massage, regular low impact aerobic exercise and moderate levels of physical activity (particularly walking) can be of great assistance in retaining good muscle strength, bone density and general health.

---

**Box 6.1** Patient education for skin care.

Discuss:

- The physiological factors that result in the normal ageing process
- The decline of the ability of injured tissue to provide functional moisture and protective sebum
- The factors that lead to skin cell decline that may result in skin tumours
- Factors that can accentuate skin cell decline such as high ingestion of alcohol, cigarette smoking and long-term or excessive exposure to sun or excess cold
- Methods of evidence-based skin care, including massage, adequate intake of water, diet and exercise.

---

See recommended websites at the end of this chapter.

## 2. SKIN LESIONS – OVERVIEW

### Background

Particular aberrations of body tissues in the skin, are usually referred to as **neoplasms**, **tumours**, or lesions, and are further defined as **benign**, **pre-malignant** or **malignant**.

In reconstructive plastic surgery the most common tumours are present as lumps under the surface of the skin (e.g. benign simple cysts) or externally, as a benign mole, various types of naevi, ageing wart-type lesions, and malignant tumours that are visible at level of the skin. There is a known genetic propensity with certain types of skin 'moles' which appear in excessive numbers and body distribution, that is also suggested to contribute to the development of malignant changes.

Other relatively common conditions, seen in the older age group are:

- Bowen's disease: an intra-epidermal squamous cell, low grade malignant lesion that does not invade into the basal layer. It is seen most often on the lower limbs in multiple numbers, requires surgery (excision or excision and skin grafting) as lesions are resistant to radiotherapy and chemotherapy.
- Keratoacanthoma: a benign, rapidly-growing flesh-coloured lesion of the skin with a central plug or horn-like formation of keratin, seen commonly on the back of the hands, arms or face. It requires biopsy or excision to differentiate from squamous cell carcinoma.

Space does not allow for a more detailed description of the large range of skin lesions observed in both children and adults, but common types of benign and malignant lesions and those with the propensity for changes from benign to malignant are outlined concisely and with photographs in most plastic surgery and dermatology textbooks[6–11].

An extensive range of photographs and descriptions are outlined at plastic surgical and dermatological websites – see examples at the end of this chapter.

## Ultraviolet radiation and its effects on the skin

In addition to light and heat, the sun emits invisible ultraviolet radiation. Excessive exposure to UV damages the skin permanently and may cause skin cancer, including the dangerous malignant melanoma.

The three types of ultraviolet (UV) radiation, based on their wavelength, are UVA, UVB and UVC.

The Earth's atmosphere absorbs nearly all of the most single dangerous rays, i.e. UVC, before it reaches the ground. UVA and UVB radiation are both involved in sunburn, but skin reacts differently to each one. The invisible ultraviolet spectrum makes up one specific portion of sunlight and this unique portion accounts for 3% of all solar radiation reaching the earth. UV light is measured as wavelengths of light, in units of nanometres (nm). Three types of UV light have been identified and are outlined in Box 6.2.

---

**Box 6.2** Identified UV light – examples.

**UVC** Many scientists rate wavelengths in the C range of the ultraviolet (UVC) solar spectrum, between 200 and 290 nm, as the most carcinogenic. The ozone layer absorbs most UVC rays. However, recent research indicates that the ozone layer may be depleted in certain areas by chlorofluorocarbons (CFCs, chiefly used in refrigerators, air conditioners, and foam insulation)

**UVB** Wavelengths in the B range of the ultraviolet (UVB) solar spectrum, measured at between 290 and 320 nm, cause most sunburns. UVB affects the skin surface and the skin responds by releasing chemicals that dilate blood vessels. This causes leaking and inflammation, better known as sunburn

**UVA** Wavelengths in the A range of the ultraviolet (UVA) solar spectrum, between 320 and 400 nm, may be up to 1000 times more intense than UVB. UVA light can penetrate to underlying tissues of the skin and cause photo-ageing or long-term skin damage.

---

See recommended websites at the conclusion of this chapter.

### The skin's reactions to UV radiation

Including the effects previously described in the previous section (photo-ageing), the skin is subject to cellular changes that are precursors to skin tumours, benign and malignant. Box 6.3 outlines the common malignant skin lesions seen presenting for reconstructive plastic surgery.

## Box 6.3 Common malignant skin and mucous membrane tumours.

**Basal cell carcinoma** (BCC), arising out of the basal cells of the skin:

- The most common malignant tumours in white populations
- 75% of patients are older than 40 years
- Male to female ratio (except in lower limbs) 3 : 1
- Rarely seen in non-Caucasians
- Do not metastasise, infiltrate along tissue lines (Figures 6.1–6.4)

**Squamous cell carcinoma** (SCC), a malignant epidermal tumour, the cells of which show maturation toward keratin formation:

- Uncommon in dark skinned races (except in keloid scars)
- Common in the oral cavity
- Common from middle age onward
- Male to female ratio is stated to be 2 : 1
- Highly malignant tumour, metastasises, secondaries occur in the lungs, brain and bones (Figures 6.5–6.8)

**Malignant melanoma** (MM) a malignant tumour of the epidermal melanocytes:

- 5% of all skin cancers are malignant melanoma
- MM causes 75% of all deaths from skin cancer[1–5]
- Metastasises – secondaries occur in the lungs, brain and bones (Figures 6.9–6.11)

**Kaposi sarcoma**

- Malignant tumour, often multiple sites, commonly associated with AIDS
- Mainly seen in males
- May be associated with diabetes mellitus and malignant lymphoma
- A metastasising condition spreading via the lymph nodes to major body organs (Figures 6.12 and 6.13).

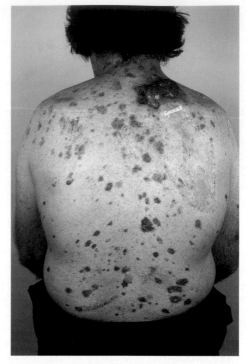

**Figure 6.1** Gorlin syndrome (genetically inherited condition; becomes malignant (basal cell carcinoma) after puberty; multiple associated anomalies.

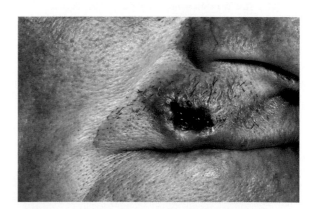

**Figure 6.2** Basal cell carcinoma – upper lip.

## Basic aetiology and pathophysiology of malignant skin lesions

Fifty per cent of all individuals who reach age 65 will develop at least one form of skin cancer, making skin cancer the most common of all cancers. Furthermore, one in five adults alive today in the United States will develop skin cancer during his or her lifetime, and more in Australia. The most common cancerous lesions are basal cell carcinoma, squamous cell car-cinoma and malignant melanoma. Australians, particularly those who live in the northern state of Queensland, have the highest incidence of skin cancer in the world[7–11].

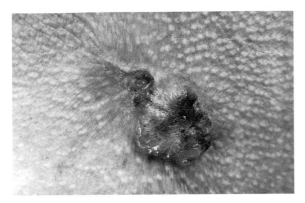

**Figure 6.3** Basal cell carcinoma – neck.

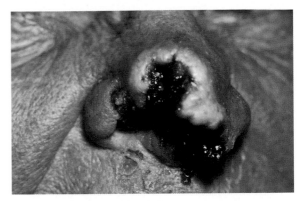

**Figure 6.5** Squamous cell carcinoma – nose.

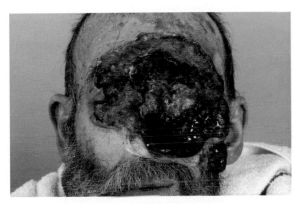

**Figure 6.4** Infiltrating basal cell carcinoma – face.

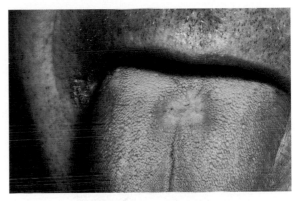

**Figure 6.6** Squamous cell carcinoma – tongue.

Australia is a country with large numbers of very fair-skinned individuals (northern European derived) living in mainly rural country environments and coastal regions with the highest level of sunshine for the most hours per year.

Typically, with community education, the majority of lesions in human cells are diagnosed early, and are removed and repaired, with a relatively high rate of cure, but wide zones of cell death and cell mutations in the skin also occur, leading to recurrences if not adequately excised. This requires more extensive tissue excision and reparative surgery.

Living human tissue is made of complex molecules and cells that include proteins and DNA. Electrons hold all these complex molecules together. When ultraviolet radiation shines on living tissue, photochemical reactions, DNA lesions and other types of damage occur. UV radiation produces DNA lesions characteristic of ionising radiation (e.g. X-rays).

It is believed that the major contributor of solar radiation damage to the skin can be attributed to intermittent and/or long-term exposure to UVB rays, of a wavelength of approximately 290–320 nm. This is thought to have the capacity to both initiate and promote skin tumours. There is no definitive scientific proof, but recently it has been suggested that there is increasing research evidence that UVA rays are similarly dangerous.

A hole in the stratospheric ozone layer is considered to have increased the incidence of skin cancers, particularly melanoma, by allowing increasing levels of UV rays to enter into our atmosphere. This is the subject of a considerable amount of controversial scientific research.

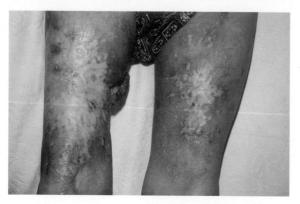

**Figure 6.7** Marjolin ulcer (squamous cell carcinoma) in old keloid burns scar.

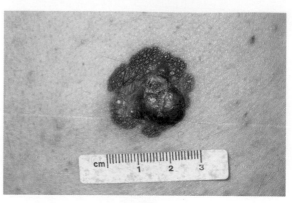

**Figure 6.9** Malignant melanoma.

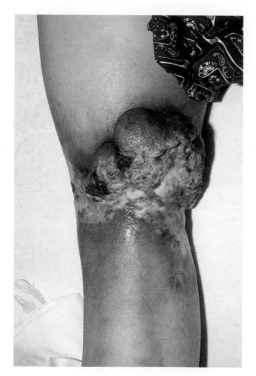

**Figure 6.8** Marjolin ulcer (squamous cell carcinoma) in old keloid burns scar.

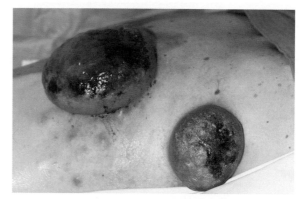

**Figure 6.10** Untreated fungating malignant melanoma of the back.

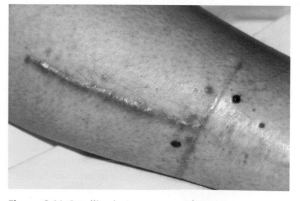

**Figure 6.11** Satellite lesions – secondary recurrent malignant melanoma lesions.

UVB rays are suggested to be largely impeded by the stratum corneum of the epidermis (by about 90%) but 10% can penetrate the basal layer, and this has been demonstrated to significantly affect the DNA of the basal cells, initiating basal cell carcinoma.

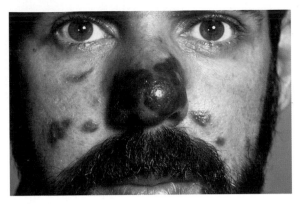

**Figure 6.12** Nasal Kaposi sarcoma (malignant) secondary to AIDS.

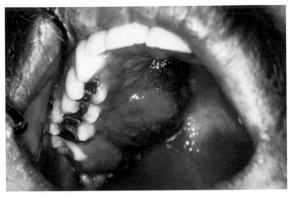

**Figure 6.13** Oral Kaposi sarcoma (malignant) secondary to AIDS.

In most instances where 30+ UV protective cream is applied as medically prescribed, or protective clothing is worn, the minimal effects on the basal cells are repaired relatively quickly. As previously stated, the presence of melanin in the epidermis is also suggested to be a protective factor but in extremely fair persons the potential for the skin to burn from the Sun's rays is high.

General skin ageing continues due to constant exposure to the sun, resulting in an ongoing and gradual degradation of the dermal cells, slowly destroying the normal protective and restorative cellular functions and increasing the risk of tumours developing.

With constant long-term exposure, and ageing skin becoming thinner, the protective ratio alters in favour of an increased capacity for penetration, with higher numbers of people presenting for assessment of a range of skin changes (lesions). These are collectively referred to as benign (non-cancerous), premalignant (potential for change to malignant), or malignant (cancerous) lesions.

Some researchers suggest that with both constant exposure, and short bursts of the Sun's rays over the long term, with little or no protection from the UVA or UVB rays, there is the potential for UVB rays to be a significant precursor to the development of premalignant and malignant skin lesions, particularly malignant melanoma, although there is no scientific evidence to support this theory.

In dark skinned persons who work in the open environment, skin cancer is not a common occurrence, but there are exceptions. Malignant melanoma of the pink cuticle skin under the finger, toenails and the eye has been observed and reported in the medical literature.

Because of the high incidence of keloid scars in the dark skinned races, squamous cell carcinoma may occur if the scar is constantly exposed to the sun (for example, on the lower limb) or becomes cracked due to the mechanical forces imposed by walking or movement on the surrounding fixed skin or contracted scar tissue skin, causing ulceration to develop. Constant shear and friction of the scar due to the wearing of rough work clothing can also be a cause of recurring ulceration. Squamous cell carcinomas do not usually develop for many years (30–50 years in some cases) after the original keloid formation, and do not occur in all individuals, black or white. Large affected areas require major reconstructive surgery with skin flaps. There is a significant potential for the recurrence of keloid scarring at the flap edges.

Individuals born with forms of collagen aberrations are at high risk of skin cancers within the first 30 years of life, particularly squamous cell carcinoma and malignant melanoma. Each of these cancerous lesions is pathologically different with significantly differing clinical outcomes. This appears to be largely dependent on the area of the body they present and timing of presentation.

## The importance of early diagnosis and treatment

Early diagnosis and curative treatment of malignant skin tumours, particularly melanoma and squamous cell carcinoma, are important as tumours are opportunistic and seek to exploit the blood supply to the region of presentation. Their further growth, recurrence and potential for spread to other body organs is highly possible if not removed early and adequately managed with adjunctive therapy if required, and regularly followed up with consultations and skin inspections.

Increased education in the causes and prevention of skin cancer has seen many patients present much earlier for diagnosis, appropriate treatment and therefore increase their potential for cure or long-term survival. Special private dermatological diagnostic and assessment clinics have been established to enable early and long-term/lifetime checks and documentation on patients thought to be in the 'at risk' groups.

## Basal cell carcinomas, squamous cell carcinomas and malignant melanomas

A basal cell carcinoma and a squamous cell carcinoma may appear similar in their very early stages of presentation. An accurate diagnosis is made based on age of the patient, history of UV exposure, clinical history, examination for specific features under optimal lighting and magnification, following high-level microscopic examination of a biopsy, or examination of the full specimen. Some tumours may require examination by more than one pathologist if doubt exists as to the true nature of the lesion. Accurate diagnosis is important if the treatment required is to match the preferred clinical and aesthetic outcomes.

Should surgery be the choice of treatment following biopsy, the extent of the excision and reparative surgery will depend on accuracy of diagnosis and existing or potential tumour spread. The extent of surgery and, if necessary, additional adjunctive therapy (radiotherapy, chemotherapy, immunotherapy) will be tailored to the type of lesion, early or late stage of diagnosis, potential for recurrence, metastatic indices, and life limiting potential.

Basal cell carcinomas very rarely metastasise (0.025%) or spread to other organs of the body, except when basal cell and squamous cell carcinoma form a combined tumour. Basal cell carcinomas are not considered life-threatening when diagnosed early and well managed. They are tumours that infiltrate rather than spread. In the facial area (Figure 6.4) (typically the inner canthus of the eye, nose upper lip) they may infiltrate locally into the surrounding soft tissue and bony anatomy tracking, for example, into the maxillary sinuses and into the brain. Because of the infiltrating nature, cause of death is usually by severe haemorrhage as large feeding vessels are penetrated and destroyed. Following early diagnosis, when spread is increasing or recurrence occurs, skin grafts and flaps may be appropriate. Aesthetic outcomes are variable because of the potential for multiple occurrences, the poor condition of the surrounding skin (which is now not available for reconstruction due to its poor vascular properties) or the existence of adjacent lesions.

Squamous cell carcinomas have a varying potential to become metastatic (suggested to be 1%) dependent on their anatomical site. Squamous cell carcinomas occurring on the lower lip, nose, tongue (Figures 6.5 and 6.6) or mucous membrane of the oral cavity, have a higher potential for recurrence and spread. This is suggested to be due to the lesion being in a highly vascular region. This may cause secondary lesions, for example by spreading to the neck lymph nodes via the blood supply, and subsequently to other important areas of the body such as the lungs, brain or spinal bones, eventually leading to the patient's death.

It is often stated that malignant melanomas do not occur in children prior to puberty, but some cases have been reported in the literature. Most lesions are referred to as a **Spitz naevus**. The differential diagnosis is very important and the specimen should be viewed by expert pathologists in the field.

Malignant melanomas in adults have a relatively high potential to become metastatic and recur, with secondary lesions occurring locally (referred to as satellite lesions) (Figure 6.9), with spread to the lymph nodes and, via the blood supply, to other areas of the body, for example, the lungs, brain or spinal bones, eventually leading to the patient's death. Early diagnosed low-level malignant melanomas have excellent survival outcomes (Box 6.4). The general population requires regular education regarding the dangers of exposure to the sun, to be observant for changes in lesions, and advised to notify their physician about any changes in these factors.

**Box 6.4** The ABCD rule is a convenient guide to the usual signs of melanoma.

| A is for ASYMMETRY | One half of a mole or birthmark does not match the other |
| B is for BORDER | The edges are irregular, ragged, notched, or blurred |
| C is for COLOUR | The colour is not the same all over, but may have differing shades of brown or black, sometimes with patches of red, white or blue |
| D is for DIAMETER | The area is larger than 6 mm (about $1/4$ inch – the size of a pencil eraser), or is growing larger |

Other important warning signs of melanoma include changes in size, shape or colour of a mole, or the appearance of a new spot. Some melanomas do not fit the ABCD rule described above, so it is particularly important for individuals to be aware of changes in skin lesions, or new skin lesions, and seek medical advice.

### *Aetiology of malignant skin tumours*

The aetiology of malignant melanoma is widely researched and discussed, but it is generally thought that, as opposed to basal cell carcinoma and squamous cell carcinoma which are usually the result of long-term UVB exposure, malignant melanoma is more common in younger people, particularly those who have short bursts of high levels of UVB intensity. Any suspicious lesion that changes colour, becomes nodular, feels itchy, or bleeds, requires examination by an expert surgeon immediately.

Treatments, through skin excisions, grafts and flaps, are repair options applied parallel to the level and spread of the tumour, with adjunctive chemotherapy or radiotherapy also a consideration. Malignant melanoma may arise out of Hutchinson's melanotic freckle, often seen on the face of the elderly, particularly women.

Plastic surgical medical textbooks outline the staging (American Joint Committee on Cancer (AJCC)) of malignant melanomas, and pathological variables (levels of invasion) devised by Breslow, and Clarke & McGovern, that statistically demonstrate expected survival rates[7–11].

Because the natural history of cancer is not known, it is important not to generalise, as every malignant tumour that presents for examination and management is relatively peculiar to the individual patient. The time of presentation, life history of the lesion, the area of the body, morbid and co-morbid medical factors, and the potential for long-term survival must all be taken into consideration before treatment modalities are determined.

### Nursing issues of safety, comfort and independence

Whilst the largest number of the presenting tumours are benign or are low-grade cancers, and curative outcomes using evidence-based management are the norm, a relative number are not.

For patients diagnosed with malignant melanoma, early diagnosis and corrective surgery can alter the prognosis significantly, particularly Level 1, and in otherwise well patients.

For reconstructive plastic surgery nurses, a basic knowledge of the most familiar skin tumours, their aetiology and potential for local and systemic spread is important. This provides the opportunity to anticipate the degree and extent of the surgery, and thus the nursing implications for the care of the patient.

Familiarity with the tumour presentation, the approaches to surgical or non-surgical procedures and experience of what treatment pathways may be appropriate or can be expected, comes over time. For example, the nurse clinician should be aware of the clinical importance of accurate diagnosis (benign or malignant), the range of treatments that can be offered (simple or aggressive surgery, chemotherapy, radiotherapy, palliative measures or a combination of approaches), variable chances of survival for different types of tumours, and support the patient as decisions are made. Some basic reading on the pathophysiology of skin tumours will assist clinicians who are working in this area.

Perhaps the best advice that can be offered is to learn to question the surgeon as to the name and type of tumour, anticipated prognosis, the extent of the surgery to be undertaken and if any post-surgery treatments are planned. From this, nursing risk management can be assessed and addressed and the setting of clinical nursing outcomes can be formulated proactively, rather than reactively.

## Safety and comfort

Surgeons will discuss the best curative and/or functional maintenance regime possible, least destructive/reconstructive approach, and anticipated prognosis, with the patient. Some patients with particularly aggressive or advanced tumours may be offered a combination of surgery, radiotherapy and chemotherapy.

At the end of the day it is the patient's decision, particularly if a cure cannot be assured, and many patients will prefer palliative management through radiotherapy and chemotherapy in preference to surgery, and a choice for a particular quality of life. Their choice must be respected by all team members and support provided to ensure the best quality of life is possible.

Should major reconstructive surgery be the primary choice of initial treatment, the nurse clinician should proceed with the pre-assessment and pre-operative preparation of the patient and these should reflect directly to the anticipated clinical medical and nursing outcomes (see Chapter 15).

When major reconstructive surgery is undertaken (e.g. for squamous cell carcinomas, head and neck surgery) nursing morbidity and co-morbidity is high. The patient will usually present with a highly dependent need for clinical safety, comfort and independence, such as for respiratory management (e.g. tracheostomy) nutritional issues, oral hygiene, pain management, mobility issues and specific complex wound management. The adjunctive therapies of chemotherapy and radiotherapy are added burdens for the patient and their significant carers.

## Independence and psychosocial issues

Regardless of the size, type or anatomical site, the term 'cancer' remains one of the most emotive, and elicits a wide range of human emotional responses. The fear and apprehension of having 'cancer', which may or may not lead to death, often accompanies the discovery of lesions which may be simple and benign, or existing spots that begin to grow, spread, change colour, bleed, etc. Whilst this diagnosis (cancer) may not be the situation, the initial patient presentation should alert the nurse to the patient's sense of fear, mortality, disability and aesthetic changes.

The overall management of malignant tumours includes an ongoing and high level of listening to the patient and counselling during every discussion on aspects of the disease process, selection of treatment options, and the likely prognosis. Making specific and uninterrupted time for the patient and their carers to discuss the situation, and ask questions, is essential. Life-limiting/threatening, disabling conditions raise issues of grief, loss and fear for patients and carers, and these fundamentally important human areas should not be forgotten during the flurry of the preparation and undertaking of surgery, and pre- and postoperative nursing management.

There will also be the psychosocial issues associated with aesthetics, with the fear of an unpleasant and prolonged period of disability, the appearance following surgery, fungating wounds, ongoing pain, and finally dying. Patients often compare their condition and outcomes with someone else they believe has had the same tumour. These are understandably quite devastating thoughts for patients and their carers.

For malignant tumours, regardless of the medical treatment that is prescribed, it is essential to address the ongoing issues of patient safety, psychosocial needs, wound care, pain management and assistance in retaining a high level of personal health control and assisted self-care. This often requires professional nursing, combined with allied health personnel, to provide a level of assistance and reassurance to the patient at a time where grief, loss and powerlessness may be profoundly disturbing, temporarily, or in the longer term[2,3].

## Benign skin lesions

In the benign group of skin lesions, solar keratosis, keratoacanthoma cysts (in the elderly), lipoma, skin tags, and fibroma form the most common of those presenting in adults.

In children, included in the benign group are skin tags, cysts, haemangioma (vascular birthmarks that usually resolve as the child approaches 7–9 years of age) and vascular malformations that grow proportional to age and do not resolve. Vascular malformations are often associated with neurological disturbances (e.g. epilepsy) and complex syndromes that have been identified but which may be rare, inherited and bizarre in their combinations. Vascular malformations are often referred to as low, medium, or high blood flow malformations, and some that travel close to the skin can result in major ulceration

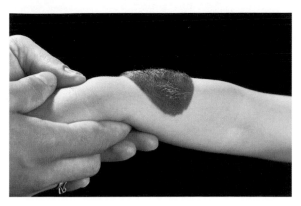

**Figure 6.14** Giant hairy naevus (benign lesion) – usually removed in staged procedures or utilising tissue expander in adjacent tissue.

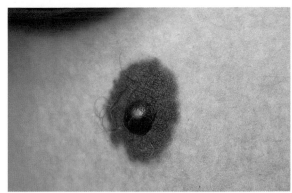

**Figure 6.15** Juvenile melanoma (benign lesion).

that may lead to a severe loss of blood and, for some patients, death.

Specialised wound bed maintenance is essential as operative procedures for treatment are often fraught with danger and should be avoided, if possible, due to the unknown and complex vascular source and pathways, particularly in the head and neck region.

Parents with children who have these lesions require a high level of support due to fear of an ulcerated lesion bleeding. Physicians will investigate any child with a lesion that appears to be part of a syndrome and educate the parents as to any physiological or psychological issues arising out of the diagnosis. Education about the lesion(s) and first aid regarding emergency measures must be provided without frightening the parents. They should be aware but not alarmed.

Examples of other lesions that may be seen are benign hairy naevus (Figure 6.14) and juvenile melanoma (Figure 6.15) but these represent only a small number of single lesions and combinations of conditions described in medical textbooks. These can be removed with minimal complications and may be excised in stages to reduce the tension and scar outcomes. Tissue expansion may be undertaken to minimise the scar. Each presentation is considered on its merits, potential for safe management, and the need for any intervention.

Increased knowledge and understanding can be acquired by accessing suggested websites, following the reference section, selected as relevant to this chapter.

## References

(1) Larsson N-G. Mice against Methusela. *Nature*, 2004 (May 27); 417–423. http://info.ki.se/article_en.html?ID=1399
(2) Brierly E.J., Johnson M.A., James O.F. & Turnbull B.M. Mitochondrial involvement in the ageing process. Facts and controversies. *Molecular and Cellular Biochemistry*, 1997 (Sept); **174**(1–2):325–8.
(3) Muller-Hocker J. Mitochondria and ageing. *Brain Pathology*, 1992 (Apr); **2**(2):149–58.
(4) http://www.cellsalive.com/apop.htm
(5) http://users.rcn.com/jkimball.ma.ultranet/Biology Pages/A/Apoptosis.html
(6) http://www.emedicine.com/plastic/topic423.htm
(7) McCarthy J.G. (ed.) *Plastic surgery, volumes 1–8*. Philadelphia: W.B. Saunders, 1990.
(8) Aston S.J., Beasley R. & Thorne C.N.M. *Grabb and Smith's plastic surgery*, 5th edn. New York: Lippincott & Raven Publishers, 1997.
(9) Ausher B.M., Erikson E. & Wilkins E.G. *Plastic surgery: indications, operations and outcomes*. St Louis: Mosby, 2000.
(10) Ruberg R.L. & Smith D.J. *Plastic surgery – a core curriculum*. St Louis: Mosby, 1994.
(11) Stone C. *Plastic surgery: facts*. London: Greenwich Medical Media Limited, 2001.
(12) Peacock, E.E. Jnr. *Wound repair*, 3rd edn. Philadelphia: W.B. Saunders, 1984.

## Recommended websites

**The ageing process**
http://www.actionbioscience.org/evolution/ingman.html
http://www.healthandage.com/html/res/primer/primer2.htm

http://www.umm.edu/patiented/articles/what_occurs_
    when_skin_ages_000020_1.htm

**Photographic atlas of common skin lesions**
http://www.medscape.com/px/dermatlas
http://www.centexderm.com/html/cancer.htm
http://www.dermalscreen.com/Types.html
http://dermatology.about.com/cs/scc/index.htm
http://www.skin-cancers.net/

http://www.skincancer.org/
http://www.doc.mmu.ac.uk/aric/eae/Ozone_Depletion/
    Older/Skin_Cancer.html

**The effects of solar radiation**
http://ohioline.osu.edu/cd-fact/0199.html
http://www.bom.gov.au/info/about_uvb.shtml (excellent)
http://askbillsardi.com/sdm.asp?pg=cancer_regimen

# Chapter 7

# Wound Bed Repair

## Introduction

The natural healing pathway (**wound bed repair**) of human tissue is an exquisite example of the complexity of the physiological responses provided by human structural anatomy and physiology, perfectly orchestrated and balanced in ways that are consistent with the homeostatic maintenance of life itself[1-8].

Optimal wound management outcomes are both the results of an exact science (research based), and inexact science (based on expert experience, psychosocial issues, and the indispensable co-operation of the patient).

Prior to determining the treatment pathway it is important to identify the type of wound that is to be managed, undertake a critical patient and wound assessment, address the risk factors that exist which have the potential to retard or inhibit the healing process, and set out preferred clinical wound and patient outcomes.

This chapter outlines the principles and fundamentals of the normal wound bed repair process prior to addressing wound management practices, described in Chapters 9–12. The rationale for this is that in order for nurse clinicians to identifying abnormal healing, they must first have a clear basic knowledge and understanding, of the pathological phases that are essentially predictable in a clean surgical wound.

Understanding of the repair process provides the clinician with the knowledge and skills to identify and address the principal adverse events that may occur during the complex pathway between injury and a healed wound. Boxes 7.1–7.7 outline the differences between principal wound types through to the identification of a healed wound.

## Principal wound types

### Box 7.1 Acute wounds.

- Heal in predictable phases in the absence of medical morbid factors and risk factors controlled
- Have excellent potential to heal despite dressings choice
- Pain control easily managed when treated proactively, and compliance optimal
- Complications are uncommon if existing actual or potential medical morbid factors are prevented or controlled
- Clinical, and patient, functional and aesthetic outcomes usually highly acceptable[1-8]
- Patients are normally compliant with treatment regimes.

### Box 7.2 Chronic wounds.

- Do not follow an expected normal or predictable sequence of wound bed repair due to pro-inflammatory stimuli, trauma, shear, friction, infection
- Complications are common mainly due to medical and nursing morbid and co-morbid factors
- Continuous or recurring pain a common feature with continuing inflammatory activity, increasing tissue oedema and presence of wound toxins, and exposure of nerve endings further compounding wound complications, retarding or inhibiting the repair process if untreated
- Patients frequently depressed due to retarded or inhibited healing, and increasing potential for mediocre clinical outcomes
- Poor patient compliance due to failure of wound to improve regardless of treatment[3-16].

**Box 7.3** Palliative wounds.

- Wounds that do not heal, or heal temporarily, and frequently recur
- Mainly arise from primary or secondary malignant tumours of the skin, or orifices
- Complications common, and wounds frequently are suppurating and painful
- Treatment complex and does not always meet the preferred clinical and patient outcome
- Compliance difficult due to the disabling factors of the disease process[10,12–15].

**Box 7.4** Basis for current evidence-based data on wound bed repair.

- The currently accepted knowledge of normal human anatomy, pathophysiology, microbiology and pharmacology
- The concepts and principles of moist wound healing based on normal wound bed repair[11–16]
- The contemporary *in vivo* applied functional anatomical studies of the total microcirculatory system, and nerve supply to the skin[17]
- Emerging results of studies based on research related to the fundamental place of stem cells for wound repair at all tissue levels[5]
- Reports of applied clinical experience by acknowledged experts in the field
- The results of a range of clinical trials reviewing dressing products and wound repair outcomes.

**Box 7.5** Terminology of types of wound healing.

- Spontaneous healing: superficial, partial thickness wounds (e.g. skin grazes, thin split thickness skin graft donor sites)
- Primary intention: normal healing in a closed surgical wound
- Delayed primary intention: wound remains open for 48–72 hours (may be longer in some cases) and then formally closed by surgical suturing
- Secondary intention: open wound allowed to granulate and resurface
- Tertiary intention: skin grafts, flaps.

**Box 7.6** Clinical practice principles of wound bed repair.

- Define the aetiology of the wound, including the mechanism of the injury
- Assess the status of the wound and potential for an uninterrupted repair pathway
- Control the pain and discomfort proactively/pre-emptively
- Control the adverse physiological and psychosocial factors that may retard or inhibit the healing process
- Set short, medium and long-term goals in order to achieve outcomes
- Select the appropriate treatment modality through a multidisciplinary approach (e.g. surgery, wound dressings, combined techniques, include allied health professionals and community nurses where appropriate)
- Evaluate the wound and patient outcomes, and plan to maintain the healed process[1–6].

**Box 7.7** When skin wounds are physiologically healed.

- When the highest level of integrity of the epidermis and dermis possible for the individual patient, is restored
- When the patient is pain free
- Tissues exhibit their ability to withstand injury by demonstrating optimal strength, stability and function under reasonable stress and wear and tear
- Mobility of the injured part and the patient's independence is restored to optimal level
- When the wound exhibits a preferred aesthetic scar result acceptable to both surgeon and patient[1–7].

## Physiological definitions

Box 7.8 provides some definitions commonly referred to in the wound repair process and required to be understood when addressing and applying wound healing principles.

## Box 7.8 Definitions in wound bed repair.

| | |
|---|---|
| **Fibrin** | exudate resulting from fibrinogen liberated from blood that forms as a clot following injury |
| **Fibroblasts** | tissue growth cells present in normal tissue and essential for wound repair |
| **Angiogenesis** | the growth of cells from pre-existing capillaries |
| **Arteriogenesis** | the growth of arteries from pre-existing arterioles (the term angiogenesis is loosely applied to all forms of vascular growth that develops at the micro level in response to arterial injury, stenosis and occlusions) |
| **Myofibroblasts** | specialised form of fibroblast cell with the ability to assist the healing dermis to contract |
| **Granulation tissue** | produced by newly formed capillaries in response to injury. Granular or rough in surface appearance for easier cellular adhesion. |
| **Epithelialisation** | regeneration or resurfacing of the epidermis providing a protective layer to underlying dermis, soft tissue and bony structures. |
| **Collagen** | 13 types identified but function of many remain unknown. They are secreted by fibroblasts and require the presence of macrophages to function properly. |
| **Contraction** | forces initiated by development of collagen (structure) and elastin (flexibility) |
| **Contracture** | the end process of contraction and resurfacing |
| **Scar tissue** | external view of the end stage of skin wound repair[3,5,9]. |

## Options and practice principles for wound bed repair

Contemporary research provides a range of options that can allow for wounds to be closed in order that the protection of the organism can be maximised. Figure 7.1 outlines the principal options available for skin closure to protect the organism. The advantages and disadvantages of different techniques are outlined in Figure 7.2.

In principle, it is stated that skin wounds heal by dermal contraction (bringing strength and resilience) and by epidermal resurfacing (restoring the protective body envelop) working in tandem, with the outcome being a matured scar[3,5,9].

All skin wounds produce visible scar, and for plastic surgeons one of the Holy Grails of wound repair in humans, following surgery, trauma or disease, is an observable scar-free outcome[3,5,9]. This outcome has been shown to be attainable in the skin with pre-birth intrauterine repair (regeneration) of congenital malformations of, for example, cleft lip. In the extra-uterine environment children heal more quickly and with least adverse events[3,5,9].

Stretch marking in scars is more commonly seen, as opposed to raised scars, in the wounds of children who do not have the factors that produce hypertrophic or keloid scarring. Matured scars are referred to as a contracture and the final result may vary, from an almost invisible line to an unacceptable functional and aesthetic mixture of contracted skin[1-6,16-21].

The availability and use of suture material, modern wound dressings, artificial skin products, skin grafts and skin flaps, as a routine component of wound closure options, provides an expanding array of possibilities to meet the closure needs of almost any wound.

Figure 7.3 outlines the projected phases of normal wound bed repair (i.e. based on a clean surgical wound in a healthy person) on which the clinician can base a judgement as to whether wound progression is satisfactory or adverse events may be occurring. Each of these phases is essential, and some acute (trauma-based) or chronic wounds may move back and forth before finally achieving the desired outcome.

## Clinical principles required for a wound to heal

In contemporary reconstructive plastic surgical wound care, the recognition of a need for a holistic and individual patient approach, by treating medical, nursing and allied health clinicians, has been significant in improving wound repair and/or quality of life outcomes in acute, chronic and palliative care wounds[1-10]. The principles in Box 7.9 are currently accepted for optimal and achievable wound outcomes (the order is not in priority, each is of equal importance).

---

**Spontaneous/secondary epithelialisation – open repair**

Abrasions
Superficial wounds – burns – superficial and superficial partial thickness
Laser therapy – dermabrasion
Split skin graft (SSG) donor sites

Moist wound healing – normothermic

---

**Direct closure by suture – primary/secondary intention**

Surgical wounds – immediate closure of all tissue layers
Clean post-trauma wounds – immediate or at 48–72 hours
Delayed primary skin closure at day 2–6
Secondary skin closure at day 10–14 (uncommon)

Moist wound healing – normothermic

Topical sub-atmospheric (negative) pressure therapy (TSA(N)PT) as primary treatment for reduction of oedema, assisting in a degree of *contraction* prior to secondary suture, application of skin graft or skin flap

---

**Split or full thickness skin grafts**

Superficial to partial thickness donor skin to wounds (epidermis and upper dermal layer)
Partial-thickness donor skin to wounds (epidermis and deep dermal layer)
Full thickness skin (epidermis and dermis) graft – i.e. upper eye lid to lower eye lid (epidermis and dermis)

SSG may be used as temporary wound dressing prior to major reconstruction
– usually following compound trauma or wide spread tumour
TSA(N)PT as primary dressing to recipient and/or donor site

Moist wound healing – normothermic

---

**Skin and soft tissue flaps**

**Local random (blood supply not identified) flap**

Full thickness skin locally relocated as a replacement (adjacent to primary wound site) to excised tissue

Moist wound healing – normothermic

**Regional flap (identifiable source and territory vascular supply)**

Axial pattern based tissue replacement for loss of regional tissues
Singular or composite tissue reconstruction of skin, fascia, muscle (blood supply intact) – donor site usually requires skin gaft for closure
May include TSA(N)PT

Moist wound healing – normothermic

---

**Distant flap**

Vascular pedicle flaps (delayed) – donor flap raised and distal end located at recipient site – blood supply left intact at proximal end for 10–21 days – cut from original primary source as blood supply re-established at recipient site (i.e. delto-pectoral flap to face)

Free vascular tissue transfer to distant site (i.e. latissimus dorsi to lower limb; blood supply detached with donor flap and microsurgically reattached at recipient site)

Moist wound healing – normothermic

May include TSA(N)PT

---

**Tissue expansion**

Replacement of full thickness skin defect with incrementally expanded adjacent local tissue by balloon technique – procedure may take upto 3 months to complete – modern extension of the fasciocutaneous flap technique

Moist wound healing – normothermic

---

**Figure 7.1** Principal wound closure options.

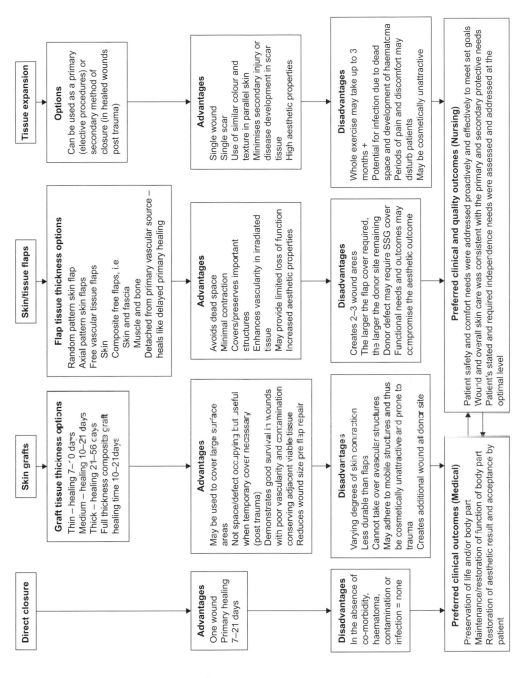

**Figure 7.2** General advantages and disadvantages of principal wound closure options.

| **Average inflammatory phase, days 0–5** |
|---|
| Blood vessels damaged – release of platelets into the tissues |

Blood vessels damaged – release of platelets into the tissues
Fibrin clot
Short period of hypoxia, then restoration of oxygen in the area (essential in establishment of new capillaries – angiogenesis – arteriogenesis)
Release of histamines and enzymes
Capillaries dilate allowing serum and white blood cells to leak into the tissues and bathe the injured area
Polymorphonuclear leucocytes and macrophages begin the repair
Due to all this activity the wound and immediate surrounding area is red warm/hot, swollen, often painful and with loss of function. It is important not to mistake this phase for infection if, e.g., pyrexia is absent.
Restoration of increased blood flow and oxygen
Polymorphs and macrophages clear the wound of devitalised tissue
Fibroblasts commence the reconstruction work depositing collagen
Angiogenesis = early initiation of granulation tissue via sprouting of new capillaries
Due to great cellular activity and increased protein more water is attracted to the area by osmosis, creating marked oedematous swelling
Subsequent reducing swelling (after 48–72 hours) as protein reabsorbed from interstitial spaces by lymphatics
In limbs, swelling may continue if dependent oedema not treated by compression and/or gravity via elevation above heart level

**Granulation, epithelialisation and contraction phase, days 3–24**

Development of pink granulation tissue = new and fragile capillary loops supported on a scaffolding of collagen fibres and matrix proteins
Development of basement membrane
Epithelialisation commences from uninjured wound edges
Presence of myofibroblasts with early dermal contraction and wound strengthening process beginning
Swelling reduced as extracellular proteins return to circulation taking water with them
Without adequate vitamin C intake collagen synthesis is suggested to be inhibited

**Maturation phase**

Scar remodelling days 24–365+
Decrease in capillary vascularity
Restoration of normal circulatory function
Shrinkage of fibroblasts, enlargement and reorientation of the collagen fibres and augmentation of the tensile strength
Wound remodelling and increased strengthening of dermal tissue
There are, however, two other important mechanisms to be considered in wound healing:

| **Contraction** | **Epithelialisation** |
|---|---|
| (Dermis) | (Epidermis – resurfacing) |
| The process of wound contraction is still not fully understood. However, there are some known facts. | Epidermal cells, squamous epithelial cells renew not only from the edge of the wound, but also from hair follicles and other deep dermal appendages lined by squamous cells still in the wounded area |
| Contraction is not a feature of normal surgical wounds in mobile tissue | A basement membrane must be developed to assist in movement of epithelial cells across granulation tissue |
| Collagen is not essential for contraction | |
| Myofibroblasts are special contractile cells having attributes of both fibroblasts and smooth muscle cells (myo = muscle) | Epithelial cell adhesion aided by granular surface of fibroblast cells |
| The motive for contraction comes from a cell's need to be in contact with other cells for survival by interaction | Assisted by process of (contractile forces) contraction moving the sides of the dermal tissue towards the centre of the wound |
| Any event that interferes with the viability of cells (loss of blood flow and delivery of oxygen) at the wound edge or within dermal appendages will inhibit contraction | In medium sized wounds should be completed in 7–14 days |
| Contracture is the outcome of completed wound contraction | |

**Figure 7.3** Projected phases of normal wound bed repair.

---

**Box 7.9** Principles of applied clinical nursing management for wound bed repair – the patient.

- A scientific, evidence-based physiological methodology, and psychosocial approach to all patient wound care needs
- An acceptance of the importance of developing a skilled multidisciplinary case management team for an individual case management approach to wound healing at all levels of care required that is based on addressing the individual person's physiological and psychosocial stated needs
- A broad knowledge base of the pharmacology and application of modern wound and skin care products
- Addressing clinical risk management including the setting and auditing of short, medium and long-term wound and patient preferred outcomes.

---

**Box 7.10** Principles of applied clinical management for wound bed repair – the wound.

- The acceptance and application of the scientific concepts and principles of moist wound healing[11–13] and moist wound dressings as the foundation on which normal biological tissue healing treatment modalities are currently based
- The application of the concept of wound bed assessment, preparation and maintenance practice principles as essential if the optimal outcome for wound repair is to be achieved[16]
- The importance of an uninterrupted microcirculatory system within, and surrounding, the wound for cellular recovery/replication for repair to be initiated and completed[17]
- An understanding of the significant effects of critical contamination and infection within the injured area and on the host. This requires the necessity of 're-balancing' wound bed/host bacteria levels significantly in favour of the host[9,10]
- Recognition of the damaging effects of ongoing tissue oedema on cellular function[18]
- An acceptance that the application of science-based compression therapy, and negative pressure therapy as treatment modalities, can clinically address localised oedema, manage wound exudates and promote rapid angiogenesis and granulation tissue[4,7,19–22]
- The recognition that there is a significant relationship between unresolved acute and chronic pain and the failure of wounds to repair[15]
- The importance of primary wound immobility to avoid shear and friction, at the wound site[3,5].

---

## Hyperbaric oxygen therapy

Empirical trials have indicated that the use of hyperbaric oxygen is beneficial, for example:

- Where previous injury has occurred and healing is anticipated to be potentially compromised
- Pre- and postoperatively in patients undergoing major flap surgery, particularly where disease is an issue
- Failing skin graft and skin flaps
- Crush injuries
- Replant surgery
- Necrotising fasciitis.

See recommended websites at the end of this chapter.

## Clinical nursing risk management issues

Addressing clinical risk issues that impede or inhibit wound bed repair increases the potential for clinical and patient preferred outcomes to be met with minimal physiological or psychosocial problems.

Boxes 7.11, 7.12 and 7.13 outline the principal issues for clinicians to consider when undertaking wound bed care.

---

**Box 7.11** Addressing patient safety issues.

- An inadequate critical assessment of the whole patient, and the wound, has the potential to lead to adverse patient and wound repair outcomes
- The principal cause of failure of wounds to repair are disturbances in systemic, regional or local blood flow regardless of the aetiology, which leads to the development of breakdown of cellular function, local tissue necrosis and/or local, and life-limiting/threatening infection (septicaemia)
- Failure to critically address ongoing oedema leads to cellular dysfunction and wound breakdown

*Continued*

- Continuing failure of chronic wound beds to repair or respond to palliative wound bed management may lead to life-limiting/threatening, local and systemic infection (septicaemia)
- Inappropriate wound assessment, wound bed preparation, and mismatching dressing products to wound needs can damage the existing normal tissues, compromise the initiation of tissue regrowth and be a persistent source of pain and discomfort
- Ineffective initial wound repair outcomes have the potential to lead to extended treatment regimes that usually include expensive dressings, rehabilitation and/or additional surgery, further contributing to a decline in the patient's safety
- Failure to restore normal function and aesthetics may be life changing and present immediate and long-term issues of individual safety, comfort and independence.

**Box 7.13** Addressing patient independence issues.

- Independence may be addressed as a partnership between clinicians, allied health professionals, patients and significant others, until patients are prepared to undertake full responsibility for themselves
- Adverse changes in levels of short or long-term independence and ability for self-care may present unanticipated issues relating to an overall decline in physical and psychosocial independence. Sometimes this loss of independence results in total reliance on the health service provider or carer
- Loss of independence at any level may compromise the potential for maintenance of a normal financial income, and cause detrimental changes in personal relationships, and attitudes to social integration
- Adverse exit outcomes of patient safety and pain management may lead to varying degrees of loss of short and long-term individual independence with negative psychosocial implications, such as depression and social isolation.

**Box 7.12** Addressing patient comfort issues.

- Failure to address the primary cause and management of patient pain and discomfort at all stages of wound care may lead to failure of the wound to heal
- Continuing pain or discomfort disables the patient and may compromise the patient's participation in initial and ongoing treatment regimes and rehabilitation
- Failure to address acute pain needs may lead to chronic and debilitating pain outcomes that affect local and general functions, and potentially lead to permanent physical disability
- Failure to address acute pain needs may lead to chronic and debilitating pain outcomes with the additional possibility of psychological disturbances, including depression.

## Setting clinical and patient needs outcomes

Clinical and patient preferred outcomes can be addressed following identification of the physiological and psychosocial risk issues (safety, comfort, independence) specific to the wound type (i.e. acute, chronic or palliative) and patient presentation. This allows for the clinician, in co-operation with the patient, to set short, medium and long-term actual or potentially achievable goals and outcomes, as appropriate.

**Review**

Boxes 7.11, 7.12 and 7.13 above.
Chapter 2 (Figures 2.1 & 2.2, Boxes 2.1 & 2.2) to assist in developing clinical and patient outcomes.

# Wound bed repair – pathophysiology

## Moist wound healing

An unhindered circulatory blood flow delivers oxygen and warmth from arterial blood and removes toxic wastes. Heat is also generated by cellular function[11–13]. Under normal physiological conditions, the human organism maintains a fine balance between intravascular, intracellular and extracellular fluid that contain the essential biological elements for a normal general and local homeostasis to be sustained. Significant internal or external injury, to the skin and underlying tissues alters this homeostatic state.

The establishment of the concept and principles of moist wound healing, and the utilisation of moist wound dressings, is the contemporary physiological foundation on which all levels, and approaches, to clinical applied wound management, are currently addressed[11–13].

The concept of physiological moist wound healing is essentially based on:

- The **acceptance** that this concept is the scientific basis on which normal clean surgical wounds repair
- The principle that an open wound will only heal through the application of a treatment process that restores and mimics the normal biological processes exhibited in the presence of the optimal internal environment of a clean, layer-closed surgical wound.

The adoption of the concept of moist wound healing was originally based on experimental wound healing studies in animals, based on what occurs under a clean eschar or a scab (collection of dead cells)[11–13]. It was observed that in the presence of specific levels of 'clean' (normal low levels of contamination) moisture, the dermis would contract, the epidermis would resurface unhindered, and the scab simply became detached. This had been witnessed countless times on prior occasions. However, on close observation of the phenomenon, it was realised that if the internal milieu was covered by an artificial barrier to the external environment that allowed the internal wound to retain its warmth and moisture in the normal oxygenated environment, uninjured, it healed, a crust did not form and the natural warmth and moisture promoted faster healing.

## Box 7.14 Conditions for moist wound healing.

Moist wound healing is stated to be occurring when:

- Pain has been controlled
- An adequate general and local circulation is in place, including control of excess levels of oedema
- Oxygen saturation and gaseous exchanges are occurring within the wound that facilitate the removal of cellular by-products and wound toxins
- There has been an initiation of growth factors within uncontaminated moisture and local tissue warmth (normothermia)
- Local homeostatic mechanisms have been restored sufficiently to allow replications of cells, initiation of dermal contraction and epidermal resurfacing
- Wounds are initially adequately splinted to avoid shear, friction, and disturbances in the primary functions necessary for the repair process to be initiated and maintained.

Healing wounds will pass through a largely unseen series of phases or stages that are built on, and overlap each other, to complete a total process for ensuring the integrity of the skin and underlying tissues[2–6].

When medical and nursing morbid factors already exist in the patient and complex wounds are present (e.g. in trauma or disease) unforeseen adverse events or complications can and will occur. The principal goal for all treating clinicians is to assist proactively in restoring stability in the patient's general systems and the local wound environment. The clinician should also engender a confidence in the patient that the care provided is conducive to re-establishing the optimal repair pathway, by whatever medically/nursing prescribed method deemed appropriate. This should be reinforced by evidence-based or expert experiential general nursing practices that will allow clinicians to assess nursing risk management, and to put into place those practices that protect the patient physiologically and psychosocially.

## Application of the moist wound healing theory

One of the first practical applications of the moist wound healing theory was the use of a commercial grade 'cling' plastic film – a polythene-based, inert, non-toxic material used to cover and store food. It does not contain plasticisers or PVC. Cling film was applied as a primary dressing over skin graft donor sites. It retained wound moisture, warmth, and protected the exposed nerve endings from external contact and repeated injury. The film-covered wound demonstrated the ability to resurface more quickly, and relatively painlessly, even on movement. The days of Vaseline®-impregnated gauze overlaid with combine/wool dressings was about to be superseded by a more scientific and pain-free approach. Because of the problems of leakage and film retention, the combine/wool dressings and crepe bandage continued to be applied.

This technique was followed by the development of comparable medical/pharmacological products which were surgically sterile and delivered in different sizes to suit various wound sizes. Manufacturers added surrounding adhesive edging to secure the plastic film dressings to the skin outside the wounded zone. This revolutionised the approach to split skin graft donor site dressings.

Although there have been many new moist wound healing products produced that meet wound needs, the use of these products continue to be varied. Many of the previously basic products are now multipurpose, that is, they may be applied as a primary or secondary dressing (e.g. semi permeable films). Their use has been expanded to IV sites, postoperative keyhole sites following endoscopic surgery as both a protective primary and/or secondary dressings allowing patients unprecedented independence for showering and self-care.

Moist wound healing management concepts and principles are the mantra on which an entire modern pharmacological industry of wound dressings for normal physiological replication has developed. Thus the requirement to balance the temperature, moisture levels, oxygen availability and pain control is incorporated into the majority of modern wound dressing products.

For superficial and superficial partial thickness wounds, recent scientific advances have seen the emergence of absorbent, flexible, waterproof, soft silicone-based dressing materials suitable for direct application to the skin. These materials have the all the physiological qualities required of many existing minimal or low exudating/absorbent moist wound healing dressings. They provide pain control, are waterproof, have adequate degrees of flexibility,

retaining relative skin and wound splinting qualities as they have adhesive retention properties with inbuilt 'membrane memory' (they return to their original position when minimally stretched), allowing for some skin and body movement[21].

For reconstructive plastic surgeons and nurse practitioners these new generation dressings are particularly useful on the chest wall, hands, following surgery, where wounds are closed, and where early mobility is essential, and as dressings for areas of the face or body following dermabrasion, and thin split skin graft donor sites.

See Chapter 12 for a comprehensive discussion of wound dressing selection.

## The biological process of wound repair

Normal wound repair follows a relatively predictable pathway (Figure 7.3). The completion of each specific phase (although stated to be an overlapping process) is singly important if the progression of repair is to advance uninterrupted. If a vital phase is interrupted, physiological disorder within the wound results, progress is impeded or halted and healing complications begin to emerge.

Because of the significance of the skin as the principal protective body organ, the individual phases of wound bed repair are of intense research interest to wound clinicians. Should it be observed that a repairing phase is under challenge, evidence-based interventions can be applied for restoring normality, and allow the complex process to continue. Two particular events of interest to plastic surgeons are the contraction and remodelling phases.

### Primary wound bed contraction

Two forms of **mesenchymal** cells, **fibroblasts** and **myofibroblasts**, are principally responsible for epidermis and dermal wound bed repair. The principal cell responsible for tissue contraction in the dermis and connective tissues is the myofibroblast, a specialised form of fibroblast with contractile forces[3]. This contraction is in parallel with the gradual restoration of the underlying forces of negative pressure in the healing wound, closing off any dead space.

---

**Review**

Chapter 5 and Figure 7.3.

---

**Box 7.15** Basic principles of primary wound bed contraction.

- In normal wounds at about 24–48 hours post injury, the inflammatory response and the instigation of wound/tissue growth factors occurs
- A primary hypoxic state initiates arteriogenesis and angiogenesis (production of new blood vessels), which is responsible for the production of new loop structured capillaries
- With restoration of blood flow and oxygen and capillary formation, the fibroblasts convert to myofibroblast and establish contractile forces
- Under normal circumstances, these fibres are then collected and arranged in bundles. These bundles assist in providing the normal strength to the tissues but this is a slow process, and in some wounds, a lengthy timeframe
- Contraction involves the movement of existing tissue at the dermal wound edges, not the formation of new tissue
- Wound contraction is the same in all normal clean surgical wounds, regardless of size – approximately 0.6–0.75 mm per day.
- In normal wounds, the main contraction time is from days 5–10, after this there appears to be is a significant slowing as the complex process of collagen maturation and remodelling of the collagen matrix begins
- In abnormal wounds the main contraction is even slower, often contributing to the conversion of an acute wound to a chronic wound[3]
- Circular wounds contract disappointingly and significantly more slowly than rectangular or stellate wounds, due to the normal method contracting movement
- The excessive tension placed on the dermis to move to the centre exceeds the ability of epidermis to resurface in a timely manner. This is why plastic surgeons prefer to convert the defect to an elliptical wound, utilise a split skin graft, or undertake a local skin flap to close a circular wound[3,5].

- The extra force to close a circular wound, as opposed to an elliptical wound, can be likened to the effort required to close a drawstring bag
- If capillary growth exceeds collagen fibre deposition, it may result in hypergranulation tissue, also called 'proud flesh'
- Epithelialisation cannot take place over this form of granulation tissue, and it must be removed by surgery and/or dressing management[4]
- Mechanical means, based on the principles of the developing contracting forces within the granulating wound bed, may be used for the temporary or permanent closure of a large open wound. These are cases where primary surgical closure is inappropriate due to oedema, excess exudate, the patient is ill, or too fragile
- In some medium/large acute open trauma wounds, and sacral pressure ulcer wounds, negative pressure by the VAC® method is now commonly applied, with excellent results[19–22]
- The removal of the excess exudate allows for arteriogenesis and angiogenesis (formation of new blood vessels)
- This initial restoration of a vascular flow allows new wound fibroblasts to convert to myofibroblast and establish their important contractile forces[3]
- Disorganised contracting processes may result in tissue distortion, potential dysfunction, and poor aesthetic outcomes – burn scar contractures are an example of this
- Stretching of the scar is seen initially more in relatively fixed skin, and major contractions in skin under tension, such as the face, back, or over joints such as the elbow or knee
- In mobile or loose skin that is subject to weight gain, pregnancy or gravity, contraction may take longer but the stretching often gives a flatter appearance[3]

---

**Review**

Figures 5.9–5.12.

---

## Maturation and remodelling in wound bed repair – the final process

With the increasing restoration of the wound circulation, primary dermal contraction, and epidermal resurfacing, relative negative pressures in the tissues are restored, providing an increasing level of normalcy within the cells/tissues. Increasing maturation of the wound and, in particular, wound strengthening is ready to begin its final phase.

## Contraction

**Contraction** is the biological process that occurs in the dermis and/or connective tissue which is responsible for decreasing the overall dimensions of an open or closed wound[3]. The principal components of connective tissues are three fibrous proteins: **collagen**, **reticulum** and **elastin**, aided by other supporting complex proteins. All of these proteins are of particular interest to the cosmetic industry in attempts to formulate pharmaceutical products to halt or slow down the loss of collagen and elastin, associated with the normal ageing process and other issues.

---

> ## Review
>
> Chapter 6.

---

Collagen, the main protein, is a complex type of protein substance that is insoluble in water and is the principal constituent of connective tissue. It is synthesised by several types of cells but the most important is the fibroblast. Collagen is a white fibrous structure and forms complex bundles with a woven (matrix) arrangement providing the appropriate body strength relative to the needs of specific body regions[3,5].

**Remodelling** is the pathway by which collagen matrix is synthesised and matures to obtain the maximum structural integrity of a healed wound[3]. This complex process may take from three weeks to 18+ months to finally complete. Total remodelling and maturation of the collagen fibres, within the developed matrix, is the final process of wound bed repair.

The outcome of the wound contraction process is a contracture and this is referred to as a scar. All normal healed wound can only gain up to 85% of the original wound site integrity. This is a problem for chronic wounds, particularly on the lower limb, where secondary injury occurs and may then progress to ulceration. Adverse events related to altered repair pathways, intermittent periods of contamination or infection, short but persistent phases of secondary disturbances in blood flow, distorted development of the collagen matrix tissue, and secondary injury interrupting the fragile collagen fibre development, can all contribute to extending the maturation phase and fragility of the final tissue/scar.

It is important for nurse clinicians to comprehend how scar tissue forms, and the varying degrees of aberrations that may occur in all patients, but particularly in elective cosmetic surgical patients. Some scars may be structurally, functionally, aesthetically disruptive, or unacceptable to the patient. The potential for scar anomalies should be discussed extensively with the patient prior to surgery as the patient will often judge the success of the surgery by the scars. Observation of the tissues for the outcomes of any existing wounds on the body is a useful guide[3].

### *Genetic conditions in collagen development and synthesis*

One of the more complex hereditary conditions is Ehlers-Danlos syndrome, of which more than 10 types have been identified. This condition is represented by varying degrees of hyperelasticity of the skin, from moderate to severe, often requiring removal by plastic surgeons[6]. Specific medical disorders and their treatment modalities may also cause disturbances in all stages of strengthening forces, for example, in rheumatoid arthritis[3].

## Risk factors governing wound remodelling

The influence of long-term treatment with corticosteroids on collagen deposition and synthesis is not completely understood at this time. It is known that in patients who are on therapeutic steroids, deposition may take place but cross linking for tensile strength may not occur. Giving vitamin A is suggested to reverse the effect of corticosteroids on the important primary inflammatory stage of healing without interfering with the progress of the normal pathway[3].

Corticosteroids may be prescribed for many medical reasons. In rheumatoid arthritis, patients undergoing reconstructive surgical procedures may remain on medication so as not to alter therapeutic levels. In the absence of any adverse factors, postoperative short courses of corticosteroids do not appear to interfere with the long-term repair process in any wound (in fact these may also be prescribed in certain inflammatory ulcers) but neither have the benefits been scientifically demonstrated in objective clinical trials. Their use is becoming more common in elective plastic surgery such as craniofacial, upper and lower limb, and cosmetic resurfacing procedures, to reduce postoperative oedema.

## Avoidance strategies for adverse wound bed repair outcomes

Clinicians are familiar with the external sight of wounds that appear closed at the epidermal level, but break down once a certain level of stress is exerted (e.g. stretching and constant pressure as seen in some back, breast and abdominal wounds) beyond the tissue tolerance of the dermis and the epidermis. This occurs because, although the integrity of the epidermis appears intact, healed or restored to its previous appearance, at the dermal level wounds in particular regions may not have reached the expected initial tensile strength even after 24+ days.

Most normal closed acute wounds can be expected to reach their primary tensile strength and be quite resilient at about 21–28+ days. Breakdown may occur due to the special nature of the skin zones. Examples of this are:

- Fixed skin areas
- Thick epidermal/dermal skin areas on the back
- Palm of the hand
- Sole of the foot.

In addition to this there may be a range of complicating and competing biological factors that are attempting to address a particular adverse episode within the closed wound and invisible from the outside (e.g. underlying haematoma, or ischaemic fat tissue causing wound contamination)[3]. Specific protective measures can be instituted:

- Wound protection
- Observation for unexpected swelling, pain, fever
- Patient education for understanding and compliance
- Immobilisation of the part, or limits on movement in the early stages – important to prevent or minimise problems.

## Difficulties in fixed skin zones

In regions where the skin is essentially thin and relatively fixed to the strong underlying connective tissues over, for example, the anterior surface of the tibia[4], the lack of dermal mobility reduces the movement of contraction that can occur. Wounds heal more slowly, with greater difficulty, and break down more easily. In addition, wound healing rates in fixed skin areas can be slower simply because of the complex fine vascular structure in the particular anatomical position, the effects of an unstable circulation if the wound is contaminated or under tension, and the constant normal body movement causing shear and friction across any fragile vessels[17].

Healing may be prolonged through secondary healing by using a granulation and re-epithelialisation technique, often resulting in thin fragile scar tissue, and an overall surrounding wound tension which is easily susceptible to secondary injury, infection and potential development of ulceration[3]. The further development of objective wound bed assessment and wound bed preparation algorithms could be of assistance in these particularly difficult wounds, that are often a feature of the older person with vascular problems.

'Intelligent' contemporary dressings have inbuilt memory that are capable of assessing the wound moisture requirements, retain cellular warmth, and allow oxygen into the wound at an optimal regulated level.

Tissue engineered products that are changing the clinical culture by which clinicians approach specific areas of wound management, for example, the goal to produce an inexpensive dermal matrix on which skin grafts can be placed for accelerated wound closure[6]. The 'Holy Grail' in this field is the development of different thicknesses of artificial dermis and epidermis, free from tissue rejection, which responds similarly to the patient's normal skin in the presence of a clean surgical wound.

## Adjunctive modalities for wound closure

In wounds under tension or that are widely open/exposed, reconstructive plastic surgeons will predominantly use negative pressure therapy (VAC® system) to reduce the size of the wound prior to secondary reconstructive surgical procedures, or apply meshed split thickness skin grafts and the VAC®

system to reduce fluid accumulation (Figures 5.9–5.12).

Where lack of dermal tissue or remaining tissue bulk (usually muscle) is an issue, surgeons may use split thickness skin grafts (STSGs) and/or flaps in areas of known poor contractile forces to obtain temporary or permanent skin closure, and thus reduce tension on the existing wound and surrounding skin[3,5,22–25].

## Examples of special problems in wound bed repair

### The oral/alimentary epithelium

Because the functional needs of the organism vary, repair and recovery of the squamous epithelium (epidermis) in body areas including the skin are achieved by the specialised programming of the tissue cells[3].

Oral and external epidermal wound repair is essentially by a regenerative process of the parenchymal (labile) cells through the constant turnover of used cells. Some areas of the oral mucous membrane may be restored with little or no scar tissue, ensuring smooth surface integrity of oral and gut lining. But other oral and alimentary areas may heal with scar tissue, causing significant strictures or reduction of the normal circumferences of the tubular digestive system (e.g., the lining of the oesophagus, external orifices, or trachea). This presents new problems in maintaining the required size of the openings by the use of regular artificial dilation or further surgical procedures[3,14].

### Issues of wound instability

Following some procedures (e.g. hand surgery), for many patients the restoration of even basic tissue strength may require an early professional hand therapist assessment and staged plans for rehabilitation. In addition, patients may need to be able to manage potentially difficult or aberrant scar development such as hypertrophic or keloid scars that occur on the neck and over joints.

Scar management experts such as physiotherapists and occupational therapists will usually grade these according to the anatomical site, type of injury

and/or operative procedure, and surgical intervention, prior to planning a management programme.

Wound instability or breakdown is psychosocially disruptive, may cause loss of income and result in multiple operative procedures.

## Psychosocial issues and wound bed repair

For many patients, the development and healing of a wound may involve three principal temporary or long-term changes or lifestyle phases. Patients may not consistently move in one direction on this descriptive scale but will move in and out of each phase depending on the skill of the attending clinician/s, the motivation of the individual, and the contextual quality of the care provided. Box 7.16 briefly outlines these phases.

---

**Box 7.16** Addressing patient levels of dependence.

| | |
|---|---|
| **Dependent** | The patient will be dependent on the skill of professionals to assess and indicate the optimal course of management. The vulnerable patient, the acutely ill, the unconscious, the cancer patient or individuals with some recent chronic or palliative care wounds may fall into this category. Clinicians require excellent communication skills and the ability to help the patient to accept a temporary handing over of some control without a sense of complete loss of personal power or identity. |
| **Interdependence/ co-dependent** | The patient and the professional will work together to set mutually attainable goals, to be met through education, communication and a sense of safety and comfort. Compliance in the context of management of extremely complex wounds (e.g. wound breakdown following |

*Continued*

|  |  |
|---|---|
|  | abdominal lipectomy) requires encouragement of the patient and the ability for the clinician to demonstrate positive results when treatment regimes are adhered to closely. |
| **Independent** | The patient regains control of their life through preferred clinical and quality outcomes being met within a safe context where decisions are essentially made by the patient, but also recognises that assistance is available as required. In the overall approach this available assistance is essential. Focus on objective but manageable interim and exit goals/outcomes through a process that the patient can understand and undertake. |

## Auditing outcomes of wound bed repair

With the completion of the wound bed repair process, auditing or evaluating the short, medium and long-term clinical and patient goals set prior to, during, and at the completion of the repair process, is essential. The patient must have a sense that a professional and caring approach by clinicians was undertaken, regardless of the wound type. Box 7.17 outlines the basic areas required to be audited at the completion of the overall treatment period.

### Box 7.17 Final audit of wound bed repair process.

- Clinical patient and wound assessment provided the optimal environment for wound bed repair to occur and was consistent with achieving the stated and preferred wound bed repair outcomes through the process of risk management
- Clinical decisions for treatments were based and evaluated on the criteria of patient safety, comfort and independence

- Planned wound repair outcomes were as consistent as possible with the preferred clinical and patient's goals and the application of research and/or expert experience
- The rationale for the failure of any wound to positively respond or heal whilst utilising the concept and principles of moist wound healing were clinically identified
- Continuing retardation of wound repair was addressed through clinical patient and wound reassessment, appropriate pathological examinations, and wide consultation with experts in the field where applicable
- The patient's physiological concerns and psychosocial issues affecting wound bed repair outcomes were always discussed and considered when decisions on surgery were considered, or treatment regimes were deliberated upon
- The wound repair process produced a functional and aesthetic outcome consistent with the normal recognised biological pathway and a timeframe appropriate for the presenting anatomical wound site.

## References

(1) Dubay D.A. & Franz M.G. Acute wound healing: the biology of acute wound failure. *Surgical Clinics of North America*, 2003 (June); **83**(3):463–81.

(2) Moy L.S. Management of acute wounds. *Dermatology Clinics*, 1993 (Oct); **11**(4):759–66.

(3) Peacock E.E. Jnr. *Wound repair*, 3rd edn. Philadelphia: W.B. Saunders Company, 1984.

(4) Bryant R.A. (ed.) *Acute and chronic wounds: nursing management*. St Louis: Mosby Year Book, 1992.

(5) Robinson J.B. & Friedman R.M. Wound healing and closure. *Selected Readings in Plastic Surgery*, 1996 8(1):1999–2000.

(6) Lazarus G.S., Cooper D.M., Knighton D.R., Margolis D.J., Pecoraro R.E., Rodeheaver G. & Robson M.C. Definitions and guidelines for assess of wounds and evaluation of healing. *Archives of Dermatology*, 1994 (Apr); **130**(4):489–93.

(7) Dealey C. *The care of wounds*, 2nd edn. Oxford, UK: Blackwell Science, 1999.

(8) Bates-Jensen B.M. Chronic wound assessment. *Nursing Clinics of North America*, 1999 (Dec); **34**(4):799–845.

(9) Pain and trauma at wound dressing changes: report on an international study. Website: http://www.world widewounds.com/News/News.html

(10) Bowler P.G., Duerden B.I. & Armstrong D.G. Wound microbiology and associated approaches to wound

management. *Clinical Microbiology, Review* 2001 (Apr): 244–69.

(11) Robson M.C. Wound infection. A failure of wound healing caused by an imbalance of bacteria. *Surgical Clinics of North America*, 1997 (June); 77(3):637–50.

(12) Vardaxis N. *Pathology for the Health Sciences*. St Yarra, Australia: MacMillan Education Australia Pty Ltd, 1994, reprinted 1998.

(13) Naylor W., Laverty D. & Mallett J. *Handbook of wound management in cancer care*. Oxford, UK: Blackwell Science, 2001.

(14) Winter G.D. Formation of the scab and the rate of epithelialisation of superficial wounds in the skin of the domestic pig. *Nature*, 1962; **193**:293.

(15) Winter G.D. Epidermal regeneration studied in the domestic pig. In: Hunt T.K. & Dunphy J.E (eds). *Fundamentals of wound management*. New York: Appleton-Century-Crofts, 1979.

(16) Bolton L.L., Monte K. & Pirone L.A. Moisture and healing: beyond the jargon. *Ostomy Wound Manage*, 2000 (Jan); **46**(1A Suppl):51S–62S; quiz 63S–63S.

(17) Taylor G.I., Palmer J.H. & McManamny D. The vascular territories of the body (angiosomes) and their clinical implications. In: McCarthy, J.G. *Plastic surgery: volume 1, general principles*. Philadelphia: W.B. Saunders, 1990.

(18) Guyton A.C. & Hall J.E. *Textbook of medical physiology*, 9th edn. London: W.B. Saunders, 1996.

(19) McCance K.L. & Huether S.E. Pathophysiology: the biologic basis for disease in adults and children, 3rd edn. St Louis: Mosby, 1998.

(19) Smeltzer S.C. & Bare B.G. *Brunner and Suddarth's textbook of medical-surgical nursing*, 9th edn. Philadelphia: Lippincott, Williams & Wilkins, 2000.

(20) Mallett J. & Dougherty L. (eds). *The Royal Marsden Hospital manual of clinical nursing procedures*, 5th edn. Oxford, UK: Blackwell Science, 2000.

(21) Vowden K. & Vowden P. *Wound Bed Preparation*. http://www.worldwidewounds.com

(22) Morykwas M., Argenta L.C., Shelton-Brown E. & McGuirt W. Vacuum-assisted closure: a new method for wound control and treatment: animal studies and basic foundation. *Annals of Plastic Surgery*, 1997; **38**:553–562.

(23) Argenta L.C. & Morykwas M. Vacuum-assisted closure: a new method for wound control and treatment: clinical experience. *Annals of Plastic Surgergy*, 1997; **38**:563–577.

(24) Thomas S. *An introduction to vacuum assisted closure*, 2001. http://www.worldwidewounds.com/2001/may/Thomas/Vacuum-Assisted-Closure.html

(25) Banwell P., Withey S. & Holten I. The use of negative pressure to promote healing. *British Journal of Plastic Surgery*, 1998; **51**(1):79.

## Recommended websites

**Hyperbaric oxygen**
http://www.uhms.org/Indications/indications.htm
http://www.baromedical.com/newsletter/010202.html

## Chapter 8

# Clinical Issues in the Causes of Wound Breakdown and the Failure of Wounds to Repair

1. Principal clinical issues in the causes of wound breakdown and the failure of wounds to repair
2. Applied nutritional issues in wound bed repair

---

**Review**

A review of Chapter 7 (Wound Bed Repair) covering normal blood flow to the skin, and the clinical principles of restoration of inadequate blood flow, may assist in a better understanding of this chapter.

---

## 1. PRINCIPAL CLINICAL ISSUES IN THE CAUSES OF WOUND BREAKDOWN AND THE FAILURE OF WOUNDS TO REPAIR

### Background

Despite contemporary physiological knowledge, every effort is exerted to anticipate and pre-empt adverse events. But many known and unknown clinical factors may actually, or potentially, place a clean surgical wound at risk, and impede the expected wound repair outcomes[1–10].

The management of clinical risk, such as stability of morbid and co-morbid factors, prevention of infection, management of general and wound pain, and having the co-operation of the patient, require a disciplined, knowledge-based holistic approach. Thus inadequate attention to detail in wound bed assessment, preparation and management are principal reasons that many areas of wound bed repair are retarded, and wounds may move to chronic, painful and debilitating states, or simply fail to heal. Some may even become life-threatening, with major cellular changes leading systemic unresolved infective states.

The key morbid and co-morbid factors that affect the normal repair process in all wounds have been described in a wide range of surgical and wound care literature, as collectively outlined in Table 8.1.

The localised clinical risk factors impeding the normal wound bed repair and maintenance processes are generally known in plastic surgery and plastic surgical nursing as the **Nine Deadly Ds** (Table 8.1), based on known complications[6].

In elective surgery, it is expected that clinical and psychosocial factors that can affect the preferred clinical and patient outcomes are identified, addressed, and stabilised prior to surgery being undertaken. The value of specialist pre-admission clinics cannot be underestimated here.

The presentation of emergency patients requires an immediate patient and wound bed assessment process to address the risk factors that relate to the patient's short, medium and long-term safety and comfort. Failure to address these risk factors as a whole, and initially prioritise in terms of patient safety, has the potential to retard or inhibit the total process of repair.

### Pathophysiology 1 – wound infection

#### The skin, wounds and the importance of pH maintenance

The pH value of blood averages about 7.4. Less than this value is considered acidic, greater is defined as alkaline. With the exception of minor deviations such as in gastric juice and urine, the pH is similar in all fluid compartments, with the major exception of the intracranial fluid, which has a pH of 7.0–7.2. Blood

**Table 8.1** Localised clinical risk factors impeding the normal wound bed repair process.

| Clinical problem | Potential causes | Suggested clinical action |
|---|---|---|
| Discomfort/pain | Inadequate arterial and venous blood flow<br>Physiological and psychological response to injury, unresolved, leads to poor healing, re-injury to delicate cells, and patient non-compliance<br>Presence of infection | Objectively assess pain source and level<br>Provide specific and adequate analgesia aimed at the root cause |
| Dead tissue | Inadequate blood supply<br>Necrotic and devitalised tissue providing an environment for further bacterial entry and ongoing infection<br>Interference with surrounding blood flow<br>Presence of contamination or infection | Debride<br>Flush wound with normal saline solution<br>Provide specifically targeted antibiotics if infection is confirmed or anticipated by aetiology |
| Debris | Foreign material contamination, e.g. dirt, road debris<br>Foreign materials such as implants | Debride<br>Flush wound with normal saline solution<br>Clinically observe for indications of infection |
| Development and ongoing presence of oedema | Inadequate venous and/or lymphatic circulation allowing for dependant oedema and displacement of extracellular fluid which thus inhibits normal cellular contact and function at capillary level | Negative pressure therapy or compression bandaging and/or appropriate elevated position for gravity to reduce excess fluid<br>Early controlled mobilisation where appropriate |
| Dislocation | Friction and shearing forces | Provide adequate immobilisation, splinting and wound protection and support |
| Disease | Diabetes mellitus<br>Vascular syndromes altering circulatory integrity and impeding normal peripheral blood flow<br>Immune compromise<br>Previous or existing tumours<br>Previous or current irradiation treatment | Stabilise co-morbid factors where possible |
| Decrease in the patient and wound environment temperature | Wound temperatures less than 35°C, or more than 39°C are not conducive to optimal cellular function, and may result in cellular dysfunction, leading to tissue death | In hypothermic states, keep patient physically warm to meet core temperature demands<br>Use occlusive moist wound healing principles<br>Provide wound and local cellular warmth care |
| Drugs | Medications used in controlling immune disease processes including steroids for rheumatoid arthritis<br>Other medical conditions where circulatory compromise is a local/regional issue | Be aware of the intrinsic factors that can alter the timeframe for the progress of the healing stages |
| Deficits in nutritional status | Inadequate dietary habits<br>Disease processes that alter normal metabolism<br>Injury such as major trauma and burns that deplete energy stocks and are not adequately replaced – protein converted for energy | Assess nutritional status, particularly in the acutely ill, cancer patients, the elderly, chronically ill, psychologically disturbed, disabled, poorly mobile<br>Undertake risk management for nutritional deficits related to development of pressure ulcers in these patients |

pH values outside the range of 7.0–7.8 are incompatible with life as the permeability of cell membranes is totally disrupted and all cellular processes cease to function[1-5].

Specific bacteria residing on human skin are at a more positively acidic value (pH of skin is 4.5–5.5) and in the normal epidermal environment this acidic mantle is an effective barrier to the multiplication of external bacteria[1-5].

When skin integrity is damaged, surface pH levels can alter. These levels may be restored in surrounding skin, and the wound, by the use of occlusive moist wound healing dressings that remove excess contaminating and diluting exudate, or by rehydrating a dry wound through restoring normal biological exudate. Restoring normal skin hydration with moisturisers restores the barrier function of skin.

Accurate wound bed assessment and preparation to remove the excess exudate that can promote maceration, alterations in pH, and the development of infection, can be an important adjunct to protecting the wound from environmental and opportunistic bacteria.

Although primary hypoxia is known to initiate particular growth factors following wounding and create a healing environment, in areas of damaged tissue and blood vessels, some regions will become hypoxaemic, then hypoxic and finally anoxic[3-5]. Changes in oxygen levels within the cells produce an increasing lowering of the pH. Granulocyte cells are sensitive to a lowering pH and respond negatively through a biochemical process to further damage and/or destroy surrounding local tissue[3,4].

With inadequate, or absent, vascular circulation in the area, a destructive inflammatory reaction is established, highly conducive to the development of fat and tissue necrosis, multiplication of bacteria and high influx of neutrophils, which leads to discharge of the collected purulent material pus[3].

## Blood supply and oxygen needs of the wound

In a normal wound, a short period of hypoxia exists paralleling a primary physiological inflammatory response, with an adequate blood flow and cellular exchange of fluids and nutrients. This initiates a preparatory process for the wound to heal through the dynamics of moist wound healing[1-8]. An inadequate general, local, and surrounding circulatory mechanism that cannot provide oxygen, nutrients, the exchange of gases, and the biochemical agents required for the lysis, or breakdown, of foreign material, initiates a destructive process that provides an ideal environment for increasing levels of contamination and potential infection.

Many components, such as neutrophils, monocytes, macrophages and cellular nutrients, are oxygen sensitive and there is a high risk of development of infection when opportunistic bacteria gain an advantage over the host. Many intrinsic chemical agents that are capable of destroying particular low or moderate levels of bacteria are oxygen-dependent. If there is an ongoing absence of oxygen at sufficient levels ($PaO_2$ must be greater than 15 mm Hg)[3], this stabilising action may not be available, and even the least active areas of the tissue repair process may be completely halted, resulting in avascular tissue necrosis. An objective assessment of the patient, and the wound, can allow a prioritising of clinical needs to be established and set in motion.

This information is important in understanding the clinical observation of flaps and wounds as the use of external or internal probes display the macro level of oxygen in the flap/wound. It allows clinicians to determine the level of arterial flow bringing oxygen to the flap zone but as most problems in flaps are venous, this information is not complete (see Chapter 18). Supplementary oxygen in the normal patient may be useful to boost the circulatory levels, but in patients with respiratory disease or heavy smokers, this must be prescribed by a medical officer.

## Pain and discomfort in wounds

Although pain or discomfort is an ever-present actual or potential factor in open or closed wounds, apart from life-threatening haemorrhage, or the loss of airway control, the control of pain takes a very high precedence in patient care.

In wound care, the importance of assessing all pain for its specific aetiology and its control/management is a dominant requirement that must not be underestimated and cannot be stated too often[1,2].

Acute or chronic pain can be a clinical indicator of minor or major physiological disturbances within or surrounding the wounded region. Expected pain, due to surgical procedures, or trauma, can be preemptively managed but an unexpected severe or uncontrolled episode within and adjacent to the wounded zone may relate to emerging complications that have the potential to be detrimental to the patient, and the wound. In addition, unresolved pain and continuing discomfort can disturb and disrupt all attempts by the clinician and the patient, to move forward in assisting the wound to repair at all stages of patient recovery (see Chapter 11).

## Wound contamination and infection in the skin and soft tissues

> **Box 8.1** Definitions of the four principal categories of wounds of the skin.
>
> - Clean wounds have minimal contamination and are less than 12 hours old (infection rate of approximately 0.5%), usually elective surgical wounds[3,9]
> - Clean-contaminated wounds have increased level of contamination but will usually heal, primarily with proper debridement and irrigation and primary closure. The mechanism of injury is often a sharp, clean blade or glass
> - Contaminated wounds with $10^5$ or less bacterial count require substantial debridement, irrigation and secondary closure and the patient will usually be given prophylactic antibiotics. These wounds are commonly seen following road accidents and superficial human or animal bites, in chronic wounds including leg ulcers and pressure ulcers
> - Bacterial counts over $10^5$ demonstrate the high propensity of a wound to become infected[9]
> - Heavily contaminated or infected wounds will have a bacterial count of $10^6$ or above. Regardless of aetiology or mechanism of injury, this indicates the clinical presence of infection
> - There are exceptions (for example, beta-haemolytic streptococci $10^3$) and the nurse should have clinical knowledge of these and be able to identify them[9].

### General pathophysiological issues

The body is replete with organisms and bacteria that normally live on the skin surface, in the mouth, vagina, gastrointestinal tract, etc.[1–9].

Postoperative clean surgery infection rates vary greatly according to the type of surgery, institutional populations, and methods of data collection, but are generally accepted to be about 1.5–2% in clean

elective surgery and about 27% in contaminated wounds[9].

Bacteria and other organisms are highly opportunistic[3,7–9]. They are constantly alert for a specific medium on which they can nourish, survive, replicate, and generally work out ways of deceiving and destroying the normal function of tissue cell membranes. They are constantly vigilant for avascular tissue, openings in the skin, mucous membrane, or bloodstream through which to enter, and seek out an environment that provides for their immediate and long-term survival needs.

In the immunocompromised or high-risk patient, these organisms can alter their membrane structures, multiply quickly, avoid identification and destruction, and become resistant to virtually all antibiotics, setting up the potential for life-threatening septicaemia[1–4,7–10].

### *Issues in elective reconstructive plastic surgery*

In elective and post-trauma reconstructive plastic surgery, the principal initiating local complications affecting overall wound outcomes, including function and aesthetics, are the development and presence of haematoma preceding the development of infection, seromas, oedema, and continuing inadequately treated pain[6].

Patients who present for surgery with, for example, a suppressed immune system, regardless of the aetiology or known diagnosis, frequently require multidisciplinary specialised medical and nursing care, and constant observation for potential infection or life-threatening systemic co-morbid factors.

In reconstructive surgery, infection may be significantly higher following surgery for cancer of the head and neck, following multiple injury, and in anatomical regions where the bacterial count is normally high (e.g. oral cavity) but not deemed a problem until the skin is broken, or the wound environment provides an opportunity for replication, e.g. haematoma[6].

### *Multiple wound site issues and issues relating to special life-threatening medical conditions*

Meningococcal infections, or staphylococcal tissue infection (necrotising fasciitis) may, and frequently do, cause major physiological systems to shutdown. The consequence of this is significant skin and soft tissue loss, with patients frequently requiring amputation of limbs and/or major skin grafting.

Significant and ongoing insults to the premier physiological systems often result in major physical debilitation, or a loss of life. These patients are nursed similarly to major burns in intensive care units co-jointly by reconstructive plastic surgeons and intensive care unit physicians. Those who survive are moved to plastic surgery units for care by experts in wound management, and allied health professionals for ongoing rehabilitation.

### The 'golden hour' – wounds

In major burns and trauma management there is a period of time referred to as the **golden hour** (the hour immediately following the primary injury)[1-3]. Patients who have access to specialist overall assessment, expert resuscitation and primary wound management during this period are known to have a higher potential for recovery than those who do not.

Many specialist plastic surgery trauma surgeons apply this theory to patients with extensive soft tissue injury and state that use of this initial hour is essential to reduce the period of time vital anatomical structures are deprived of a blood supply. With bone and skin essentially reliant on a stable circulation at muscle level, the subsequent consequences (avascular necrosis of muscle) is a major episode leading to significant complications – see below.

The following 24–72 hours are the second step on the ladder to repair and recovery, as the physiological and wound needs may significantly alter in either direction, and these requirements must be anticipated and addressed as a matter of some urgency[3,4,9,11].

Following significant burns, trauma or major reconstructive surgery, a typical and expected post-injury immune suppression (at about days 5–14) has been described[3,9]. This is also observed in partial and full thickness burns, and where multiple wound sites are involved.

A suppression of the immune system is caused by the convergence of all the overwhelming physiological 'assaults' placed on each of the major biological systems. These relentless 'onslaughts' may require ongoing responses, due to the consistent high levels of biological protective demands. The potential for devastating infection due to avascular necrosis of the tissues, including muscle, and/or leading to renal failure, may require the need for renal dialysis or may lead to death of the patient. Knowledge of this phenomenon and being alert for any signal of adverse events must be a high priority.

The level of suppression of the normal immune response appears to be relative to the degree and extent of the response to the injury, and may be exacerbated by additional morbid factors (e.g. age, previous, current or increasing emerging medical or nursing morbid factors).

Elective reconstructive surgery, particularly head and neck for malignancy, may increase the number of major wound sites to three: the original wound, a donor flap wound and a skin graft. In addition, a donor vein graft may be taken, creating a fourth site. There may also be wounds associated with intravenous and arterial lines, a central venous line, tracheostomy, and insertions of percutaneous gastric tubes, or a nasogastric tube for feeding, and a urinary catheter[1,2,10].

### Results of avascular necrosis

Because the blood supply to any muscle is complex, vessels will infarct, or thrombose, according to the efficiency rate of the macro and microcirculation. Any resulting avascular necrosis is an idyllic medium for both aerobic and anaerobic bacteria. This can potentially lead to life-threatening systemic infectious conditions, with ultimate renal failure and untimely death of the patient.

Initially, the loss of soft tissues or limb(s) for life-saving purposes, is the primary, with a loss of functional mobility and aesthetics being secondary considerations. But, for the cognitively aware patient, this often has devastating psychosocial outcomes. For this reason, inadequate primary and secondary debridements can contribute to the necessity for multiple surgical procedures. As a general rule, the surgeon debrides back until the muscle bleeds adequately to demonstrate a circulation is in place. This has been demonstrated in, for example, post-compound trauma, free flap muscle transfer, compartment syndrome, full thickness burns, electrical burns and spider bites. Negative changes in the patient's overall physiological status can disturb the circulatory blood pressure and general circulatory flow, particularly at the micro level. Expert wound care then becomes complex, intense and extremely significant for the final result.

*Staphylococcus aureus* is the most common bacterial offender cited in post-traumatic surgical and burns wounds, although *Pseudomonas aeruginosa* (also called *Pseudomonas pyocyanea*) a Gram-negative non-sporing motile bacillus, is also becoming a major problem[9].

The longer wounds remain open or exposed (including time taken for surgery) or unhealed, the wider the range of organisms that have the opportunity to find a medium in which to multiply. This, on one hand, increases the range of special antibiotics required, on the other hand significantly limits what antibiotics are available to destroy the most recalcitrant organisms – and subsequently means that the patient's overall condition may deteriorate to a life-threatening state[9].

Regular counts of white cells, especially lymphocytes and T cells, should be undertaken and monitored closely[9]. This will include assessment of physical muscle loss by physiotherapists, and professional dieticians to assess and address intrinsic nitrogen balance to ensure protein levels and essential additional nutrients are adequate to support the high cellular energy demands. The high metabolic needs of the organism will continue whilst physiological adjustments of homeostasis are in progress, and this should be anticipated, particularly as unexpected major local and systemic infection can occur or recur.

## Assisting the immunological system by addressing nutritional needs

For elective patients at risk, adequate preoperative oral nutritional regimes, and preoperatively inserted percutaneous endoscopic gastrostomy (PEG) with introduced dietary needs and supplements, have been demonstrated to improve the patient's overall response to major elective surgery, and significantly increase positive patient outcomes. Although there some complicating factors regarding the insertion of PEGs, when properly inserted and managed, they have also demonstrated significantly positive patient outcomes prior to chemotherapy and/or radiotherapy for cancer, reducing nausea and vomiting, and sustaining a relative nutritional status (see applied nutritional issues for wound repair, later in this chapter).

---

**Box 8.2** Clinical modalities for the avoidance of potential life-threatening infection.

- Recognition of the physiological factors that precipitate increasing wound contamination and wound infection
- Timely and proactive general resuscitation/stabilising measures
- Removal of avascular and necrotic tissue
- Removal of excess and highly contaminated exudate
- Strict adherence to the matching of dressings to specific wound needs
- Skin cover/replacement as required
- Scientific identification of offending organisms in the light of presenting signs and symptoms of high levels of contamination or infection
- Intravenous systemic antibiotic cover for both aerobic and anaerobic organisms as identified
- Addressing primary and secondary nutritional issues as a matter of some urgency to prevent malnutrition that further contributes to compromising the immune system.

---

## Nursing risk management issues – avoiding adverse wound outcomes

Nurse clinicians should be vigilant and critically observe for any general changes in the patient's overall systemic condition and in all localised wound sites that may indicate impending adverse events. Box 8.3 outlines the principal modalities available to avoid adverse wound outcomes.

---

**Box 8.3** Early clinically visible signs of wound infection.

- Increasingly painful cellulitis surrounding the wound
- Increasing heat in and around the wound
- The colour of the tissue – increasing redness
- An increase in the volume and type of exudate
- A fluctuation or spiking of temperature is also an important early systemic response of a rise in the number of organisms present
- Gradual loss of local or regional function as swelling increases
- Often there is also a decline in mental capacity of the patient, with restlessness and alternate periods of loss of interest in self and the surroundings.

---

The patient should be fully examined to ensure that there are no other clinical indicators for negative changes in their condition, for example: the development of pressure ulcers, local or regional cellulitis, extravasation or thrombosis at intravenous (IV) and central venous pressure (CVP) sites, reactions to PEG insertion sites, or urinary tract infection due to catheter insertions.

The next section discusses the common microbiological methods for diagnosing wound infection.

> **Box 8.4** Guidelines for identifying levels of organisms following tissue biopsy specimens[9].
>
> | | |
> |---|---|
> | + | 1 plus ($10^2$–$10^3$ CFU/g of tissue) |
> | ++ | 2 plus ($10^3$–$10^4$ CFU/g of tissue) |
> | +++ | 3 plus ($10^5$–$10^6$ CFU/g of tissue) |
> | ++++ | 4 plus ($10^7$ CFU/g of tissue) |
>
> CFU = colony forming units

## Differential diagnosis – contamination and infection

Despite substantial microbiology research over many years, there remains some difference in interpretations of what various methods and numerical scales mean. Nurses with a professional interest in uninterrupted wound repair can only be guided by the analysis of the best available research, expert experience, microbiologists, clinical observations and clinical assessment[7–9].

### Wound swabs

The use of wound swabs is suggested to provide only an indication of surface contamination or infection in acute wounds, and is considered totally unsuitable for chronic wounds because of the types of offending organisms that may be responsible for the chronic nature of the wound[9].

Inadequate clinical understanding of the proper techniques for obtaining wound specimens is believed to contribute to inaccurate identification of the contaminating organism and, in particular, inaccurate concentration levels[9,12,13]. Microbiology lectures, applied clinical teaching sessions, and consultations with experienced microbiologists on their preferred method of obtaining a swab and tissue biopsy specimen establish a good professional relationship and a greater accuracy in scientific reporting when procedures are undertaken correctly.

Swab reports often describe the result as '+' *signs* on a range of 1+ to 4–5+, providing a diagnostic accuracy rate stated to be 65–98% depending on the organism identified[9].

### Using tissue biopsy

Rather than the use of cotton wound swabs or wound fluid, accurate and properly obtained biopsy specimens of wound tissue provide the most accurate guide to the presence and concentration levels of organisms in a wound, with a stated accuracy rate of 90–100%[9]. This technique is considered best practice, but whilst accuracy is high, obtaining specimens and a report can often take days and surgeons may prefer not to injure the wound further. Several researchers have demonstrated the use of the rapid Gram stain smear technique, where organism identification was required quickly, to be of value. Results showed reliability of the technique with, for example, a single organism sighted on the slide preparation being equivalent to $10^5$ CFU/g of tissue[9].

Attempts to objectively quantify concentration levels of organisms that cause infection may vary slightly between organisms, but with the presence of organisms at $10^5$ it is advocated that wound closure should be delayed until surgical measures of debridement and antibiotic therapy are undertaken, and the wound count is substantially less than $10^5$. Concentrations of $10^6$ or more of organisms per gram of tissue are clinically accepted to indicate infection and this must be correlated with the specific identification of the organism(s) and the clinical signs and symptoms[9]. In most cases, the initial use of the correct IV antibiotic(s) is considered standard to establish and maintain a high therapeutic or serum concentration level in the blood to combat the potentially spreading bacteria. The assessment of a wound and the choice whether to use antibacterial dressings, and topical antibiotics, is a medical decision as their efficacy remains very controversial amongst leading microbiologists.

## The exception

As established earlier, the one exception to the numerical count rule is beta-haemolytic *Streptococcus*. It has been demonstrated that, with $10^2$ or significantly fewer organisms per gram of tissue[4,9], it is sufficient to cause wound breakdown and retardation of wound bed repair. Such is the power of this particular bacterium, as an example, donor graft skin placed on a recipient site in the presence of this organism will simply disintegrate within 24 to 48 hours as the organism voraciously ingests and destroys the graft's dermal substrate and the epidermis. This particular bacterium is highly destructive to cells and tissue in pressure ulcers, as the wound will not begin the stages of repair until the bacteria has been eliminated, and any grafts or flaps which have been applied to cover the defect will also fail. It must be reinforced that the accurate diagnosis of beta-haemolytic *Streptococcus* can only be made with wound tissue specimens and not with wound swabs[4,9].

## Sutures and foreign implant material

Wound assessment and setting up a practice framework to address adverse events is fundamental to establish the problems that may emerge. Internal suture material, external skin sutures, small foreign bodies, and implant materials, can be responsible for the development of inflammatory reactions and infection. The terms 'stitch abscess' or 'implant response' are familiar to plastic surgical nurses. Observation of an emerging pustule with redness, heat, pain and swelling at a single or multiple suture site(s) indicate an impending wound problem. Underlying reactions to specific foreign materials, preservatives, or avascular necrosis from tight sutures, particularly in the fat tissue, are examples of causes.

It is usually necessary to initiate the removal of the suture(s) or implant material and identify the bacteria with a clinical tissue bacterial count. The wound may then require cleansing with warm sterile normal saline, application of active debridement, and the application of an appropriate moist wound healing dressing. IV or oral antibiotics may be required but should not be instituted unless there is a clear clinical diagnosis of infection and the infecting agent has been identified[4,9].

## Conversion from acute to chronic wound status

Scientific reports indicate that the absence of an adequate circulatory blood flow, the presence of continuing critical levels of wound contamination and the development of infection will retard every level and stage of wound bed repair and, in some cases, convert acute wounds to chronic wounds[4-9]. Failure to provide the optimal physiological wound environment that continually removes foreign contaminating material, reduces existing colonisation, and prevents infection, will directly affect normal healing responses in acute wounds. The current concept and principles of wound bed preparation are based on this hypothesis.

There is some difference of opinion regarding the definition of a chronic wound, with a wide range of views from the failure of a wound to heal within three to four weeks, to failure to heal greater than 40% surface area within one month. None of these definitions seems to be truly scientifically based, but arise from experience and attempts to quantify a complex, and often contextually based physiological event. This area requires objective and user friendly scientific criteria for clinicians to utilise.

## Who is at risk in reconstructive plastic surgery? Some principal areas of concern

In addition to the usual suspect bacterial groups identified prior to elective surgery, all acute or emergency patients or those who are referred/transferred for reconstructive plastic surgery consultation and management should be considered at medium to high risk of infection until proved otherwise. Lack of time to assess and stabilise many chronic medical conditions, nutrition etc., are issues to be addressed if the wound repair pathway is to be initiated and sustained at a level that is acceptable.

Existing entry levels of hospital and patient environmental contamination added to any known morbid and co-morbid factors can raise the potential for infection unless the primary and secondary risk factors are removed or minimised and strict patient and staff hygiene practices (e.g. hand washing) are adhered to. Wound bed preparation (see Chapter 10) requires optimised and timely stabilisation of any intrinsic medical risk factors and of any conditions in the immediate wound region that may prevent wound bed repair.

Hospital-acquired (nosocomial) wound infections are common, costly and very debilitating for the patient[1,2,10]. Despite every clinical effort, some patients are in hospital for longer than a few days, and may have an open wound associated with a major trauma, or a debilitating illness. This compromises the systemic integrity of the body, having the potential to acquire, for example, methicillin-resistant *Staphylococcus aureus* (MRSA), *Pseudomonas aeruginosa* (Gram-negative), or beta-haemolytic *Streptococcus* in open wounds, particularly in pressure ulcers[14].

Within plastic surgery, the presence of nosocomial infection can also be devastating to the healing process – for example, in patients with oral reconstructive surgery, major upper or lower limb bone and soft tissue injury, burns, skin grafts, and complex skin flaps[6].

In elective plastic surgery some procedures may have a higher index of suspicion for potential infection than others[11,15,16]. These include major breast reduction surgery, abdominal lipectomy in obese patients (e.g. fat necrosis), reconstructive flaps in the elderly, and patients with co-morbid factors (e.g. malignancy, diabetes mellitus, vascular disease and major nutritional deficits) that all have the capacity to interfere with the basic wound repair process.

The exudate that comes from fat necrosis[11,15,16], due to disturbances in blood flow (e.g. in abdominal lipectomy patients), presents an ideal environment for bacteria to multiply and for significant wound infection to develop, particularly if dead space exists.

Dead or failing cells or tissue not removed by physiological or active processes (wound dressings, debridement), regardless of their aetiology, with loss of blood supply, oxygen and changes in local pH, attract opportunistic bacteria and other organisms.

Although wounds can be observed to heal slowly in low oxygenated environments, damaged vessels, cells and tissue surrounding diabetic ulcers, or major accidental wounds, can be very unforgiving. This provides little in the way of vascular assistance to secondary wound healing or the application of local skin flaps or grafts, but very conducive to the entry of both aerobic and particularly anaerobic bacteria.

The astute wound expert may observe the presence of a bio film or thin slime-like cover over what appears to be an excellent granulating wound[3]. This should raise suspicion not only of the presence of beta-haemolytic *Streptococcus*, but also of potential early contamination by *Pseudomonas aeruginosa*, or MRSA. This clinically relevant observation requires clear diagnostic confirmation, a science-based wound management plan, with possibly wound dressings (e.g. silver-based dressings, slow release iodine dressings, wet to dry normal saline dressings) and targeted systemic antibiotics before procedures such as skin grafting are undertaken or the wound is closed by a skin or tissue flap.

Wounds that fail to heal, non-healing pressure ulcers, infected skin flaps, or grafts that fail to exhibit what appears to be a normal granulating bed, are highly suspect and should be checked for the presence of beta-haemolytic (Group A) *Streptococcus pyogenes* as well as any of the usual suspect organisms, for example, MRSA or *Pseudomonas*[4,7].

The wound tissue biopsy technique, not just surface swabs, must be used wherever possible if the accuracy of microbiological diagnosis is to be a principal determinate of wound bed preparation for its ultimate repair[7].

Additional mitigating factors (see Box 8.5) and the overall consequences can be extremely devastating for the patient who expects an uncomplicated outcome to what was understood to be a relatively straightforward procedure.

---

**Box 8.5** Additional clinical factors affecting wound bed repair.

- Extended periods of surgical time
- Multiple operating procedures
- Multiple sites increasing the extent of injured tissue
- Inadequate pain management, basic wound, and surrounding skin care
- Failure of early recognition of the primary or secondary development of a haematoma, seroma, or oedema can further contribute to the risk of injury or extended disease[2,6].

## Pathophysiology 2 – oedema, dead space, haematoma, wound serum and seroma

### Oedema and its adverse effects on wound repair

'Oedema' comes from the Greek word *oedema*, meaning 'a swelling' and in science is described as a presence, or abnormal accumulation, of an excessive amount of fluid in the tissues. It excludes serum (seroma), and lymph or blood (haematoma)[4,5]. Ongoing and abnormal presence of oedema within the tissues is one of the leading causes of failure of wounds to heal, wound recurrences in chronic lower limb venous disease, a principal cause of acute and chronic pain, restricted mobility, disability, and patient distress[1–10].

Wound-based tissue oedema is seen following all forms of injury that go deeper than the epidermis[3]. It is a fundamental component of the initial response of the normal acute inflammatory process but, in some adverse circumstances, this state may also become long-standing and chronic in nature. It occurs when the formation of extracellular fluid in the tissue exceeds the rate of normal reabsorption, and this can be intracellular or extracellular. Oedema that is concerned with congenital malformations or major burns is not discussed here.

**Box 8.6** Three principal grades of oedema.

| | |
|---|---|
| **Primary** | post-injury and until the wound is healed |
| **Secondary** | continuing to present for a period after wound is healed but can be resolved |
| **Tertiary** | chronic in nature regardless of aetiology and unable to be completely resolved. |

**Box 8.7** The four principal categories of tissue oedema.

| | |
|---|---|
| **Local, regional or generalised** | may be localised within a small zone of tissue, or a particular region, e.g. a hand – generalised tissue oedema may be related to a range of system dysfunctions (e.g. cardiac or renal), or major burns, etc |
| **Dependent** | related to immobility – main areas: pelvis and lower limbs – major contributor to development of pressure ulcers |
| **Chronic** | swelling that exists long-term, for example in a wound such as leg ulcers – usually due to continuing breakdown of tissues |
| **Lymphostatic** | if the lymph system becomes sluggish (e.g. due to local infection or injury) or is damaged by surgical removal of lymph nodes, oedema can develop in the affected limb or surrounding wound tissues. |

**Box 8.8** Principal causes of chronic wound-based oedema.

- Systemic medical conditions and chronic disease processes
- Primary and secondary wound complications
- Inadequate resolution of primary oedema due to circulatory disturbances in the post-injury phase, including 'reperfusion injury' within the wound and surrounding tissues
- Inadequate mobility leading to swelling and joint stiffness in the limbs
- Rehabilitation that excludes active deep tissue and passive skin massage following injury
- Inadequate patient compliance during rehabilitation.

**Box 8.9** Principal clinical risks and outcomes of unresolved oedema.

- Acute and chronic pain requiring long-term to lifetime management
- Unsatisfactory wound outcomes (e.g. in function, mobility, aesthetics)
- Increasing levels of immobility
- Reduced levels of independence
- High levels of patient dissatisfaction.

## Addressing potential primary adverse outcomes – clinical nursing risk management

As a part of professional observation practices, it is also within the nurse's province to establish collaborative clinical protocols that may assist in the reduction of excessive oedema, particularly in acute wounds of the face, upper and lower limbs. These can be based on the concepts and established practice principles using the acronyms in Box 8.10 to address individual patient basic wound needs.

**Box 8.10** Primary practice modalities for the management of local or regional oedema.

**The RICE acronym**

| | |
|---|---|
| Rest | comfort measures |
| Immobilisation | of the zone of injury above and below (with or without the use of ice or heat) |
| Comfort | systemic pharmacological or alternative methods such as transcutaneous electrical nerve stimulation (TENS) or passive skin massage for the control of discomfort and pain |
| Elevation | of the part above the heart where possible. |

**The RACE acronym:**
Rest
Alignment
Compression
Elevation

## Pathophysiology of oedema

Figure 8.1 provides an excellent diagrammatic example of normal microcirculatory pressures at the dermal level. These are required to be in place to address the physiological changes that happen when injury occurs[7].

Homeostasis with normal circulatory function is dependent on controlled and regular vascular function, uninterrupted levels of circulating water and blood volumes, the presence of plasma, adequate blood pressure within the arteries, arterioles, capillaries, venules and veins, and a satisfactorily functioning lymphatic system to deliver, and return, fluid to the normal circulation[1,3–5].

Two major circulatory systems are primarily responsible for the resolution of oedema. The venous system and the lymphatic system function through intermittent muscle operations. This creates a pumping action, assisted by changes in gravity (physical position of the limb/body). In addition, the suggested normal presence of negative pressures (created principally by lymphatic function) within the tissues, act as a suction mechanism, forcing the blood upwards. These fundamental and simultaneous actions are essential to counteract the low pressure gradient at the venous end, and the forces of gravity in the standing position[1,3–5].

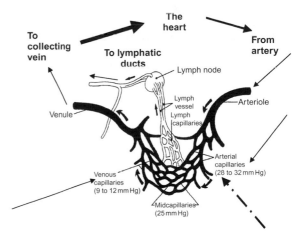

**Figure 8.1** Circulatory pressures within the capillary bed. Reprinted from: Bryant R.A., 1992, with permission from Elsevier.

Following any form of trauma, because of their fragile architecture, the regional or local capillaries and venous and lymphatic systems are easily injured. This contributes to the development of a state of primary localised oedema and is essentially a part of the primary or continuing inflammatory response.

The regional significance of this can be seen in massive third space shifts following major burns and major trauma of the upper and lower limbs or face[1-6]. Depending on the initial degree of injury, resolution of primary oedema, rate of the repair process, level of scar or fibrous tissue, and post-injury level of mobility, the potential for secondary and tertiary oedema may be significantly transformed (see also Boxes 8.5 and 8.6).

## Intracellular and extracellular fluid movement

Water makes up about 60% of the total weight of a 70 kg human body. For example, in a 70 kg male the total water load of 42–45 litres is contained within two principal spaces, intracellular (about 30 litres), and extracellular (about 15 litres). The extracellular fluid is divided into the intravascular (plasma) space and the interstitial spaces (spaces that support the cells), also called the third space. The latter contains the tissue fluid that moves between the cells, bathes and nutritionally sustains them, and aids in the removal of waste products created by the metabolic functions of the cells[1].

At the arterial (arteriole) end of the capillary, the pressure of blood flow is about 28–32 mm Hg and as the capillary membrane is permeable (porous) to water and very small protein molecules, these are forced into the tissues, forming the basis of the normal interstitial tissue fluid. As the arterial pressure moves the blood along, the arterioles and capillary vessels become smaller to facilitate precisely measured levels of glucose inflow and allow gaseous exchange within the cells. This causes the arterial blood pressure within the capillaries to fall to about 25 mm Hg at the venous end, but this is still sufficient to force water out into the tissue spaces[1,5] (see Figure 8.1).

The high level of intravascular plasma protein (higher than tissue fluid) extracts some water from the tissues back into the intravascular circulation (by osmosis) but, because there is a difference in pressures at work at this level, more fluid escapes to the tissues than is absorbed[1,7] – this is normal. Although the capillary membranes are said to be relatively impermeable to proteins, small amounts do escape into the tissue spaces – even more, and larger in form, when tissue is injured. As these proteins and particulate substances appear in the tissues, even in minute amounts, they are quickly picked up by the lymphatic system, broken down further, and offloaded into the thoracic and lymph ducts, enter the jugular and subclavian system and then enter the right ventricle and back to the general circulation[1,5].

This supporting function to the capillaries is an important action and is said to be the single most important function of the lymphatic system, as accumulation of these larger proteins in all of the body's interstitial tissues would see a mass transfer of water into the third space and the body would literally drown within 24 hours[1,5]. This pumping action is important as it also internally sustains the negative pressure within the tissues[5].

Any dysfunction of the lymph system or removal of lymph glands allows the large proteins in the interstitial tissues to accumulate, further trapping water and leading to the formation of gross oedema that is often observed in legs and arms (lymphoedema). This is often seen, for example, following lymph gland dissection of the groin or axilla at the time of, or after, the removal of particular malignant tumours that demonstrate the potential to spread[1,2,4,5]. This requires external and mechanical methods of fluid removal that mimic the local internal physiological pumping mechanisms, the muscles and internal negative pressures.

Finally, under normal circumstances, at the venous end of the capillaries, with pressures moving from approximately 25 to 12 mm Hg (Figure 8.1) the osmotic suction force created by the intravascular proteins is higher than the overall capillary blood pressure, and excess fluid returns to the capillaries, into the veins and lymphatics, and circulatory equilibrium is maintained[1,5].

## An example of the destructive process in wounds

Under normal circumstances the control of fluid movement between cells, tissues and the general circulation is governed by negative feedback. That is, it is automatically regulated to meet the needs of the organism. But sometimes this feedback system is overwhelmed and external control (by pharmacology or clinicians) is required[1].

Normal cells are stabilised into their required position to form tissues by an extracellular gel[5]. Oedema causes this gel to become increasingly dilute, and escalating numbers of cells become mobile, disordered, in collision and, finally, dysfunctional[1,5]. Unless control is restored, the large numbers of cells that are separated from each other become chaotic and the colliding forces cause injury to the outer cell membrane, initiating leakage of cytotoxic agents, further exacerbating wound disturbances.

The cells also move or are forced away from the capillaries, so exchange of gases and nutrients reduces, causing the death of many cells[1,3,4,5]. This abnormal presence of dead cells further results in the leakage of unremoved cellular toxins from the local and regional wound environment and leads to further cellular destruction. Consequently, the normal capillary and lymphatic action (negative pressure dynamics cease) is overwhelmed, reduced, and in some cases, rendered dysfunctional. The normal fluid equilibrium is not re-established until the conditions that have contributed to the formation of oedema are significantly reduced or removed. The continuing presence of oedema thus substantially interferes with cellular function and wound bed repair, and its removal is imperative if tissue destruction is to be ceased, and wound bed repair reestablished. This potentially leads to secondary and tertiary states (see Box 8.5).

The clinically assisted control of oedema, aberrant interstitial fluids, critically contaminated or infectious exudates, and the related pain and discomfort, are some of the principal functions of wound bed preparation and wound bed maintenance.

Application of the concept and practice principles of restoring normal negative or positive tissue pressures is one of the primary steps to wound repair, and the use of gravity and/or the application of negative pressure therapy[17] provides a mechanical reinforcement for the important restoration of interstitial fluid stability, in both compromised and potentially compromised wounds (see Box 8.11).

## The dynamics and effects of disturbances in intracellular oedema in wound bed repair

**Box 8.11** Principal reasons for the occurrence of intracellular oedema.

- Continuing depression of circulatory function (for example, coronary/vascular disease and/or heart failure) directly affects the integrity of blood flow and blood pressure. This in turn disturbs gaseous exchange and nutritional distribution to the cells, slowing down the metabolic activity required for the normal creation of energy and movement of fluid
- Generalised disturbances of blood flow can ultimately lead to cellular metabolic dysfunction, particularly by the mitochondria, which is the powerhouse for all cellular function[1-4]
- Alterations in the sodium/potassium ionic pump may cause retention of intracellular sodium. This draws in additional water and causes abnormal swelling of the cells. Finally, complete intracellular pump failure occurs and cell death follows[1-4]
- Disturbances in the normal movement of sodium, potassium, chlorides and calcium levels can also add to the accumulation of cytotoxic matter in the wound bed exudate
- The extended presence of inflamed tissue usually has a direct and disrupting effect on cell membranes
- Inflammation alters permeability of cell membranes leading to increasing diffusion of glucose, sodium and associated ions into the cells
- This increases water retention and a build up of potassium, chloride and calcium in the extracellular spaces
- Continuation of this atypical process beyond normal parameters and timeframes also leads to cell dysfunction and ultimately cell and tissue death[1-4].

## Reperfusion injury

**Necrosis**  a pathological response to cellular injury.

**Apoptosis**  a normal physiological cellular response to specific cellular suicide signals, or lack of cell survival signals.

Intracellular oedema principally occurs when the cell's outer membrane is breached due to injury and disturbances in extracellular activity. This causes chaos within the cellular structure leading to the emergence of toxic substances leading to surrounding cellular/tissue necrosis and/or apoptosis (see Box 8.10).

Reperfusion injury is suggested to be caused by an intermittent restoration of high blood flow pressure into a wound bed of minimal or no flow circulatory pressure. This pressure can force the accumulated cytotoxic cocktail of dead cells, and their contents, further into the wound bed and immediate surrounding tissues, resulting in the ongoing destruction and apoptosis of viable cells. Unrestrained destructive cellular and tissue process may lead to widening areas of avascular necrosis and further tissue loss[1,3,5].

With the disordered function of the microcirculation, there is an urgent need to mechanically remove the toxic wound bed exudate and stabilise blood flow, if normal cellular function is to be restored and further tissue loss is to be minimised through wound bed preparation and management.

## The dynamics and effects of disturbances in extracellular (third space) oedema in wound bed repair

Several principal factors may be working alone or in concert to hasten interstitial and third space oedema. These are outlined in Box 8.12.

### Box 8.12 Principal factors that instigate interstitial and third space oedema.

- Oedema causes separation of normal cellular formation, causing loss of contact with the capillaries – their important source of oxygen, nutrients and exchange of gases. This may result in increasing pressure within the capillaries, for example, excessive retention of sodium and water by the kidneys, heart failure and venous dysfunction[1–5]
- Decreased intravascular plasma proteins (for example, as a result of major burns, severe traumatic wounds, liver disease or malnutrition) result in increased capillary permeability, which may cause leakage of larger protein to the interstitial spaces. This may also be related to, for example with bacterial infections, reactions to toxins, immune responses, local venous occlusion or inflammation associated with wounding. This has the effect of completely overwhelming the capacity of lymphatic system to respond adequately[1–5]

- Lymphatic blockage/dysfunction (e.g. lymph node block as seen in cancer, infection and congenital lymphatic conditions/malformations, the critically ill) can result in a chronic and disabling condition that can significantly alter patient safety, comfort and independence[1–5]

## Clinical disturbances of fluid movement in postoperative plastic surgery patients

When circulatory volumes are altered significantly, and third space fluid shifts are expected, fluid balance must be critically managed during all phases of the operative procedure and in the patient postoperative recovery phase, particularly for the first 72 hours.

Initially, following major injury or procedures, some patients receive artificial replacement of lost intravascular fluid products and proteins lost due to wound bleeding, or protein leakage into the interstitial spaces to protect the injured cells and tissues. This replacement may include the patient's own preharvested blood prior to surgery.

The undertaking of major and multiple surgical interventions, or major body trauma significantly increase the developing level of oedema. Some major aesthetic surgery (e.g. liposuction) and some specific flap surgery may be undertaken as day surgery or require a stay of 24 hours[3,6].

At about 72 hours, with the relative intravascular fluid balance restored, and in the absence of infection, the increased level of intravascular proteins will attract water to move back into the intravascular circulation (via capillaries and veins) through a process of reverse osmosis[1–3,6]. Where substantial fluid shifts have occurred, care must be taken to ensure that the overzealous use of fluid replacement does not cause hypervolaemia or intravascular flooding, which may develop into, for example, pulmonary oedema[1–3,6].

Research reports, and the author's clinical experience, indicate that in the early days of free flap procedures, digital replants and major reconstructive procedures, hypovolaemia was a frequent problem intraoperatively and immediately postoperatively. This initiated an increase in circulatory problems at the operative site with postoperative complications, and, frequently, wound breakdown. An increasing awareness of this particular physiological and observable fact paralleled with prevention of hypothermia has significantly reduced this complication.

Plastic surgery nurses must be aware of these particular risk factors, especially where substantial fluid shifts have been surgically or traumatically initiated and inadequately corrected and managed. Examples include: major/total body liposuction procedures, multiple injury patients, major reconstructive free flaps of the lower limb, craniofacial, breast, burns and major upper limb and severe hand injury.

### Secondary clinical adjuncts

For nurse clinicians, blood pressure within microcirculatory flow (from distributing artery to collecting vein and lymphatics) has important significance in understanding the effects of, for example, wound oedema, the initiation and timing of passive skin massage, the accurate application of pressure and compression bandaging in wound zones such as fixed skin, and the pathophysiology of the development of pressure[7,8].

It also has importance in the clinical postoperative management of tissue flaps for congenital malformations, and following injury and disease (see Chapter 18).

### Application to wound bed maintenance practice

The acute and protective phase of normal fluid movement within the inflammatory process, into extracellular spaces, can be observed following any wounding. As discussed in Chapter 7 (Wound Bed Repair), in a clean, closed wound fluid resolution is relative to the gradual restoration of sufficient arterial, capillary, venous and lymphatic circulation and this can generally be observed at about 72 hours post-injury[1-5]. This allows for the normal wound repair processes to be initiated in parallel with an increasingly regulated fluid formation and reabsorption to take place.

Negative pressure is gradually restored as the lymphatic system recovers, interstitial gel is reformed, and cells re-orientate close to the capillaries[5]. The level and timing of resolution is anatomically specific, related to the region of functional anatomy, degree of injury and mobility (e.g. upper and lower limbs take longer with loss of their muscle 'pump'), morbid and co-morbid factors.

When the injury is substantial and other co-morbid factors that impair healing are present and ongoing, the repair process is held back by intrinsic medical disturbances or varying levels of loss of arterial, capillary, venous and lymphatic circulatory function. If the reconstitution of overall and sufficient blood flow is slow or does not occur, much of this exudate remains in place and may move the injury from an acute to a chronic state with the increasing demise of otherwise healthy tissue areas[3-5].

In some wounds, such as those healed after trauma, major reconstructive surgery or chronic venous disease, the resolution of oedema may never be absolute (e.g. in the lower limbs[3-8]). In the upper and lower limbs, the presence of complex dermal and aberrant scar tissue, presence of thick fibrous tissue, and microvascular changes, may require long-term assistance and each presenting injury or condition requires individual professional assessment.

Active intervention may be necessary, utilising manual soft tissue massage, layered bandaging techniques, pressure support garments, mechanical massage pumps, intermittent elevation and management of any presenting pain[1-3,7,8].

A professional vascular assessment, which includes ankle brachial pressure index (ABPI), is essential before any specialised compression bandaging treatment regimes are instituted to prevent adverse outcomes, particularly if the patient has associated arterial and/or cardiac disease, and/or to protect the vascular integrity of reconstructive surgery[7,8]. No treatment should be instituted without medical discussion (particularly if the patient has heart pump problems), advice to the patient, and referral to expert wound nurse clinicians or physiotherapists, specifically trained in the application and risk management of this area of care.

### Introducing manual massage therapy as a intrinsic part of clinical nursing practice for oedema management

Given the evidence of the close physiological relationship between oedema, the venous and lymphatic systems and the normal and assisted resolution, special techniques for gentle skin massage are highly indicated and advocated. Evidence exists to support the introduction of soft tissue massage, particularly in preoperative work up and immediately postoperatively. This is discussed more fully in Chapter 12 (Wound Bed Maintenance) as a modern approach to overall skin care, pain management and increasing the patient's mobility for independence.

## Discharge education – management of oedema

For plastic surgery nurse clinicians the formation of oedema within local and regional wound environments can present challenges for optimal postoperative management, and preferred wound outcomes.

It is necessary for the patient to accept the education and importance of proper elevation of the body part in the initial and healing repair phase and during rehabilitation. Following primary discharge, patients will often discard slings, are tardy in maintaining gravity elevation of limbs, and they may fail to understand the true value of minimising oedema and its significance in the cause of postoperative pain.

The application of three-inch (7.5 cm) cohesive bandages over the existing limb bandages can significantly reduce the problems of poor co-operation and loss of bandage compression that are responsible for oedema, particularly in children. This must be applied with minimal to moderate stretch, with reinforcement of prior education regarding neurovascular observations by the patient or significant carers. If oedema does occur under this type of bandage there is a major risk that distal blood flow may be lost, subsequently creating new problems.

It is essential to remember that under normal and uninjured flow circumstances, it is suggested that fluid is prevented from accumulating in mobile tissue by an established negative pressure effect/force[6], as long as the epidermis and underlying dermal layers of the skin remain intact, sealed and minimally injured. If excess fluid removal is not, or cannot be, accomplished by early restoration of the normal functional attributes, dressings, gravity, skin massage and so on, mechanical[15] and/or professional assistance from a physiotherapist is required.

## Dependent oedema – clinical nursing risk issues

Immobility is one of the principal causes of nursing co-morbidity. The lack of patient mobility and increasing levels of dependence requires a critical assessment of patient safety, comfort and level of ability for self-care[1-5].

The formation of 'dependent' oedema is principally the result of immobility because the movement of extracellular and intracellular fluids (particularly venous and lymphatic blood flow) is 'dependent' on part or all of the body being mobile, or appropriate gravity levels of the upper and lower limbs and some body parts[1-5].

Prolonged or extended periods of immobility may result in thrombosis of the microcirculation, causing fluid to become trapped in the interstitial spaces in regions of the body that are physiologically dependent on gravity, and the physical movement of the muscles, for example in the pelvis, limbs and face.

The continuing use of gravity flow in the limbs, by elevation above the level of the heart, temporarily relieves this situation for immobile patients/limbs before more active mobilisation commences as part of the rehabilitation process.

In the limbs, some cases of partial or total immobility due to severe compound injury and the formation of fibrous and scar tissue may cause a permanent and unresolved level of oedema, joint stiffness, and, ultimately, regional dysfunction and overall physical disability. This may necessitate a wide range of deep and soft tissue massage techniques, long-term physiotherapy/occupational therapy strategies, palliative pain management and/or subsequent surgical procedures.

## Pathophysiology of dependent oedema in development of pressure ulcers

All medical, surgical and/or immobile patients are at risk of developing pressure ulcers unless risk management is practised proactively and pre-emptively. The research figures available for the prevalence (those at high risk, or those who have pressure ulcers at a specific stage) and incidence (the number of cases reported over a period of time, for example, one month, six months, etc.) that are reported, are significant and appear somewhat alarming[1-5,7].

The heels and sacrum come under the category of relatively fixed or specialised skin regions with compact cell structure and an accompanying complex microvascular system of blood supply to the skin, which is necessary to meet the specific functions of the sites. Figure 8.2 demonstrates the complexity of the microcirculation within the heels and thus their vulnerability to injury caused by dependent oedema in the presence of diabetes mellitus (see Chapter 5).

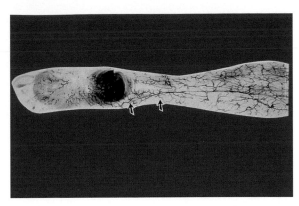

**Figure 8.2** Injection studies demonstrating the microcirculation of the heel. With permission: Professor G.I. Taylor.

When dependent oedema develops in areas where the skin is comparatively fixed and tightly adhered, only small amounts of protein fluid are required to escape from the stressed capillaries to create an increased level of fluid and positive pressure levels, causing subsequent tension within the tissues. This internal tissue tension (versus the external pressure exerted by the patient lying dormant on a hard surface), with the shear and friction of inappropriate positioning, creates enormous levels of internal tissue loads and frequently results in microthrombosis within the capillaries, venules and venous capillaries[1 5,7].

Cells lose their compactness, are forced away from each other and the capillary blood flow lifeline, and tissue integrity is at risk of ongoing injury. Arterioles and capillaries are further compressed, blood flow slows, toxic metabolites accumulate in the cells and the tissue fluid and cells begin to die. As pressures are increasingly exerted in both directions this results in imposed vascular stresses leading to avascular necrosis and ulceration of the region. This is dominant in areas such as the heels (8%), sacrum (23%), over the ischium (24%), and trochanter (15%)[7]. Although the statistical evidence for the heels appears low, patients' independence is directly related to their ability to be mobile.

These statistics support the application of 30° body/pelvic tilts and removal of pressure on the heels to reduce unnecessary pressure over bony prominences, and the application of research-based pressure-relieving devices and techniques[7].

Some texts and research papers quote small variances to these statistics, nonetheless with the current evidence available even these figures should be considered too high. Life-threatening infections (previously discussed in this chapter), such as osteomyelitis may develop, being the major causal factor leading to significant systemic infection, ultimately leading to the patient's death.

The external manifestation of damaged tissue that leads to ulceration can be slow to emerge[3,5]. The reason for this may become clearer with the application of research into the architecture of the blood supply to fixed and mobile skin regions of the body and the combined effects of varying levels of direct (external pressure) and indirect (pressure from within, i.e. oedema) compression. A review of the complex three-dimensional structure of the blood supply to the skin (arising from muscle – see Figures 5.6 & 5.7) demonstrates the complexity of this process, and as muscle dies slowly, why the external manifestation at the level of the skin is slow to emerge.

Despite the multitude of pre-emptive external or systemic factors, some research has demonstrated that the external expression of a pressure ulcer can take up to five days[7], with initial damage occurring during long journeys in an ambulance on a hard stretcher, extended periods in the operating theatre and/or ICU before transfer to the surgical or clinical medical area. This information is poorly understood and not readily acknowledged in clinical discussions. Clinical surgery or medical units are often held responsible, but the explicit external signs may only be observed after the patient has passed through these initial acute care areas, emerging in the surgical or medical unit about three to five days later.

### Dependent oedema – clinical nursing risk management and outcomes in the clinical unit

In patients who cannot control their individual mobility, the use of appropriate pressure-relieving mattresses and two-hourly repositioning, or repositioning according to the individual needs, alternating 30–40° body tilts should be performed with soft pillows[7].

Patients should not be completely turned on their side as the whole lower abdominal and pelvic area is then subjected to increased fluid retention in the tissues (dependent oedema). In addition, intrathoracic pressures may be altered and adequate expansion of the lungs put at risk. Turning the patient completely on their side will also increase the weight/pressure load ratio on the perforating vessels over the hip region, increasing the risk of pressure damage on the local muscle tissue. Additional movement accentuates the risk of shear and friction to the skin and underlying vessels. This is reflected in the statistical incidence quoted above, particularly when paralleled with Figure 8.1 outlining what pressure loads arterial, venous and capillary vessels can tolerate, before thrombosing or rendering the tissues avascular.

As previously stated, the head should be elevated at 30° (unless medically ordered otherwise) and the heels elevated at 15°–30°[4], or enough to ensure the heels are free and off the bed surface, by placing pillows under the calves (lengthways). This action should be checked with the doctor for patients with arterial disease (elevation reduces peripheral blood flow) or arthritis of the knees (causing hyperextension of the knees) who are thus at greater risk of complications.

Contrary to previously held views, there is no scientific evidence that soft pillows placed under the calf cause or increase the incidence of deep vein thrombosis (DVT). DVT is principally caused by immobility and other intrinsic vascular issues, as described within Virchow's Triad[1–4,7,8]. This is accentuated by hereditary factors, previous vascular injury and failure to instigate pre-emptive risk prevention strategies in suspected, or known at-risk patients.

## Dependent oedema – problems related to limb splinting

In addition to elevation for gravity flow, for those patients who are unable to move their feet resting splints will be needed to prevent foot drop, caused by the increasing contraction of the relaxed/unused flexor tendons.

Common risk problems are inadequately padded splints, splints bandaged too tight, and failure of a daily check of the heels for injury, because of the potentially increasing dependent oedema. Constant vigilance to detect swelling of the toes is essential, particularly for the severely ill or unconscious patient, as this is an excellent clinical indicator of underlying oedema. Splints should be removed daily, and checked. The tissues can then be gently

moisturised with a stroking massage applied (no rubbing) to assist venous and lymphatic return for approximately five minutes. Repadded splints are then replaced. Remember, wool padding flattens out under normal immobile pressure, so too much padding is much better than not enough, unless it creates pressure itself.

If the patient is required to be in the sitting position (for example, post reconstruction of the head and neck) the bed should be broken in the middle and the legs elevated to stop slippage. Constant slippage causes shear, friction and increased pressure loads on the sacral area and the heels and, in the presence of dependent oedema that has developed due to immobility, tissue injury develops. Alternate side-to-side body tilting as outlined above should be maintained at two-hourly intervals, ensuring that there is also no pressure on the face or ears, which should also be protected with foam/gel pads. Failure to do this also increases the potential for pressure ulcers on the back of the head, particularly in the unconscious patient deprived of sensory perception.

Traditional forms of vigorous rubbing of the skin 'to stimulate circulation' must be avoided, if reperfusion injury is to be avoided. The accumulation of cytotoxic material from dead and dying cells may increase damage to the local area by further aggravation of partially damaged, dying or recovering cells[2,8].

See massage therapy in Chapter 12 – Wound Bed Management.

Conscious but immobile patients who complain of pain or muscle spasm in the legs or feet should have splints removed immediately and their feet checked thoroughly. This spasmodic movement may cause shear and friction over fragile skin and oedematous tissues.

## Managing involuntary muscle spasm in post-surgical patients

Some patients may require injections of Botox® to treat the spontaneous emergence of muscle spasticity or spasms. Botox® is a drug made from *Botulinum* toxin type A, the bacterium associated with food poisoning. Given in small doses, Botox® blocks release of acetylcholine, a neurotransmitter that activates muscle contractions. Botox® is known to temporarily inhibit the uncontrolled firing action of the local or deep nerves and nerve activity of the injected zone by acting on neuromuscular junctions and neural endplates. These injections weaken muscle activity enough to reduce a spasm, but not enough to cause paralysis. This therapy reduces and in some cases eliminates painful muscle spasms and tremors.

Botox® has been used successfully to treat involuntary muscle spasm in many patients suffering from cerebral palsy. The use of Botox® in aesthetic surgery has the effect of reducing the effects of frowning and thus wrinkles, etc., on the skin.

## Discharge education

Whilst, in specific cases, regional or limb immobilisation is an important part of wound repair, particularly in the first 72 hours, failure to recognise the actual and potential relationship between the continuing presence of unresolved wound tissue oedema, pain and the increasing risk of infection, can impede wound repair. As discussed in Chapter 7, postoperative dilution of dermal and epidermal sebum by the continuing presence of wound oedema, increases the potential for infection.

Regardless of the aetiology of oedema, a longer than expected physiological state within the tissues can alter cellular functions, and cause secondary and tertiary tissue injury. This can lead to joint stiffness, pain, increasing levels of immobility and decreasing levels of independence.

Nurse clinicians must be firmly resolved in their attempts to ensure patients with limb injuries understand the necessity for specific compression bandaging techniques and 24-hour disciplined gravity elevation, whilst the potential for reactionary postoperative injury oedema is anticipated. Reinforcement of discharge education for patient compliance is essential to avoid adverse events.

Nursing clinicians who practise in acute surgery areas and wound management need to understand their responsibility to recognise how oedema develops, how it can be minimised, and the consequences of inadequate clinical management by both clinician and patient.

See Chapter 14 for suggestion on the transfer of discharge education advice.

## Dead space and its relationship to wound infection

The terms 'space', 'dead space' and 'space occupying' are commonly used in all surgery and particularly in plastic surgery[3–5]. 'Dead space' essentially describes an area that is not occupied with tissue within its normal anatomical limits.

In the normal human body, every anatomical area is theoretically occupied by, for example, a diversity of tissues, organs, air, water or blood, but physiologically some areas are described as having potential, or actual, 'dead' space[1–3,6]. Clinicians will be familiar with this term in relation to several areas: the physiology of respiration, compensating for dead space in tubing during the provision of oxygen therapy, or the potential for air to occupy or create dead space in an IV tube.

Dead space may be 'artificially' created in several ways, some examples are: surgery (inadequate closure of tissue layers within any surgical wound), space remaining when tumours are removed, loss of soft tissue and/or bone due to trauma, disease or infection.

Dead space may also be artificially created to allow for an object (for example a breast prosthesis, or artificial joints in the hand) to be inserted[11–15]. In mobile skin regions, significant removal or loss of normal tissue can result in a space being left that may not be completely filled by surrounding tissue due to inadequate wound closure of the wound layers and loss of normal negative pressures[6].

## Clinical risk management and potential outcomes

Dead space is one of the principal reasons given for the development of a collection of fluid (particularly haematoma or seroma) following injury and surgery, which can lead to an infection. Hence, measures are undertaken to eliminate the space[3–5]. This allows the host to regain control of the balance, allowing development of a healing environment and for the inner tissue layers to heal by normal contracting forces, and epidermal resurfacing processes, unhindered by collecting contaminated fluid.

Closure of dead space can be achieved by the use of normal wound repair, if the size of the space does not exceed the ability of the tissues to come together, without tension. Skin grafts, skin/soft tissue flaps, internal (closed negative pressure drainage systems) or external, mechanically applied negative pressure techniques can be used to eliminate dead space which cannot be primarily closed (Figures 5.9–5.12).

Fistulas and sinuses are abnormal forms of dead space usually caused by local infections attempting to expel foreign material (e.g. foreign bodies, dead tissue)[1,2,7,8]. These will track from within a wound to the surface, usually requiring surgical excision to remove the connective tissue canals, and specialised dressing regimes, orchestrated according to restoring the healing process. With the smooth connective walls excised, and apposition of the 'raw' wound edges along the tract, they heal by a slow process of granulation from the bottom of the wound, contracting inwards, obliterating the dead space, and finally undergoing epithelialisation.

The absence of critical contamination or infection must be sustained or wound breakdown of the fragile granulation will occur, increasing the size of the dead space and re-establishing the chronic nature of the sinus or fistula[1,2,7,8]. It is stated that negative pressure therapy set at high settings is useful in these wounds by ensuring firm apposition of the edges of the wound's internal walls and thus preventing the accumulation of exudate attractive to opportunistic bacteria.

External concave wounds (e.g. absence of partial thickness or full thickness skin, where skin grafts have been applied) have special requirements for securing the donor skin, such as wound packing with foam padding, or selected dressing materials with the application of securing techniques to prevent shear and friction across the wound (e.g. tie-over dressings, retention tapes, negative pressure therapy). The application of compression bandaging can also provide a temporary measure but must be regularly reapplied, or firmly secured in place, to maintain a reasonable and constant level of effectiveness. This is discussed in Chapter 17.

## Space occupying lesions

Abnormal or artificial pressure within mobile or relatively fixed tissue zones may be created by the growth or development of benign or malignant tumours. These are commonly referred to as 'space occupying' lesions[4].

These 'space occupying' lesions may be seen in any part of the body but are more dangerous in areas where they can exert pressure on critical anatomical structures, causing injury and pressure on blood vessels and nerves. This can be observed particularly in regions where tissues are enveloped in relatively tight or fixed structures, for example, within the upper or lower limbs, upper facial bones, or the brain itself. In plastic surgery, the most common examples would be maxillary tumours, ganglions, dermoid cysts and benign and malignant tumours within the muscle of the upper or lower limbs.

## The development of a wound haematoma

**Haematoma** is described as a collection of blood that is the result of a haemorrhage or slow leaking of blood into a normally enclosed tissue space or any anatomical dead space[1–9]. It may be due to leaking blood vessels, ruptured and bleeding tumours, accidental primary or secondary trauma, or surgery. It usually stays within an enclosed space and the collection of blood causes increasing swelling and pain within the immediate site. Extravasation of some blood may leak into surrounding tissues, disguising the extent of the primary underlying collection, and may give the appearance of superficial swelling and bruising.

Clinical signs to be observed include the external presence of unilateral or bilateral swelling, hardness of the area, and pain, particularly increasing pain not relieved by analgesia. The presence of sharp, or dull and throbbing pain is caused by unrelieved pressure on the immediate and surrounding blood vessels and nerve endings, in response to the potential impending cessation to the normal vascular supply.

Superficial haematoma (within the dermal region) may form as a small but increasing swelling and be identified easily and early, in minutes or hours, regardless of the anatomical region. Haematoma may also form deeply within the muscle tissues but particularly largely mobile tissues, and remain undetected for long periods. These may only be identified when attention is focused on them when the volume of collected fluid causes major discomfort or severe pain, the haematoma becomes infected, or ultrasound is undertaken to identify a persistent swelling and discomfort. Initial lack of detection, continuous bleeding in areas such as the abdomen, may become a life-threatening episode in some patients, because of slow, concealed exsanguination, or provide the medium for the development of major infection.

In tight, fixed skin regions, a minimal level of haematoma can exert sufficient pressure on wound tissues to disturb or occlude normal circulatory flow, and on local nerve endings, causing increasing pain. This can result in early reactive ischaemic pain and avascular necrosis of local soft tissue, and the skin.

The increased flow of blood into muscle (usually due to injury or tight plasters) encased in tight fascia, and development of reactive oedema also causes severe ischaemic pain, muscle death and nerve damage. This condition can occur in any part of the body, but is usually identified and observed in the upper or lower limbs and is referred to as **compartment syndrome**[1-4].

Compartment syndrome is common in major burns, with the extravasation of fluid into the third space of the wounded and surrounding tissue zones. Both conditions constitute a surgical emergency and fasciotomy by incision into the fascia that encloses muscle compartments may be required as a matter of urgency to relieve the pressure on vital structures, particularly vessels and nerves responsible for muscle, and ultimately skin, viability[2].

## Haematoma – clinical risk management and outcomes

In elective plastic surgery, any wound has the potential to develop a postoperative haematoma. The presence of a haematoma is seen as a disaster because of the potential for infection with resultant adverse functional and aesthetic outcomes[3]. It is not uncommon for haematomas to develop following breast, facial and abdominal surgery and to be responsible for the loss of prosthesis, skin grafts and skin flaps. They can cause disturbances in microcirculation, separation of cells and tissues and disruption of wound edges leading to wound dehiscence.

When a significant haematoma develops, and is not evacuated immediately, it is thought that the development of necrotic tissue and entrance of bacteria blocks the migration of normal fibroblasts and thus the formation of new capillaries and granulation tissue[3]. Consequently, wound breakdown is initiated, infection is a further complication and the wound and the patient are both compromised.

Ability to identify a potentially destructive haematoma is essentially related to the anatomical position of a wound. For example, the presence of a haematoma of 2–20 ml in mobile skin areas such as the abdominal wall or large breasts may not be recognised or overly painful until normal inflammatory oedema has subsided. Many small haematomas may resolve over time without any residual complications, though others may become infected. The presence of this volume of fluid (2–20 ml) in fixed/firm skin areas such as the palm of the hand, side of the nose, the ear or around the eye may be extremely dangerous, causing avascular necrosis and loss of important structural anatomy.

An important element within reconstructive plastic surgical procedures is attention to detail by surgeons in obtaining strict haemostasis before any wound is closed. In many wounds, this attempts to minimise or eliminate the need for the introduction of invasive drainage systems that have the potential to introduce destructive bacteria. In medium or large wounds (open or closed) the application of negative pressure therapy is becoming a common protective measure to avoid the development of a haematoma.

Some open wounds can be equally well managed with moist wound healing dressings with or without compression management (e.g. various layer bandage techniques). Each wound must be individually assessed and evidence-based wound care applied to meet the need of the wound and the patient's needs.

For nurse clinicians, recognising 'at risk' procedures, and the wound observations that alert early diagnosis and reporting, are important nursing functions[15-17]. Timely reporting can allow evacuation of a haematoma by the removal of sutures, surgical incision and drainage, or by needle aspiration as necessary. This is a matter of urgency if important tissue structures are not to be lost. For example, in the case of the eyes following blepharoplasty, failure to recognise a developing haematoma may result in pressure on the orbit/optic nerve. The consequence of this may be unilateral or bilateral loss of vision, unless the pressure is immediately released. In addition, the aesthetic outcomes of even small unresolving swellings on any part of the body can be aesthetically unacceptable to the patient.

## The development of wound serum

Initially, the presence of **serum**, a light yellow-coloured protein fluid, plus some water related to osmosis, is a normal part of overall inflammatory response[3-5]. In a wound, it is the fluid that remains after the coagulation phase as the constituents of blood are solidified or broken down by haemolysing agents.

Blisters following superficial thickness burns are of a more watery, serous, type as the germinative layer of the epidermis contains more water, and the dermis has a more protective microcirculation that thromboses quickly, reducing the level of protein leakage. The leakage is greater in the reticular layer of the dermis. This reflects the term 'the reticuloendothelial system', a primary functional protective response within the dermis. With its larger sized mixed microcirculation vessels, thrombosis may be slower, but the higher leakage of protective protein attracts greater volumes of intra- and extracellular water (i.e. exudate forming oedema). This clear or yellow coloured fluid is usually referred to as lymph fluid[3-5].

## The suggested function of serum

Serum is suggested to be an independent medium with short-term antibacterial properties, that kills some resident or invasive bacteria but for how long this is physiologically active (diluted by oedema, secondary injury, failure to heal wounds due to medical factors) has not been scientifically established[3-5].

Following acute injury this serum has a lysing or destructive (breaking down) effect on Gram-negative bacteria. Other intrinsic humoral or proteolytic enzymes mechanisms can also directly kill Gram-negative and Gram-positive organisms[3-5]. This is proposed to be one of the two frontline forms of immunity but is suggested to overlap the immediate response of 'the reticuloendothelial system' that sustains the primary response to the presence of foreign material and bacteria.

It is important to understand that the human organism has primary and secondary protective response systems. Plastic nurses involved at all levels of wound care should have a clear understanding of these response systems as tissue repair management is intrinsically paralleled to how wounds are managed achieving set short, medium and long-term wound goals/outcomes.

## The resolution of wound serum

Under normal circumstances this serous fluid and its associated water should be slowly absorbed by about day 5 postoperatively, in line with the normal resolution of fluid[3-5].

See normal wound healing data in Chapter 7 – Wound Bed Repair.

After about day 5, the efficacy of the serum as a protective medium appears to become weakened as, at about this stage, proteolytic enzymes have been observed to begin to enter the tissues and break down the fibrin within the fluid[3-5]. The ongoing presence of serum, regardless of the level of oedema, should put clinicians on red alert for a potential risk of development of increasing levels of contamination in the wound and ultimately infection[3-5]. Patient wound assessment and management will need to be reviewed as the presence of an area of dead space may be factor.

The immediate bactericidal attributes of protein serum exudate as part of the normal inflammatory process has been described in relation to recipient skin graft beds[3]. Its normal presence in the dermal or muscle recipient wound bed (it is sticky and acts like a form of glue) during the first 24–48 hours is partially attributed to skin graft take. Its declining absence in the wound bed during that specific (24–48 hours) period, is stated to be directly related to partial or total failure of skin graft to take[3,5]. It has also been suggested that closing off the wound from the external environment initiates the negative pressure normally observed in the specific wound zone[5]. The internal negative pressure draws the donor skin inwards to the recipient tissue and holds it securely in place.

## The development of a wound seroma

A **seroma** is the ongoing accumulation of a yellowish or clear coloured fluid arising from the serosa or lining of body cavities[1-4]. An example is in the breast cavity, related to an extended inflammatory response, which may be related to a 'foreign body' such as a synthetic prosthesis. The serous fluid fails to be absorbed back into the normal circulation and remains as a collection walled off in a capsule form, within the wound. Its continuing presence has high potential for development of increasing levels of contamination in the wound, infection and, ultimately, wound dehiscence[3].

## Nursing management issues regarding seromas

Serous fluid must also be distinguished from pus, or the fluid that accumulates as a result of dead adipose/fat cells[3,4]. The latter fluid demonstrates a fatty, glistening consistency. One of the principal actions of modern dressings is to absorb serous and fatty exudate and trap it within the dressing layers, leaving the internal dressing layer free from any irritating material over the surface of the wound[7,8].

Dead fat cells have a very high incidence of bacterial invasion (almost a magnet type attraction) and the use of modern fluid-absorbing moist wound healing dressings significantly reduces the level of wound site contamination, assists in denying the bacteria this medium and any early opportunity for development of infection[1-4,7,8].

In plastic surgery, seromas may be observed postoperatively within the breast or abdomen (mobile tissue areas) and may be loosely described as a 'mobile encapsulated fluid collection'[3]. This may be seen on about days 3 to 4 as the final remaining exudate following cessation of blood flow in the drainage bottle. Volumes greater than 20 ml per day may require drainage systems to be continued until the volume reduces to 10 ml or less per day. This is a surgical decision and failure of the collected exudate to reduce should be documented and reported. Surgical intervention may be required, for example large bore needle aspiration, followed by compression to minimise the redevelopment of the encapsulated seroma.

If exudate via a drainage tube continues unabated at more than 20 ml per 24 hours, an ultrasound examination is commonly undertaken for diagnostic purposes to determine the exact position and size of the suspected seroma. This provides a differential diagnosis and decisions can be made regarding ongoing treatment modalities.

Many surgeons view the continuing use of drainage tubes as a foreign body causing an inflammatory response, which is the source of continuous exudate, so will remove the drainage tubes and observe for any adverse wound events. This clinical observation has contributed to the rise of negative pressure therapy as an external system exerting negative pressure within a totally enclosed environment that mimics normal physiological processes whilst ensuring the integrity of the wound/skin.

Although many small seromas will probably be absorbed in time, some appear to be encapsulated by fibrous tissue, significantly reducing an opportunity for the serum to be absorbed back into the capillaries or lymphatic system, and these require surgical drainage[3].

Regardless of the aetiology of fluid that accumulates within a wound, the surgeon will exercise judgement as to whether to do nothing, undertake needle aspiration or surgical evacuation, or apply wound compression by external means such as layered bandages, individually fitted elasticised tubular bandages or negative pressure therapy. Nurse clinicians must ensure patients are observed closely, until the wound is healed, for signs of inflammation and pain over the site, fever, lethargy or general malaise that may indicate impending infection, leading to major short to long-term wound disturbances.

## 2. NUTRITIONAL RISK MANAGEMENT FOR RECONSTRUCTIVE PLASTIC SURGICAL PATIENTS

### Protein and wound repair

**Protein** is the building block of cells, supported mainly by vitamins and trace elements[18-22]. The absence of adequate protein in the body means that the replication of cells required for tissue repair (and normal replacement) is substantially reduced. **Mitosis** is the process by which the body produces new cells, for both growth and repair of injured cells[1-5,7-10,18-22].

It is stated that, in the seriously injured person who was previously well nourished, protein stores begin to significantly decline after 72 hours. This is a critical time in wound repair as maximal mitotic activity has been observed to occur after 48–72 hours. In addition, protein depletion is suggested to significantly alter the ability for angiogenesis to take place, and angiogenesis is required for the proliferation of fibroblasts, which are essential for the instigation of new vessels in wound repair, and also for the replacement of collagen Types 1–5. Excess intake of protein in some medical conditions (renal disease) can result in fluid imbalance[1-5,7-10,18-22].

All age groups are at risk of dehydration, malnutrition, and the basic or complex consequences of inadequate fluid and dietary intake. The incidence of malnutrition can be high in many low socio-economic groups, persons with poor dietary habits, the elderly, cancer patients, the medically sick, the infirm, and many who live alone. It has been reported that **protein energy malnutrition** rates of 25–50% are recorded in patients upon admission[19]. Of patients who are well nourished upon admission, approximately 25–30% will develop a malnourished state, exponential to their disease and immobility status during their inpatient stay. These figures are largely determined by the hospital's assessment criteria and the case mix of the patients within the population of the hospital.

Protein energy malnutrition is stated to be one of the most common reasons that wounds fail to heal. That being so, clinical nurses must be scientifically educated to understand basic protein–caloric calculations and the significant risks associated with dietary imbalance. Clinicians should also be able to identify those patients who are at risk, prepared with an assessment and strategic management pathway to rectify any actual and potential problems[1–5,7–10,18–22].

Nutritional risk assessment is a proactive approach to evaluate the actual or potential of caloric malnutrition and identifies patients who would otherwise go unrecognised and untreated. Two principal tests are utilised, albumin and pre-albumin. For surgical and wound management, pre-albumin is suggested to be the most effective, the most simplistic to undertake, speedy and reliable[19].

---

**Box 8.13** Indication for protein analysis in at-risk patients.

- Preoperatively as part of the pre-assessment prior to major surgery
- Critically ill or chronically ill patients
- During major surgery or major injury, recovery phase and postoperatively
- Postoperatively following surgery for malignancies, chemotherapy or radiotherapy
- Patients with a life-threatening disease
- Patients with chronic wounds or high volume exuding wounds
- Patients in institutions
- Patients with AIDS or immune deficiencies
- Patients who live alone.

---

## Laboratory testing for albumin – risk management issues

Laboratory tests for indications of stored protein include albumin, pre-albumin and transferrin.

### Albumin

Normal adult blood protein (a traditional nutritional marker) levels are 6–8 g/dl. Albumin is a test used to determine the presence of liver or kidney disease or if sufficient protein is being absorbed by the body.

Albumin has an expected half-life of approximately 20 days and this can lead to the false belief that all is well, when in fact a significantly low level of albumin exists[18–22]. Levels of albumin below 3.0 g/dl are associated with oedema in the tissues, and levels of 2.5 g/dl are accepted as indications of severe protein deficiency. Low levels of albumin (2.0 g/dl) are commonly seen in the elderly and severely burnt people[1,2,10,18–22].

Clinical trials indicate that albumin levels of less that 2.0 g/dl are responsible for major impairment of tissue repair[20–22]. Above this level, injured tissue can be expected to heal, but with marked and increasing difficulty unless adequate replacement is instituted. In addition to all other existing problems, these patients (regardless of age) are at high risk of developing pressure ulcers, which produce additional complications and increase the risk of a range of life-threatening conditions, particularly intractable infection[18–22].

With identification of low albumin levels, it is expected that the level of vitamins and minerals will also be depleted. This also needs to be investigated and professionally managed. The test's principal disadvantage is that it does not detect the protein energy malnutrition status in the short term (i.e. pre-albumin results available in two days[19]) although it does monitor nutritional status[19]. Albumin has a half-life of 20 days so nutritional markers take much longer to present for management to begin[19].

### Pre-albumin

A test utilised as a clinical indicator for assessing the nutritional status and nutritional risk in the management of many disease processes, but demonstrated to be very effective in pre-surgical screening to identify patients at risk, nutritional assessment during recovery from major surgery and major trauma, and in wound repair[19].

**Box 8.14** Principal advantage of undertaking pre-albumin testing[19].

- In the USA, the Joint Commission on Accreditation of Healthcare Organizations (JCAHO) specifies all patients must be nutritionally assessed immediately following hospital admission
- Early identification of nutritional status (two days) – normal range 17–40 mg/dl and a half-life of 1.9 days
- Biochemical marker is extremely sensitive to changes in nutritional status
- Less sensitive to changes in hydration, liver and renal function
- Patients can be monitored, ongoing, post surgery and trauma
- Quick interventional responses with nutritional replacements sustaining life support systems.

See recommended websites at the end of this chapter

**Box 8.15** Assessment risk levels – pre-albumin.

| | |
|---|---|
| 100 mg/l | severe |
| 100 to 170 mg/l | moderate |
| 170 mg/l | no risk[19]. |

## The importance of nutritional management in wound repair

It is an old but fundamentally important adage in wound care that *'if you starve the patient, you starve the wound'*. This can be translated into a physiological imbalance of nutritional need and energy requirements for wound bed repair.

With some exceptions (e.g. major burns, severe trauma, major head and neck surgery, gastrointestinal surgery), for patients who cannot orally digest adequate food after three days, the introduction of parenteral or nasogastric feeding, must be considered. Until this time in fit healthy patients, IV fluid feeding (providing only essential electrolytes, glucose and water) are usually sufficient to meet nutritional needs in the short term.

If there are issues of previous, existing or increasing illness due to, for example, systemic medical morbidity (disease) or infection, that affect nutritional levels, arising in the previously averagely nourished person, proactive nutritional replacement should also be considered. Interventions should be made on the basis of existing and ongoing patient and wound repair needs (e.g. enteral feeding, PEG or nasogastric feeding[1,2,10]).

As the body is continually renewing many used tissue cells within different timeframes, a ready availability of an optimal fluid and food supply is fundamental for restoration and the ongoing function of cells. This means an adequate nutritional protein intake is required for the energy demands of the normal reparative process. This is relative not only to the physiological responses required to meet normal cell replacement, but also to the increased cellular needs of adequate water, nutrition and oxygen that are essential for cellular repair and systemic responses in, for example, unexpected secondary injury, or diseases such as cancer, excessive exposure to inhaled cytotoxic agents, heavy smoking and overuse of alcohol.

Cigarette smoke and excess use of alcohol are high among those agents argued to be capable of destroying squamous alimentary tract cells through cytotoxic and constant irritating actions. These are also responsible for the destruction of essential vitamins required for metabolism, particularly the B group[1–4,6–8,10,23–25].

## Nutritional risk management in reconstructive plastic surgery nursing care

As with other surgery, within reconstructive plastic surgery practice a range of circumstances may indicate patients who are potentially at nutritional risk (see Boxes 8.13 & 8.14). Preoperative assessment allows timely referrals to professional dieticians to facilitate nutritional supplements to be provided in preparation for major illness periods, and wound bed repair.

For inpatients who are considered to be at risk (see also Boxes 8.16 & 8.17), it is crucial that testing for malnutrition by medical nursing staff, and professional dieticians is undertaken.

---

**Box 8.16** Major wounding – at risk patients.

- Severe injury (adults and children) following major trauma, including burns
- Unconsciousness for more than 72 hours
- Facial surgery (elective or post trauma) that alters normal dietary intake
- Major reconstructive surgery to the head and neck for cancer, with or without tracheostomy
- Elderly patients undergoing surgery that limits their physical mobility
- Children with major craniofacial deformities that inhibit normal mastication and nutritional intake.

---

**Box 8.17** Morbid and co-morbid conditions – at-risk patients.

- Major sepsis with extended periods of wound repair
- Co-morbid conditions that alter normal metabolic functions (e.g. diabetes mellitus, diseases affecting absorption)
- Medications, such as steroids, that alter metabolism
- Prolonged history of cigarette, substance and/or alcohol abuse
- Extended fasting times prior to and after multiple surgical episodes
- Psychological-based conditions that may precipitate starvation regimes
- Extreme dieting prior to surgery for removal of excess tissue
- Age – increasing inability to sustain normal metabolism
- Patients who live alone and have inadequate nutrition, physical or psychological support
- Patients who are admitted for reconstructive surgery for pre-existing wounds and pressure ulcers, with pre-existing major nutritional deficits.

---

**Box 8.18** Principal nursing risk management issues.

- Inadequate, or failure to undertake, assessment of baseline nutritional status
- Inadequate response to, or failure to address, unexpected nutritional deficits
- Delay in initiating pre-emptive nutritional replacement strategies

---

- Inappropriate use of nutritional formulas required for replacement of specific deficits
- Inadequate attention to poor digestive compliance by the patient (e.g. bowel disturbances)
- Failure to ensure that discharge management includes nutritional support
- Development of pressure ulcers in patients who have not been appropriately assessed for risk[2,8,18,19].

---

### Dehydration and nutritional risk management issues – elective reconstructive plastic surgery patients

Most patients who undergo elective plastic surgery will have maintained an adequate pre-operative level of nutrition and exercise, allowing for an uneventful episode of normal wound repair.

The average inpatient's short term (0–72 hours) nutritional and circulating volume fluid requirements can be supplied via intravenous infusions that provide electrolytes and glucose, proportional to physiological and energy needs. Pre-operative fasting times should also be part of this equation, particularly if the time between initial fasting time, time of surgery, period of surgical time and the return to the unit when fluids/nutrition can be taken, is long. Patients who have postoperative nausea and vomiting are at an added disadvantage of dehydration (and potential malnutrition in those 'at risk'). These issues should be addressed by the nurse clinician in association with the medical staff and dietician.

If blood or serum protein is lost, this too is replaced according to circulating volume requirements. Should the patient's condition unexpectedly decline (e.g. due to haemorrhage, infection, medical illness) earlier or around 72 hours postoperatively, further nutritional assessments (pre-albumin testing) should be conducted to address the potential loss of essential protein, water, body electrolytes, glucose and ultimately muscle bulk.

Chronic wounds may develop and divert general energy needs toward the systemic and local needs of the wound. Patient and wound bed assessment can assist in pre-emptively determining any consultations with dietary professionals for pharmacologically prepared electrolyte and nutritional supplements.

Initiating a risk assessment process, as part of preadmission protocols to obtain baseline nutritional scores, can significantly increase the potential for gradual restoration of tissue integrity and the psychological status of the patient. Simply asking a patient about their physical activity and what they eat each day can provide a good indication of the patient's nutritional status and exercise regime (although sometimes the reality is hard to obtain). Results of full blood examination determine levels of haemoglobin, protein and clotting factors, and nutritional risk appraisal can also help to build a whole picture of the patient and significantly ward off or minimise adverse events.

In addition, because of the relationship between protein deficits, malnutrition, and the emergence of pressure ulcers in the seriously or critically ill and immobile patients, the appropriate pressure-relieving devices and nursing protocols, can be put in place pre-emptively.

### Avoiding adverse clinical outcomes

As outlined, inadequate basic nutrition is a major precursor to the development of clinical malnutrition, poor wound repair, infection, pressure ulcers and, equally significantly, psychosocial issues. These are important factors as they may increase the development of infection, pain, life-threatening morbidity and mortality.

As an example, patients who are to undergo major head and neck reconstruction for cancer, may be admitted in a negative protein status. Physically and psychologically they are in a very highly dependent phase, particularly if they have a long history of cigarette and alcohol use, and have long-term inadequate nutrition.

In selected cases when pre-surgical admission time permits, oral nutritional regimes should be initiated[11-17]. Professional dieticians can detail an objective regime that the patient can afford, and will probably be prepared to undertake in their home setting. Some patients may benefit from nasogastric or PEG feeding as preparation prior to surgery, particularly when disease states are early and malnutrition is a risk in postoperative and healing phase. Both these regimes have their advantages and disadvantages, and should be conducted under the management of experienced and competent physicians, nurse clinicians and nutritional experts[19-22].

### Dietary supplements to increase protein energy levels

Available supplements include oral supplements in the form of packet drinks with complete food provisions (protein, fat, carbohydrates) or energy drinks or foods that provide glucose, fats, proteins, minerals and vitamins[18,19]. Non-oral supplements include those given via the enteral route, or via tube, such as nasogastric feeding or PEGs. Jejunostomy (tube inserted into the jejunum) may be necessary in specific cases of gastrointestinal surgery where surgical reconstructive flaps are based on mesenteric vessels[11-15].

Parenteral supplements or non-oral supplements, for example a central venous line via the subclavian vein, are additional options[10]. In pre-prepared supplements the principal components of nitrogen, glucose, fat, electrolytes, vitamins and trace elements are pharmacologically and hygienically prepared to meet the critical energy needs of the patient[18,19].

Varying levels of bowel irritation may occur when antibiotics and/or pharmacologically prepared supplements are used. Natural yoghurt containing *Acidophilus bifidus casei* is often suggested as a natural remedy and is extremely useful for assisting in the restoration of an acceptable level of bowel flora.

### On discharge

On discharge, patients who, for example, have had surgery for major tumours, should be checked regularly in the community by their general practitioner and community health nurse. Regular pre-albumin and weight reports should be requested from both, and the progress reports of the patient should be sent to the hospital and/or surgeon managing their care.

Ongoing visits to the surgeon or outpatient clinic should be undertaken and should include weight, nutritional and fluid intake. This can also be confirmed by a basic assessment and undertaking full blood examinations that include pre-albumin.

General regular oral examinations for mouth ulcers, checking the smell of the patient's breath, alimentary excretion including bowel regularities, and skin moisture, are also important in assessing the patient's progress or early diagnosis of disease recurrence. Continuing weight loss can be an early indicator of both physiological (tumour/disease recurrence) and psychological problems[1,2,10,21–23], thus regular weighing of the patient in the community and at each outpatient visit is essential.

Nutritional needs for major burns or major infections (e.g. necrotising fasciitis) are not discussed here and clinicians should refer to specialised texts that provide expert research-based formulas for all levels of injury and patient requirements.

See recommended websites for evidence-based nutritional assessment and management at the end of this chapter.

## The place of vitamins in wound bed repair

In addition to protein, it is acknowledged that the principal vitamins, A, B, C, K, and zinc and copper are essential for wound healing, but there are no specific scientific data to describe the specific therapeutic oral doses required for the artificial replacement of vitamins, particularly vitamin C, or B complex[21–23].

Scientific testing of vitamin body levels is expensive and said not to be very reliable because of the time interval between the test and the results, in view of the changing status of patient needs and the fact that inflammatory diseases will falsify the results. Although studies have shown that wound healing in animals is increased when vitamin supplements are given, stated dosages in humans have not been scientifically determined. The *ad hoc* high or low dose use of most oral vitamins is expensive, and rarely useful, as the body excretes amounts in excess of its needs of particularly water-soluble vitamins.

Nurse clinicians should be familiar with the indications, known pharmacology and contraindications of multiple doses of vitamins. The regular and excessive ingestion of vitamin tablets and other supplements is contraindicated, and as such, they should be treated similarly to drugs.

Medical and pharmacological knowledge is important if adverse reactions are to be avoided. For example, the overuse of vitamin C is known to produce oxalate stones in the kidney and, in some patients, renal dysfunction. Giving vitamin A may be useful in temporarily nullifying the actions of oral steroids in patients who are to undergo surgical treatment related to the long-term management of rheumatoid arthritis, but overdosage of vitamin A

may lead to adverse effects on the liver and cornea[1–3,10]. Too much zinc inhibits absorption and function of copper in the system.

For patients who have good chances of survival, pre-emptive nutritional programmes assist the patient with optimal recovery, wound bed repair, and a positive quality of life. In these times of extreme stress and grief, it is important to provide the patient with avenues of crucial support that will increase the patient's mobility and ability to deal with real or perceived impending catastrophic life events, such as a diagnosis of cancer with the potential for severe disability, or early death.

See recommended websites on nutrition at the end of this chapter.

## Smoking and wound healing issues

The long-term systemic toxic effects of smoking, such as lung and chronic respiratory diseases, are widely acknowledged and cigarette smoking is also acknowledged as having an adverse effect on blood vessels and platelets, and ultimately wound repair at cellular level. This recognition is based on animal studies that have looked at the individual components and adverse effects of nicotine, carbon monoxide and hydrogen cyanide[1,2,23–25].

Long-term local skin effects of smoking (using a pipe, cigarette holder, etc.) are associated with the development of leukoplakia or white, pre-cancerous patches on the lip. All forms of smoking, including marijuana, are suggested to be a major precursor to lip, oropharyngeal and lung cancer[1,2,23–25]. Smoking has also been shown to have major detrimental effects on the major and microcirculation and skin tissue, accelerating the development of wrinkles and aberrations of the skin[1,2,23–25].

Risks associated with the development of deep-vein thrombosis and vascular ischaemia increase the potential for a range of life-threatening medical complications and significant wound problems, and every effort to minimise these risks should be instituted[1,2,23–25].

### Nicotine – risk management issues

Nicotine has been shown to cause vasoconstrictive actions that may last for up to 50 minutes following the smoking of a cigarette. A smoke-free period of more than three to six weeks is required to significantly lower the risk of reduction in blood flow and high levels of tissue ischaemia in the macro and microcirculation[23–25]. Nicotine results in platelet adhesion, promoting blood clotting, particularly in the microcirculation, and is accepted to inhibit the proliferation of red blood cells, macrophages and fibroblasts, thus retarding the initiation of wound repair and increasing the potential for conversion to a chronic wound[23–25].

As indicated above, the injurious effects of cigarette smoking on wound repair caused by a major interference in blood flow, blood clotting, restricted oxygen flow and cellular dysfunction are seen not only in the skin but at all tissue levels, including bone.

Should the patient also have peripheral vascular disease, be on long-term steroid therapy, consume large volumes of alcohol, or have diabetes mellitus, the healing process is profoundly disturbed. Many elective patients who arrive for surgery with, for example, major skin or oral malignancies, will present with these morbid factors[23–25].

Some large institutions have professionals on staff (in cardiorespiratory units) trained to prepare and provide support to patients attempting to cease smoking prior to surgery. Clinicians should use any available avenues to assist the patient and to reduce wound complications[24,25].

### Carbon monoxide

Carbon monoxide produces hydrogen cyanide, which severely retards the process of oxygen transport and cellular respiration required for metabolic activity at cellular level. Increasing levels of carbon monoxide decreases normal transport of oxygen as it competes for transportation on the haemoglobin molecule. Carbon monoxide's low binding affinity means that it overrides the oxygen molecules[1,2,23–25].

For patients undergoing elective surgery, wound bed preparation prior to surgical intervention should include education encouraging the patient to reduce or cease smoking. Some surgeons decline to operate on patients requesting aesthetic surgery who refuse to cease smoking. For the patient with trauma or chronic wounds, every effort should be made at least to indicate the benefits of ceasing to smoke until the wounds have healed, particularly with the use of nicotine patches[1,2,23–25].

### Patient-based discharge issues

The universal move to community-based postoperative care, or self-care in the home environment, has seen the early discharge of patients following many major procedures[16–19]. In some instances there is an unrealistic reliance on the patient's ability to objectively observe wounds, recognise impending complications, and intelligently report possible harmful signs and symptoms. The patient's culture, educational status, readiness to learn and ability to manage new information must be assessed, so that suitable and important information can be given to the individual or significant providers, at an appropriate time[1,2,10].

## Audit of preferred wound and patient outcomes

### Box 8.19 Safety.

- The patient's physiological condition was initially assessed in order to identify, address and stabilise any relevant medical/nursing morbidity and co-morbidity that had the potential to compromise the desired repair processes and healed outcome of the wound
- The patient's general physiological condition was an ongoing focus and actual and potential adverse events were addressed in a timely manner during the total repair process
- Individual actual and potential adverse episodes were identified and addressed to prevent/minimise any detrimental wound or patient outcomes
- The presentation of any existing open wounds was perceived to present actual and potential complications during the repair process unless assessed and addressed in a timely manner
- Any expression of unexpected pain or discomfort was immediately assessed/investigated to ensure the safety of the patient and the wound was not compromised
- Any dissatisfaction or difficulty expressed by the patient was professionally assessed and addressed immediately, documented and reported as appropriate
- The patient expressed satisfaction with the professional management of his or her infirmity at all stages of the wound repair process.

## Box 8.20 Comfort.

- The assessment and practical management of pain and discomfort at all stages of wound care was a primary consideration in the provision of patient comfort and ensuring the repair process was not compromised
- Any statement of unexpected pain or discomfort was immediately assessed/investigated, documented, and reported appropriately
- Any dissatisfaction or difficulty expressed by the patient was professionally assessed and addressed immediately, documented and reported as appropriate
- The patient expressed satisfaction with the professional management of his or her pain or discomfort at all stages of the wound repair process.

## Box 8.21 Independence

- The management of the patient was a collaborative progression that allowed the maximum level of self care without compromise to the repair development and outcome
- The education received was understood and patient was able to feedback the information correctly
- Any dissatisfaction or difficulty expressed by the patient was professionally assessed and addressed immediately, documented and reported as appropriate
- The patient expressed satisfaction with the professional management of his or her general nursing care at all stages of the wound repair process.

## References

(1) McCance K.L. & Huether S.E. *Pathophysiology: the biologic basis for disease in adults and children*, 3rd edn. St Louis: Mosby, 1998.

(2) Smeltzer S.C. & Bare B.G. *Brunner and Suddarth's textbook of medical-surgical nursing*, 9th edn. Philadelphia: Lippincott, Williams & Wilkins, 2000.

(3) Peacock E.E. Jnr. *Wound repair*, 3rd edn. Philadelphia: W.B. Saunders Company, 1984.

(4) Vardaxis N. *Pathology for the health sciences*. St Yarra, Australia: Macmillan Education Australia, 1994, reprinted 1998.

(5) Guyton A.C. & Hall J.E. *Textbook of medical physiology*, 9th edn. London: W.B. Saunders, 1996.

(6) Morris A. McG., Stevenson J.H. & Watson A.C.H. *Complications of plastic surgery*. Baillière Tindall: London, 1989.

(7) Bryant R.A. (ed.) *Acute and chronic wounds: nursing management*. St Louis: Mosby Year Book, 1992.

(8) Dealey C., *The care of wounds*, 2nd edn. Oxford, UK: Blackwell Science, 1999.

(9) Bowler P.G., Duerden B.I. & Armstrong D.G. Wound microbiology and associated approaches to wound management. *Clinical Microbiology Review*, 2001 (Apr); 244–69.

(10) Mallett J. & Dougherty L. (eds) *The Royal Marsden Hospital manual of clinical nursing procedures*, 5th edn. Oxford, UK: Blackwell Science, 2000.

(11) Donovan S. Wound infection and wound swabbing. *Professional Nurse*, 1998 (Aug); **13**(11):757–59.

(12) Cutting K.F. Identification of infection in granulating wounds by registered nurses. *Journal of Clinical Nursing*, 1998 (Nov); **6**:539–46.

(13) Smedley F., Bowling T., James M., *et al*. Randomized clinical trial of the effects of preoperative and postoperative oral nutritional supplements on clinical course and cost of care. *British Journal Surgery*, 2004; **91**:983–90.

(14) Andenaes K., Amland P.F., Lingaas E., Abyholm F., Samdal F. & Giercksky K.E.A. Prospective, randomised surveillance study of postoperative wound infections after plastic surgery: a study of incidence and surveillance methods. *Plastic Reconstructive Surgery*, 1995 (Sept); **96**(4):948–56.

(15) Armstrong M. Obesity as an intrinsic factor affecting wound healing. *Journal of Wound Care*, 1998 (May); **7**(5):220-21.

(16) Soper D., Bump R.C. & Hurt W.G. Wound infection after abdominal hysterectomy: effect of the depth of subcutaneous tissue. *American Journal of Obstetrics and Gynecology*, 1995; **173**:465–71.

(17) Banwell P., Withey S. & Holten I. The use of negative pressure to promote healing. *British Journal of Plastic Surgery*, 1998; **51**(1):79.

(18) McWhirther J.P. & Pennington C.R. Incidence and recognition of malnutrition in hospital, *British Medical Journal*, 1994; **308**: 945–48.

(19) http://www.beckman.com/resourcecenter/literature/default.asp

(20) Gray D. & Cooper P. Nutrition and wound healing: what is the link? *Journal of Wound Care*, 2001 (March); **10**(3):86–9.

(21) Flanigan K.H. Nutritional aspects of wound healing. *Advances in Wound Care*, 1997; **10**(3):48–52.

(22) Osak M.P. Nutrition and wound healing. *Plastic Surgical Nursing*, 1993 (spring); **13**(1):29–36.

(23) Netscher D.T. & Clamon J. Smoking: adverse effects on outcomes for plastic surgical patients. *Plastic Surgical Nursing*, 1994 (winter); **14**(4):205–210.

(24) Silagy C., Lancaster T., Stead L., Mant D. & Fowler G. Nicotine replacement therapy for smoking cessation. *The Cochrane Database of Systematic Reviews* (England), 2000 (2) pCD000146.

(25) Lancaster T. & Stead L.F. Self-help interventions for smoking cessation. *The Cochrane Database of Systematic Reviews* (England), 2002 (3) pCD001118.

## Recommended websites

**Nutritional assessment and management**
http://www.cgsupport.nhs.uk/Resources/Eurekas/Older _People/Nutritional_Status.asp http://www.jcaho. org/accredited+organizations/hospitals/standards/h ospital+faqs/provision+of+care/assessment/ nutritional_functional_painassess_screens.htm http://www.cancerresource.co.uk/nursing%20 developments/nutritionprotocol.htm http://www. mkgeneral.nhs.uk/redtrayproject/RedTrayProject.pdf

# Chapter 9

# Wound Bed Assessment

## Background

Wound care is a holistic, dynamic undertaking where the wound bed assessment process[1-4] is not completed until the short, medium and long-term goals have been achieved and the preferred clinical and patient outcomes have been met.

For nurse clinicians, it also carries increasing responsibility and accountability as nurses increasingly become primary decision-makers based on the wound bed assessment undertaken, and plan treatment for wound bed repair or whatever outcome is realistically possible to achieve. Failure to accurately assess the type of wound to be managed, inappropriate decision-making and inadequate use of a case management focus can compromise the entire wound repair process, and potentially endanger the patient's life.

## Wound bed assessment – basic principles

### Box 9.1 Essentials of wound bed assessment.

- Comprehensive and formal patient assessment
- Establishing medical and nursing morbid and co-morbid factors that prevent the wound repair process
- Describing the specific location of the wound and its immediate surroundings
- Establishing normal wound boundaries against which atypical findings can be measured
- Establishing protocols that allow for the selection of dressings to parallel the objective needs of the wound and its surroundings
- Establishing protocols that prevent the unnecessary changing of dressing, increasing the opportunity for the wound to repair, preventing patient discomfort and significantly reducing nursing downtime
- Addressing the overall risk of failure to achieve healing, and setting up protocols that can provide an acceptable quality of life
- Setting short, medium and long-term goals
- Setting wound outcomes
- Auditing wound outcomes.

## Elective and clean wounds

Elective surgery wounds that are clean and closed by primary closure, skin grafts, or skin flaps, require appropriate dressings, ongoing clinical observation for wound perfusion and wound bed assessment of progress until healing has been accomplished[1-4]. But if adverse events do occur, clinicians must be able to assess, evaluate, report, and document changes through an objective process. Observing for the development of circulatory problems, haematoma, excess swelling, pain and patient psychosocial issues, demand a plan of care as an inpatient or outpatient.

## Wounds related to trauma

Following significant trauma, any actual or potential risks to or alterations in life support systems (e.g. airway, circulation, neurological) should be primarily stabilised before determining the most appropriate approach to repair of the wound(s), although this may be closely allied to patient stabilisation, e.g. multiple trauma[5,6].

Short-term protection of injured tissues can be achieved by applying wet normal saline dressings covered with occlusive dressings such as semi-permeable film to retain warmth and moisture, and protect the entry of environmental bacteria or organisms until a decision is made regarding primary treatment for the wound(s).

Immobilisation and elevation of limbs is determined by their vascular status but, in the absence of arterial compromise, elevation will assist venous return, reduce oedema, help to reduce the level of pain, and protect cells and tissues against further injury.

## Addressing the process of wound bed assessment

The ability to observe and assess any wound, analyse the data, set wound care goals and preferred outcomes requires a high level of understanding of the topics in the previous chapters.

Ongoing evidence-based and expert experiential practice, allows what initially appears to be a long and daunting wound assessment to be undertaken in a short span of time[1-9].

For example, in assessing acute open wounds, or chronic wounds, identifying wound zones where it is obvious that there is a range of viable or non-viable blood flow is an important skill. Setting goals of care to increase the vascular flow to wound zones that have a vascular/oxygen compromise is fundamental to increase circulatory and cell function (see Chapter 7) and further improve the potential of tissue healing in adjacent compromised zones. These techniques can be applied to any wound.

## What are the initial important questions?

Initially, and wherever possible, the patient should be asked to state the reason for their presentation in their own words – nothing should be assumed.

In traumatic wounds that present as acute or delayed, a thorough history of the mechanism of injury is fundamental, as knowledge of how the injury was caused and in what context may help in recognising problems that are not immediately visible. For instance, small holes caused by a thin sharp instrument (e.g. a knife) may cause significant injury to vessels, nerves and/or tendons. These questions and an examination of the wound(s) can provide an initial plethora of information that may ultimately determine the primary and secondary course of management[1-19].

---

**Box 9.2** Primary assessment – information to obtain.

Ask the patient to describe, in their own words:

- How did it happen?
- Where does it hurt?
- When did it occur?
- Do you have any other wounds?

If it is a chronic wound or a referred patient, elicit any previous and existing treatments.

Are there any medical, nursing, occupational or personal deterrents to retard or slow the repair process?

---

**Box 9.3** Wound bed assessment areas to be addressed – overview.

- Wound type(s)
- Wound sites/location
- Wound description – using tissue colour as an integral wound assessment tool to determine healing/non-healing status
- Wound depth
- Description by exudate – colour, type and volume
- Wound dimensions and overall extent
- Assessing the vascular and cellular integrity of an open or closed wound.

---

## Wound types – general definitions

There appears to be no universal consensus on how wounds are objectively described. In general, the terms in Box 9.4 are commonly used.

---

**Box 9.4** Wound types – general definitions for assessment.

- Acute or primary healing (clean, with primary closure or granulation) = potential to fully heal within 7–21 days
- Post-acute non-surgical (highly contaminated, becomes infected, maintained by dressings) = determined by control of bacteria and loss of viable tissue, may take up to 21–56 or more days to heal
- Post-acute surgical secondary healing (clean, surgical, post-reconstruction with primary closure or allowed to granulate) = potential to heal within 7–21 days
- Chronic wounds treated, not healed by 21 days or 40% surface area (indicating whether following trauma, acute surgery, or disease-based) = appears contaminated, may be infected, may be odorous
- Wounds with large areas of dead fat, *Pseudomonas* infection or with gas gangrene (anaerobic infection) have a distinctive odour
- Chronic wounds with arterial compromise will lack visible moisture and may be extremely painful
- Original clean wounds not completely healed by days 14–21 (depending on the wound site) should perhaps be classified as chronic, regardless of their aetiology, in order that some delineation between normal and abnormal wound repair/recovery can be described[10]

*Continued*

---

- Palliative wound = recurrence of chronic or cancer-based wound which has no potential to heal – may require ameliorating dressings, or surgery for pain, wound management, hygiene, and aesthetics (see Chapter 13)
- Satellite wounds = lesions secondary to the original tumour – cancer-based local wounds related to recurrences of original tumours

Wounds begin as small pimples, slowly enlarge, become ulcerated, often leading to fungating sites that meet up to become large, odorous, frequent exudate (inflammatory reaction), and painful wounds.

## Wound sites

It is acknowledged that some wounds heal more easily than others, or fail to heal, for a range of reasons, as outlined in Chapter 8.

Clear descriptions of the site(s) of the wound(s) is essential and the use of original photographs, diagrams, digital photos or drawings, can assist all interdisciplinary clinicians to have a clear understanding of the geographical and structural wound site. *Note, however, digital photos are not legally accepted as they can be changed or enhanced.*

By understanding the geographical locations of fixed and mobile skin[5,6,11–14], the anatomical site of the wound can provide information on the flexibility or extensibility of the skin, skin thickness, blood supply, and potential for uninterrupted healing and help to initiate the 'best practice' treatment modalities to be applied.

## *Risk management issues*

**Box 9.5** Wound bed assessment issues to be considered in relation to wound sites.

- The wound will close primarily with sutures, or other means, or without assistance, and protect the tissues beneath, without tension
- The wound requires moist wound healing dressings, negative pressure therapy, or an artificial skin cover to provide a moist wound healing environment and introduce healing without tension
- The patient's safety is at risk, and surgery to close a wound by, for example, skin graft or skin flap, would be in the patient's best interests.

**Box 9.6** Risk management issues.

- In some wound sites, the potential of large, wide zones of scar tissue to withstand secondary injury is markedly reduced, as most scar tissue does not possess the same degree of elastic flexibility as do normal epidermis and dermis, and lacks a true blood supply[5,6,11–14]
- Resulting scar tissue, following healing in fixed skin zones, can easily place significant tension over the area. For example, secondary injury is quite high over the tibial region. Clinicians must ensure patients are aware of this and encourage regular application of simple, inexpensive but effective moisturising lotions (e.g. Sorbolene and glycerine combinations, vitamin E cream, oatmeal or aloe vera). Gentle stroking skin massage to the scar and surrounding areas increases local venous and lymphatic flow (see Chapter 12)
- Wounds that fail to completely heal by day 21, or have only a 40% recovery through normal dermal contraction, and epidermal resurfacing, require a total reassessment of the wound, any underlying pathophysiology and the current treatment modality. There may be a need to consider surgical intervention, for example, the need for surgical debridement and an alternative covering (e.g. different dressing approach, negative pressure therapy, a skin graft or a skin flap) to protect 'at risk' anatomical areas and tissues
- Fixed skin zones or skin with limited mobility resulting from scarring related to previous injury require special attention.

## Wound description by colour

Describing wounds within zones and by colour is the most visible format available to clinicians. Figures 9.1, 9.2, 9.3 and Table 9.1 outline method of using colours as an important assessment tool to demonstrate and confirm the physiological status of a wound. Table 9.2 provides information for use of colour in assessment and identification of vascular perfusion and oxygen available to the wound and surrounding tissues. Table 9.3 discusses wound depths, potential problem, healing times and scar outcomes in acute wounds.

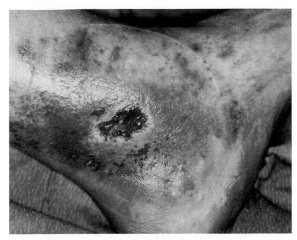

**Figure 9.1** Leg ulcer wound presenting for wound bed assessment. From: Dealey C., 2000.

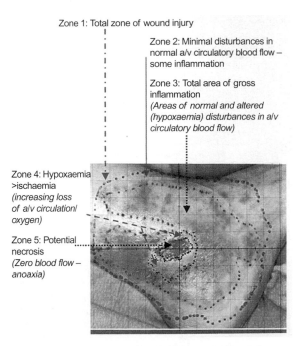

Zone 1: Total zone of wound injury

Zone 2: Minimal disturbances in normal a/v circulatory blood flow – some inflammation

Zone 3: Total area of gross inflammation *(Areas of normal and altered (hypoxaemia) disturbances in a/v circulatory blood flow)*

Zone 4: Hypoxaemia >ischaemia *(increasing loss of a/v circulation/ oxygen)*

Zone 5: Potential necrosis *(Zero blood flow – anoaxia)*

**Figure 9.3** Outlining zones of cell/tissue potential viability according to blood supply – selection of dressings for specific zones as required. Adapted from: Dealey C., 2000.

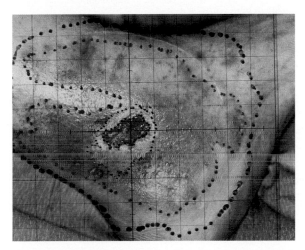

**Figure 9.2** Defining zones of cell/tissue injury. Adapted from: Dealey C., 2000.

## Assessing vascular integrity

Colour can be applied in both open wounds (the tissues) and closed wounds (the skin). It can also be extended to observation and descriptions of actual and potential loss of vascular integrity in wound surrounds, which may be due to arterial infarction or venous thrombosis, causing the loss of capillary function at a local level.

Evidence-based wound management is a slowly developing scientific discipline in which universal objective assessment, analytic and diagnostic techniques are gradually being developed. The use of wound colour computer diagnostic tools that analyse photographs, and vascular Doppler sensors and oxygen saturation sensors are some of the basic and common tools available to clinicians in very modern settings. Because of cost, computer programs that allow for scientific analysis of the wound status are available to only a few institutions, mainly those involved in research.

For reconstructive plastic surgery nurses, the visual colour of the skin, examination of capillary integrity and, in an increasing number of institutions, Doppler probes and external skin (dermal) oxygen measuring probes are emerging as the basis on which the vascular and oxygen status of a surgical flap wound is analysed, in parallel with regular vascular observations.

Despite the sophistication of technical adjuncts, in a skin flap or a flap with an attached skin paddle, it is the colour of the blood from dermal pricking that remains the gold standard.

**Table 9.1** Use of basic colours to illustrate the important vascular status of an open wound.

| Colour | Description | Vascular and oxygen status |
|---|---|---|
| Pink/red zones | Granulating wound, principally free from any contamination with angiogenesis and potential arteriogenesis in progress.<br>'Islands' of pink/red may be seen in previously non-healing wounds, indicating a potential to proceed to epithelialisation process.<br>Potential for spontaneous healing with aid of occlusive moist wound healing dressings and/or negative pressure therapy.<br>Healing may be accelerated by STSG in selected wounds.<br>Excessive and raised redness will indicate hypergranulation. | Excellent vascular integrity, high level of incoming circulation and gaseous exchange.<br>Islands indicate fibroblast development only possible in the presence of oxygen and growth factors.<br>Significant recalcitrant organisms may be present if a film or a form of 'slime' is observed over the red tissue or skin graft fails to take on what appears to be an optimal wound. |
| Green zones | Contaminated tissue may also be infected (*Pseudomonas aeruginosa* or *Staphylococcus aureus*).<br>Can be odorous.<br>Infection status determined by bacterial count according to specific bacteria by wound culture.<br>Potential to compromise blood flow to surrounding tissue, increasing the size of the whole wound.<br>May require active surgical debridement in association with moist wound healing dressings and/or negative pressure therapy.<br>Healing may be accelerated by STSG in selected wounds once clear of heavy contamination or infection and environment allowing for angiogenesis to be established. | Increasing loss of vascular integrity, hypoxaemia and hypoxia uneven in surrounding tissue, inadequate gaseous exchange.<br>Oxygen and nutrition to functioning cells reduced and, in some areas, absent.<br>Potential to change to the colour black if not debrided. |
| Yellow zones | Contaminated and/or infected tissue.<br>May be necrotic fat or congealed fibrin.<br>Infection status determined by science-based bacterial count.<br>On a continuing pathway to central and peripheral wound necrosis through significant loss of tissue cells.<br>Wound often malodorous.<br>May require active surgical debridement down to bleeding level and moist wound healing dressing. Healing may be accelerated by STSG in selected wounds once clear of heavy contamination or infection and environment allowing for angiogenesis to be established. | Loss of vascular integrity, wide areas of hypoxia with no gaseous exchange possible, potential to increase wound size by loss of blood flow through increasing loss of dermal tissue.<br>Potential to change to the colour black if not debrided. |
| Black zones | Necrotic tissue, multiple dead and dying cells, dehydrated, may or may not be malodorous.<br>May be surrounded by 'yellow' and/or 'green' tissue.<br>Infection status in surrounding tissue determined by bacterial count beneath eschar.<br>Requires active surgical debridement down to bleeding level followed by moist wound healing dressings and/or negative pressure therapy.<br>Healing may be accelerated by STSG in selected wounds once clear of heavy contamination or infection and environment allowing for angiogenesis to be established. | Total loss of vascular and healing integrity, anoxic tissue, increasing risk of cytotoxic and destructive forces affecting wide area of surrounding tissue. |

**Table 9.2** Identifying zones of tissue injury with altered tissue perfusion.

| Zone | Colour | Description |
|---|---|---|
| Total wound zone of injury – oxygen levels disturbed according to different zones | Multiple colours – pink, dark blue, white, yellow, black relates to vascular integrity of injured tissue | Lower limb injury (venous ulcer) demonstrating major blood flow disturbances interrupting any potential for normal wound recovery<br>Availability of oxygen and nutrients varied by circulatory status in wound zones. |
| Zone of inflammation – oxygenation presumed at adequate level | Red/pink | Protective physiological actions, increased/variable blood flow, increased metabolic activity<br>Disturbed vascular integrity – circulation may be in process of loss/recovery<br>In chronic wounds, circulation may be chaotic and intermittent causing tissue damage from cytotoxic effects arising from damaged cells<br>Potential to move to hypoxaemia but retrievable. |
| Zone of hypoxaemia – oxygenation varied | Blue = venous compromise<br>White = arterial compromise (may be yellow or green if situation has existed over an extended period) | Increasing loss of vessel integrity, variable/reducing blood supply, severely inhibiting/interrupting the normal arterial flow of oxygen and nutrition to cells<br>Potential venous thrombosis due to poor flow<br>Exchange of gases reduced and increasingly inadequate<br>Potential for local region to move to ischaemia but may be retrievable<br>Potential for cytotoxic effects high from increased load of dead cells<br>Contamination level increasing – potential for infection. |
| Zone of ischaemia – oxygen levels inadequate | White (primary cessation of arterial flow) → black (dead cells). Blue/purple may exist if problem is ongoing venous thrombosis | High level of circulatory incompetence, unpredictable/absence of adequate blood supply due to infarction/thrombosis of immediate and surrounding vessels<br>Increased cellular dysfunction, cytotoxic activity high with tissue destruction also increasing in adjacent areas<br>Local situation irretrievable without debridement<br>Contamination level increasing – high potential for infection (*Should not be confused with macerated tissue*). |
| Zone of anoxia leading to necrosis – oxygen levels zero | Black from arterial cessation of flow<br>Dark blue to purple to black with ongoing venous thrombosis | Blocked arterial or venous vessels, circulation to the region ceased, ultimately leading to anoxia and tissue necrosis (dead tissue). Irretrievable without debridement down to bleeding level<br>Cytotoxic to surrounding cells – increasing loss of immediate and surrounding tissue<br>Critical contamination levels increasing – high potential for infection |

## *Clinical assessment outcomes*

As discussed, the colour of open wound tissue can be equated with the status of vascularity, contamination, infection and the potential to heal or to progress to an increasingly chronic state.

Wound colour can also predict the potential for:

- 'Take' in split skin graft recipient sites (Figure 17.32)
- Monitoring of the skin of flaps (Figure 19.22) – dermal pricking to visualise the colour of the blood to determine vascular status
- Capillary refill, an essential tool in the assessment of burns – pricking the skin to check for normal dermal bleeding which indicates actual and the potential for dermal destruction.

Wound dressing companies have excellent teaching aids, photographs and videos that demonstrate

**Table 9.3** Wound depths, potential problem, healing times and scar outcomes in acute wounds.

| Wound depth described by tissue layers | Potential problem, healing times and scar outcomes |
|---|---|
| Normal intact skin | Closed wound, normal intact skin, some bruising, blanching erythema with capillary bed intact, significant internal tissue damage zero<br>**Goals** avoid swelling and pain<br>**Outcome** normal – zero scarring |
| Abrasion superficial – surrounding skin appears normal | Simple wound – relatively intact skin that is only superficially abraded (loss of 2–3 cell layers of epidermis)<br>Some inflammatory oedema, usually resolves within 72 hours<br>Heals quickly (5–7 days) if kept clean and occluded by moist wound healing dressing to prevent contamination and secondary injury. No scar tissue as dermis intact<br>**Goals** wound hygiene – wound protection – pain management<br>**Outcome** normal healing |
| Superficial – partial thickness skin | Simple/complex wound – superficial partial thickness level with loss of epidermis and the superficial layer of the dermis including some areas of the basement membrane – inflammatory oedema increased, resolves 72 hours+<br>In the absence of complicating factors, epidermis and dermis are capable of self-repair<br>Heals relative to the site, approximately 7–10 days, if kept clean and occluded by moist wound healing dressing to prevent significant contamination and secondary injury<br>**Goals** wound hygiene – no maceration – pain management<br>**Outcome** scar tissue least as dermal injury minimal |
| Deep partial thickness skin with zones of potential full thickness | Complex wound – partial thickness level with loss of the epidermis and some portion of the dermal layer<br>Not all micro vessels injured, and skin is capable of self-repair/recovery<br>In clean wound, may be expedited by direct closure if minimal skin lost, or application of moist wound healing dressings, negative pressure therapy or a split thickness skin graft<br>In untidy/contaminated wound, need to debride any unhealthy tissue to exclude infection<br>Healing time relative to closure method, absence of infection, approximately 10–21 days, more if left to contract and resurface<br>**Goals** wound hygiene – avoidance of increasing wound contamination and potential infection – pain management – patient support<br>**Outcome** scar tissue comparative to dermal contracting forces, relative to increasing dermal depth/level |
| Full thickness skin | Full thickness level with loss of the epidermis and the dermal layer usually includes superficial layer of subcutaneous tissue or hypodermis (fat cells) and may extend to the underlying fascia<br>Immediate surrounding skin demonstrates non-blanching erythema, oedema, indicates vascular insufficiency/compromise with capillary bed injury and may indicate substantial loss of vascular integrity at muscle level<br>This type of wound may require debridement, negative pressure therapy with early secondary closure, thick split thickness skin graft, full thickness skin graft or skin flap<br>Healing time is relative to closure method, 10–21 days in the absence of heavy contamination or development of infection<br>**Goals** achieve closure ASAP – avoid infection – pain management – patient support<br>**Outcome** scar outcome relative to the closure technique and patient normal response to injury |

**Table 9.3** *Continued.*

| Wound depth described by tissue layers | Potential problem, healing times and scar outcomes |
|---|---|
| Skin to muscle and/or including bone | **Compound wound** <br> Full thickness with loss of the epidermis and the dermal layer, includes superficial layer of subcutaneous tissue (fat cells) – extends to the underlying fascia, muscle and possibly bone; Referred to as 'compound wounds' as they are composed of many tissue layers <br> In post-traumatic wounds where vascular integrity is adequate, the application of negative pressure therapy for several days can reduce the level of oedema (and promote angiogenesis) and thus decrease the overall size of the wound <br> Many wounds can then be secondarily sutured or skin grafted <br> If wounds remain open following use of some temporary occlusive technique (moist wound healing, negative pressure therapy or split thickness skin graft) they are prone to infection and muscle necrosis, and this may lead to osteomyelitis, a potentially life-threatening condition <br> Usually a large complex wound that requires a tissue flap to restore vascular integrity <br> Difficult to predict exact healing time, outcome goal would be a minimum of 14 days, maximum of 28 days <br> Skin grafts and/or skin flaps may be considered if overall wound dimension is substantial and to reduce overall healing period <br> **Goals** prevent infection – pain management – patient support <br> **Outcome** scar outcome relative to the closure method absence of contamination or infection and patient normal response to injury |

single and multicoloured wounds and these are extremely useful for all clinicians involved in wound management.

## Wound depth

In describing wound depth, there is frequently an inconsistent use of the words **depth**, **stages** and **levels**, depending on the specialty areas. The terms 'stages' and 'levels' may also be used to describe the vertical depth of a tumour within the skin and soft tissue, and to describe the degree or extent of the spread of the tumour – the stage in, for example, breast cancers and malignant melanomas.

The term 'stage' may be used to describe the level of exposed tissue within, for example, pressure ulcers. Some nursing clinicians use the term 'level', as they believe that 'stage' implies an irreversible process moving towards an expected endpoint (i.e. healed).

Within accepted wound-based terminology, open wounds are not 'reversed staged'. Wounds heal upwards (**granulation**), inwards (**contraction**) and resurface (**epithelialisation**). Reverse staging is also not applied to describe traditional wound healing, for example partial full thickness skin graft donor sites. Reconstructive plastic surgeons will, however, often refer to the fact that a wound was 'deep partial' thickness, and that it is granulating and resurfacing rather than describing it as now, a superficial partial thickness wound.

In some wounds, plastic surgeons may use the term 'level' to describe the anatomic depth or thickness of tissue injury, and vice versa. For example, a wound may be described as being at the 'level' (depth) of the dermis, fascia, muscle or bone. When describing burns to the skin and skin graft donor sites, surgeons will describe wound depth as superficial thickness to full thickness.

These descriptive variations demonstrate how important it is to clarify what exact layer of skin is involved, and then include deeper structures by name to avoid any misunderstanding by other staff and the patient. Thus, as a clinical practice, to avoid confusion and in parallel with the current thinking, it seems reasonable to describe wound depth according to:

- the layered level of the skin in epidermal and dermal wounds
- stages 1–4/5 as described in modern texts related to the tissue type from skin to the base of the wound, as in pressure ulcers.

Table 9.3 provides an overview of wound depths using skin tissue layers, potential problems, healing times and scar outcomes.

## Describing a wound by exudate – type/colour/volume

With the exception of blood flow or frank pus, **exudate** is the general term used for the fluid that is discharged from a wound (i.e. clear, green, yellow), regardless of its aetiology, constituents and measured amount.

Although accuracy is important, traditional measurement of exudate in dressings is by subjective volume measurement. For example, nil, minimal moisture, moderate, or heavy exudate are common descriptions but other than nil, are relatively meaningless. Clinicians should establish what these generalised terms designate, as confusion regarding management modalities may occur unless some objective parameters are established.

The objective questions regarding fluid(s), their source, their site and effects on the wound to be addressed are shown in Box 9.7.

---

**Box 9.7** Assessment of fluid/exudate.

- Colour and suspected type of fluid
- Fresh or old blood, amount of loss
- Mixed blood/serum, intermittent or continuous
- Transparent fluid (cerebrospinal fluid) emanating from the ear or nose, diagnosed by glucose test
- Lymphatic fluid – thin opalescent (semitransparent white) colour – may also resemble a yellowish colour
- Pus – amount, consistency, odour
- Faecal material.

---

**Box 9.8** Exudate volume – estimating by objectivity.

| | |
|---|---|
| Dry | no exudate |
| Low exudate | 5 ml of exudate per 24 hours – wound bed moist – only surface contact marks on removed dressings |
| Heavy exudate | 5 ml or greater volume per 24 hours. |

---

**Box 9.9** Wound location – wound surrounds – the patient.

- The anatomical location of the wound and the source of the exudate:
  - Breast, abdomen, oral cavity
  - Fat layer, muscle layer or tissue combinations
- Peri-wound assessment – dressing choice may also need to reflect surrounding state of the skin, for example, uncontained incontinence, maceration of peri-wound and its edges, strike through on moisture managing dressings, effects of shear and friction
- Wound location may be difficult to sustain dressings
- Pain in and surrounding the wound – pain related to oedema and/or altered mobility
- Self injury – Munchausen's syndrome
- Co-operation and commitment of the patient to dressing changes
- Effects on patient safety, comfort and level of independence.

---

## *Selecting dressings to parallel exudate*

In many wounds, a single dressing will be appropriate from wound presentation to healing but there are many exceptions, and a regular objective wound bed assessment can assist.

Most moist wound healing dressings are described, in their accompanying literature, principally by the way in which they interact with the wound tissue and absorbency capacity. Selection of the dressing can be made by estimating the amount to be absorbed, naming the specific dressing used, and suggesting the regularity of change in relation to the dressing. This may assist in reducing unnecessary dressing changes and in observing reducing or increasing exudate movement, adjusting treatments appropriately.

One method of attaining relative accuracy of exudate volume is to weigh the dressings required for moderate to large volumes before application and after removal, documenting each change. In heavily draining wounds, a drainage bag similar to a stomal drainage bag is often used in order to reduce dressing intervention and patient discomfort. The container is then emptied daily or as required.

Objective clinical assessment of the patient and wound and its surrounds, allows for an evaluation of the wound status at any given time. Morbid, or co-morbid patient factors, or local wound conditions that affect wound repair can also be addressed in a timely manner.

## Wound dimensions and overall extent

One of the ongoing problems during any form of wound care is the number of clinicians that may be involved. It is useful to take photographs (normal SLR cameras or professional) on presentation and at specific intervals. *Digital photos are currently not legally accepted because of the ability for evidence to be tampered with, but they can be extremely useful clinically and for teaching.*

Photographs can act as a continuing record for the patient history, record of recovery for the individual patient, clinical teaching and legal implications. Plastic sheeting with grid marks to demonstrate mathematical dimensions is very useful, particularly for chronic wounds to demonstrate incremental increase, or resolution of size[1-6,13,14].

Two-dimensional plain hand drawings indicate dimensions for large wounds, using a clock face as a general guide to problem areas. Templates/photocopies of common anatomical zones are useful (e.g. arms, legs, the back or the face). These charting processes, including those of operative procedures, are used extensively in plastic surgery.

Computer programs for digital mapping of wounds in 3-D are now available in some hospitals, and used by an increasing range of community professional wound clinicians on laptop computers, for maintaining records, consulting with other colleagues, and education. Regardless of the type of objective records used, they provide important information to be contained in the patient's record, rationales for treatment changes, reminders for wound changes, information for court evidence if required, and for clinical teaching purposes.

## Summary

Every aspect of wound bed assessment determines wound care planning, including:

- Choice of in-patient or outpatient management, including overall control of co-morbid factors, level of mobility, potential for infection, pain and nutritional management
- Specific needs of each wound area, for example:
  - Need for debridement, wound cleansing, moist wound healing dressings to remove exudate and encourage tissue growth, normal contraction and epidermal resurfacing
  - Negative pressure therapy to remove excess oedema and allow the wound edges to more closely appose, or allowing wounds to heal by secondary intention or surgical intervention such as primary closure, delayed closure, skin grafts or skin flaps
  - Psychosocial issues including status of immediate and ongoing patient independence.

## *Addressing wound bed repair based on the wound bed assessment process*

Wound bed assessment takes into account the original aetiology of the injury, the type of tissue in the current bed of the wound, the type of tissue required in order to complete healing, and indicates the clinical interventions required to reach this position.

Apart from tissue in the wound bed, the specific location of wound, the volume of exudate, depth of injury, condition of surrounding (peri-wound) and any other factors which may impact on the total outcomes, must be considered. It is of primary importance that the wound is not assessed in isolation but as a fundamental part of the whole person. The overall management process (Figure 4.1) directly impacts on positive physiological and psychosocial outcomes required for safety, comfort and independence[1-22].

## Review

*Setting goals of care and preferred clinical and patient outcomes,* Chapter 2, Boxes 2.7–2.9. Adapt according to risk management issues and clinical patient needs.

*Auditing preferred clinical and patient outcomes,* Chapter 2, Boxes 2.10–2.12.

## References

(1) Dealey C. *The care of wounds*, 2nd edn. Oxford, UK: Blackwell Science, 1999.

(2) Flanagan M. A practical framework for wound assessment 1: physiology. *British Journal of Nursing*, 1996; **6**(1):6–11.

(3) Flanagan M. A practical framework for wound assessment 2: methods. *British Journal of Nursing*, 1996; **5**(22):1391–97.

(4) Carville K. *Wound care manual*, revised edn. Osbourne Park, Western Australia, Silver Chain Foundation, 1995.

(5) Naylor W., Laverty D. & Mallett J. *The Royal Marsden Hospital handbook of wound management in cancer care*. Oxford, UK: Blackwell Science, 2001.

(6) Schultz G.S., Sibbald R.G., Falanga V., Ayello E.A., Harding K., Stacey M.C., Teot L. & Vanscheidt W. Wound bed preparation: a systemic approach to wound management. *Wound Repair and Regeneration*, 2003 (Mar); **11** Suppl 1:S1–S28.

(7) Vowden K. & Vowden P. *Wound bed preparation*. http://www.worldwidewounds.com/

(8) Enoch S. & Harding K. Wound bed preparation: the science behind the removal of barriers to healing. *Wounds*, 2003; **15**(7):213–29. http://www.medscape.com/viewarticle/459733

(9) Bryant R.A. (ed.) *Acute and chronic wounds: nursing management*. St Louis: Mosby Year Book, 1992.

(10) http://www.wounds1.com/woundcareguide/WoundCareGuide10b.cfm (interactive wound assessment guide)

(11) Robinson J.B. & Friedman R.M. Wound healing and closure. *Selected Readings in Plastic Surgery*, **8**(1), 1996.

(12) Peacock E.E. Jnr. *Wound repair*, 3rd edn. Philadelphia: W.B. Saunders Company, 1984.

(13) Cutting K.F. & Harding K.G. Criteria for identifying wound infection. *Journal of Wound Care*, 1994 (June); **3**(4):198–201.

(14) Bowler P.G., Duerden B.I. & Armstrong D.G. Wound microbiology and associated approaches to wound management. *Clinical Microbiology Review*, 2001 (Apr): 244–69.

(15) Thompson P. The microbiology of wounds. *Journal of Wound Care*, 1998 (October); **7**(9):477–78.

(16) Robson M.C. Wound infection. A failure of wound healing caused by an imbalance of bacteria. *Surgical Clinics of North America*, 1997 (June); **77**(3):637–50.

(17) McCance K.L. & Huether S.E. *Pathophysiology: the biologic basis for disease in adults and children*, 3rd edn. St Louis: Mosby, 1998.

(18) Vardaxis N. *Pathology for the health sciences*. St Yarra, Australia: Macmillan Education Australia, 1994, reprinted 1998.

(19) Ausher B.M., Erikson E. & Wilkins E.G. *Plastic surgery: indications, operations and outcomes*. St Louis: Mosby, 2000.

(20) Morris A. McG., Stevenson J.H. & Watson A.C.H. *Complications of plastic surgery*. London: Baillière Tindall, 1989.

(21) Mallett J. & Dougherty L. (eds). *The Royal Marsden Hospital manual of clinical nursing procedures*, 5th edn. Oxford, UK: Blackwell Science, 2000.

(22) Dowsett C. The role of nurses in wound bed preparation. *Nursing Standard*, 2002 (Jul 17–23); **16**(44):69–72, 74, 76.

# Chapter 10

# Wound Bed Preparation Incorporating Wound Dressing and Bandage Management

1. Wound bed preparation – principles
2. Wound dressings – a basic approach to selection in reconstructive plastic surgery nursing

---

**Review**

Section I, Chapter 2, Tables 2.1 and 2.2
Section II, Chapters 8 and 9

---

## 1. WOUND BED PREPARATION – PRINCIPLES

### Background

In current times, there has been an increasing focus on scientific approaches to address the precise reasons for breakdown within normal wounds, and a failure of existing wounds to heal.

Wound bed preparation is a developing research-based concept that has been recently proposed to address the management of chronic wounds. Its genesis is based on the premise that wound bed preparation allows the clinician to address specific biological and psychosocial components whilst at the same time maintaining a global view of what outcome is desired to be achieved, and is acceptable to the patient[1-4].

Three principal clinical and patient outcomes are aimed for:

- Obtaining an unhindered research-based pathway towards normal wound repair
- Restoring the integrity of the integument through evidence-based approaches
- Restoring, or permitting, a preferred level of patient independence that delivers a quality of life acceptable to the patient.

These desired outcomes should be addressed through the setting of collaborative patient/clinician goals that are seen as practically achievable.

---

**Box 10.1** Proposed clinical application of wound bed preparation.

- Preparation of the patient prior to elective surgery through the risk management process to prevent adverse wound events from occurring
- Wound breakdown following elective surgical procedures
- Following accidental trauma
- Wound breakdown following traumatic wounding
- Chronic non-healing, or recurrent wounding
- Preparing malignant wounds to provide an optimal quality of life.

---

### The rationale for addressing wound bed preparation

Although a common clinical expression used in reconstructive plastic surgery (particularly in relation to recipient beds for split skin grafts), the term 'wound bed preparation' has recently begun to take on greater significance in general wound management[5,6].

Wound bed preparation is suggested to be a significant advancement in improving wound repair outcomes, as a central component of a total approach to science-based wound management towards wound bed repair. It can also be an approach to tackle the minimising of exudate, pain and odour and increase mobility to restore or provide an acceptable and stabilising quality of life.

An increasing understanding of the developing science of wound bed repair, the focus on costs to the patient and the community, the pain and disabling nature of chronic and cancer-based wounds, an outlining of the principles of wound bed preparation has recently assumed an even greater importance following any form of injury or disease.

With the advent of the increasing medical breakthroughs related to hygiene, microbiology, genetics, cellular biology, micro blood flow, antibiotics and modern science-based wound dressings, the goals set by wound bed preparation are now more achievable than ever.

Wounds that fail to respond to healing are as would be expected:

- Chronic or frequently recurring
- Highly debilitating, psychologically depressing for the patient and socially incapacitating
- Costly, transferring costs from preventive programmes to maintenance treatments
- Frustrating for the clinicians responsible for the patient's care.

They require:

- A professional healthcare enculturation that is expensive to fund
- Extensive multidisciplinary professional healthcare time
- Vast costs in surgery and wound products, to the patient and community
- Psychosocial care related to a quality of life that is acceptable to the patient.

Significant areas of biological concern are observed to be increasingly dominating wound care discussion and these are listed in Box 10.2.

**Box 10.2 Biological goals of wound bed preparation.**

- Restoration of an adequate circulatory blood flow
- Correction of cellular dysfunction
- Restoration of biochemical balance
- Restoration of bacterial balance in favour of the host
- Management of exudate
- Management of necrosis
- Maintenance of achieved wound repair goals[1-12].

**Box 10.3 Principal approaches to wound bed preparation.**

- Identified genetic aberrations, disease predispositions and lifestyle processes
- Identification of medical and nursing morbid and co-morbid factors
- Increased understanding of the blood supply to the skin
- Recognition of the implications of poor nutrition
- Application of the moist wound healing concept and principles to the development of modern dressings as an adjunct to addressing patient's physiological disturbances including pain management
- Increased understanding and application of scientific and adjunctive therapies as total approaches to the pain management processes
- Increased understanding of the science of compression techniques to reduce oedema, including the development of negative pressure therapy
- Understanding the pharmacology, advantages and disadvantages of wound cleansing solutions
- Understanding the psychosocial effects of disability, immobility, and loss of independence
- An understanding of the consequences of a failure to recognise and address the risks of a non-science based approach.

**Box 10.4 Advantages of a multidisciplinary approach to wound management.**

- Mobility – improving levels of mobility for greater independence by, for example, physical balance, provision of physical aids in the home or living environment
- Significant issues of acute and chronic oedema[13] can be managed by clinical nursing experts and allied health professionals
- Ability to undertake treatment(s) within the community (at home or as outpatient)
- Nutrition – assessing and managing important dietary needs
- Pharmacology – managing appropriate timing for medications (e.g. patients on diuretics), in relation to the timing of treatment modalities
- Experts to address psychosocial issues (body image disturbances, financial problems, as appropriate).

**Box 10.5** Significant areas of wound bed disturbances requiring wound bed preparation.

- In general terms, addressing the principle that *'what is missing needs to be restored or replaced'*
- A wound lacking an adequate blood supply and all the biological circulatory benefits (e.g. oxygen, nutrients, removal of toxic waste products, and the initiation of subsequent repair events), must have circulation restored or replaced[8,14]
- Wound bed disturbances which result in the normal host bacteria balance being tilted in favour of the bacteria will result in an increasing dominance of the host by the bacterial invasion
- The outcome of this is a wound bio-burden and systemic infection, wound tissue necrosis, and failure of the wound to heal unless the balance is restored in favour of the host[1–4,6–12]
- The substantial issues of wound bed and surrounding tissue pain must be resolved as a primary consideration
- The continuing presence of abnormal levels of oedema secondary to the normal inflammatory process of primary injury, or an existing disease process[13]
- Failure to address this atypical condition and to achieve a curative or palliative status, sets up a continuous cycle of unrelieved tissue hypoxia, ulceration, pain and infection, leading to patient disability, dysfunction, and depressive states[1–70]
- The problems of the mismatch of the treatment regime to a specific wound, due to clinical knowledge deficits in pathophysiology, and misunderstandings of what is observed and assessed
- Inaccurate wound bed assessment, preparation and management clinical modalities will result in intermittent and final adverse outcomes.

## Summary

The old adage of, *'preparation is the key to success'*, is unquestionably appropriate in wound management, to address interim goals and to deliver preferred outcomes, regardless of the wound type or site.

With the core concept of moist wound healing aiming to describe an optimal healing environment in clean wounds, further research is continuing to expand the important initial theoretical framework, and the transitional evidence-based application of wound bed preparation to chronic wounds, and wounds that require palliation, or ameliorating care.

Currently, research is centred into the identification of the principal wound growth factors, stem cells, and methods of applying synthetic growth factors, that appear to be absent in chronic wounds. The practical outcomes of these research areas appear years from the feasible use of placing the exact physiological growth products into, for example, wound dressings, to parallel the exact needs of each patient's wound.

## 2. WOUND DRESSINGS – A BASIC APPROACH TO SELECTION IN RECONSTRUCTIVE PLASTIC SURGERY NURSING

**Review**

Chapter 7 (Wound Bed Repair)

## The principles of applying moist wound healing to wound bed preparation

As previously discussed, the concept and principles of moist wound healing have been extensively researched and evidenced in acute wounds, but despite effective wound outcomes, its application has not been clearly demonstrated as the principal ingredient in the healing of chronic wounds.

What is known is that the removal, or stabilisation of known deterrents (e.g. patient morbid and co-morbid factors, oedema, contamination, infection, pain), and the application of moist wound healing dressings, have been very effective in many cases. Many questions remain unanswered, for example, 'what is the ratio of volume and type of moisture that is optimal?' The answer to this question may largely lie within a greater understanding and control of the dynamics and stabilisation of fluid movements for initiating wound bed repair and providing an optimal milieu for the initiation, or scientific application, of specific growth factors[1–4,7–10].

The physiological term 'moist wound healing' has largely taken on a life of its own in wound bed repair. It has also been adopted to describe most modern dressing products and these are referred to as 'moist wound healing' dressings.

One of the most common errors in wound care is the mismatch of wound bed assessment and the treatment/dressing selection prescribed for wound bed preparation and repair. Unless the manufacturers' instructions for use are carefully read and understood, there can be a misinterpretation that the product contains many (or all) of the essentials of what is required to remove the abnormal wound fluid and/or tissue, and to reproduce the desired milieu for the wound to heal.

Unfortunately, it is not always that simple, and for wounds other than most clean closed surgical wounds, a comprehensive assessment process of the patient and the wound, often necessitates a combination of interdisciplinary interventions. This latter approach may be necessary to restore the wound to the state where the 'optimal' milieu for undergoing moist wound healing can initiate the dynamics of the repair process. Parallel to this practice approach is the adoption of a wound care product that reflects atraumatic principles[9,10,16–23]. The removal/minimising of pain is a primary consideration when selecting any form of clinical management.

## Addressing wound drainage management

A normal open and healing wound is red, surrounded by pinkish tissues, with an exudate of a watery consistency, in minimal volumes, and readily removed by low exudate management moist wound healing dressings.

In a normal non-injured tissue environment, any fluid in excess to cellular requirements, fluid containing minute cytotoxic agents or dead cells, are removed by physiological feedback dynamics, and mechanisms aimed at maintaining continuity of a relative state of homeostasis.

Win an increase in abnormal fluid level states within the tissues, this requires mechanical removal until equilibrium is restored. Failure to do this results in adverse primary, secondary and tertiary wound instability, cellular breakdown, potential infection and a chronic wound bed state. The concept of the current dialogue on wound bed preparation is principally based on restoring equilibrium of fluid levels and the resolution of pain leading to the initiation of the wound bed repair process[1–4,6–27]. This is undertaken by approaches outlined in Box 10.6.

---

**Box 10.6** Wound drainage – appliance/mechanical applications – dressing applications.

- Surgical incision allowing for free drainage by tubes or wicks with the assistance of gravity (not advocated unless based on moist wound healing principles and sealed against outside environment)
- Application of an ostomy-type device that allows free drainage into a closed receptacle/bag
- Drainage tubes inserted into a wound, sealed and attached to mechanical suction devices or pre-vacuumed bottles
- Science-based compression bandaging and elevation of the part where possible
- Application of a range of specific science-based wound dressings (hydrophilic – hydro-selective) that contain factors that have the capacity to physiologically attract exudate (water, cytotoxic 'soups' and/or fatty exudate) into the dressing material
- The application of a mechanically driven topical (external) negative pressure device
- The use of soft tissue massage to assist lymphatic drainage.

---

**Review**

Figures 7.4–7.7

---

## Selecting a wound care product

As stated previously, many approaches in wound management remain based on expert experience or independent discretionary judgement, rather than scientific fact. In addition, much of current modern clinical practices are based on 'transitional' research (i.e. medical, nursing and allied health research that is increasingly providing research-based pathways to clinical applications).

The choice of a wound care product, dressing or bandage to be applied to a wound is not a random decision, rather it must be a science-based exercise that follows an accurate wound bed assessment[9,10,16–27]. For this to be achieved, certain criteria need to be considered.

**Box 10.7** Wound care products – important aspects to consider.

- No one dressing will meet all of a wound's requirements
- As the wound changes, so the tissue needs change, requiring a further wound bed assessment and potentially a change of product to meet the goal of care and wound repair outcomes
- Which group of products for which type of wound(s)?
- Which brand is the most appropriate, due to cost, availability and ease of use?
- How often does the dressing need to be changed?
- Does the patient have sufficient mobility to undertake dressing changes independently, or require assistance?

**Box 10.8** Ideal basic criteria for a wound care product.

- Safe to use
- Non-adherent
- Pain control is effective
- Absorption appropriate to the wound's needs
- Properties remain constant
- Cost effective to institutions and the patient
- Able to be sterilised
- Capable of standardisation
- Provide mechanical protection
- Freely available within the community
- Long shelf life.

**Box 10.9** Biological functions of modern wound care products.

**Function 1** protects the wound and surrounds, assists in correcting the problem within the wound, controls pain, has aesthetic qualities without altering the dressings function – dressing is acceptable to the patient

**Function 2** fluid donating (debriding) or fluid absorbing

**Function 3** products which actively promote debriding and moisture management

**Function 4** retention (fixation sheet) dressings have both primary dressing applications (protect superficial injured tissue) and secondary dressing properties (hold primary dressings in place).

**Box 10.10** Biological requirements of modern wound care products.

- To assist in controlling low level haemorrhage
- To assist in a normal and uninterrupted wound repair continuum in a pain-free environment in the optimal timeframe
- Provision of a normothermic moist wound healing environment that aims to simulate a normal wound bed milieu
- To provide thermal insulation by maintaining a constant temperature of 36.8°–37°C for optimal mitotic activity
- A drop of 2°C at the wound surface may take up to four hours to return to previous level of optimal activity – cells are suggested to cease to function in temperatures less than 30°C
- To maintain an optimal wound humidity to prevent the wound from becoming dry and forming eschar, preventing direct cell migration across the wound bed
- To allow gaseous exchange by increasing the level of oxygen and nutrients to the wound via the microcirculation, reducing the level of wound contamination arising from dead cells
- To provide optimal patient comfort and pain relief during the healing phase and allow removal without pain and discomfort during dressing change by selecting a dressing that requires reduced frequency of dressing changes
- To be free of particles and toxic wound contaminants by selecting dressings that do not shed fibres (gauze, cotton wool) that cause irritations, leading to infection, or cause sinuses or lead to wound granulomas
- To be impermeable to bacteria by providing a barrier to airborne bacteria from entering the wound, and wound bacteria from escaping from the wound
- To remove excess exudate by selecting a dressing that absorbs in parallel with the level of exudate, and prevents maceration of surrounding skin
- To provide odour control, by managing the bacterial bio-burden – particular odours distress the patient, significant carers and staff
- To protect the wound from secondary physical damage, and minimise discomfort/pain by restoring and correcting anatomical form through realigning tissues, and providing temporary immobilisation
- Provision of aesthetic properties to reduce the distress of patients and others from the visual effects of a wound.

## Classification of wound products

There are several methods of describing wound care products but as clinicians learn and understand more about their scientific constituents, two classifications dominate[9,10]:

- Products described through their **pharmacology**
- Products described by their **function**.

### Box 10.11 Wound care products by pharmacology.

- Natural fibre dry dressings – gauze, cotton wool, combinations
- Synthetic fibre gauze – woven or spun-bonded synthetic gauze fibre
- Non-adherent, non-absorbent dressing – knitted synthetic viscose rayon
- Dry non-adherent or film coated
- Tulle Gras dressing
- Tulle Gras with impregnated antiseptics or antibiotics
- Semipermeable films – polyurethane film dressings
- Polyurethane foam dressings
- Hydrocolloid products
- Calcium alginate products
- Hydrocolloids – hydrocolloid (absorbent – paste/powder)
- Hydrogels
- Odour absorbing
- Pressure relieving dressings
- Silicone gel sheets
- Haemostatic agents
- Hydro-fibre products
- Fixation sheet dressings.

### Box 10.12 Wound care products described by function.

- Wound protection products
- Wound rehydration products
- Moisture retention products
- Wound debridement products
- Compression therapy products
- Skin-care/protection products.

## Risk management in the selection of dressing/retention tapes

### Box 10.13 Contemporary adhesive backed retention tapes.

- Many of the modern semipermeable film dressings or fixation sheet dressings may themselves be used as wound dressings where there is little or no exudate
- Superficial skin thickness donor sites for skin grafts and superficial burns are examples of situations where, for example, film dressings, fixation sheet dressings and the new generation soft silicone-based dressings can be used as primary or secondary dressings
- They can themselves act as superficial epidermal substitutes for enclosed moist wound healing and wound protection, until epidermal resurfacing takes place
- Thus contemporary and scientifically designed fixation/retention dressings may be used to secure a wound dressing in place, or imitate/mimic the epidermis as a protective cover over minimal/non-exudating superficial wounds to aid the moist wound healing process and minimise/prevent pain
- They can maintain wound dressings in position by providing a low level splinting effect, increasing the level of comfort, and reduce/prevent secondary injury.
- Wound tapes and, specifically, dressing fixation/retention tapes/sheets, come in a variety of sizes and scientific components
- They have the ability to conform to body contours that allows them to be utilised in a range of wound situations (e.g. in plastic surgery, particularly the hand for early mobility)
- They must not be stretched and used as pressure or medical compression dressings
- Should some pressure be required, this may be achieved by the application of crepe or elastic-based bandages, alone or over retention dressings/tapes
- Synthetic medical adhesive backed 'paper' type products are available in skin colour and these are popular with surgeons and patients as they assist in disguising the presence of a wound
- They have particularly advantages for their clinical, adhesive and aesthetic qualities for supporting/maintaining wound edges in apposition following small excised and sutured wounds
- They are also useful for additional epidermal wound support following suture removal, scar management and their application may assist in the prevention of local secondary injury by temporarily reminding the patient of their wound.

**Box 10.14** Clinical nursing risk management issues.

- Certain adhesive tapes are contraindicated in particular areas such as highly sensitive irradiated or excoriated skin
- Because of the extensive range available, all dressings and retention tapes, regardless of their type, must be applied according to the manufacturers' specific indications and instructions and the patient's allergy status should also be ascertained
- Retention/fixation tapes must not be stretched prior to application to the skin, as their function is to hold a dressing in place, or act as an artificial epidermal substitute
- All retention/fixation tapes have a minimal degree of stretch and 'memory' built in, but the purpose of this is to allow for normal conforming movement of the skin with a splinting effect
- When additional restriction of movement is required, different approaches are taken to ensure a true splinting effect, for example, slings, the use of moulded plaster of Paris, thermoplastic materials or Zimmer® metal-based splints
- When wounds expand and swell beyond the tape's capacity to conform, the tape should be removed immediately. Otherwise, shear and friction caused by overstretching of the tape will cause erythematous rashes, blisters and subsequent distress to the patient
- Despite manufacturers' instruction for use, inappropriate applications of a tape frequently occurs, and the above adverse outcomes continue to be mistaken for allergic reactions to the adhesive component of the dressing/retention tape (particularly Elastoplast®)
- Many excellent adhesive retention tapes have subsequently been labelled 'flawed' and clinically discarded because of inadequate knowledge of the value of the products when applied according to the manufacturer's instruction
- Adhesives tapes and dressings must never be applied to overlap onto themselves, specifically on a limb or digit, as any oedema/swelling may produce a tourniquet effect and cause catastrophic avascular outcomes
- Even tightly applied Band-Aids® may cause problems of reduced blood flow (i.e. acts as a tourniquet), particularly in children
- Adhesive tapes tightly applied over the chest region can cause restricted ventilation of the lungs, leading to respiratory complications in addition to skin irritation due to shear and friction
- Firmly applied tapes and bandages are contraindicated following breast surgery, with the use of bandages or circular taping of the rib cage/chest wall having fallen into disrepute
- The objective management of potential postoperative bleeding by disciplined intra-operative haemostasis, and control of postoperative pain, has been made the primary focus in providing proper pain-free chest/lung expansion
- For this reason the use of most previously called 'chest strapping tapes' has been confined to only securing/retaining dressings in place in this region
- Fixation sheet dressing materials or elastic-based mesh/net tubular bandages are best suited to these areas to allow free movement of the chest wall
- Following abdominal surgery, elasticised and adjustable Velcro binders, used as external garments to support the primary dressing of choice, are the most appropriate
- Medical grade polyurethane film wipe products are now widely available for application prior to the retention tapes
- These act to protect the patient's skin, and to enhance adhesion/bonding by the tape. Medical grade adhesive solvents are also available, enabling the removal of tapes to be relatively pain-free
- Some non-medical grade adhesives continue to be used by many surgeons to secure retention tapes, to enhance tape bonding to the skin, and to prevent early curling of the retention tape edges that may be caused by friction on clothes, etc.
- These can potentially cause skin damage, are not accredited for medical use in wound care, and should be avoided by nurse clinicians
- Surgeons who wish to use them should apply them personally
- The potential for litigation, in the non-medically accredited use of these agents, should be considered prior to application.

See recommended websites (wound dressings, retention and tubular retention dressings) at the end of this chapter.

# Bandaging, compression and dressing retention

Prior to the application of any dressing or compression bandage, the first principle is to ask the question *'exactly what do I want this dressing or the exerted compression to scientifically and/or clinically achieve?'* (see Tables 10.1 & 10.2).

As surgical compression by elasticised products has an expected and decreasing effect over about 30 minutes when pressure or compression is applied for bleeding, should the bleeding continue, the wound should be investigated[11]. Continued low level post-surgery wound bleeding (longer than 30 minutes) commonly means that the leaking vessels are too large to be stopped simply by compression, dressings, or externally applied pressure by the hand, and

**Table 10.1** Bandage actions and rationale.

| Bandage action | Rationale |
| --- | --- |
| Extensibility | Determines the change in length that is produced when the bandage is subjected to an extending force (extended in both directions at the same time) |
| Power | Determines the force that is required to bring about specific bandage length |
| Elasticity | Determines the ability of the bandage to extend related to the force applied |
| Compression | Implies the deliberate level of compression in order to produce a desired pressure effect, improving venous flow and the movement of extracellular fluids |
| Support | The retention and control of tissue immobility without application of compression |
| Conformability | The ability of the bandage to follow the contours of the limb or body part – governed largely by the density and extensibility of the fabric |
| Aesthetic properties | Visual effect<br>As a wound cover to conceal disfigurement |

**Table 10.2** Rationale for bandage use.

| Bandage function | Purpose/outcome |
| --- | --- |
| **Retention** of dressings | Assist in moist wound healing by maintaining dressing stability |
| **Protection** of the wound | Assist in prevention of wound shear and friction that may result in secondary injury at or around the wound site |
| Support | Restrict movement to prevent unintended secondary injury |
| Fixation | |
| Immobilisation | |
| Compression<br>Moderate to high = 18–35 mm at the ankle<br>Extra-high = 35–50 mm at the ankle | Aid in re-establishing and maintaining circulation<br>Immobility<br>Reduction of oedema essential for cellular maintenance |
| **Correction** of deformity | Restore, correct and maintain anatomical form |
| **Relief** of pain | Provide wound splinting that decreases the degree of movement and increases the level of comfort |
| Patient **recognition** of the injury | Provide additional wound protection |
| **Aesthetic** properties | Patient and community acceptance of visual difference |

this will require surgical intervention[6]. Such bleeding may occur where diathermy, sutures or sub-atmospheric drains have not been wholly effective.

Where continuous oozing of micro vessels occurs, with a rise in postoperative blood pressure and pain, there may also be increased risks of slow haemorrhage and formation of haematoma. This is particularly relevant in those patients who are taking medications such as aspirin, prophylactic anti-stroke medication, warfarin, therapeutic heparin, anti-inflammatory medications, or some herbal preparations.

When vasoconstricting agents (such as adrenaline) have been added to local anaesthetic agents, and begin to lose their efficacy, this may initiate slow but continuous ooze from vessels, causing the formation of a haematoma.

This is a danger when local anaesthesia and adrenaline (either in small or large volumes) are used, as they are commonly in reconstructive plastic surgery and aesthetic surgery. This could require return of the patient to the operating room, surgical control of the bleeding, and the need for an internal negative pressure drainage system inserted for the first 24 to 48 hours. Clinicians should be fully conversant with the range of medication currently being taken by the patient or added/used during the surgical procedure.

Wound observation and ongoing pain assessment are important in evaluating whether a haematoma is developing, or the dressing is too tight and causing ischaemic wound pain. Haematoma is the principal precursor to infection in otherwise clean wounds. To reduce the potential development of dead space, haematoma, significant or excess serous fluid, swelling and oedema, the use of short term internal or negative pressure drainage systems, plus dressing and bandage application, with elevation to assist in gravitational flow, is considered standard practice.

## Applied clinical risk management principles

Before selecting a bandage, the following questions should be asked:

- Is a bandage required?
- Does this bandage do what is required?
- What are the risks?

- Could some other product be more effective and less costly? (See Tables 10.1 & 10.2).

Principally, in wounds that require a secondary dressing (e.g. bandage), these will usually be described under the headings in Box 10.15.

**Box 10.15** Common types of bandages – examples.

| | |
|---|---|
| Non-extensible | e.g. cotton |
| Extensible | e.g. cotton, rayon, synthetic, elastic |
| Adhesive or cohesive | e.g. cotton or synthetic material – may stick to itself |
| Orthopaedic casts | e.g. plaster of Paris, fibreglass, plastic |
| Orthopaedic padding | cotton and/or synthetic |
| Medicated paste or gel | e.g. cotton gauze or crepe bandages impregnated with medications combined with zinc base. |

### Crepe bandages

The quality of 'crepe' and other forms of elastic non-cohesive bandages differs. For example, crepe elastic bandages (commonly used by reconstructive plastic surgeons) differ in the quality of material, of the elastic material woven in, how and in which country they are made, and the level of hygienic conditions under which they are manufactured.

Reconstructive plastic surgical nurses should be familiar with differences in bandage quality, as this dictates the method of application and the effect following application. The rationale for purchasing cheaper crepe or elastic bandages should first be evaluated. Cheaper elasticised bandages can be used to maintain splints (i.e. for retention purposes) but they will usually need additional external securing tapes to stop slippage and ensure a degree of conformity.

Elastic-based tubular retention garments can be applied over these cheaper bandages for children, in order to maintain immobility and reduce slippage, shear and friction.

Applying poor quality crepe elastic bandages in an attempt to gain the same effect as a high quality bandage can result in these lower quality bandages acting as tourniquets because of the lack of uniform properties.

Inferior quality crepe or elastic bandages should also not be used on fingers, hands or limbs, or over the eye or ears, as there is the high potential for vascular damage. For example, any attempt to exert compression over the eyes following upper or lower lid surgery is fraught with risk because of the potential for excessive pressure on the globe or damage to the cornea[14].

Any bandages applied by the surgeon should be monitored for pain or any comment from the patient that the eye feels itchy or they feel 'something' in their eye[14]. This should be reported immediately and the bandage removed. It is stated that 30–40 minutes of corneal abrasion can result in permanent scarring and potential blindness[6,14]. Any bandages over the eyes should be removed on return to the surgical unit, or prior to the patient being discharged if admitted as a day patient. Ongoing clinical skills by clinicians in the use of top quality bandages, develops as the uniformity of the product becomes more reliable and precise.

Surgeons should be informed when the crepe bandage brand is changed for any reason. There is a truism here: *you get what you pay for*. High quality, medically graded crepe bandages remain the choice of the majority of plastic surgeons.

---

**Box 10.16** Methods of soft tissue compression – examples.

- Medical grade crepe bandages
- Cohesive bandage techniques (e.g. Coban™)
- Negative pressure therapy (VAC® Therapy)[16–20]
- Commercial adjustable compression garments (e.g. abdominal binders, upper or lower limb splints such as Zimmer®)
- Graduated tubular compression garments (e.g. Tubigrip®)
- Application of silicone sheeting or gels to reduce scars (e.g. Spenco® Silicon® dressing, Cica-Care®)
- Tie-over dressings used to secure skin grafts or scalp dressings in place.

---

## Compression techniques – the principles

The term compression essentially means 'pressing together'. In respect of surgical wounds, the overall goals of compression are to provide a level of pressure not greater than 22–28 mm Hg maximum pressure at capillary level to ensure the integrity of the microvascular system[11].

Several methods of compression, or approaches for exerting desired levels of pressure, are commonly used in reconstructive plastic surgery (Box 10.15).

Note: It must be pointed out that the above stated pressure gradient is not related to the scientific studies and medical-based grading for levels of compression which have been advocated to manage the oedema related to venous ulceration and lymphoedema.

---

**Box 10.17** Rationale for expert-based compression techniques in surgical wounds.

- Protection of the microcirculatory system
- To assist in the removal of oedema or excess interstitial fluid in the wound bed and surrounding tissue
- Suggested to minimise/reduce the degree of scar tissue forming following burns, for example, in applying a downward force to the immediate and peripheral surrounds of a wound, a compression effect is obtained by mechanically exerting a prescribed level of a uniform energy
- The use of the term 'pressure' dressing is perhaps an anomaly in modern wound care, and may be better applied where occlusion of arterial blood flow is required to halt a haemorrhaging vessel and exsanguination
- The goal of attaining a constant compression through a wound dressing (when applying a sustained degree of pressure) is essentially a misnomer unless it applies to a wound in a fixed skin anatomical area (the upper or lower limbs)
- Counter pressure can be exerted by a fixed structure in the centre (e.g. solid bone[5]) and the limb remains completely immobile.

---

## *Risk management in compression by bandage technique*

Exerting exact levels of effective uniform pressure or compression cannot be sustained for extended periods because of the gradual loss of elastic integrity in the bandage or tape through regional or local normal movement.

The pressure initially produced gradually reduces to zero over 30 minutes as the dead space in the gauze/wool itself collapses and flattens out and the compression dressing will gradually lose any elastic qualities it may have had[6]. With this in mind, the use of gravity (elevation of the part) has the potential to override this loss of compression and aid in the removal of oedema, by reducing the arterial flow, and assisting the venous and lymphatic return.

Unfortunately, in an effort to exert semi-rigid compression, the bandages or tapes applied in an attempt to attain a desired pressure level can effectively become a tourniquet, or result in shear and friction to the skin with even the slightest movement of the region.

This tourniquet effect can often be seen in the digits of the hand following surgery where crepe bandages are applied in an unnecessary and potentially dangerous effort to reduce oedema or postoperative bleeding (e.g. a tourniquet outcome leading to ischaemia of the part). In the limbs, the most effective method is to use a dressing, plaster wool, crepe bandage and immobilising plaster splint, with elevation of the limb above the level of the heart, and a pain-free environment. Bleeding in other parts of the body requires uniform pressure or surgical intervention.

Many surgeons remove crepe bandages and/or dressings from closed 'straightforward' wounds after 24–48 hours, particularly in elective hand surgery when early mobilisation is part of the rehabilitation programme. Surgeons may then request the application of adhesive soft silicone dressings, or fixation sheet dressings, to reinforce and protect the wound and suture line.

For regions of mobile skin/tissue such as the chest wall and abdomen, modern retention dressing tapes (as outlined above) are appropriate for increasing levels of mobility in the early stages of recovery. Oedema in these regions is subject to the normal dynamics of gravity and the early restoration of blood flow that includes the re-establishment of the dynamics of intrinsic physiological negative pressures, or the use of negative pressure therapy.

It is important not to impede cardiorespiratory function by the use of compression tapes. Brassières and medical graded abdominal binders should be applied with firmness, not at levels that restrict normal respiratory function, but rather provide support, comfort and protection.

## Cohesive bandages

The term *'cohesive'* means *'sticking together in a consistent manner'*. In bandage terms this means the bandage will remain firmly in its applied position (not sticking to the skin but to itself), providing strong resistance to increasing internal swelling.

The early 1970s saw the introduction of Coban™, a new generation of bandage called a *'cohesive'* bandage. These gained popularity with neurosurgeons to maintain difficult cephalin head dressings, and with plastic surgeons to secure outer bandages on the limbs. Coban's™ benefits were marred by a lack of understanding of the difference between it, a cohesive (solid, consistent) bandage and a crepe (cotton with added lightweight elastic fibres) bandage. Because of this there was incorrect application, resulting in some reported cases of wound ischaemia in the scalp and limbs.

Coban's™ true value was reinstated when the medical benefits of reducing oedema were realised when it was applied according to the manufacturer's advice. This was particularly in the ongoing exclusion of oedema in fingers/hands during rehabilitation by hand therapists and in the treatment of venous ulcer oedema by securing 3–4-layer bandages. With its scientific quality of manufacture, Coban™ has excellent 'memory' and self-adhering properties over much longer timeframes than ordinary crepe bandages when applied according to the manufacturer's instructions.

Cohesive or compression bandages are used extensively by limb therapists particularly those involved in hand and lower limb rehabilitation. Sustained compression significantly aids in reducing oedema in these fixed skin regions and enables increasing normal movement of the digits. This is important in minimising joint stiffness, and internal fibrous tissue scarring, which is suggested to take place at approximately week 3.

Because of the ability of a cohesive bandage to maintain long-term elastic compression properties, it is also used to protect bandages in children. Again, it must be applied strictly in accordance with the manufacturer's instructions, keeping in mind the risks of vascular compromise associated with inappropriate application. Although cost may be somewhat prohibitive for some institutions, this ability to sustain compression combined with hand or leg movement provides a pumping action to assist venous return, which accelerates recovery time and provides cost benefits. The benefits of modern cohesive bandages far outweigh the costs when used selectively and judiciously, and the risks are safely managed.

Medically designed graduated compression bandages and garments that provide specific amounts of compression are also available for burns, long-term scar management and ongoing oedematous limbs. Expert wound care clinicians and allied health professionals are trained to measure and fit these garments to gain their best effect and protect the patient from secondary adverse events, for example, injury.

## Specific risks in the use of surgical retention tapes, compression and retention bandages in plastic surgery

The primary function of any elasticised adhesive tape (e.g. Elastoplast®) is the retention of a dressing in place. In addition, they can provide a minimal splinting effect. Their principal advantage is to allow for some expansion in the presence of normal swelling following application and to retract when swelling recedes (bandage memory). This memory is 'short' in that the elastic qualities, as in crepe bandages, are lost when unrestricted mobility is allowed or is constant.

To secure head and limb dressings and external bandages:

- One inch (2.5 cm) skin coloured Elastoplast®
- Half (1 cm) or one inch (2.5 cm) zinc oxide tape (zinc oxide has no elastic qualities)
- Coban™, still preferred by many plastic surgeons (see Chapter 24).

Tapes must not be applied directly from their roll, as uniformity of application cannot be guaranteed. Regardless of the type of tape selected, it should be cut to appropriate lengths from the roll prior to application, and applied firmly but without stretch.

The purpose of using adhesive retention tapes is to prevent the bandages from slipping and retaining the dressing in place, not an attempt to exert pressure or compression. Tapes applied too tightly may cause pain and discomfort and, rather than meeting their designated purposes can easily have a tourniquet effect and compromise blood flow (e.g. following limb surgery or ear reconstruction). This can occur particularly when normal inflammatory wound oedema and swelling is present in the first 48 to 72 hours post-injury or post-surgery.

## Importance of a scientific selection of tapes/bandages

One of the most common mistakes made in bandaging techniques is a mismatch between the bandage size and the region to be bandaged, and thus the accuracy of application and absence of the desired effect. Because patients and the sites to be bandaged vary in size, the width of the bandages should be carefully chosen to provide uniform and secure relative compression. For example, applying a wide bandage to a narrow leg means that no effective conformity or compression can be gained even in the short term, as the bandage wrinkles with movement, and will soon become dysfunctional.

A narrow bandage on a wide area will usually lose its integrity, and either fall off or act as a tourniquet. The selection of finger bandages to match the dimensions of each finger is an important example. The bandages may be furthered secured by cohesive retention tapes, or over bandages of an appropriate size, to secure the fingers collectively, for extra protection and to minimise movement.

Combinations of cotton and elastic supports (e.g. Surgifix®) that are constructed in a tubular form with a range of compression and sizes, are extremely useful in retaining crepe bandage dressings or basic loose dressings in both children and adults. The elastic fibres adhere very firmly to the crepe bandage, preventing early slippage and reducing the problems of poorly applied tapes and the reduced firmness of the compression bandage. These tubular dressings are useful for the first 72 hours in securing facial dressings that are used to absorb copious level of exudate sometimes experienced by the patient following laser or dermabrasion surgery to the face. They should be selected so as not to place undue pressure, but rather provide dressing conformity.

The use of single or double-layered elasticised tubular garments can be quite useful in place of bandages where very low levels of compression are required in association with maintenance of a dressing beneath, remembering that double layers double the compression applied. Objective goals must be set for what is required to be achieved by the application of dressings and bandages before selection is made. Failure to undertake an objective assessment that includes risk management means that preferred clinical outcomes will not be achieved and the patient may incur unnecessary injury and cost.

## Physiological risk management issues for plastic surgery nurses

Like many otherwise effective treatments, if used inappropriately, and in 'at risk' patients, compression that exceeds arteriole, capillary and venous pressures can cause serious injury or tissue necrosis and in some cases may lead to limb or digit amputation. Children and the elderly are in the high-risk category. It should be remembered that patients with lower limb venous disease and cardiac conditions where there is generalised oedema or lower limb oedema due to gravity and immobility, may not be suitable for compression bandaging in the limbs. This is because an increased cardiac load may occur and initiate a shift of the circulating fluid volume, putting increased stress upon the right side of the heart leading to pulmonary stress.

Diabetes mellitus and peripheral vascular disease patients also fall into the high-risk category. Before the application of 'firm' compression to the lower limb, ankle brachial pulse index (ABPI) measurement is an essential tool to clinically demonstrate any existing arterial problems. Proficiency in taking an ABPI measurement is a skill that all nurses involved in wound care should acquire and maintain.

The use of compression therapy is contraindicated in patients with suspected or known arterial disease. Medical advice must be sought before commencing treatment. Compression in excess of 22–28 mm Hg exerted on wounds with vascular fragility, following upper or lower limb flap reconstruction or skin grafting procedures, is also contraindicated[24–27].

## Tie-over wound dressings

A variation of the compression technique is referred to as a 'tie-over' dressing. The decision to use this type of dressing is to secure grafts in regions where patient movement results in inadequate donor/recipient bed contact (e.g. on movement/mobility the graft falls off), graft movement, to exclude dead

space in the wound, to facilitate general mobility of the patient, and to allow home management.

The most important factor in utilising this type of dressing is to gain initial uniform pressure over the grafted wound sufficient to prevent the collection of fluid of haematoma under the donor skin, which would prevent skin adhesion. Donor skin may be mechanically meshed, or multiple holes may be inserted by sharp scissors or a sharp scalpel blade. This attempts to serve two purposes:

• Prevent the accumulation of blood or fluid under the donor skin
• Allow blood or serous fluid accumulating under the graft to escape to the surface[1,14]

A non-adherent dry, or film-coated dressing should be placed over the donor skin after it is placed in the wound to avoid adherence and lifting of the graft at the time of primary dressing.

One, or half-inch sterile porous polythene foam is the choice of most surgeons and this is determined by the size of the area to be grafted. Wet wool, or acriflavine wool (a mixture of acriflavine and paraffin oil emulsion in which cotton wool is soaked, and the excess emulsion expunged), are examples of less scientific alternatives. The two principal dressing techniques currently in favour are polythene foam or the VAC® system.

Again, the pressure exerted should not be greater than the wound capillary pressure (22–28 mm Hg) or the fragile blood flow to the grafted area and the donor skin will be blocked.

The height of the dressings, within the dead space, is important for initial wound compression, and should be about 30–50% or 20–30 mm higher than the level of the normal skin margins to obtain the required degree of overall compression. Judgement is necessary in relation to the depth of the wound and this will often require the use of more than one piece of polythene foam, usually cut in decreasing sizes to meet the required height at the centre of the wound, which is the most difficult zone to sustain equal compression.

Polythene foam may be secured with the edge of the skin and the foam sutured together, tied over with holding sutures from opposing wound corners, or attached with staples. The specific positioning of the staples (e.g. star-like formation) is important to obtain uniform pressure. Acriflavine wool is secured with sutures tied over from opposing edges.

Pain within the first 24 hours is a common clinical indicator of pressure that causes local ischaemia and, if reported, should be investigated immediately[6]. Pain after this time is likely to be caused by the early development of wound infection. (Prior to discharge, patients should be educated to observe for any of the cardinal signs of excess inflammation or infection, particularly pain.)

Regardless of the material used, retention tape or gauze and a bandage may then be gently applied to produce additional compression, retention of the dressing and overall comfort and protection from secondary injury. The bandage may be removed and a retention tape applied after 48 hours, for comfort and aesthetics. Tie-over dressings on the limbs are usually splinted (with plaster of Paris or commercial splints) for up to seven days to prevent shear and friction.

In some cases (e.g. larger wounds), the application of negative pressure therapy (VAC® system) is fast superseding other forms of skin graft bed immobilisation for achieving successful skin graft management. The technique is particularly applicable for patients with complex wounds, difficult wounds to immobilise, and patients who are hospitalised, or confined to bed. The availability of small mobile VAC® units is also allowing patients to be managed in the community, reducing the necessity for inpatient care and increasing patient mobility and independence.

### Tie-over dressing on the scalp

On the scalp, bleeding comes from the wound edges. Compression and appropriately placed sutures or skin clips provide methods to achieve haemostasis. This does not necessarily reduce the incidence of haematoma, as a degree of dead space will exist between the skin and scalp fascia where blood can accumulate.

To minimise the initiation of a haematoma a tie-over compression dressing similar to the securing of a skin graft is frequently applied. For example:

- Following initial suturing or stapling of the wound, additional wound sutures are inserted approximately 1–1.5 cm outside the primary suture line, without initially being fixed

- Gauze or polythene foam is folded into a firm roll (like a tampon or large dental roll) and placed along the length of the primary suture line
- The secondary sutures are tied over the gauze, exerting firm, but not tight, compression
- Usually no other dressing is required
- If the patient complains of any pain, the dressing should be checked to ensure the tie-over sutures are not exerting excess tension or pressure, causing ischaemia of the wound edges, or that a haematoma has not formed adjacent to the suture line.

## Preferred outcomes of wound bed repair through wound bed preparation

- Accurate assessment and stabilisation of the patient's physiological and psychosocial status including the needs of the wound was undertaken prior to setting goals to achieve optimal wound bed preparation
- Achievable wound bed preparation goals for wound bed repair were set to realise the optimal steps towards wound bed repair
- Ongoing clinical risk management and process audits were undertaken to prevent/minimise adverse events during the process of wound bed preparation
- Achievable patient, comfort, independence, and wound repair outcomes were set to be achieved within a realistic time frame and to the patient's satisfaction.

## Guidelines for the current principles of best practice

In 2004, the World Union of Healing Societies, at an international conference in Paris, France, formulated and published a research-based document, *Principles of Best Practice – minimising pain at wound dressing-related procedures – a consensus document*. See website: http://www.wuwhs.org/consensus/index.html.

This is a significant and very timely document for all clinicians involved in many facets of wound management, and could form much of the foundation for current pain management in wound care practices[29].

Also in 2004, a position document on *Wound bed preparation in practice* was launched at the EWMA (European Wound Management Association) meeting. This document is available from http://www.mepltd.co.uk/oneoffs.html, in a range of languages.

## References

(1) Vowden K. & Vowden P. *Wound bed preparation*. http://www.worldwidewounds.com/

(2) Enoch S. & Harding K. Wound bed preparation: The science behind the removal of barriers to healing. *Wounds*, 2003; **15**(7):213–29. http://www.medscape.com/viewarticle/459733

(3) Dowsett C. The role of nurses in wound bed preparation. *Nursing Standard*, 2002 (July 17–23); **16**(44):69–72, 74, 76.

(4) Schultz G.S., Sibbald R.G., Falanga V., Ayello E.A., Harding K., Stacey M.C., Teot L. & Vanscheidt W. Wound bed preparation: a systemic approach to wound management. *Wound Repair and Regeneration*, 2003 (Mar 11); **Suppl 1**:S1–S28.

(5) Montandon D. *Clinics in plastic surgery: an international quarterly. Wound healing*. Philadelphia: W.B. Saunders Company, 1977.

(6) Robinson J.B. & Friedman R.M. Wound healing and closure. *Selected Readings in Plastic Surgery*, 1996, **8**(1).

(7) Robson M.C. Wound infection. A failure of wound healing caused by an imbalance of bacteria. *Surgical Clinics of North America*, 1997 (June); **77**(3):637–50.

(8) Bowler P.G., Duerden B.I. & Armstrong D.G. Wound microbiology and associated approaches to wound management. *Clinical Microbiology Reviews*, 2001 (Apr): 244–69.

(9) Dealey C. *The care of wounds*, 2nd edn. Oxford, UK: Blackwell Science, 1999.

(10) Carville K. *Wound care – manual*, revised edn. Osbourne Park, Western Australia, Silver Chain Foundation, 1995.

(11) Peacock E.E. Jnr. *Wound repair*, 3rd edn. Philadelphia, W.B. Saunders Company, 1984.

(12) Bryant R.A. (ed.) *Acute and chronic wounds: nursing management*. St Louis: Mosby Year Book, 1992.

(13) Guyton A.C. & Hall J.E. *Textbook of medical physiology*, 9th edn. London: W.B. Saunders, 1996.

(14) Ausher B.M. Erikson E. & Wilkins E.G. *Plastic surgery: indications, operations and outcomes*. St Louis: Mosby, 2000.

(15) McCance K.L. & Huether S.E. Pathophysiology: *the biologic basis for disease in adults and children*, 3rd edn. St Louis: Mosby, 1998.

(16) Kendall Healthcare Systems: The VAC® System (Vacuum Assisted Closure) http://www.kci1.com/products/vac/index.asp/ and http://www.medtech1.com/companies/kci.cfm

(17) Argenta L.C. & Morykwas M. Vacuum-assisted closure: a new method for wound control and treatment: clinical experience. *Annals of Plastic Surgery*, 1997; (38):563–77.

(18) Thomas S. *An introduction to vacuum assisted closure*. 2001. http://www.worldwidewounds.com/2001/may/Thomas/Vacuum-Assisted-Closure.html

(19) Banwell P.E. Topical negative pressure therapy in wound care. *Journal of Wound Care*, 1999 (Feb); **8**(2):79–84.

(20) Mullner T., Mrkonjic L., Kwasny O. & Vecsei V. The use of negative pressure to promote the healing of tissue defects: a clinical trial using the vacuum sealing technique. *British Journal of Plastic Surgery*, 1997, **50**(3):194–99.

(21) Thomas S. *A user's guide to the selection of dressings*, 1997. http://www.worldwidewounds.com

(22) Thomas S. *Atraumatic dressings*, 2003. http://www.worldwidewounds.com

(23) Morgan D. *Setting up wound dressing guidelines: avoiding the pitfalls*. September 2000. http://www.worldwidewounds.com

(24) Thomas S. Bandages and bandaging: the science behind the art. *Care Science & Practice*, 1990 (2):56–60. http://www.worldwidewounds.com

(25) Thomas S. *Compression bandaging in the treatment of leg ulcers*. 1998. http://www.worldwidewounds.com

(26) O'Hare L. Scholl compression hosiery in the management of venous disorders. *British Journal of Nursing*, 1997; **6**(7):391–94.

(27) Maylor M.E. Accurate selection of compression and anti-embolic hosiery. *British Journal Nursing*, 2001, **10**(18):1172–84.

(28) World Union of Wound Healing Societies. *Principles of best practice*. The document is available from http://www.wuwhs.org as a downloadable PDF. For further details contact Medical Education Partnership Ltd, 53 Hargrave Road, London N19 5SH. http://www.mepltd.co.uk

(29) European Wound Management Association Positioning Paper. *Wound bed preparation in practice* 2004. http://www.woundbedpreparation.com/

## Recommended websites for wound dressings, retention and tubular retention dressings – examples only:

http://www.blackwell-synergy.com/links/doi/10.1046/j.1322–7114.2003.00417.x/abs/

3M Healthcare http:/www.3M.com/intl/UK/uk-english/
Smith and Nephew http:/www.smith-nephew.com/
US/Wound/
http://www.woundcare.org/newsvol2n4/prpt2.htm
http://www.footamerica.com/drestubban.html

http://www.medifoam.co.kr/Eng_Sub01(s)ale_skin02.
htm#
http://www.greenfingerslandscaping.com/wounds/html
/moist wound healing.html http://www.kci1.
com/products/vac/index.asp

# Chapter 11

# Pain Associated with Wounds and Dressing Changes – Principles of Patient Care

## Background

'All pain is real, regardless of its cause. Pain is what-ever the person experiencing it says it is and exists whenever he says it does. Unfortunately, some health-care professionals erroneously believe that if emotions cause or perpetuate pain, pain is imaginary and thus not real. But calling pain imaginary won't make it go away. No pain sensation is truly imaginary – certainly not to the patient. You must believe that his pain is real before you can help him.'[1]

The word 'pain' comes from the Latin poena meaning 'punishment'. Acute and chronic pain may be caused by a wide variety of healthcare, traumatic and disease-based events.

Regardless of the aetiology of a patient's physical pain it is often suggested that there are distinct psy-chological aspects to the experience, for example, there may be a sense of 'personal' punishment or ret-ribution (i.e. a sense of personal responsibility (guilt) for the accident or disease), and it can often be the 'fear' of pain that is so disquieting to the patient[1,4-7].

This fear can also be translated into both a psy-chological and physiological sense of expectation for the patient – for example, the mere thought, or sug-gestion, of a medical procedure, changes of dress-ings, increasing mobility, or the remobilisation of an area that is, or has been, painful on movement. For the patient, the actual experience, potential for, or perception of, pain is one the principal influences on, and risk to, one's quality of life[1-9].

There are considered to be two basic forms of pain – physical and psychological[1]. Pain is a protective response to a potentially harmful stimulus. Once a primary assessment and provisional diagnosis is made, pain no longer serves a useful physiological purpose. At this point, pain must be treated uncom-promisingly and there can be no justification for allowing a patient to suffer.

Such is the modern healthcare concern for patients with unresolved acute physical pain, that it has been labeled 'the fifth vital sign'[2-5].

> **Box 11.1** Pain as the fifth vital sign[2-4].
>
> - Respiratory rate
> - Pulse/heart rate
> - Blood pressure
> - Body temperature
> - Pain.

For nurses, the pathophysiology and the application of pain management modalities must now be studied and understood at the same level as other life-supporting physiological systems (i.e. respiratory, circulatory, neurological and immunological) which are responsible for sustaining life itself.

The primary reasons given by individuals seeking primary or ongoing healthcare treatment is stated to be pain, major discomfort, or ongoing physical sore-ness. This may or may not be associated with other significant physiological events or conditions.

Pain associated with acute wounds, and not relieved by medication post discharge from hospital or day surgery units, is equally a significant reason for return to a healthcare facility or the seeking of medical/nursing assistance.

## Significant pain management issues identified in wound care

'The brain surgery (I had two procedures to remove tem-poral lobe tumours) wasn't terribly painful, it was the removal of the staples that really hurt. For each opera-

*tion there were over 40 staples sealing the incision. They'd sit me down, hand me a disposable tray and set to work with the pliers and no anaesthetic. It was excruciatingly painful.'*

Emma Miall, now in her early 20s, describing part of her surgical experience of two brain tumour removals during her teens in *Inside my head*, The Health Report, Australian Broadcasting Commission – Radio National, 9 June, 2003, http://www.abc.net.au/rn/talks.

---

**Box 11.2** Nursing risk management – primary practice principles.

- It is acknowledged that increasing the attention to objective pain management in all phases of in-patient bed-days, outpatient care, and during rehabilitation, will reduce hospital stay, and readmission episodes[1–7]
- Pain management is only effective when it is understood that pain is the individual's experience, what the patient states is unconditionally accepted, and the patient's fears and expectations of safety are identified
- The clinician must have a sensitive/empathic approach to pain management, based on adequate objective knowledge of pain pathophysiology, and an understanding of the consequences of inadequate pain control[1]
- Overall care needs to be co-ordinated and proactive, rather than fragmented and reactive
- A case management approach, through a model, such as 'safety, comfort and independence', or similar, is essential
- Inpatient or outpatient management planning must include the actual or potential for pain during wound care and dressing changes
- The principal preferred outcome of objective pain management is to achieve zero pain experienced, or minimal discomfort
- There is a recognition of a patient's potential fear for primary or recurring adverse events:
  - Wound breakdown
  - Background or breakthrough pain
  - Incidental pain associated with stages of mobilisation
  - Loss of personal control – recall of prior significant psychological and physiological stress
  - Reduced concentration
  - Loss of ability to co-operate, and fear of general safety

- The inadequate evidence-based selection by clinicians of the appropriate wound dressings to match the specific wound, and the wound dressing process itself, can be the basis of a painful experience
- Recognition that pain associated with long-term wound care, in particular frequent dressing changes (i.e. chronic wounds), can be intense
- Unresolved pain may lead to psychological disturbances, fear, anxiety and depression and, in long-term care, sometimes amputation of limbs, and/or ultimately suicide
- An understanding of the profound effects of patient pain should alert nurse clinicians to the need for regular continuing education in relation to their clinical approach to pain management
- The professional clinician must be prepared to act as the patient's advocate for:
  - Ensuring that an objective pain management assessment and management programme is in place
  - Ensuring the correct pharmacological type and dosage of medications that provide pain control is delivered[1–9]
  - Ensuring that the patient is satisfied with the treatment programme and the level of pain/discomfort control.

---

## Contemporary studies of pain

It is a reality of contemporary clinical experience that many wound dressing changes are often undertaken under less than optimal conditions, time available, an inadequate understanding of the wound and its specific needs, and the dressing process itself.

For the patient, the outcome of this experience can be pain, or major discomfort, and a clear and present fear that during following dressing changes, similar experiences, will occur again. The following provide examples of recent studies undertaken that demonstrate the importance for improved education (clinical, ethics, legal) and an empathic approach in this fundamental area of clinical nursing care.

### Study 1

Reviewers of data in Study 1[10] (reviewing attitudes to general pain) pointed out that 'invisible barriers'[12] and misinterpretations appeared to exist between clinicians and each patient's sense of experienced pain. The study concluded that clinicians required education that put a greater emphasis on the acceptance on the patient's expressed view of their pain[10].

## Study 2

A national survey[11] conducted to review nurse views related to pain and trauma at dressing changes reinforced the complexity of planning and delivering integrated pain management.

## Study 3

In one institution[12], following clear evidence that overall patient pain was not effectively being addressed, a subsequent study was recently undertaken to evaluate the efficacy of a hospital-based procedural pain-monitoring programme (PMP)12 which had been put in place. The principal components underpinning the programme were:

- Recognition that pain assessed (as stated by the patient) and its overall treatment was a principal component of patient care
- The recognition of pain as a very significant issue in healthcare:
  - Short and long term cost factors involved of unresolved pain
  - Acknowledgement of the legal responsibilities related to professional practice at all levels of care, and treatment outcomes.
- The necessity of targeting clinical education that regarded pain as a biological concept of un wellness that requires treatment
- The importance of an evidence-based assessment for the underlying aetiology of the individual's pain
- The specific targeted matching of pharmacology to pain sites, and the single or combined use of traditional and alternative modalities.

The study outcomes clearly demonstrated that with the disciplined use of these components as guiding principles for clinical practice, pain management was significantly improved.

## Study 4

Concerned by previous studies[13] and continuing anecdotal evidence that indicated an inadequate focus on pain management in wound care by clinicians, an international community of wound care specialists conducted a survey to explore how the problems associated with pain, particularly during

dressing change, could be scientifically addressed[13]. The results of the survey were presented at the 12th annual conference of the European Wound Management Association in May 2002.

The significant clinical outcomes of this report were:

- The time of dressing removal constituted the time of greatest pain
- The principal cause was the use of gauze dressings
- Moist wound healing dressings were stated to be responsible for the fewest pain problems.

---

**Box 11.3** Additional causes of wound pain identified (Study 4).

- Differences in dressing availability in various countries
- Inadequate knowledge regarding the dressing materials
- Inappropriate selection or mismatch of dressing material for the wound in question
- Inadequate knowledge and understanding in the scientific assessment and the specific dynamic needs of a wound on presentation, and during the healing stages.

---

The survey group recommended an educational programme should be established and this should form a prescribed component of evidence-based wound care. Two central areas would need to be addressed:

- An evidence-based ongoing pain assessment and monitoring programme
- Nurse/client communication to be placed at the centre of the care plan for all wound care[13].

## Study 5

Following a clinical trial conducted in 2004, pain management during dressing care for burns was reported[14]. Intranasal fentanyl was given to one group and intramuscular morphine to another. No statistical difference was found between the effects of the two analgesics.

Noteworthy, and somewhat disturbing, was the very significant statistical differences between the nurses', and the patients' assessments of the pain levels that were experienced during the wound care procedures. Nurses reported a significantly lower level of perception of the patient's pain experienced than was reported, on an objective scale, by the patients.

A reviewer of the study suggested that this negative response perhaps represented a self- protective strategy adopted by nurses during the most painful period of dressing removal and dressing change. Further studies are needed to explore this proposition.

---

**Box 11.4** General conclusions that may be drawn from these studies.

- A lack of recognition of the true reality of patient pain experienced/expressed during and after wound changes
- A lack of professional empathy shown by some clinicians in relation to the patients expressed level of pain
- An educational (science-based) gap that exists in objectively assessing and addressing the source and scale of pain
- A lack of understanding of the effects of pain on the biological wound repair process including that caused by dressing/wound mismatch
- Inadequate evidence-based wound bed assessment, preparation and maintenance and in overall case management planning by many clinicians charged with wound care.

---

## Addressing the issues of pain management at an international level

With the increasing recognition of the objective and subjective effects of untreated/inadequately treated pain, the World Health Organization (WHO) has set out a three-step relief ladder of recommended analgesics for pain management. This is based on the correlation of pain severity with recommended medications.

---

**Box 11.5** Outline of three-step pain relief ladder.

| | |
|---|---|
| **Non-opioid** | ± adjuvant |
| **Opioid** | for mild to moderate pain ± adjuvant |
| **Opioid** | for moderate to severe pain ± non-opioid ± adjuvant. |

---

In 2004, the World Union of Healing Societies, at an international conference in Paris, France, formulated and published a research-based document *Principles of Best Practice*, in relation to minimising pain at dressing-related wound bed preparation procedures. This is a significant and very timely document for all clinicians involved in many facets of wound management, and could also assist in forming much of the foundation for current pain management in wound care practices.

---

## Risk management in addressing patient pain in wound management

---

**Box 11.6** Principal clinical and patient risks associated with wound bed repair in the presence of pain.

- Inability to identify root causes and address different forms of pain (i.e. sharp, dull, throbbing) within presenting wounds
- Failure to pre-empt, recognise and address actual or potential adverse pain events in a timely fashion
- Inadequate pharmacological knowledge and application of analgesics through evidence-based therapeutic guidelines for specific applications
- Mismatch of dressing(s) to specific wound(s) types
- Failure to identify the early presence and effects of wound disturbances (i.e. haematoma, significant oedema, infection)
- Inability to define contamination versus infection
- Failure to control physical movement in the primary wound by utilising adequate primary immobilisation of the tissues.

---

**Box 11.7** Overall physiological and psychosocial effects of pain on wound bed repair.

- Inclination of patient to remain immobile, initiating postoperative systemic (pulmonary, circulatory, immunologic, endocrine) complications including 'the stress response', particularly in the elderly, and those with multiple trauma and major injury
- Unconfirmed (but suggested) effects on the function of white blood cells within the wound, probably related to circulatory disturbances in and surrounding the wound site

*Continued*

- Pain may also be the overall effect of a compromised general circulation within the wound and if this is the case wound bed repair may be very inferior or lead to avascular necrosis
- Cellular dysfunction related to the introduction of enzymes and fluid that inhibit the initiation of the repair process
- A desire by the patient to interfere with the dressings, and non-compliance with treatment modalities
- Issues related to clinical nursing morbidity and co-morbid factors:
  - Immobility leading to pressure ulcers, major joint stiffness
  - Fatigue, sleep deprivation, disorientation, depression
  - Stress, frustration, anger and depression leading to significant non-compliance, loss of work time and financial deprivation.

## Adverse effects of inadequately treated pain – legal issues

Failure to address pain, pre- and postoperatively and particularly at times of dressing changes in an inpatient or outpatient setting, is a significant contribution to poor patient co-operation in rehabilitation, a continuing sense of anger, grief and loss, ongoing disability.

It is stated that in many cases of reported and treated chronic pain, there is a parallel between prior inadequately treated acute pain management, and the disabling outcomes of chronic pain. In addition, cancer pain can present additional legal and ethical issues in the provision of adequate and appropriate pain management[1]. The ineffective treatment of pain regardless of the aetiology can be the source of legal compensation or damages.

For example, during the 1990s the nursing press in the USA reported a case of a professional nurse being sued by a patient for withholding the prescribed dosage of pain medication to match the patient's stated needs. In addition, there was a failure to report to the physician that the patient's pain had remained uncontrolled. Internet medico-legal sites report this and a number of cases of nurse clinicians being successfully sued for a failure to adequately assess and deliver an adequate level of prescribed pain management.

Clinicians are encouraged to explore the Internet for sites outlining a range of interesting discussions on this contemporary and topical subject.

See recommended websites (evidence-based legal responsibilities in relation to pain management) at the end of this chapter.

### Box 11.8 Risk management and legal responsibilities – questions to be addressed.

- What are the laws governing the prescribing and administration of pain relieving drugs in the state/country where clinicians are practising?
- What is the clinicians' legal responsibility towards the patient in the prevention and management of pain?
- What will be the risk to this patient, and the wound, if pain management is not optimal?
- What are the goals and outcomes to be established for pain management that is required to ensure the patient's safety, comfort and independence?

## Addressing wound care needs within a pain management framework

### Box 11.9 Suggested practice principles for improving pain management outcomes.

- Application of evidence-based, expert experiential and current best practice principles[1–29]
- Increasing knowledge and understanding of research-based practices applied to the use of wound solutions becoming readily available[16]
- Utilising therapeutic pharmacological guidelines designed to objectively focus on specific areas of pain management[17]
- Providing adjunctive pain management during wound care as deemed appropriate
- Objective based wound dressing selection designed to meet the needs of the specific wound, from primary to tertiary needs
- Specialist use of atraumatic dressings and, in particular, soft silicone interfaced dressings that assist in the problem of pain where wound protection and early mobility are essential.

**Box 11.10** Application of the principles of pain management in wound care.

- Know the laws governing the prescription and administration of drugs used for pain management in your sphere of practice
- Understand the aetiology and pathophysiology of the pain
- Understand the tissues involved and their healing process
- Have a science-based understanding of all wound dressing types and the clinical indications for application
- Listen to and believe what the patient says his/her pain level is or believes it will be
- Importance of a genuine display of empathy
- Review with the patient past wound or injury experiences, and record any previous negative experiences
- Ensure an objective wound assessment process and parallel this to the patient/wounds needs – utilise objective numerical scales and document accordingly
- Involve the patient in all aspects of the pain assessment and management proposed
- Set realistic and achievable goals and outcomes for pain management
- Use a scientific pharmacological and multidisciplinary approach wherever possible[17]
- Utilise adjunct therapies during treatment period as assessed (i.e. distraction methods, local soft tissue and body massage, music, etc.)
- Evaluate the preferred clinical/patient outcomes – review for changes to care approach as required
- Anticipate pain/discomfort during wound care and dressing changes so that fear and apprehension prior to each dressing change may be proactively addressed
- Explain the entire procedure to the patient, eliciting their assistance where appropriate
- Ensure the wound surrounds are managed to exclude maceration, allergies, itchiness that cause discomfort and eventually pain.

See recommended websites at the end of this chapter.

## Applied pharmacological interventions

Only 3 principal classes of drugs are considered mainstays for acute pain treatment[17,18]:

- Opioids – opioid derivatives
- Non-steroidal anti-inflammatory drugs (NSAIDs)
- Acetaminophen (paracetamol).

Other classes of drugs, such as antidepressants and anticonvulsants, are sometimes used as co-analgesics or adjuncts.

Although a variety of pharmacological approaches to acute pain management are available, many of these require the services of a pain specialist. Fortunately for most patients, NSAIDs, acetaminophen and opiates can provide adequate basal analgesia. However, incident or breakthrough pain often requires a different approach.

Although the initial prescribing of narcotic pain management drugs (IV, IM, patient-controlled pumps, epidermal patches or intranasal sprays i.e. fentanyl) requires medical staff intervention, pre-emptive patient assessment and decisions for objectively advising the medical staff of the patient's specific and anticipated need for pain control are components of professional nurses' responsibility.

As the decision to administer prescribed pharmacological products for pain management is largely within the responsibility of professional nurses, clinicians have an ethical and legal responsibility to understand, pharmacologically and clinically, the specific actions of pain control medications:

- In what areas of pain experienced they optimally work
- Peak time effectiveness
- Half life
- Any adverse effects and methods of reversing the effects[1-7,17].

Proactive assessment and pre-emptive administration of a suitable category and dosage of an opioid or non-opioid analgesia, combined with a mild sedation (anti-anxiety medication, for example, low dosage of diazepam/lorazepam) prior to dressing treatments, should be options available to the nurse clinician. These modalities can form an important component of an overall armamentarium for addressing acute and wound dressing pain[17].

The postoperative/discharge instructions given to the patient should be based on a pre-emptive protocol that parallels an inflammatory and normal or extended healing process, and prescribed medications must be taken by the patient strictly as ordered, if the pain is to be controlled effectively. It is important to stress to the patient the clinical need for effective pain control, not only as a comfort measure, but one of physiological safety, essential for the healing process, and allowing for greater independence.

Although in a large area of wound dressing changes and wound care, oral analgesics specifically targeted to meet the individual patient's needs are generally adequate, for a number of patients their comfort needs are greater than particular oral analgesics are able to meet. General anaesthesia, intermittent or continuous systemic narcotics, with bolus dosages for breakthrough pain, strong oral analgesics containing high levels of codeine, or analgesic gases (i.e. Entonox which is 50% oxygen and 50% nitrous oxide) may be necessary prior to and during removal of, or change of dressings in some wounds – for example, those patients with large areas of deep tissue loss, such as burns, necrotising fasciitis, meningococcal infections, or similar wounds. Many of these patients are initially critically ill, intubated and ventilated, but following post-extubation the reality of the pain situation becomes obvious as dressing changes can be a major and often a very painful exercise, if they go unplanned.

## Setting preferred clinical patient and nursing outcomes

- The goal/outcome of pain control, wherever possible, should be set at zero, and patient management should be focused around this
- Pain or varying degrees of discomfort will be expected when interventions, or physical actions, are undertaken, that have the potential to stimulate pain receptors (i.e. open wounds, complex wounds), or psychologically instigate a sense of anticipated pain, discomfort, or fear
- Patients will often articulate their fear, particularly if previous dressing changes have been a negative experience
- Whenever possible, pain management must be proactive and pre-emptive if the normal homeostasis is to be maintained and optimal patient and wound outcomes are to be achieved. It must also be equally focused on the physiological and psychological aspects of the patient's experience[1]
- Identification of the risks of not undertaking and treating acute and chronic pain associated with wounds and dressing changes procedures and should be addressed through setting realistic and achievable patient goals, and end-outcomes[4-7]

- Pain, or continuous and disruptive discomfort that cannot be minimised (and accepted by the patient), or prevented, is not an acceptable result for the patient, regardless of the procedure or disease[28]
- Unexpected, breakthrough, incidental, uncontrolled pain by adequate proactive measures requires a medical and a nursing reassessment to ensure that tissue damage, or other adverse events are not occurring
- The process of setting up a formal data collection (i.e. the use of pain assessment charts) for ongoing analysis of acute, chronic, and palliative pain care can provide a database for objective evidence-based pain management, and patient and staff education
- Following discharge, community healthcare nurses could be requested to maintain a database for evaluation of the patient's pain/discomfort
- Multidisciplinary (and pain management team) assistance may need be called upon to provide a care model to suit the individual patient that includes a palliative approach to improve the health, lifestyle and psychosocial needs of the patient.

## Focusing on pain in plastic surgery wound dressing management

The average length of hospital stay is reducing annually. Currently in plastic surgery up to 80% of elective surgery and large numbers of trauma patients will be discharged within 12–48 hours. Anecdotally, many surgical nurses engaged in home discharge postoperative patient care, indicate the presence of poorly controlled pain as the primary reason they receive calls from patients in the first 48 hours.

Age, gender, culture and the actual or perceived extent of the injury to the tissues will all contribute to a person's perception of pain. Pain may be experienced due to initial trauma, in the immediate postoperative period after surgery, following discharge, and during dressing changes, regardless of whether the patient is in a hospital or being treated in the community as an outpatient. The patient's initial experience of pain management is their self-reference for further treatment modalities and this may set the scene for compliance issues and return for ongoing dressing changes.

Previous experiences and anxiety caused by preceding negative management of pain may add to the distress of the current experience. This is particularly observed in burns dressing and skin graft care in all age groups.

If the primary experience in a doctor's rooms or the emergency department has been distressing, this sets an emotional precedent and an anticipated poor experience of any additional treatments proposed or undertaken.

According to the objective pain management studies previously discussed, wound care pain is inadequately treated at all levels of care and across all age groups. As previously discussed, it is also stated that professional nurses have a range of perceptions regarding an individual's pain, tending to:

- underestimate actual levels of pain
- overestimate the effectiveness of pain medications.

## Physiological implications for the wound

Wound repair is a complex and dynamic process and is not always as clear-cut and predictable as might be expected even in the most well prepared patient and elective surgical conditions.

Following tissue injury, initial chemical responses to cellular and tissue trauma alert biological systems to tissue damage, and these systems work in an attempt to protect the cells, by reducing the pain cycle.

The biological systems aim to satisfy all the competing physiological interests for the repair processes, and unless the additional primary and ongoing treatment modalities for circulatory needs, reducing oedema, and timing of immobility, are accurately matched to the needs of the wound, pain will continue.

In addition, physiologically, tissue will not heal if it suffers continual cellular damage from repeated procedures and dressing changes where the developing, fragile and highly sensitive granulation tissue is continually traumatised, and peripheral nerve endings are exposed with pain as the principal signal of injury[8]. Repair timeframes are increasingly prolonged as the granulation tissue repeatedly struggles to recover from secondary injury and, finally, acute wounds may become chronic wounds.

## Recognised effects of pain in reconstructive plastic surgery

As previously stated, pain is a significant indicator that the patient's homeostasis is under strain. The presence of pain or major discomfort must not be a factor which is to be 'tolerated' by the patient or discounted by the staff as it may be an indicator that vascular compromise is occurring, which may result in the loss of flaps, grafts, digits, etc.[8]. The pain exhibited following major hand injuries is an excellent example of the physiological and psychological effects of pain on the individual.

Constant restlessness, movement or friction may result in poor immobilisation of the wounded zone, with anxiety resulting in peripheral vascular shutdown, reducing blood flow, oxygen delivery and nutrition for cellular recovery[8]. In addition, pain may induce patient immobilisation resulting in the potential for respiratory compromise, and deep vein thrombosis.

Assessment involves appraisal of intrinsic factors (the patient's general condition, the wound injury, patient pain threshold, anxiety, status of peripheral vascular circulation) and extrinsic factors (mechanical reasons for pain, such as tight bandages causing excess pressure on fragile blood vessels reducing capillary blood low, inappropriate elevation of the limb or body part leading to wound oedema)[8].

## Effects of the application of cold wound solutions and pain

Normal saline (NS) gauze packs and irrigations constitute a large part of wound care in plastic surgery wounds and wound care practices. The effect of applying unwarmed NS dressings or irrigation on the exposed cells of an open wound (which in itself can be painful or uncomfortable), increases the period of repair by up to an additional four hours following each procedure. Over a period of days or weeks, this adds up to a significant time period. This is related to the effects on the fibroblast cells and red blood cells within the wound[8].

In addition, fragile, developing fibroblast cells do not tolerate temperature changes that have the potential to alter their own homeostasis, and the exposure of an open wound to hypothermic conditions is contrary to the concept of moist wound healing which includes the need for physiological warmth.

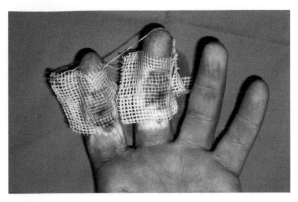

**Figure 11.1** Vaseline® gauze dressing adhering to lacerated fingers.

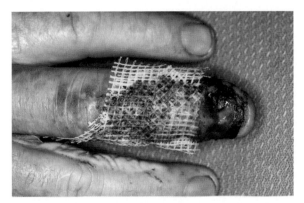

**Figure 11.2** Vaseline® gauze adhering to toxic spider bite wound oedematous – painful.

## Avoiding adverse outcomes in plastic surgical dressing changes

Plastic surgery patients with their extensive range of wounds and wound dressing needs, present significant challenges to all clinicians who are charged with the responsibility of anticipation and assessment of pain, postoperative pain management, dressing selection, dressing changes and the education of the patient in inpatient and outpatient settings. Added to this is the psychological anticipation of the aesthetic outcome of procedures undertaken.

A scientific and pharmacological knowledge of pain, its effects on different targeted tissue and body sites, matching medication to management require-

ments, the use of risk management and pain assessment/management charts, must become essential tools of the professional nurse[1].

Pain control can be effective when an individual person's wound management criteria include pain as a parallel aspect of care and as a central measurement of clinical outcomes, at all discrete stages of the wound bed repair process.

For instance, on discharge, day surgery patients will require prescribed administration of oral analgesics for the first 72–96 hours to parallel the inflammatory process where pain and discomfort is an expected result of injury/surgery, and reflect the patient's needs. If the pain is not resolved by oral medications and surgical site elevated as ordered, it must be suspected that adverse events may be occurring and this must be reported to the surgeon.

Patients who are free from pain have significantly reduced complication rates[1]. They are able to listen and understand requests, are more co-operative, and have the ability to maintain adequate respiratory function, aiding general and peripheral perfusion and oxygenation to the injured areas, and significantly higher levels of mobility.

Non-adherent forms of oil-impregnated or synthetic material based types of dressings are freely available and should be the first choice. The use of the adhering dressing types, as seen in Figures 11.1 and 11.2, should be diligently avoided.

On inspection varying degrees of tissue can be seen pushing through the open weave of the gauze. Tulle gras is extremely painful to remove, and induces bleeding by injuring the fragile capillaries, and each dressing change strips the outer layer of epidermal cells, significantly retarding resurfacing, prolonging the healing timeframe.

## Removal of fixation/retention wound dressings

The primary selection of the primary wound dressing is usually made by the surgeon in the operating room and will reflect the nature of the surgical procedure. Fixation sheet dressings are commonly used to secure the primary dressing. In some instances, skin coloured Elastoplast® may be used by plastic surgeons and others, to secure the primary wound dressings (i.e. non-adherent gauze) following the removal of small to medium skin lesions – this is becoming less the case with modern retention/

fixation dressings being applied to secure specifically selected primary dressings.

The removal of inappropriately applied Elastoplast® (in attempts of tissue compression) has probably been one of the most common sources of pain/discomfort expressed by plastic surgery patients, and in many instances remains so. The old adage of *'just rip it off quickly and it won't hurt as much'* is no longer clinically or legally appropriate when modern alternatives are available. Its incorrect application (causing shear and friction on movement) is also one of the most common causes of so-called 'allergic' reactions at the dressing site.

Many surgeons are now moving towards modern fixation/retention dressings and experienced practice nurses can advocate for change to these by demonstrating the advantages to the surgeon when assisting in the application of the primary dressing in the operating theatre, and when the postoperative dressings are undertaken.

Complex dressings, such as those for multiple small skin grafts on the hand, or oral dressings, may be uncomfortable to remove. Care must be exercised by:

- Not compromising on practice excellence
- Good planning prior to removal
- Pre-emptive analgesia
- Reassuring the patient
- Informing the patient of what is occurring
- By ensuring the patient is lying down and comfortable, and working without appearing to be in a hurry, pain can usually be avoided
- Using distraction therapy techniques, such as basic conversation, or headphones for patients to listen to music, are also useful.

## Special issues

Some children require analgesia or anaesthesia for dressing changes and suture removal, for example, major grafted areas or burns, following major facial and hand surgery, urogenital reconstructive procedures, or free flaps.

Adults will usually require a bolus dose of narcotic analgesia and/or general anaesthesia for primary and secondary dressing changes in major burns, fungating wounds, and major lower pelvic wounds that have grafts and/or flaps.

In general, for most wounds there are sufficient choices of modern dressings available to ensure that,

although some minor or moderate discomfort is initially felt, pain on removal is rarely experienced if good planning is a principal element of care.

Significant soreness or discomfort related to the overall wound, rather than the pain of dressing change may be the sensation expressed by the patient, but this can also be a source of fear for the patient and should be discussed with them and addressed with reassurance and analgesics, as the patient requires. But if the patient says it is painful, then it is pain he or she feels.

If there has been an inappropriate selection (i.e. dressing materials mismatched to the wound bed assessment on, for example, skin graft donor sites), the issue of some anticipated discomfort should be discussed with the patient – pre-emptive analgesics may be deemed necessary.

A second example is alginates (left on too long) which may sometimes be painful to remove in sensitive areas such as fingertips, as the limited fluid that escapes is easily drawn from the delicate sensitive tissues, leaving a hard, dried-out lump of dressing material.

Pain has also been reported/implicated in the use of hydrocolloids and low adherent dressings, and again these are usually a case of mismatch between wound and dressing, or the patient's previous experiences. The inappropriate application of dressings outside the prescribed zones, as indicated by the manufacturers, can also be a source of discomfort on removal, with hairs and epidermal surface cells adhering to the dressing material, or maceration.

Adherent dressings such as films used to secure other dressings in place (e.g. on skin graft donor sites) will cause pain on removal if hair is not removed prior to application. Fixation/retention dressings may be removed with almost no discomfort if, prior to removal, commercially available tape remover (most comfortable to the patient), citrus oil or a fine olive oil is poured over and left for a few minutes before the dressing is gently removed (more oil may need to be applied during the process). Soaking in warm soapy water is not advocated as this usually leaves the adhesive on the skin in a sticky form.

In patients on long-term steroid treatment, redressing using dressings with adhering properties can cause loss of the epidermal layer because of the poor integrity of the tissue, so these should be applied judiciously and skilfully, removed in the same way, or avoided completely.

A method worthy of note, and use, is the concept of a 'window framing' of the wound. A non-macerating type dressing is applied around the wound leaving the actual wound exposed. The wound can be dressed and an external securing tape attached to the 'window frame', which remains *in situ* for a number of days or often up to one week. This is a common feature of mixed superficial and partial thickness burns dressings. Its genesis is based on the principles of stoma management.

For outpatients, suggesting that they take adequate pre-emptive analgesia, of type and dosage that is normally acceptable to them, prior to dressing changes, can provide a good basis of trust in the process, and minimise expected discomfort or pain.

---

**Review**

*Setting goals of care and preferred clinical and patient outcomes*, Chapter 2, Boxes 2.7–2.9. Adapt according to risk management issues and clinical patient needs.

---

## Dressing changes in clinical practice

### Box 11.11 Assessment of existing dressings.

- What primary dressing was applied?
- Were the primary dressings applied according to the manufacturer's directions?
- Were there any adverse events/effects during the period the dressing has been on the wound(s)?

### Box 11.12 Patient safety and comfort – pain/discomfort management.

- Assess the patient and address any patient immediate needs
- Does the patient require pre-emptive analgesia and/or mild sedation prior to the dressing change?
- Ensure that analgesic medications have been pre-emptively administered according to the patient's wound care needs and peak effect will match the dressing change time
- Ensure the patient is not physically cold prior to commencing the procedure.

### Box 11.13 Dressing change preparation.

What new dressings are proposed to be applied, if any?

- In your mind's eye, consciously walk yourself through the steps you propose to undertake in order that you can prioritise the importance of each, select the appropriate equipment required, and estimate the time needed to be set aside
- Prepare all the dressing change needs/equipment (prior to attending to the patient) away from the sight of the patient
- Ensure you have the correct instruments for the job
- Excellent direct/focused lighting is essential
- Fine instruments are essential to remove fine sutures and prevent local injury, particularly around the eyes
- Be prepared for the unexpected – and maintain a professional approach by not commenting until you have assessed the wound, and if appropriate, sought the surgeon's or an experienced clinician's advice
- Do not frighten the patient by making negative comments on any aspect of the surgery or the wound
- Clinicians should use sterile gloves and their hands to undertake dressings, as fingers are more sensitive than inappropriate general plastic moulded forceps, which can cause tissue damage and pain.

### Box 11.14 Patient preparation.

- Find an appropriate venue and explain/discuss with the patient exactly what is going to happen, in what order, and why
- Be reassuring, answer any relevant questions and secure the patient's trust and confidence in your competence to undertake the proposed procedure and manage any adverse events
- Provide a beverage if the patient is thirsty or needs an early diversion.

## Box 11.15  Patient independence.

- Secure the patient's physical and psychological independence by respecting the patient's privacy, and providing safety, a secure position, warmth, calmness and quietness
- If the area is cold and the patient is to be exposed, ensure that extra blankets are available
- Remember that if the patient is frightened, peripheral vascular circulation will shut down to preserve internal warmth, leaving the patient peripherally cold, and shivering may occur
- The physical area where the dressing is being undertaken may be air-conditioned and colder than the environment the patient has come from.

## Box 11.16  Dressing change procedures.

- Appropriate access to the patient may require certain physical positioning, such as using a reclining chair (useful if the patient faints), surgical table or, in the case of the hand, a resting table to enable ease of dressing care
- Have diversionary tactics available, suitable for children or adults (e.g. reading material, television, games, music or relaxation therapy via tapes and earphones)
- Lighting must be adequate to clearly see fine sutures and undertake simple wound cleansing and debridement of dead tissue/skin
- Sit, whenever possible, as if the arms can be rested in a comfortable position, this helps to minimise the clinician's normal physical tremor, particularly when removing children's sutures or fine sutures on the face, etc.
- Give the patient your undivided attention, ensuring the procedure will not be constantly interrupted by other distractions (hold/divert phone calls)
- Maintain a skilful technique with attention to detail – don't hurry!

## Box 11.17  Minimising/preventing adverse events through the dressing procedure.

- All fluids used for open or closed wound irrigation or soaking of limbs, such as normal saline or sterile water, must be pre-warmed – cold fluids may be unpleasant/frightening, particularly to children and the elderly, and may exacerbate pain in open wounds with sensitive nerve endings exposed[16]
- Wound irrigation should be used according to best practice guidelines as new granulation tissue is fragile and easily damaged[16]
- The soaking of dressings has been clinically and experientially demonstrated to have very limited effects on reducing pain on removal
- Gentle irrigation has been demonstrated to have some positive effect during the removal of contaminating wound debris which can become caught in wound dressings, and dressing products such as hydro-polymers which are water-attracting
- Irrigation with hydrogen peroxide is damaging to viable tissue cells and surrounding skin, and has been known to cause fatal air embolism[8]
- Bleach-based products (e.g. Eusol) are painful when used as a dressing and are injurious to viable cells at all stages of application and removal
- The scientific place for these products is extremely questionable (clinically and legally) and there are no evidence-based data for their use in the current modern approaches to wound dressing management[16]
- Many topical applications may cause pain on application and removal, such as aerosol skin sprays frequently used on superficially healed, surgically sutured wounds
- The adhesive potential of hydrocolloids and semipermeable dressings is at maximum when the product is first applied and gradually reduces over a few days
- Pain can be minimised by leaving these products on for the maximum time possible, and incrementally reducing their size by cutting off the excess over a period of days
- Film dressings should be removed by being stretched parallel with the skin, rather than 'pulled' at an angle
- Occlusive dressings can reduce pain, as interactive products, including hydrocolloids, hydrofibres and alginates, react with wound exudate to form a moist gel at the wound interface and therefore are virtually pain-free at dressing changes, but this only occurs if sufficient fluid was present in the wound to sustain the moisture

*Continued*

- Problems exist if moisture exceeds the uptake capacity of the dressings. This causes maceration and subsequent discomfort
- Alginates and hydrofibres provide an excellent alternative to traditional products for packing cavities and there is considerable evidence to support the use of these agents
- Polyurethane foam dressings indicated for moderate to heavy exudate have a moist wound contact, which reduces tissue adhesion and disruption to new granulating tissue.
- Soft silicone products are the latest generation of low wound adherence dressings[24–26]. They are extremely useful for fragile or sensitive tissues causing nil or minimal pain on removal, and are frequently used following dermabrasion and laser treatments to the face
- Many plastic surgical nurses will apply them after the primary dressing for wound protection and the final stages of moist wound healing and for easy secondary removal
- The selection of atraumatic dressings for the minimisation of pain during use and changes of dressings, without compromising the healing requirements, contributes to patient satisfaction and significant compliance in rehabilitation
- When the dressing change is completed, reassure the patient, and answer any additional questions regarding hygiene management, showering, and suggested level of mobility
- On conclusion of the dressing change procedure, ensure the patient is satisfied and comfortable
- Provide verbal and written instructions regarding for any further dressing care particularly if wound changes are to be undertaken by the patient, or primary carers
- Send a copy to the local treating doctor and if a community nurse is to be involved, send a copy to him/her
- Ensure the patient has a clear understanding regarding the need to seek medical or nursing attention should adverse events occur, particularly pain not relieved by the patient's preferred normal medication.

---

**Review**

*Principles of nursing discharge management and ambulatory care following reconstructive plastic surgery, Chapter 14.*

---

## Auditing clinical nursing outcomes in pain management for wounds and dressing changes

### Box 11.18 Safety.

- Evidence-based data and expert experience for the management of pain were the foundations for determining the process of patient needs and treatment modalities throughout the period of dressing change(s)
- The presence of unresolved pain was clinically assessed, addressed and professionally managed
- The patient's physiological and psychological safety was addressed through scientific and experiential-based principles in the preparation and conduct of all levels of wound dressing changes.

### Box 11.19 Comfort.

- The presence of physical pain or some degree of discomfort was anticipated to occur during dressing changes, but this was objectively assessed and managed to the patient's satisfaction through evidence-based pharmacological principles
- The patient was included in all aspects of pain assessment and management where possible
- Pain management was successfully applied in order that the movement to wound bed maintenance and repair could be achieved at a comfort level acceptable to both clinician and patient.

### Box 11.20 Independence.

- The level of interdependence and independence desired by the patient was respected and reflected in all aspects of treatment planned and undertaken
- The patient expressed confidence and satisfaction in the total pain management process and clinical outcome of their wound care.

## A specialty focus for all wound types

With the increasing focus on wound pain, the traditional fields of pain focus (i.e. acute, chronic, malignancy) could also be expanded to include education and protocols directed at clinical fields such as 'pain associated with wound management', and include interventions such as insertion of intravenous lines, primary mobility and rehabilitation modalities associated with wounds.

Specific protocols (e.g. algorithms or flow charts) based on WHO guidelines, clinical research and expert experience could be very useful reference charts for reliability, consistency and accountability in clinical practice.

Setting pain management practice goals and outcomes (safety, comfort, independence) is an essential element of nursing practice and is gaining more importance as the initial and ongoing presence of pain places the wound, and the patient, at risk in both safety and quality of life[28].

As can be seen from the references and sample of websites provided, the issue of unresolved pain is becoming a major crisis in the whole area of healthcare, and significantly increasing the overall costs of healthcare within all categories of patient management.

## References

(1) McCaffrey M. & Beebe A. *Pain: clinical manual for nursing practice.* St Louis: Mosby, 1989.

(2) American Society of Pain Management. *Pain: the fifth vital sign.* http://www.ampainsoc.org/advocacy/fifth.htm

(3) Jackson M. *Pain: the fifth vital sign.* Canada: Random House, 2002.

(4) Taylor D.R. Improving outcomes in acute pain management: optimising patient selection. *Medscape Neurology and Neurosurgery,* 2004 (2). http://www.medscape.com

(5) Smeltzer S.C. & Bare B.G. *Brunner and Suddarth's textbook of medical-surgical nursing,* 9th edn. Philadelphia: Lippincott, Williams & Wilkins 2000.

(6) Mallett J. & Dougherty L. (eds). *The Royal Marsden Hospital manual of clinical nursing procedures,* 5th edn. Oxford, UK: Blackwell Science, 2000.

(7) McCance K.L. & Huether S.E. *Pathophysiology: the biologic basis for disease in adults and children,* 3rd edn. St Louis: Mosby, 1998.

(8) Peacock E.E. Jnr. *Wound repair,* 3rd edn. Philadelphia: W.B. Saunders Company, 1984.

(9) Dealey C. *The care of wounds,* 2nd edn. Oxford, UK: Blackwell Science, 1999.

(10) Mann E. & Redwood S. Improving pain management: breaking down the invisible barrier. *British Journal of Nursing,* 2000 (Oct 26—Nov 8); 9(19):2067–72.

(11) Hollingworth H. & Collier M. Nurses' views about pain and trauma at dressing changes: results of a national survey. *Journal of Wound Care,* 2000 (Sept); 9(8):367–73.

(12) de Rond M.E., De Wit R., van Dam F.S. & Muller M.J. A pain monitoring program for nurses: effects on communication, assessment and documentation of patient's pain. *Journal of Pain Symptom Management,* 2000 (Dec); 20(6):424–39.

(13) Molnlycke Health Care. *Pain and trauma at wound dressing changes.* Multinational survey report, 2002. http://www.tendra.com

(14) Finn J., et al. A randomised crossover trail of patient controlled intranasal fentanyl and oral morphine for procedural wound care in adult patients with burns. *Burns,* 2004 (30):262–68.

(15) Gould D. Wound management and pain control. *Nursing Standard,* 1999 (Oct 27—Nov 2); 14(6):47–54.

(16) The Joanna Briggs Institute. *Best practice – evidence based practice information sheets for health professionals: solutions, techniques and pressure for wound cleansing.* 7(1). Adelaide, South Australia: Blackwell Science, 2003. http://www.joannabriggs.edu.au

(17) Hawthorn J. & Redmond K. *Pain: causes and management.* Oxford, UK: Blackwell Publishing, 1998.

(18) Department of Human Services. Victorian Drug Usage Advisory Committee. Interprint Services. *Therapeutic guidelines: analgesics,* 3rd edn. Victoria, Australia: Department of Human Services, March 1997/98.

(19) Acute and post operative pain management for children: http://www.spineuniverse.com/displayarticle.php/article392.html

(20) Dobson F. The art of pain management. *Professional Nurse,* 2000 (Sept); 15(12):786–90.

(21) Allcock N. Physiological rationale for early pain management. *Professional Nurse,* 2000 (March); 15(6):395–7.

(22) McDowell K. Wounds and pain management. *Nursing Standard,* 2000 (Feb 23–29); 14(23):47.

(23) Bucknall T., Maniaas E. & Botti M. Acute pain management: implications of scientific evidence for nursing in the postoperative context. *International Journal of Nursing Practice,* 2001; 7(4):266.

(24) Thomas S. *A user's guide to the selection of dressings,* 1997. http://www.worldwidewounds.com

(25) Thomas S. *Atraumatic dressings.* 2003. http://www.worldwidewounds.com

(26) Morgan D. *Setting up wound dressing guidelines: avoiding the pitfalls.* Sept 2000. http://www.worldwidewounds.com

(27) Kendall Healthcare Systems: The VAC® System (Vacuum Assisted Closure). http://www.kci1.com/products/vac/index.asp/ and http://www.medtech1.com/companies/kci.cfm

(28) Stark P.L., Sherwood G.D. & Adams-McNeill J. Pain management outcomes: issues for advanced practice nurses. *International Journal of Advanced Nursing Practice*, 2000 **4**(1). http://www.ispub.com/ostia/index.php?xmlFilePath = journals/ijanp/front.xml

(29) *Principles of best practice: minimising pain at wound dressing-related procedures. A consensus document.* London MEP Ltd, 2004. (A World Union of Wound Healing Societies Initiative). http://www.wuwhs.org/consensus/

## Recommended websites

**Postoperative pain management within the care of wounds**

World Health Organization (WHO) – three-step pain relief ladder recommendations

http://www.medscape.com/pages/sites/infosite/ultracet/article-whopain

http://www.ultracet.com/understanding/postop.html

http://www.medscape.com/pages/sites/infosite/ultracet/article-postsurgical

**Pain management within the general care of wounds**

http://www.wuwhs.org/consensus/ (*Principles of Best Practice*)

http://www.vnaa.org/vnaa/g/?h = html/wound_center_march

http://www.worldwidewounds.com/2001/march/Pediani/Pain-relief-surgical-wounds.html

http://www.studentbmj.com/search/pdf/03/11/sbmj406.pdf

http://www.rcna.org.au/pages/infosheets.php

http://www.woundspecialist.com/resources.htm

http://www.worldwidewounds.com/2004/september/Ryan/Psychology-Pain-Wound-Healing.html

**Evidence-based legal responsibilities in relation to pain management**

http://www.painandthelaw.org/

http://www.postgradmed.com/issues/2001/09_01/editorial_sep.htm

http://www.accc-cancer.org/publications/journaljuly03/j03legal.pdf

http://www.csdp.org/ads/painman1.htm

http://www.religioustolerance.org/euth_pai.htm

# Chapter 12

# Wound Bed Maintenance

1. Splinting
2. Suture line care
3. Wound scar management
4. Skin maintenance and massage therapy

## Background

Wound bed maintenance is a process that ensures the safety of the internal and surrounding wound tissues in the healing and rehabilitation phase. This is maintained through a range of surgical and mechanical splinting techniques, scar management and skin maintenance techniques.

In the context of wound care, the term 'splint' may be applied to any technique that restricts, retards, or governs the movement of the wound, and the immediate surrounding tissue zones.

## 1. SPLINTING

### Box 12.1 Example of suture line and wound tissue (including bone) splinting techniques.

- Wound adhesive glues (suture lines)
- Suture materials
- Wound edge securing staples
- Suture line fixation tapes
- Bandages
- Conforming tubular elastic garments
- Fixation/retention sheet dressings
- Internal plates and screws
- Surgical wires
- Orthopaedic staples
- Rigid splints (plaster of Paris and thermoplastic materials)
- External pins (with or without crossbar frames).

### Box 12.2 Wound bed maintenance – principal goals/outcomes of splint application.

- To correct the wound deformity by restoring normal anatomical alignment
- To protect the healing wound(s) by ensuring a rigidity of realignment for integrity of wound vessels, cells, tissues and surrounding skin, muscle or bone
- To control any movement that initiates pain
- To assist in restoration of the aesthetic qualities of the body part by reducing the incidence of re-injury, wound infection and wound distortions.

### Box 12.3 Wound bed maintenance – practice principles.

- Wound healing is assisted when primary immobility is practised to protect injured tissues and to allow cellular and vascular realignment to take place[1–9]
- Wounds require systemic and physical protection from complications (particularly infection and oedema) that may arise due to accidental secondary injury, or adverse local or systemic factors (e.g. age, patients on steroids, or anticoagulants, with an immune disease, or cancer)
- The evidence-based management of pain is central to wound bed maintenance
- Care of artificially created wounds such as external pin sites is important in maintaining the bacterial balance in favour of the host[10–15]
- The removal of sutures and staples requires planning and clinical skills[16–18]
- Scar management is an essential component of total wound management[7–9]

*Continued*

- Skin maintenance is an important factor in protecting the skin against superficial injury
- Therapeutic soft tissue massage therapy is an integral component of skin maintenance and wound repair
- Addressing the patient's psychosocial needs is important in gaining trust and co-operation during the period of wound recovery and rehabilitation[2–6].

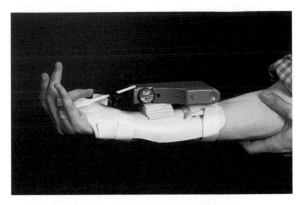

**Figure 12.1** Battery driven dynamic splint.

**Box 12.4** Factors influencing wound immobility techniques following surgery/injury.

- The anatomic structure
- The degree of injury, actual/potential formation of oedema
- The healing time required by the individual patient related to any disease processes, current medications
- The clinical treatment regime defined by the surgeon to produce the best outcome
- Unexpected adverse events – secondary injury, unresolved pain, infection – wound/dressing mismatch
- Unresolved psychosocial issues leading to negative attitude in the patient, e.g. lack of co-operation in prescribed treatment regime.

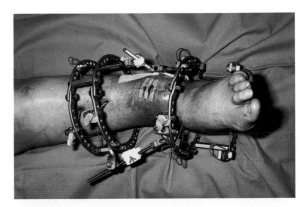

**Figure 12.2** External orthopaedic fracture stabilising frame.

## Dynamic splints

Special dynamic splints are constructed for injured flexor tendons in the palm of the hand[1,7–9] (Figure 12.1).

The extremely strong tendons (e.g. flexors of the hand) are slow to heal because of poor blood supply[1,7–9], are easily ruptured (torn) following primary injury, and require early, slow and disciplined control during passive and active pain-controlled rehabilitation.

Early, controlled, dynamic mobilisation prevents the tendon from adhering (tethering) to the internal tissue of their sliding tunnels that keep the tendon in a vertical directional line[1,7–9]. Failure to heal primarily, or rupture due to secondary injury, sets up a long process of multiple procedures (tendon grafting),

that may take over 12 months to restore some degree of acceptable function.

## External splints 1

Rigid splinting techniques may be defined as **non-invasive** (e.g. plaster of Paris, thermoplastic splints) or **invasive**. Invasive techniques include absorbable or non-absorbable plates and screws, wires, internal/external placed metal pins, or pins with connecting/stabilising frames such as the external fixator. These may be used alone or in combination (Figures 12.2 and 12.3).

These techniques are commonly used in reconstructive plastic and orthopaedic surgery following injury to significant muscles, tendons, nerves, and small and large bones.

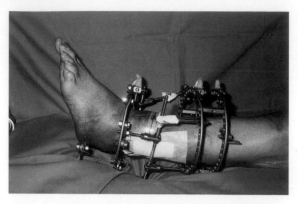

**Figure 12.3** External orthopaedic fracture stabilising frame.

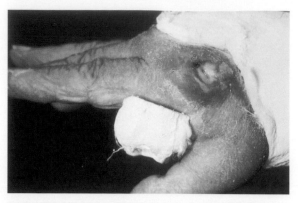

**Figure 12.4** Pressure ulcer caused by tight plaster splint.

Rigid devices are used to support, protect, conform, and totally immobilise an injured part in a specified position, but are not without their risks[10-15].

Some specialised external frames and devices allow for tension on the bone ends to be adjusted, ensuring that bone ends are firmly in alignment. Specially designed devices (similar to orthopaedic frames) may also be used to incrementally expand or lengthen the bone, for congenital shortening of long and short bones of the limbs, or the jaw[7-9].

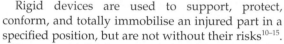

## External splints 2

Examples of non-invasive splints are externally applied plasters, wire frames and specially contoured thermoplastic moulds for hands, legs, or necks, according to the pre- and/or postsurgical needs (e.g. following burns grafting). Figure 12.4 shows plaster of Paris applied too tight, with resultant pressure ulcer.

In reconstructive plastic surgery, some non-invasive splints may be purpose built to meet non-surgical approaches to injury, for example thermoplastic (plastic contoured/moulded by heat) for open and closed hand and finger splints for management of distal finger fractures.

## Invasive/internal splints

Examples of invasive techniques are internally secured metal plates and/or screws applied directly to the fractured bone, internal wire, steel or titanium pins inserted through skin into the bone, either singly, or as part of a fracture stabilising frame.

Straight, suitably sized Kirschner wires (K-wires) may be inserted crossways through a finger or toe bone, or vertically through the distal end to secure a bone fracture, as an alternative to open surgery[7-9]. One (or more) end of the wire is left external to the skin and removed with relative ease, and usually painlessly (bone has no sensation, although periosteum does) with surgical pliers once the fracture is healed sufficiently. This allows rehabilitation before joint stiffness can occur.

Vaseline® should be smeared around the base of the pin and any eschar/scabs removed to increase the ease of extraction, as it is usually the tender skin of the fingertip that is highly sensitive. A small moist wound healing dressing should be applied until the hole is completely sealed to prevent any entry of opportunistic bacteria.

Internally, titanium is the optimal metal used, where available, because of its lightness and significant strength in comparison with stainless steel (high strength to weight ratio)[7-9]. Titanium's inertness causes little or no inflammatory reaction and as such, there is less need for surgical removal postoperatively. Micro lightweight titanium internal bone splinting of the facial and finger bones has allowed patients the opportunity for earlier mobility than was possible when stainless steel plates, screws or external frames were used. Although it is quite costly, titanium appears to provide superior surgical outcomes, and is less costly in the longer term[7-9].

Internal plates and screws that dissolve over time (similar to dissolvable sutures) are available on the market[18,19]. These have been developed because use of stainless steel can involve an overall higher cost, potential for infection, osteomyelitis and chronic pain, and risks associated with further surgery for removal if necessary. Surgeons report that they are selective in the areas in which the dissolvable products are used. This is probably due to their perception of the material in relation to the strength required.

## Special splinting needs

Thermoplastic splinting moulds, or dilators, may also be shaped in the form of an erect penis to be used as a series of sizing dilators following surgery for gender reassignment (male to female), or following surgery to correct congenital absence of the vagina. These splints maintain the size of the artificially constructed opening, which will readily contract down if, for example, skin grafts are used, or if vaginal sexual intercourse is not frequent[7-9].

The next section considers some of the clinical nursing risks associated with the care of splints, commonly seen in plastic surgery, such as the application of plaster of Paris, metal, fibreglass and thermoplastic splints, and surgical pins to the limbs.

## Splinting – risk management issues

### Box 12.5 Patient safety issues 1.

- All surgical wounds should be primarily/temporarily reinforced with retention tapes, surgical adhesive tapes, and immobilised (splinted-rest) for the first 4–72 hours[1,8–10,20]
- The construction and application of any splint should be consistent with what the splint is expected to achieve
- Splints should include the provision of pain control, wound protection, allow the maximum opportunity for the patient to undertake adequate personal hygiene and have optimal independence for the activities of daily living
- Inadequately made and applied splints can potentially compromise the healing and rehabilitation pathway

- Wounds over joints, and in fixed skin zones, are extremely vulnerable to breakdown when increasing stress is placed on them, as prescribed and guided remobilisation begins
- With wound breakdown there is the potential for joints to be exposed and extended healing or further surgery required
- When primary rigid plaster of Paris splints are removed, lightweight rigid thermoplastic splints are more comfortable for the patient, if full immobility is to be continued
- Following removal of rigid splints on the limbs, firm graduated tubular elastic support garments are also extremely useful to reduce oedema, provide wound support, and remind the patient that a wound exists
- Firm tubular elastic supports should be measured according to the manufacturer's instructions to ensure excessive compression is not exerted on and surrounding the wound
- Older patients, and patients with free flaps on the limbs, are at risk of vascular compromise if the application of firm tubular elastic supports is not undertaken under directions from the medical officer, or expert nurse clinician
- On the leg, an ankle brachial pressure index should be undertaken to determine arterial integrity to prevent tissue ischaemia.

### Box 12.6 Patient safety issues 2.

- The potential for inappropriate techniques of immobilising and rehabilitation to compromise the preferred clinical and patient wound outcome
- Inadequate splinting negates the primary and ongoing realignment of wound tissues and the opportunity for most favourable healing opportunities within a pain-free experience
- Failure to educate the patient in the need to maintain prescribed immobilisation of the wounded area to prevent movement, shear and friction of the tissues, generates secondary injury
- Splints should be checked 2–3 times daily for any undue pressure, or shear or friction injuries that may lead to ulceration and a painful wound
- Any pain, particularly continuing sharp pain, should be reported immediately to avoid an underlying pathology developing and increasing the risk of a pressure ulcer

- The potential for secondary injury to the wound, an extension to the repair process timeframe and the potential for undesired scarring to occur
- The potential for infection to develop, retarding the repair process, compromising the patient as a whole
- Failure to educate the patient in the primary need for reduction of oedema from within the wound and its surrounds, by elevation of the part will generate pain, discomfort, wound aberrations and the potential for infection
- Splints are important reminders to the patient to protect the wound from secondary injury.

## Box 12.7 Patient comfort issues.

- Assessment of any pain must be conducted according to scientific principles that will reflect the true nature of any adverse conditions such as swelling, pressure, emerging ischaemia or infection
- A care plan regarding neurovascular pain assessment and projected management protocols should be undertaken as part of the case supervision
- Primary strict four-hourly pre-emptive oral analgesia selected, and titrated, to the patient's needs, is essential at least for the first 72 hours post-surgery/injury
- With gravity assistance, this will be sufficient if the splint, swelling and bandaging are within normal parameters
- Sharp, or dull and throbbing pain not relieved by the prescribed analgesic require immediate investigation of the wound and splint
- An ischaemic pressure ulcer over bony prominences may develop if the splint is too tight (Figure 12.4), is too loose, or has sharp or rough edges causing pressure (skin ischaemia) and/or shear and friction (rupturing superficial vessels), and may lead to secondary injury to the wound and/or adjacent skin[2,4]
- Pressure pain is a burning type of pain that is usually felt slightly away from the site of the primary injury (referred pain)[5]
- An external splint that is incorrectly applied and inadequately padded to provide a buffer for potential swelling, oedema or accidental bleeding may cause increasing pressure and significant pain within the wound[1]
- If any avascular problem is suspected, the splint bandage and/or Velcro® should be split or completely removed

- Wound bandages and dressings should be cut down to the skin (decompressed) and the wounded zone examined and assessed for treatment
- The original padding and plaster of Paris may be contaminated and will need to be disposed of and a new resting splint constructed
- Replacement splints should preferably be thermoplastic and applied with Velcro® for ease of adjustment
- If internal compartmental muscle or bone bleeding continues and is not recognised and corrected, there is the risk of unresolved compartment syndrome[7–9]
- This life-threatening complication (mainly seen in the upper and lower limbs) can potentially result in devastating wound and patient outcomes, for example, avascular tissue leading to gas gangrene and amputation[1,4,6–9]
- In addition, compartment syndrome may occur when the splint's securing bandages and/or bandage retention tapes have been applied too firmly[1,4,6–9].

See Box 12.8 for signs and symptoms[1,4,6–9].

## Box 12.8 Principal signs and symptoms of compartment syndrome.

| | |
|---|---|
| **Pain** | sharp ischaemic type, not relieved by opioid/narcotic |
| **Pallor** | whiteness due to lack of arterial blood flow |
| **Paraesthesia** | loss of sensation due to loss of blood supply to the nerve |
| **Paralysis** | loss of motor function |
| **Pulselessness** | loss of arterial blood flow |
| **Poikilothermia** | cold skin due to loss of warm blood flow and immobility of the muscle and tissue cells. |

## Box 12.9 Principal issues regarding compartment syndrome for nurse clinicians.

- Neurovascular (sharp) pain as experienced in compartment syndrome is not relieved by narcotics, requires immediate investigation and constitutes a surgical emergency
- Tightness and swelling of the limb may also be present, and the patient may be required to undergo technical compartment pressure testing
- Measuring the calf circumference of the affected limb, with a tape measure, for internal swelling, and documenting the data may also be requested
- Surgical fasciotomy may be required to relieve the pressure and rescue the nerves, vessels and muscle
- The key to avoiding adverse events is to perform objective and documented neurovascular assessment for 72 hours on the injured/affected limb(s) and to immediately investigate the cause of constant, severe and unrelieved pain[1]
- It is important to point out that in the presence of an arm block, epidural or spinal anaesthetic, which disguises pain and sensory indicators, the three principal signs to assess for are pulse, colour and skin warmth.

## Box 12.10 General nursing issues and discharge education.

- Comfort advice and pain management should also include strategies for limb elevation when the patient is at rest in a chair and in bed
- The patient should receive effective education, in a language easily comprehended, regarding the importance of elevation of the limb above heart level
- Discharge education should also be explicit enough to enable the co-operative patient to adequately assess the origins of adverse swelling and pain and to use the appropriate reporting mechanisms for emergency care
- Following hand or upper arm injury, ambulatory supports such as slings or adjustable orthopaedic arm supports should be used in the postoperative and rehabilitation phase
- The hand should also be above the level of the heart (pointing towards the opposite shoulder) to reduce the oedema and pain in the upper limb/hand
- The use of polythene foam or combined dressings of wool and gauze at the back of the neck can reduce pain/discomfort from the weight of the splint and arm

- In injuries to the upper and lower limbs, it is very important that physiotherapy exercises for major adjacent joints are included in the discharge plan. This ensures ongoing mobility of the hip or shoulder joint, and reduces the potential for distal joint stiffness and loss of muscle power, particularly in the older age group
- In the older patient, or the patient with existing compromised mobility, it is suggested that immobility of the principal upper articulating joints for about three weeks, without specific exercises, is sufficient to compromise the mobility of the hip or shoulder joints as tissues contract, reducing subsequent movement, mobility, and causing significant pain on attempted rehabilitation
- Patient education regarding splint hygiene and care is also important.

## Box 12.11 Patient independence issues.

- Competent, clearly delivered patient education results in a sense of personal control and wellbeing for the patient
- Prior to discharge the patient's psychosocial status for self-care and potential need for home assistance must be assessed
- There is potential for accidental falls or other physical injury where education in use of crutches or other adjuncts for mobility is inadequate to meet the particular need of the patient
- The older person who may be slower to respond, on medications affecting or significantly altering their mobility status, may be at risk of falling
- Potential for loss of income and long-term lifestyle requirements may be significantly altered (e.g. disabling outcomes leading to inability to function at the same level in his/her preferred workplace, need to change workplace)
- The potential for resentment, anger and depression to frustrate the patient may reduce the patient's co-operation and engagement in a rehabilitation programme for the preferred healing outcomes.
- Potential for issues related to body image to emerge with loss of self esteem, declining co-operation and emerging depressive episodes
- On discharge, patient education sheets should be given to the patient and significant carers, outlining what the patient is and is not allowed to undertake, and timeframes, as relevant
- Emergency contact phone numbers should be provided to the patient.

**Box 12.12** Children and adolescents – safety, comfort and independence issues.

- Regardless of the precautions taken by carers, children and adolescents appear to find ways of damaging or removing bandages and splints with ease
- All of the risks to the wound and secondary injury for adults apply equally to children, but damage may occur more quickly in children as surface skin and deeper tissues are fragile and more easily injured
- In terms of available time between the onset of ischaemia and disaster, children do not tolerate bleeding into wound tissues or an inadequate blood flow to the tissues as do adults, and ischaemic digits or compartment syndrome may occur within a shorter period of time
- Visual observations with the addition of descriptions and assessment questions must be tailored to the child's language and level of understanding
- Drawings and pictures can be helpful. Comforting by cuddling, providing favourite toys and treats and so on will help the child to feel safe
- Skilful proactive and pre-emptive pain management plan is important if compliance is to be expected, as children will not co-operate at any level if they are in any pain or discomfort, or feel unsafe
- Adolescents, in particular males, put great stress on their dressings and splints
- Appealing to their maturity will sometimes help, but the boredom of immobility will often encourage patients to undertake risks which may end with split plasters, compromising infection control measures and wound healing outcomes[21]
- Adding an outer cover of coloured fibreglass to plaster splints or casts for children and adolescents can provide reinforcement and a source of interest, which may extend the life of the splint
- For small children, some plastic surgeons will automatically apply a full plaster and then split it on one side, and apply an outer cohesive bandage rather than take the risk of a splint being removed
- When the swelling reduces, children have been observed slipping their hand out of a full plaster cast if the dressings beneath are minimal
- Elevation of a limb in children with slings and orthopaedic arm supports often needs reinforcement by extra large safety pins along the line of the arm to secure the arm in the sling, and a foam pad to reduce neck soreness from weight and friction
- Discomfort is one of the main reasons for patients removing retention dressings/bandages, and in particular the sling or limb support provided, following discharge

- Because dressings applied to children's hands and feet are often bulky and fully enclosed following reconstructive surgery, fingers and toes may be masked from sight. This reduces the ability of clinicians to undertake visual neurovascular observations
- If the limb is adequately elevated, pain is the primary indicator and, in children, persistent unrelieved levels of pain may indicate pressure and vascular problems that require immediate and urgent attention by the nurse or medical officer. Parents should be informed of this prior to discharge
- An assessment of the child's general activity level is important so that additional precautions can be taken to ensure the medical function of the splint or plaster cast is not disrupted. Partial or complete destruction is not unknown in adolescents and young men, and certainly, very active boys can present challenges to any clinician
- The preferred clinical outcome is a splint that is right for the task to be done. It should be in the optimal functional position, be pain-free, not cause secondary injury and should be comfortable to wear helping to reduce oedema and assist in the healing process.

**Review**

Chapter 2, Boxes 2.7–2.9. Adapt according to risk management issues and clinical patient needs.

**Box 12.13** Splints – skin maintenance.

- Basic hygiene and protective management of the skin beneath and surrounding the splint requires attention to ensure the integrity of the epidermis is maintained
- Dry or moist washing of adjacent areas is important to the skin and the patient, and a discharge care plan should be laid out that can easily be achieved by the patient and/or primary carers
- Restoring moisture levels to the surrounding dry, flaking, exposed tissues that are immobile can be undertaken at regular intervals during the day
- Medical grade moisturisers or, for example, Sorbolene and glycerine combinations, are useful as both water and oil are available in these products. This also prevents itching from dry skin
- Exposed finger or toenails should be cut, kept clean from debris and moisturised

*Continued*

- The combination of pin sites, splints and other forms of immobility requires a plan of general nursing care that meets the combined objectives of safety, comfort and independence
- In addition, checking to ensure that exercise directions of adjacent major joints is maintained can improve the patient's general physical stability and aid in the optimal return to the activities of daily living.

---

**Box 12.14** Preferred clinical and patient outcomes.

- The splint was properly applied with sufficient padding to allow for the expected expansion of wound size in response to normal or unexpected oedema/swelling
- Clinical neurovascular observations were optimal to address the risk of adverse events
- Adverse events were identified and managed in a timely manner
- A pain management plan was pre-emptive, and unexpected pain was assessed according to its origins, being mindful of adverse clinical outcomes if it was not critically analysed and controlled
- The wound and/or surrounding area have not experienced any secondary injury
- General nursing care of the skin was undertaken as prescribed
- There was excellent patient compliance in all areas of education and self care
- The patient expressed satisfaction with the splint and level of independence made possible, and was free from pain and discomfort at all stages.

---

## External pin site wounds

Splinting with metal pins has long been used to immobilise bones, tendons and complex skin and soft tissue wounds on the limbs[10–15].

Stainless steel is the common metal used for pins/wires. As metal is a foreign agent, some degree of local irritation in addition to the normal inflammatory wound response is to be expected within the first 72 hours. This may be increased in compound and complex wounds that have a poorly recovering vascular perfusion to the immediate and surrounding skin and have high degrees of contamination.

In plastic surgery, a wide range of surgical procedures on the face and limbs may require the use of metal pins to secure fractures or immobilise a wound near a joint for short or extended periods of time[7–9].

Complex flap reconstructions are often undertaken on the limbs to replace lost tissue or bone, to supplement severely compromised vascular supply, and where orthopaedic-type frames are in place. New techniques are arising in the approach to some craniofacial malformations with lengthening of bone, by incremental bone distracting (stretching) techniques using external pins and frames[7,8].

Despite the fact that external pins sites following surgery are very common, there is no truly agreed evidence-based management protocol for their protection against critical contamination or infection[10–15].

## Clinical risk management – external pin sites

There is a consensus within reported research and experience that there are four principal risks causing clinical adverse events due to the insertion of surgical pins (exposed externally)[10–15].

---

**Box 12.15** Principal issues leading to adverse events of external pin site wounds.

- The general physiological condition of the patient
- The length of time the pin remains *in situ* within the bone
- The inadequate maintenance of pin site hygiene for the exclusion of opportunistic bacteria
- The most serious complication arising from these adverse events is the development of osteomyelitis, which has the potential for chronic wound conditions, potentially leading to loss of the limb[10–15].

**Box 12.16** Potential wound and surrounding risk issues.

- General physiological instability of the patient or poor wound status due to unstable general blood flow. This leads to chronic inflammatory responses at pin sites, and significant changes in the surrounding local tissue. This issue remains unresolved until the patient's potential for infection is resolved and the wound's normal homeostasis is restored, or the pin is removed
- Circulatory compromise by injury to the surrounding capillaries or wound tension caused by poor insertion techniques and/or swelling of the tissues and skin in fixed skin areas
- Reaction to the presence of the pin
- Signs of local clinical inflammation with minimal serous drainage after 72 hours is considered to be a normal reaction but has the potential to lead to minor or major infections at the wound site or may lead to bone infections (osteomyelitis) if wound hygiene is not practised
- Continuous and unresolved movement of the pin may be a cause of pin reaction and pain, as the normally sealed internal tissue around the pin continues to be broken, allowing exudate to flow externally
- Pin site infection related to unstable movement is usually due to long-term insertions in the bone
- Infection is usually a sign of a continuing inadequate blood supply to the periosteal region that compromises general bone and tissue healing
- Significant contamination levels or diagnosed infections can be treated with hygiene and systemic antibiotics but any signs of major pin site infection will require removal of the pins to reduce the risk of osteomyelitis.
- Pins and connecting bars should not be use as 'handles' to lift the extremity or the patient. Extreme tension on the pin(s) can lead to dislodgement or tearing of the periosteum and skin
- In the hand, pain in the fingers at the insertion site may be due to the cross pins inadvertently perforating the neurovascular bundle that runs vertically along each side of the finger.

## External pin sites – wound care

The clinician should ascertain from the surgeon if he or she has any wound cleaning or dressing preferences. Should the prescribed treatment be adverse to the current evidence regarding some topical applications, this should be professionally questioned. For example, hydrogen peroxide and iodine-based ointments can be irritating to the exposed tissue[1].

There is a lack of consensus on the removal of crusts and scabs/eschar, and some differences in definitions[10–15]. Textbooks and journal papers use the two terms interchangeably and state they are the same entity.

- **Crusts** appear to be dried exudate or old cells that lift when the healing process has taken place beneath and do not bleed on removal[1]
- **Scabs/eschar** appear to be attached to underlying cells/thin granulating tissue, are moist beneath and will usually bleed on removal leaving a divot or small defect[1]

Unless they are oozing, with signs of inflammation or critical contamination/infection, they should be moisturised with Vaseline® as required, and are best left alone to simply fall off, leaving a thin layer of new epidermis, similar to skin graft donor sites[1].

## Wound bed maintenance

There is a consensus in the literature that normal saline is the preferred wound cleansing agent and dressing[10–15]. Alcohol swabs may also be used to maintain a dry environment in a non-exudating pin site. With the immobility of the area, surrounding skin dryness and skin cracking may become an issue and this should be managed with medical grade skin moisturising liquids.

Collaboration with the surgeon and infection control team in the setting of protocols can be effective for establishing best practice pin care standards based on risk management and the current literature[10–15].

**Box 12.17** Suggested protocol based on current evidence and expert experience.

- Cleanse only with normal saline using sterile techniques
- Avoidance of the use of non-pharmacologically approved ointments at any stage unless ordered by the attending physician, as these have a high risk of irritation to the wound, which can sustain inflammation

*Continued*

- For the first 72 hours, normal saline soaked gauze should be wound around the pin, ensuring that moisture is continually maintained – it should not be allowed to dry out
- If there are increasing amounts of exudate, change the dressing as required. If not, continue to maintain moisture by, for example, a sterile ampoule of normal saline and change twice a day
- The gauze should not be cut (use half-inch ribbon gauze), as lint pieces will contaminate the exposed tissue
- After about day 2–3, continue gauze soaked in normal saline to keep pin insert areas clean from any exudates
- Semi-dry scabs can have Vaseline® applied and will usually lift after 72 hours, but part of the initial treatment must be to prevent or minimise the development of dry scabs that will bleed on accidental removal
- In the absence of crusts or scabs, low/minimal exudate dressing care can be undertaken 4–6-hourly, or once a day, when the pin sites are generally clean and dry
- Scabs/eschar that are moist, attached to necrotic tissue and have surrounding redness should be excised gently and moist wound healing dressings applied
- A dressing that reflects moist wound healing principles (e.g. a thin hydrocolloid) may be used and wounds should be continually monitored for clinical and observable signs and symptoms of unexpected exudate, wound edge irritation, inflammation or infection
- Any evidence of local critical contamination or infection with clinical signs and symptoms should be investigated and appropriate medical and nursing measures undertaken.

---

**Review**

*Setting goals of care and preferred clinical and patient outcomes*, Chapter 2, Boxes 2.7–2.9. Adapt according to risk management issues and clinical patient needs.

---

**Box 12.18** Audit of preferred clinical outcomes

- Pin wound(s) sites were cleansed to prevent or minimise the development of wet zones of eschar
- Pin wound(s) sites were continually assessed to identify any indications of clinical signs of continuing inflammation, critical contamination or infection
- Skin wound edges were maintained in close opposition to the pin, limiting the risk of bacterial entry, using normal saline gauze dressings or moist wound healing dressings as appropriate to the wound's assessed needs
- The moisture of the surrounding normal skin was maintained to ensure the integrity of the skin
- The patient's condition was not adversely compromised by any undesirable physiological or psychosocial events related to the wound pin sites.

## 2. SUTURE LINE CARE

### Surgical sutures and staples

Many simple lacerations or incisions are managed with the use of surgical sutures, for example surgical adhesive-backed paper tapes, or a biological wound 'glue'. These are useful for children in particular, to avoid the additional discomfort or pain of local anaesthetic and suturing. There are advantages and disadvantages for the use of wound glues based on variants of cyanoacrylate (e.g. Dermabond®) and it is important to follow the manufacturer's directions closely and review high-order studies undertaken for its efficacy.

See recommended websites (wound 'super' glue application and management issues) at the end of this chapter.

The most common form of wound closure is by suturing, first of all the internal tissue layers where required, for inner wound strength and, finally, the skin. This is then commonly reinforced by the application of surgical adhesive tape strips[20]. Again, following the manufacturer's guidelines for application is important if skin blistering is to be avoided. This can result from improper application to a suture line under tension in both fixed and mobile skin zones.

Suture materials are essentially of two types:

- Synthetic materials that dissolve (commonly used in/on the skin with children) and are absorbed over time and do not require removal
- Those that do not dissolve and will usually require removal (e.g. external sutures, intradermal continuous monofilament nylon).

Modern materials cause much less tissue reaction than in the past, reducing wound irritation, wound sinuses and infections. The majority of local wound problems are related to avascular necrosis of the fat layer and/or skin when sutures are inserted under tension.

It is accepted that the longer the external sutures remain in a wound, the higher the chances of major indentation/scarring effect in the skin (i.e. the 'ladder' or 'lattice' appearance) and the potential for bacterial entry through suture holes. Early removal of sutures is advocated where possible, and the wound is reinforced with securing adhesive tape strips and fixation/retention tapes. This practice contributes to improved aesthetic outcomes.

The use of subcuticular sutures in many wounds today has assisted in significantly reducing the lattice or ladder appearance of suture lines. However, these can occasionally be difficult to remove if they have been in for some time in a situation where healing may be slow due to movement, such as in the abdomen or breast.

## Technique for removal of intradermal continuous nylon suture

The knot should be cut as close to the skin as possible at one end. Then the knot at the other end is cut and the suture is gently drawn out parallel to the skin. If there is repeated moderate resistance, the suture should be gently stretched parallel to the skin again and cut off on the stretch, allowing it to spring back into the wound. This is repeated at the opposite end. This can be undertaken at approximately 3 weeks post surgery and the wound line reinforced by the use of surgical adhesive paper strips.

A general rule for external interrupted suture removal is to remove alternate sutures, commencing with the second from the end and leaving the central suture until last, as this is the area of greatest tension. If the wound does not appear to be under tension, and wound edges appear firmly opposed, the remaining tapes and sutures can be removed.

If the wound appears under strain, the remaining sutures and tapes should be left in and the surgeon informed. Some surgeons may prefer to have the sutures removed and the wound further secured with new tape strips. These should be applied in a way that does not allow the wound tension to be released and the wound to spring open.

An overlay of a fixation sheet dressing is extremely useful in these situations, as they provide an additional splinting effect. For wounds that may be expected to undergo altered tension with increasing mobilisation and rehabilitation, reinforcement with skin preparation adhesive prior to the application of wound retention/securing tape may be more appropriate for security[3,4,16,17,20]. A waterproof dressing may be applied for an additional few days to allow the patient to shower.

Suture/scar lines that remain exposed require a smearing of Vaseline® or neomycin ointment until normal physiological moisture is restored. Surrounding skin zones also require general skin maintenance.

## Children

In children (and adults with good healing properties) who are not overly active, because of the excellent blood supply to the face, external sutures can be removed by day 4–5, or earlier. Wound tapes are then gently applied to the suture lines to secure the wound edges and prevent secondary injury for a few additional days.

For wounds on the limbs in children, keeping the wound edges together with securing tapes until day 7–10 (day 10–14 in adults) depends on the wound site, mechanism of the injury, wound tension required, and the age of the patient. Each patient and wound context is different, so it is not really appropriate to make hard and fast rules about timing of suture removal.

For children it is best if absorbable subcuticular sutures are used, as these do not necessarily require active removal and will dissolve over time. This helps to remove the fear and anxiety of both child and parent and the need for a second anaesthetic and surgical procedure.

In babies and small children, unless advised, it should be assumed that, for procedures that require sutures to secure grafts or dressings (e.g. in hand surgery), for redressings and secure splinting a short general anaesthetic may need to be administered in the operating room so that the dressings can be done free from movement and in excellent lighting. Before the child is discharged, the surgeon should be consulted regarding plans for any future procedures required, so that the necessary arrangements can be made.

### Removal of staples

The use of staples is becoming more common[16]. Whilst they are timesaving at the time of the operation, extreme care must be used when removing them. Both sharp edges must be free to avoid dragging the skin edge and causing secondary injury. In skin grafts this can easily occur, and clinicians must be alert to ensure they do not accidentally lift the graft from its bed. In addition, staples should be counted before and after removal and disposed of as for all sharp objects, to prevent accidental injury to the patient or nurse.

**Box 12.19** Discharge education and patient information.

- Reinforce ongoing home dressing procedures and rationale to the patient – if possible, obtain return demonstration of care
- Give information regarding alteration to the normal pattern of expected events and reporting mechanisms if adverse events occur
- Reinforce importance of rest (i.e. elevation of limb if appropriate) and limitation of movement to prevent wound dehiscence
- Avoid pressure or rubbing on wound when wound hygiene is undertaken
- If appropriate, apply ointment or cream as instructed to maintain soft tissue environment
- Report any increasing swelling or persistent pain not relieved by pain medication as ordered
- Protect the wound from the sun – use protective cream

Patients should be advised of the need to report the occurrence of any of the following:

- pain disproportional to injury and not relieved by medication as ordered
- swelling of the immediate and surrounding area
- increasing redness and heat surrounding the primary injury
- increase in body temperature and development of a fever
- unusual odour or excess exudate
- secondary injury to the area.

## Audit of preferred patient and clinical outcomes

**Box 12.20** Patient safety.

- The selection of the wound dressing and timely removal of sutures was based on evidence or expert experience that reflected a scientific assessment of the wound
- The wound dressing produced an acceptable outcome, which reflected the goals or objectives originally outlined
- Wound and suture lines were maintained in order to protect internal tissue from secondary injury and the potential for critical contamination or wound infection
- Adverse events were anticipated and addressed in a timely manner.

**Box 12.21** Patient comfort.

- Pain and discomfort was a primary consideration and pre-emptively addressed when wound bed management was undertaken
- The patient expressed satisfaction with pain and discomfort management by nursing staff.

## 3. WOUND SCAR MANAGEMENT

### Special healing problems

Some patients, regardless of the location on the body, have the potential for hypertrophic or keloid scar development. Although the biology of these developments is poorly understood, unstable myofibroblast cells are suggested to be implicated in some phases.

In some dark-skinned people, individual areas appear more vulnerable than others, particularly the neck, chest wall, the shoulder and ear lobes. Predominance in these areas may be due to the fact that they are common zones of injury (neck and chest wall burns in children) regardless of the vulnerability of the patient to their development[7–9].

Whilst there is a basic understanding of the normal healing process of clean surgical wounds, there is continuing search for (and identification of) the principal growth factor cells that may have the potential to accelerate the healing of chronic wounds. This is in the absence of any aberrant factors such as certain medical conditions, oedema, contamination/infection and repeated secondary injury.

### Descriptions of scars

Scars are principally of four types, described as linear, widespread, hypertrophic or keloid[1,7–9].

### Linear

Linear scars are the result of a primary clean wound, producing a fine line, flat skin, not red or raised, non-irritating, with demonstration of scar stretching. They usually fade over time.

### Spreading

Spreading scars may spread minimally or widely. The primary problems are usually related to cosmetic outcomes, but may be subject to the effects of UV radiation (development of skin lesions) if constantly exposed without UV protection.

Hypertrophic and keloid scars are defined and discussed later in this chapter.

### Scar development – the principles

Disciplined wound bed maintenance that allows for the wound(s) to repair free of adverse episodes leads to contraction and epithelialisation that results in acceptable scar results.

Wound bed maintenance encompasses this phase in order that secondary injury is prevented and resolution of the scar occurs without incident. But despite the best attention in wound care, not all healing produces acceptable functional and/or aesthetic results, for a broad range of reasons[1,7–9].

Wounds that incorporate any level of the dermis heal by contraction and epithelialisation, with scar development in maturation are referred to as a contracture. The final outcome of a normal scar is approximately 85% of the area's previous strength and usually results in a mark/line relative to whether healing was normal, or disturbed by a range of adverse events[1]. A scar is described as being the result of two specific actions: mechanical and biological[1,7–9].

### Mechanical techniques of wound closure

Normal scars are principally the result of correct planning of surgical incisions, excisions, and wound closure made parallel to the line of least stretch/tension (Langer's lines). Under normal conditions, the process of wound healing can be expected to proceed unhindered, resulting in fine linear scars.

Wide or spreading scars are usually caused by mechanical stress and tension – vertical tension between the maturing and contracting dermal fibres within the wound, and the stress and stretch applied to the wound by functional needs and gravity[1,7–9].

Tissue such as skin, fat or subcutaneous layers that are closed under tension or inappropriately splinted post surgery or injury, may suffer avascular necrosis of some areas of tissue. This may potentially lead to wound infection, wound breakdown and development of disfiguring and unstable scars. In addition, failure of the patient to co-operate with immobilisation and rehabilitation pathways can be an important contributing factor[1,7–9].

## Biological disturbances in production of normal scar tissue

Keloid and hypertrophic scar development is unique to humans and, for unknown scientific reasons, aberrations in the physiological healing cascade of events can occur[1,7–9]. No valid theory or scientific explanation of what initiates development of keloid and hypertrophic scars has been put forward. Textbooks collectively agree that there is no way to diagnose with absolute certainty the difference between keloid and hypertrophic scars – some descriptions are provided but they do not have scientific confirmation. That said, careful clinical diagnosis, and constant observations by specialist plastic surgeons or skin specialists, provide the best pathway for those unfortunate enough to have these scar abnormalities[1,7–9].

Some tumours of the skin may give the appearance of a keloid scar. Tumours may arise many years later in the keloid scar area or on the margin of a burns scar (Marjolin ulcer), and this is thought to be associated with long-term exposure to UV radiation, or chronic ulceration due to ongoing irritation caused by constant stretching of the scar on movement of the body part. Any doubt about the clinical appearance of the scar requires biopsy to rule out malignancy. Severe disturbances of body image may occur with hypertrophic and keloid scars and patients often pursue fast track treatments without success[1,7–9].

**Box 12.23** Principal risk factors associated with inferior scar outcomes[1,7–9].

- Congenital or acquired aberrations (immune disorders) in the synthesis of collagen
- Systemic disease processes – diabetes mellitus, vascular disease
- Smoking
- Malnutrition
- The cause of the wound (surgical site, gross trauma, disease)
- The anatomical position of the wound (e.g. over the knee, on the back)
- The degree and extent of the injury (e.g. compound, more than one wound site)
- The surrounding and available blood supply (e.g. avulsed skin and underlying tissues)
- Co-morbidity (contamination or infection) and current medications (e.g. warfarin, steroids)
- Racial propensity to abnormal scar development (e.g. dark-skinned races)
- Inadequate recognition of the importance of early splinting, immobilisation and rehabilitation processes relative to each specific patient's injury state of general health, existing mobility, or the ability to comply
- Inadequate personal hygiene management during the use of compression garments and silicone gel pressure pads
- Inadequate patient education by the treating clinicians
- Difficulty with co-operation from the patient.

## The ideal conditions for ensuring an outcome for the best scar

Incisions and flap repairs are made in the natural skin lines, referred to as Langer's lines, which are normal crease lines observed in the line of least tension. Where the wound is clean, and skin wounds closed by the use of wound tapes rather than sutures, it will heal with minimal scarring.

- Only some wounds are suitable, and they are usually in areas of accelerated healing, such as the face. This is an example of the normal process[1,7–9].
- It is surgically acknowledged that adequate, and accurate, debridement of all contaminated material, back to bleeding zones, in trauma-based wounds, is essential before repair is undertaken.

- If a wound is closed by sutures or staples it should not be under any tension that may cause ischaemia within the tissue layers, particularly the hypodermis (fat) layer, with its fragile blood vessels
- Alternative methods of closure, for example temporary or permanent skin grafts or a skin flap, would be considered rather than risking skin necrosis[1,7–9]
- Any minimal tension within the wound should be distributed along the whole length of the wound with the use of appropriate wound closure material, giving consideration to size and type of suture material
- Any dressing material applied over the wound should reflect the moist wound healing principles, and these dressings should not allow abnormal mechanical pressure, shear or friction capable of disturbing normal blood flow within the wound.
- Wound splinting/immobilisation and reduced activity in the initial healing phase will reduce mechanical stress, which may cause spreading of the scar outcome[1,7–,9]
- Following facial lacerations (trauma), scarring is common due to ragged wound edges, and will often require secondary procedures (e.g. scar revision) to achieve better scar outcomes.

## Timing of suture removal to assist scar outcomes

The timing of the removal of suture material, and of secondary procedures to minimise or prevent the potential for scar development will enhance the cosmetic outcome. Almost without exception, the timing is based on the individual patient, reflecting all of the known risk factors, professional experience, and the scientific evidence to date[1,7].

Whatever the technique of surgical closure used (for example, direct closure, delayed closure, skin graft or skin flap), certain principles apply in the care of the wound and suture line and the timing of the removal of the sutures, staples or tapes if wound breakdown and/or the spreading of scars is to be prevented, minimised, and managed.

- To reduce/prevent indentation marks in the skin, sutures/staples should only be removed according to the known healing capacity, blood supply and mechanical stress of the area[1,7–9]

- Special conditions apply to wounds in particular areas such as the face, back and fixed skin zones
- In most patients where no tension exists, sutures on the face can be removed in 3–5 days. Patients who have sutures removed early to prevent suture line marks (e.g. on the face), should have horizontal wound tapes applied for at least 3–7 days to reinforce the wound and protect it from secondary trauma
- For the back, the insertion of continuous intradermal monofilament nylon with supporting external interrupted sutures, adhesive horizontal adhesive-backed paper tapes or equivalent, with a non-adherent dressing, retention dressing and/or adhesive film, is the most appropriate. This provides the wound with optimal support and allows the patient to shower
- Retention tapes can remain *in situ* and be dried effectively with a hair dryer on warm/cool
- In optimal conditions the external sutures can be removed after 10–14 days, leaving the intradermal suture in for up to 3 weeks for security and most favourable repair
- Adhesive moist wound healing dressings may be continued to allow for hygiene and showering and improved scar outcomes
- In wounds at risk, alternate interrupted sutures may be removed to test the tension of the wound, and decisions can then be made about the remaining sutures in relation to the anticipated patient's ongoing activities.

As stated previously, sutures left in for long periods, under stress or with a high level of inflammation during the healing period, may leave a cross-hatching scarred ladder effect. It is important to alert the patient to potential trouble in primary or secondary wounds, including unexpected pain, heat, redness, swelling and loss of function, particularly around tight suture holes. This may indicate excess tension and disturbances in blood supply to the wound or wound edges, which may be a precursor to tissue necrosis, dehiscence and subsequent infection. Any wound, regardless of the aetiology, that is primarily closed under tension is at risk of breakdown and infection regardless of the time sutures remain in place. Any clinical indications of inflammation or fever should be investigated immediately.

## Scarring in specific regions of fixed and mobile skin

Similar to the back, fixed skin areas also take longer to heal and gain tensile strength, particularly those in regions that are constantly under various levels of pressure, shear or friction, and are subject to dependant oedema when they are non-functioning (e.g. palm of the hand or sole of the foot). Regions where the strain is in a range of directions (e.g. over joints) are more likely to be subject to spreading scars.

Initially, central sutures should be left in, as these are the regions of greater tension. Commonly, a continuous non-absorbable suture (e.g. monofilament nylon) will be used to support the healing tissues for up to 3 weeks or longer. Wound securing adhesive tapes (flexible) should also be used to reinforce the suture line[21]. These should not be applied under tension or stretch, as normal shear and friction will result in skin blisters[21]. The wound can be covered with a transparent adhesive dressing to allow for normal hygiene to be practised.

Wound dressings must be properly applied as per the manufacturer's instructions. With wound splinting the surgeon should state the optimal time for the restriction of movement of the injured area and immediate surrounds to prevent stretching of the non-mature collagen fibres.

### *Reinforcing the suture line*

Wounds in those mobile tissue regions such as the breast and abdomen are at special risk with continuous movement caused by normal respiration, movement and gravity. Breast and abdominal wounds that are at high risk of stretching-type scarring because of gravity reflect that commonly seen following pregnancy (referred to as 'stria').

In active patients where it is difficult to discourage even minimal movement, for example in skin grafts and skin flaps utilised for wound closure on the back, the use of shoulder restraints in the form of an orthopaedic sling for the arm on the affected side may be necessary for the first 7–10 days to reduce the primary strain on the wound.

Suture lines may be under critical tension in skin flaps that have moderate to major swelling and this may result in avascular disturbances at the suture line site. Sutures may need to be removed immediately or within the first few days to restore vascular integrity to the flap and a skin graft may be needed to fill the gap.

No research has been undertaken to assess the scar outcomes in regions at risk when negative pressure therapy has been used, which decreases wound tension by reducing the degree of local and regional oedema and swelling.

## Wound scars – wound bed maintenance

Development of haematoma or seroma in the wound, signs and symptoms of abnormal inflammation, and potential development of infection should be observed for, and reported to the surgeon immediately. The patient should be aware of the need to report any direct pain in the wound unrelieved by normal pain control programmes, particularly after discharge from the surgical environment.

The patient who presents long term with frequent breakdowns and non-healing ulcers within scars should be directed for biopsy to exclude skin cancer. If malignancy is diagnosed, it is commonly squamous cell carcinoma, but it may also be some form of rare tumour[1,7–9].

## Care of the skin post surgery

Basic hygiene care of wounds must be undertaken regularly, particularly where pressure splints, garments and silicone gels are used, to reduce/prevent development of skin rashes and sweat irritations. Primary wound care must be attended to, and suture lines must be kept clean and free from debris, such as early scabs, and dry blood.

Dry scabs in the suture line holes need to be removed to allow dermal contraction and total epidermal resurfacing. Wound cleansing can be undertaken by the use of cotton buds soaked in normal saline, or the application of Vaseline®, as a thin eschar softener allowing the dried material to simply lift off as healing is completed.

To prevent skin allergies, only non-perfumed, natural soaps should be used. The skin should be gently massaged (see massage therapy later in this chapter) using aloe vera oil, vitamin E cream, Sorbolene® and glycerine cream, or any creams/oils that are non-irritating and contain no preservatives. This assists venous and lymphatic circulation, retains skin softness and pliability, and prevents dryness and skin breakdown that may lead to undesirable ulceration. Some surgeons believe that softening the scars and surrounding skin encourages further spreading of the scar itself. Lack of flexibility has to be weighed against the drying of the scar and potential development of skin splitting or ulceration.

Some fragile healing/healed wounds that cover wide areas of the body (Figures 12.5 & 12.6) will require disciplined, planned and ongoing wound bed maintenance. This will need to include not only bathing techniques, oil and moisture replacement and often pain management, but also education regarding appropriate clothing to prevent secondary injury. This may be time consuming, but if the wound is not to break down as physical mobility begins, it is an essential part of total wound care, and must be planned accordingly, in association with physiotherapists.

## Hypertrophic and keloid scarring

### Hypertrophic scars

Hypertrophic scars (Figure 12.7) occur in all racial groups, but are not recorded as having been seen on soles of the foot or palms of the hand, and they usually remain within the confines of the original wound. The primary clinical symptoms are irritation and change, often red and raised (up to 1 cm). They demonstrate itchiness and tenderness, and are often hypersensitive to clothes and sunlight, causing subsequent pain[1,7–9]. They can tend to regress or resolve over a long period of time but are self limiting. They have a potential to respond to pressure management over an extended period of time.

Hypertrophic scars are often disfiguring. They occur in areas of high wound tension where a wound is stretched in multiple directions, for example in the neck, shoulder, back sternum and deltoid areas.

They also occur in soft tissue areas (e.g. oral surrounds, nose, eyelids, chest, ears), causing significant functional problems. They frequently recur after excision and repair. Major contractures and development of ulceration in the scar at points of high stress (e.g. the neck, elbow or armpit) may occur, causing major restriction of movement, pain, and possible need for surgical release by Z-plasty, full thickness skin graft, or a free flap[1,7–9].

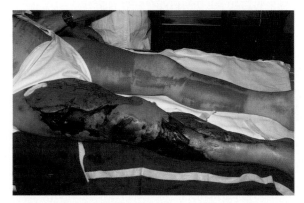

**Figure 12.5** Partially healed major lower limb injury (de-gloving) – right leg, with large zones of eschar, and healed donor site wounds – left leg.

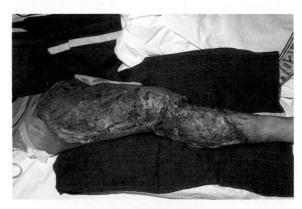

**Figure 12.6** Following eschar debridement and further skin grafting.

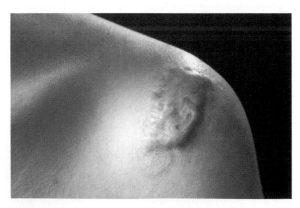

**Figure 12.7** Hypertrophic scar.

## Keloid scars

Keloid scars (Figure 12.8) are very common in dark-skinned races but are seen in all races particularly following surgery and burns. They can be disfiguring, persisting at the site of injury. They are different to hypertrophic scars as they grow outside the original boundaries of the wound and do not resolve with pressure treatment. Some respond to early pressure care and local steroid injections, but treatments cannot be guaranteed. The primary clinical indications are itching, tenderness and pain on stretching[1,7–9]. Complications often recur after excision, with continued enlargement and thickening, frequently resulting in ulceration at points of high stress.

Severe scarring, called keloid contracture, causes major restriction of movement and often there is the development of ulceration in the scar because of constant stress and tension on the contracted scar.

Life-threatening malignant skin tumours may develop in a burns scar (Marjolin ulcer/squamous cell carcinoma tumour) (Figures 6.7 and 6.8) and some rare and bizarre tumours may be disguised as an ulcerating keloid scar. The time taken for a scar to mature varies from one individual to another and one body region to another and is unpredictable. This timeframe is largely determined by the age of the patient, degree of skin mobility, degree of tension on the area and available blood supply to the area[1,7–9]. Treatment options for hypertrophic and keloid scars are discussed later in this chapter.

For children who may be susceptible to either hypertrophic or keloid scars, the outcomes are worse than for adults, as children's skin has less mobility. In burnt areas where the thickness of the injury is more than superficial, burns experts suggest that, for children, unless skin grafting is utilised, the healed skin contraction may be up to 20% of the original wounded area[1,7–9].

## Hypertrophic and keloid scars – common treatment approaches for minimising atypical outcomes

> **Box 12.24** Common treatment approaches for hypertrophic and keloid scars[1,7–9].
>
> - Pharmacological
> - Mechanical
> - Radiation modalities
> - Surgical interventions
> - Laser therapy.

Treatment of abnormal scar development is essentially based on control, in contrast to cure.

By far the largest number of patients who present for assessment and management of scars, have hypertrophic scars. Of these, most are single scars which, although not often large, may present significant cosmetic issues for the patient.

Large contractures from hypertrophic or keloid scars of the neck, chest wall and over joints, caused originally by burns, particularly in children, may severely reduce function by increasing contracture of the skin, require intermittent reconstructive surgery for scar release over joints and be cosmetically disturbing for the patient and others[1,7–9].

### *Pharmacological*

Pharmacological treatment is directed towards altering the turnover rate of protein and, more specifically, collagen utilising intradermal steroid injections, and it is recommended to be used in conjunction with externally applied scar management, for example, compression garments or soft and conforming silicone gels[1,7–9].

### *Mechanical*

Some individuals have a high predisposition for development of excess scar growth following injury

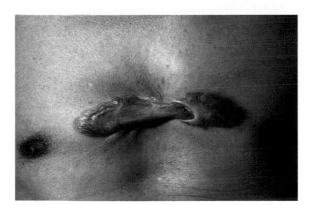

**Figure 12.8** Keloid scar.

to the skin[1,7–9]. Pressure garments that apply mechanical pressure may be used for adults and children[22,23].

The level of pressure is directed towards curtailing scar formation by reducing blood flow. This is achieved by uniform compression through an elasticised garment exerting external pressure to counter the pressure of the body surface. There is no scientific evidence to demonstrate how pressure may work or what pressure levels are optimal. Some clinicians suggest 24–40 mm Hg[22,23]. Pressure garment management should only be used under the guidance of an experienced health professional, usually a specialist burns nurse, or physiotherapist[22,23]. Custom sized garments made of specialised one-way elastic material are designed to fit the region(s) of the individual body[22,23]. They may be small enough to fit a single digit, a hand, leg, face, or whole body suits may be required for major burns victims.

In children, these garments need to be regularly resized and remade as the patient grows. Child compliance is often difficult in warm climates due to sweating, itching and discomfort, especially if garments are too tight or too hot, or if they are the subject of ridicule by other children. Adults may also be very self-conscious about wearing facial masks and gloves in public places. This long-term treatment requires practitioners to demonstrate continuity and the patient to feel confident at all stages. Children find the prospect of further long-term treatment difficult, as they have often recently experienced enduring and painful physiological and psychological effects of earlier burns treatments. Patience, reassurance and education about the benefits of wearing the garments may be useful but is not always persuasive. Nursing and professional psychological counselling for the child and family should be considered to help in overall rehabilitation. If the garments are not worn continuously, the increasing development of scar contractures (particularly over body joints) will begin to be observed, slowly reducing the overall physical function of the area[1,7,8,22,23]. Some patients have a preference to wear garments for life as a disguise of their scars.

## Spenco Silicone® gel pads

Spenco Silicone® gel pads and surgical adhesive tapes have gained widespread use in patients with superficial scars, in the hope of minimising the development of scar tissue[7–9]. These have had varying degrees of success but have shown promise in some patients.

As stated earlier, the evidence for many of the above treatments is mainly still anecdotal and based on clinical experiences but, even in the absence of scientific proof, some of these modalities appear to work for many patients. Therefore, until there is proof to the contrary, they should not be discarded if no harm is experienced by the patient.

Small areas of thickened scars may respond to the application of a conforming silicone gel pad for extended periods. The moisture and the warmth that develops under the gel, combined with lack of oxygen to the area, are thought to contribute to retarding further growth of the scar. Again, physiotherapists or occupational therapists are best placed to manage this form of treatment as it may also be combined with other rehabilitation processes.

## Special pressure clamps

Special pressure clamps have been designed for scar aberrations of the ear lobe following ear piercing. The mode of action is also unknown (perhaps reduction of blood flow to the area) but overall, results have been acceptable for many patients. Ease of application has enabled their widespread use. Again, application should be under medical or specified practitioner supervision[7–9].

## Radiation modalities

Radiation treatment is not considered to be appropriate as ionising radiation rays are non-selective and will destroy viable cells. Caution should be practised in the use of this method as, although no radiation-induced tumours have been reported to date, this risk is always considered to be a possibility[7–9].

## Surgical

Surgery is not considered a cure but may improve function and aesthetics of the area. The axilla, neck, eyelids, elbows, fingers, and infra-mammary lines in growing breasts of young women are common points of tension. In the latter case, surgery may need to be repeated according to breast growth with age or recurrence of contractures.

Surgery by excision of the region of the scar, and full thickness skin grafts, skin flaps, free flaps, or Z-plasty technique may be undertaken to release tension of contracting joints. In the area of the neck, using free vascularised flap tissue is a popular reconstructive approach that gives excellent functional and aesthetic results. Some experimentation is being done with the use of artificial dermis and the secondary application of a split thickness skin graft[1,7–9]. Tissue expansion techniques may also be used in normal tissue, adjacent to the scars.

All reconstruction in these patients has the potential to present new problems of scar development, but patients will accept this for improved functional and cosmetic outcomes in areas such as the neck, eyelids (preventing cornea damage) and major joints.

Combinations of techniques (pharmacological, pressure, surgery) may be considered depending on the anatomical area and need for additional function or desire to improve aesthetic outcomes[7–9].

### Laser therapy

If all else fails, the surgeon may consider/discuss the use of laser therapy. This is usually used in association with other adjunct therapy as described above. Results are mixed but the technique holds substantial promise and is currently undergoing further research[7–9].

### Scars and body image issues

The clinician should be alert to the effects of disturbances of body image. What may seem of little consequence to others may be a significant issue to the patient. Patient counselling may be useful and should be offered if the patient demonstrates continuing and more than average focus on specific or disfiguring scars.

In plastic surgery practice, the scar is the result of the surgery and, almost without exception the patient will judge the success of the surgery on the aesthetic appearance of the scar(s) and seek redress through litigation when expectations are not met, regardless of prior education. Adherence to the disciplined nursing principles of minimising or preventing adverse events that compromise the wound healing process can substantially assist the patient towards meeting their preferred scar outcomes.

Patients should be provided with information regarding specialist camouflage cosmetic make-up preparations available for the subtle disguising of some scars[7,8]. If additional problems begin, patients should be guided towards skilled rehabilitation practitioners, experienced in scar management.

See recommended websites (scar treatment modalities) at the end of this chapter.

## 4. SKIN MAINTENANCE AND MASSAGE THERAPY

The use of complementary modalities in addition to traditional medical treatments is gaining increasing momentum within orthodox medical and nursing practices, with manual massage therapy and music therapy, pre- and postoperatively being reported in the literature[24–28]. Although the main goal stated for their use has been for the purpose of relaxation, the application of massage therapy may have scientific advantages for wound bed repair and maintenance.

As discussed in Chapter 8 and earlier in this chapter, one of the primary principles of wound repair is an uninterrupted circulation within the wound and surrounding tissues. This section seeks to outline the important place that massage may have in the overall conditioning of the skin, and immune system, prior to and following surgery, for the enhancement of wound bed repair and maintenance.

### Oedema and lymphoedema

In the skin, the lymphatic system runs in parallel with the arterial and venous system within the dermal layer (superficial lymphatics), entering via the hypodermal layer with its primary source vessels (deep lymphatics) arising from within the muscle (Figures 5.5–5.8).

The lymphatic system is the foundation of our immune system[1]. It is primarily responsible for carrying disease fighting material to cells attacked by bacteria, transporting the bacteria away and supplying protein-rich plasma fluid back to the heart, and the general circulation. When this system is blocked, we become virtually defenceless against attacks by virus, fungi, and bacteria. As previously outlined, the mechanical function of the lymphatics produces a suction effect that generates a negative pressure within the tissues, restricting dead spaces to a minimum or zero.

The term 'oedema' refers to the accumulation of an excessive amount of fluid in tissues or organs resulting in swelling. Lymphoedema is the swelling of skin and subcutaneous tissue as a result of the local or systemic obstruction or non-functioning of lymphatic vessels, or lymph nodes, causing the accumulation of large amounts of lymph fluid in the local region, or anatomical zone, that it is responsible for[1].

There are principally two major types of lymphoedema. They are primary lymphoedema (Milroy's syndrome – a rare inherited condition), and secondary lymphoedema, which is caused by a blockage or interruption of the normal flow of lymph fluid through the lymphatic system[1].

Congenital or medically related lymphoedema can be treated by several modalities, for example, professional-based massage, intermittent bio-compression therapy, exercise and surgery.

The most common form of lymphoedema in the United States and other Western countries is secondary lymphoedema. Secondary lymphoedema commonly affects those who have survived cancer and have undergone surgery, and/or radiation of the lymph nodes[4,7,8].

---

**Box 12.25** Recognised risk factors for secondary lymphoedema – examples.

- Breast cancer surgery
- Cancer radiation therapy
- Cancer of the lymph nodes
- Infection
- Chronic venous insufficiency
- Filariasis (a parasitic infection transmitted to humans by mosquito bites)
- Minor to moderate lymphoedema associated with inferior wound healing, particularly in the upper and lower limbs.

---

## Manual lymphatic drainage

The principal lymph nodes are found in the neck, underarms, and groin. Another group of lymph nodes adjacent to the small intestine helps blood absorption and digestive fats. In addition, white blood cell production is aided and natural immunity is bolstered.

Manual lymphatic drainage was developed by the Danish physiotherapist Dr Emil Vodder in the 1930s. Today there are five recognised schools[24,25]. Manual lymphatic drainage can assist in the increase of the flow of lymphatic material within the network of lymph ducts and lymph nodes, thereby assisting the venous system in its waste removal function[24,28].

Manual lymphatic drainage involves light, rhythmical massage that aids the body in collecting and moving lymphatic fluid, which plays a key role in delivering nutrients, antibodies and other immune constituents to the tissue cells of the body and removing debris such as toxins, cell waste and dead particles which are then cleansed by clusters of lymph nodes.

It is also suggested to work on the nervous system, lowering blood pressure, reducing stress and improving sleep patterns. Massage also increases drainage of venous (deoxygenated) blood to promote the removal of waste products from the body via the skin (as perspiration), the lungs (as exhaled air vapour), and the kidneys (as urine).

The manual lymphatic drainage technique is becoming increasing acceptable in clinical practice as a procedure capable of clinically assisting in replacing any lost lymphatic functions. This is attained by the stimulation of the collateral lymphatic channels to alleviate chronic symptoms including swelling, pain and loss of function[24,25].

### Basic massage techniques

The standard massage techniques are:

- Deep tissue massage (strong longitudinal strokes are designed to promote length of tissue) commonly seen used in hand therapy – hands and feet have very little lymphatic structure, relying on the venous system stimulated by constant movement
- Effleurage massage (wide sweeping movements that clear the superficial tissues of excess lymphatic fluid)

Combined, they have a rich variety of effects that combine to treat, and then loosen muscle fibres bound by scar tissue by improving overall muscle flexibility, assisting to clear any oedema (fluid) collected, and restoring good nutrition to the muscle via an improved circulatory blood supply. Fresh oxygenated blood increases the integrity of the blood supply to muscles and organs, thereby stimulating their nourishment and metabolic efficiency and thus improving the blood supply to the skin.

### Basic motions required to achieve lymph movement

All the lymphatic drainage strokes are based on specific motions and based on the goal or outcome to be achieved. Research has found that the initial lymphatics open up and the lymphangions are stimulated by a straight stretch but, importantly, even more so with a little lateral motion.

After these two motions, there is a need to release completely to allow the initial lymphatics to close and the lymph to be sucked down the channels. In this zero pressure phase, the finger tips are not completely disconnected from the skin, but the return of pressure to one of touch. Also the skin should not be pulled back as the release is in progress – it should be allowed to 'spring' back by itself using its 'elastic memory'.

These basic motions resemble a circle, and are called stationary circles. All motions are based on this principle. In orienting this motion, the aim is always to push the lymph towards the correct nodes, so the last, lateral stretch motion should be going towards the nodes.

This may be better understood by visualising moving fluid within those micro lymphatics in the dermal layer of the skin, firstly stretching, opening up, then releasing and waiting for the lymphangions to pump–suck the lymph down the vessel. It is important to understand where the superficial lymphatic system is situated within the dermis. If muscle is felt under the skin, the compression exerted is too firm[24,25].

Some additional application techniques are outlined in Box 12.26.

---

pressure in attempting to attain lymphatic drainage massage. It is often difficult to believe that a touch so light could be so therapeutically effective
- Always remember – you are working on skin. How much pressure does it take to deform the skin? Almost nothing. Remember – pushing too hard will collapse the superficial lymphatics directing situated under the epidermis
- Direction of each stroke is of great importance, because the direction required is one of always wanting to push the lymph towards the correct nodes
- If the lymph is directed the wrong way, the action will not be effective
- Rhythm, and speed of application is very important because with the correct rhythm and speed, the initial lymphatics are opened, and then allowed to shut providing time for that lymph to get sucked down along the vessel into the deeper lymphatics
- An appropriate rhythm will also stimulate the parasympathetic nervous system, causing the client to relax – this is the foundation on which remedial massage is practised
- Sequence means the order of the strokes
- When wanting to drain an area, always start near the node and move in the direction of the node is draining to
- Always push the lymph toward the node
- Then gently stroke the skin moving further and further away from the node, but always push the fluid back in the direction of the node. In this way, a path is cleared for the lymph to move, as well as creating a suctioning effect that draws the lymph to the node.

---

**Box 12.26** Principal points to remember when performing manual lymphatic drainage.

- Correct pressure is deep enough that the fingers do not slide over the skin, but touch is light enough so that nothing is felt below the skin.
- It is very common for massage therapists trained in Swedish or deep tissue techniques to apply too much

---

**Box 12.27** Contraindication to manual lymphatic drainage.

- Generally, massage is not advised for anyone with an infectious skin disease, a rash, or an unhealed wound
- It is also wise to avoid massage immediately after surgery, or if the patient is prone to localised blood clots or deep vein thrombosis.
- Circulatory ailments such as phlebitis or varicose veins preclude the use of massage and it should never be performed directly over:

*Continued*

- bruises
- inflamed or infected injuries
- areas of bleeding or heavy tissue damage
- at the actual site of recent fractures or sprains unless prescribed by a specialist surgeon as part of an overall treatment programme to reduce swelling.
- Massage is not recommended for cancer patients immediately after chemotherapy or radiation therapy
- While there is no evidence that it actually prompts cancer to metastasise to other parts of the body, the theoretical possibility exists
- Avoid massage over any known tumour, and in any area of recent surgical incision following cancer surgery.

**Box 12.28** Auditing preferred clinical and patient outcomes.

- A healing process that was not disturbed by adverse events and was aesthetically acceptable by the patient, with any pain or discomfort addressed promptly and to the patient's satisfaction
- A linear scar that faded with time
- A scar that spread minimally in, for example, a mobile area of the body or over joints
- Surgical improvement of hypertrophic or keloid scars that had the potential to alter physical function significantly, or result in malignant tumours
- The patient was educated prior to surgery and understood the nature of the expected and actual outcomes
- The patient accepted the clinical outcomes – based on the attention given to the prevention or minimisation of adverse scar outcomes
- Wound swelling was minimised by a proactive approach through professional massage therapy undertaken by a specialist wound clinician, or allied health professional.

## Summary

The evolving use of science-based massage therapy, as an adjunct to medical treatments and mechanical aids, is becoming more widely used for oedema as the benefits of the stimulation of the immune system become more recognised and acknowledged.

The use of massage following hand surgery (the hand essentially lacks a discrete lymphatic system), has long been recognised, and is an integral component of a two-prong approach of both deep and soft tissue massage to reduce oedema and restore optimal movement.

In elective plastic surgery the use of a prescribed plan for pre- and postoperative professional massage therapy could be considered by physicians and practice nurses alike, to enhance overall health outcomes.

More research in the area of both therapeutic massage (as part of the ongoing activities of body maintenance), and clinical remedial massage (as part of a holistic approach to acute, chronic and palliative wound care within specific clinically formulated boundaries) is required if the potential advantages of manual lymphatic drainage are to be beneficial to a broad range of patients. This could be an exciting new challenge for nurse clinicians.

See recommended websites (massage therapy within wound bed maintenance) at the end of this chapter.

## References

(1) Peacock E.E. Jnr. *Wound repair*, 3rd edn. Philadelphia: W.B. Saunders/Harcourt Brace, 1984.
(2) Bryant R.A. (ed.) *Acute and chronic wounds: nursing management*. St Louis: Mosby Year Book, 1992.
(3) Dealey C. *The care of wounds*, 2nd edn. Oxford, UK: Blackwell Science, 1999.
(4) Smeltzer S.C. & Bare B.G. *Brunner and Suddarth's textbook of medical-surgical nursing*, 9th edn. Philadelphia: Lippincott, Williams & Wilkins, 2000.
(5) Hawthorn J. & Redmond K. *Pain: causes and management*. Oxford, UK: Blackwell Publishing, 1998.
(6) Mallett J. & Dougherty L. (eds). *The Royal Marsden Hospital manual of clinical nursing procedures*, 5th edn. Oxford, UK: Blackwell Science, 2000.
(7) Ausher B.M., Erikson E. & Wilkins E.G. *Plastic surgery: indications, operations and outcomes*. St Louis: Mosby, 2000.
(8) Aston S.J., Beasley R.W. & Thorne C.N.M. *Grabb and Smith's plastic surgery*, 5th edn. Philadelphia: Lippincott & Raven Publishers, 1997.
(9) Ruberg R.L. & Smith D.J. *Plastic surgery: a core curriculum*. St. Louis: Mosby, 1994.
(10) Ward P. Care of skeletal pins: a literature review. *Nursing Standard*, 1998 (June 17–23); **12**(39):34–9.
(11) Wood M. A protocol for care of skeletal pin sites. *Nursing Times*, 2001 (June 14–20); **97**(24):66–8.

(12) Sims M. & Whiting J. Pin site care. *Nursing Times*, 2000 (Nov 30–Dec 6); **96**(48):6.

(13) McKenzie L.L. In search of a standard of pin site care. *Orthopaedic Nursing*, 1999 (Mar–Apr); **18**(2):73–8.

(14) Bernardo L.M. Evidence-based practice for pin site care in injured children. *Orthopaedic Nursing*, (USA), 2001 (Sept–Oct) **20**(5):29–34.

(15) Brereton V. Pin site care and the rate of local infection. *Journal of Wound Care*, 1998 (Jan); **7**(1):42–4.

(16) Hrouda B.S. How to remove surgical sutures and staples. *Nursing 2000* (Feb); **30**(2):54–5. http://www.springnet.com/

(17) Smith L., Baker F. & Stead L. Removal of sutures. *Nursing Times*, 1999: (Mar 3–9) **95**(9):Suppl 1–2.

(18) Katz K.H., Desciak E.B. & Maloney M.E. The optimal application of surgical adhesive tape strips. *Dermatology Surgery*, 1999 (Sept); **25**(9):686–88.

(19) Eppley B.L. Zygomaticomaxillary fracture repair with resorbable plates and screws. *Journal of Craniofacial Surgery*, 2000 (July); **11**(4):377–85.

(20) Cox T., Kohn M.W. & Impelluso T. Computerized analysis of resorbable polymer plates and screws for the rigid fixation of mandibular angle fractures. *Journal of Oral and Maxillofacial Surgery* (USA), 2003 (Apr); **61**(4):481–87, discussion 487–88.

(21) Bowler P.G., Duerden B.I. & Armstrong D.G. Wound microbiology and associated approaches to wound management. *Clinical Microbiology Reviews*, 2001 (Apr); **14**(2):244–69.

(22) Stewart R., Bhagwanjee A.M., Mbakaza Y. & Binase T. Pressure garment adherence in adult patients with burn injuries: an analysis of patients and clinical perceptions. *American Journal of Occupational Therapy*, 2000 (Nov–Dec) **54**(6):598–606.

(23) Rayner K. The use of pressure therapy to treat hypertrophic scarring. *Journal of Wound Care*, 2000 (Mar) **9**(3):151–53.

(24) Dr Vodder School. The original Dr Vodder method of manual lymph drainage (MLD®). http://www.vodderschool.com

(25) McRee L.D., Noble S. & Pasvogel A. Using massage and music therapy to improve postoperative outcomes. *AORN Journal*, 2003 (Sept); **78**(3):433–42, 445–47.

## Recommended websites

### 'Super glue' treatment modalities

http://www.bestbets.org/cgi-bin/bets.pl?record=00022

http://www.fensende.com/Users/swnymph/refs/glue.html

http://www.unhinderedliving.com/wounds.html

http://www.mirage-mfg.com/html/super_glue.html

### Scars and treatment modalities

http://www.surgical-tutor.org.uk/default-home.htm?core/preop2/scars.htm~right

http://www.scarinfo.org/scar_facts.html

http://www.texasface.com/instruc_scars.html

http://www.mmhs.com/clinical/adult/english/derm/scars.htm

http://www.burnsurvivorsttw.org/hyper.html

http://www.mmhs.com/clinical/adult/english/plassurg/scar.htm

### Remedial lymphatic massage therapy within wound bed maintenance

http://www.manual lymphatic drainageuk.org.uk/index.htm

http://www.deeptissue.com/learn/modal/lymph.htm

http://cfltmassage.allarounddanville.com/

http://www.emedicine.com/med/topic2722.htm

# Chapter 13

# Palliative Wound Bed Management – Malignancy and Non-malignancy

## Modern palliative care

The definition of 'palliative' (from the Latin *palliare*, to cloak) places the emphasis on alleviation rather than cure by the use of basic human caring, analgesics, or calming[1]. Modern texts expand the term to examples of treatments to alleviate recurring, but intractable conditions that can lead to long-term painful physical and mental suffering, because there is no known cure[1-16].

Thus, the care is not meant to cure but rather to provide a palliative management programme that delivers a quality of both nurture and nature (safety, comfort, independence) and one that provides the best possible quality of life[1-16].

This chapter further raises the question as to whether the long-held concepts, principles and practice of palliative wound bed management can be scientifically advanced and applied to what is currently referred to as 'long-term chronic' (non-cancerous) wound care, in addition to wounds that are malignancy-based.

## Chronic or palliative management?

*'To occasionally cure, often relieve, always comfort'*, is an old adage that expert and experienced clinicians often quote. The traditionally held view of palliative care is the management of individuals with terminal cancer, managed under the multidisciplinary specialty practice of oncology[1-9].

Scientific advances and medical screening processes have provided early diagnosis of a range of malignancies (e.g. breast, prostate, skin). Within medicine, chemotherapy, radiotherapy, clinical trials of new 'cocktails' of drug treatment modalities are aimed at potential cure or the prolongation of life. This is aided with significant advances in pain man-

agement appearing to assist in substantially longer periods of comfortable remission, and providing a qualified, but acceptable quality of life for many people, for significantly longer than previously anticipated. Patients falling outside the traditional parameters of palliative cancer care are usually classified as chronic, invalid, long-term, care within nursing home establishments, basic nursing care only, and a range of other terms[10-16].

With the aid of scientific and humanities research, the concept of modern palliative care for cancer has been extended outside the traditional cancer treatment boundaries[10-16]. This has been approached by utilising and expanding the concept of the meaning of a patient-focused preferred 'quality of life'.

An increasing number of patients are addressing long-term disabling medical conditions with a range of non-medical approaches (e.g. remedial massage, lifestyle changes, alternative medicine, spiritual-based approaches) in order to satisfy the needs they believe are absent from within traditional healthcare frameworks.

### Psychosocial issues

For many clinicians and patients, the connotations of 'chronic' are often negative, lacking hope of any description, and express a large degree of equal fragility, powerlessness, and finality.

The lack of a specific concept and applied practice principles of multidisciplinary care approach to encompass the broad range of non-cancerous patients appears to have led to a fragmented view of what actually constitutes chronic wound bed management. Wound bed preparation for chronic wound care appears to have developed as a result of this perceived void. Various other non-malignant conditions also cannot be 'cured', and are currently categorised within healthcare as requiring long-term 'chronic' care[2–16].

For a patient, hearing the constant use of the terms 'chronic wound, chronic patient, or chronic condition' may infer an extended period, or a lifetime, living with a degraded physical and social status compounded by periods of pessimism, hopelessness, powerlessness, blame, guilt, depression and social isolation. This may make the patient reluctant to engage in treatment modalities that can provide positive degrees of safety, comfort and increased levels of independence. For some, positive efforts afforded for survival become an engaging process, and for others, such is the despair and depression that accumulates, that suicide may become an inevitable decision.

When cure is not anticipated or possible, and a 'chronic' state is inevitable, levels of safety, increased comfort and independence acceptable to the patient can be achieved in many circumstances, but require an objective case management model of care[5,15,16].

A palliative care model approach could assist to ensure that small and incremental objectives or goals that are collaboratively set and agreed upon by the patient and carer are genuinely achievable. They may be reinforced by a concept of overall care, rather than focused on cure.

It can be observed in the literature that patients are becoming more adversarial in their approach to what science and governments have told them they can reasonably expect from the application of modern research and general healthcare. Legal claims made by patients regarding objective expectations of wound care, quality of life, pain and suffering, are now a reality in modern courtrooms[8].

## Advances in the use of a palliative model

As stated at the beginning of this chapter the original term 'palliative' does not imply 'cure' or 'death' but rather a process of 'care'.

Increasing numbers of patients have need of wound care that requires complexity and a multi-dimensional focus. Much of this care falls between the traditional categories of acute and palliative oncology care.

Research and development into non-cancerous disease processes, new technology and treatments, have seen the growth of new medical and nursing approaches in almost every specialty practice area. A question that may be posed is: 'is previously anticipated early mortality in many patients beginning to become long-term morbidity, as patients are being assisted to live longer?'

Palliative care for chronic conditions outside the oncology model are based on:

- Modern treatment options and modalities
- Determining and addressing the patient's wishes
- Setting achievable goals and outcomes with the patient
- Engagement with the patient in achieving higher levels of independence
- The potential for an improved quality of life.

In wound management, this has been suggested as a 'third way' for addressing chronic or recurrent wounds[10–16].

A search of the current literature clearly demonstrates that new treatment modalities for conditions such as congenital malformations, cardiac, neurology and nephrology, to mention a few, are embracing models in which 'care' labelled 'chronic' are emerging in a new pathway of 'palliative' care – the alleviation or amelioration of the serious symptoms and disabling effects to a level that provides the most favourable quality of life available, relative to the patient's medical condition[10–16].

As an example, this emerging contemporary patient care, for the patient whose condition is currently considered inoperable, cardiology medical and nurse clinicians have begun to discuss expanding and introducing the concept of palliative care into cardiac management as a standard of modern care. These are the group of patients who may have an incurable and debilitating cardiac condition. They require a multidisciplinary-based palliative care model to enable a reasonable quality of life that may continue for a considerable or long period of time. This is being referred to as palliative cardiac management[12]. The plan is focused on the development of a specific case management approach for each patient through a multidisciplinary framework that can address the patient's safety, altered mobility, optimal control of pain, loss of body image and personal independence, in a positive and supportive manner. This approach is revolutionary in a major scientific discipline in which many patients may have come to expect a painful and, often an early, terminal state.

Box 13.1 outlines some of the more unfavourable wound outcomes that may arise as a result of a long-term breakdown in the process towards an acceptably healed or non-healing wound.

---

**Box 13.1** Risk management related to outcomes of complex (non-malignant) wounds.

- Normal healing results in optimal wound strength (85%), an acceptable scar and patient satisfaction
- Inferior quality healing results in major scar aberrations, reduced functional abilities, undesirable aesthetic outcomes and usually patient dissatisfaction[4,6]
- A totally unacceptable outcome for the patient is a complete failure of the wound to heal, or frequent recurrences – these consist of chronically ulcerated wounds, permanent fistula, persistent and often excessive oedema, lymphoedema, recurrent infections, and unresolved chronic pain/discomfort
- Some wounds/conditions (e.g. arterial and venous leg ulcers, malignant-based lymphoedema) result in delayed healing that deliver poor scarring, continuous or intermittent oedema, stiffness, pain, discomfort or potential to breakdown from secondary injury will cause significant patient frustration
- Patients with painful, debilitating arterial ulcers who are at serious medical risk of corrective surgery are classic candidates for palliative wound bed management
- Skin conditions related to diabetes mellitus present long-term wound care needs
- Wounds such as percutaneous endoscopic gastrostomy (PEG) or stomas have long-term wound care needs
- Inferior recurring painful wound outcomes are frequently accompanied by patient grief, increasing loss of independence, co-morbid factors including depression and despair, closely associated with social isolation.

---

## Advances in plastic surgical applications to provide palliative wound bed management

Within reconstructive plastic surgery, many patients with significant medical or surgical morbidity may have, for example, unresolved permanent fistulas or sinuses, associated with head and neck free flaps, tra-cheostomy, PEGs, breast wounds related to failed prosthesis procedures and an assorted range of recurring lower limb (post-trauma) wounds that have the potential to break down.

Referred patients, such as those with wounds related to both oncology and chronic aetiology, are forming an increasing number of individuals seeking relief from the debilitating effects of pain, wound breakdown and psychosocial disturbances.

With contemporary resuscitation methods, aggressive surgery, dressings and antibiotics, patients who would have died from major systemic infections are now surviving conditions such as major burns, meningococcal infections, and necrotising fasciitis[17] (Figures 12.5 and 12.6). These patients will often require a lifetime of ameliorating or palliative wound care to prevent recurring skin breakdowns that may begin the need for frequent multidisciplinary interventions for contractures, ulceration, etc.

Patients who have suffered major trauma and survived can be left with wounds that lead to severe contractures with hypertrophic, or keloid scarring, and frequent wound breakdowns that also require a lifetime of palliative scar contracture management to prevent recurrent ulceration. This is necessary if the potential for skin cancers within the scars are to be avoided many years hence. It is now seriously being discussed that patients falling into these general categories and currently classified as 'chronic' may require a reassessment of the approaches currently utilised[14–16].

Finally, within plastic surgery some long-term and painful wounds have resulted from bizarre and significant adverse reactions to silicone breast prosthesis. These wounds often require an extended or lifetime period of observation, surgery, pain management and psychosocial care[17].

## Applying modern reconstructive surgical techniques to an old problem

Surgery aims for total removal of a tumour and an optimal reconstructive outcome as the primary goal[17–20]. In patients with a local tumour recurrence (e.g. oral squamous cell carcinoma, breast cancer, melanoma) or lymph node breakdown in the axilla or groin, these are often sited in difficult anatomical areas combined with the wound itself being a significant cause of pain, discomfort, and disability.

The emergence of satellite lesions (e.g. post malignant melanoma[18]) and the delivery of optimal wound care that satisfies all the patient's needs, can be very challenging to achieve by the very nature of the wound. A high degree of focus on pre-emptive pain management, and, where appropriate, the application of modern non-adherent (odour-containing) dressings can assist in this dilemma[2-7] but are not always the complete answer.

Independence requirements, including quality of life, aesthetics and other complex life and family factors are required to be addressed by assisting the patient's wishes with professional guidance[2-8].

A shift in conceptual surgical thought appears to be emerging. Palliative flap surgery is being applied with excellent results for hygiene and aesthetics, particularly in early and advanced cancer of the breast and other areas of the body[17-20].

It has often been considered that bringing in a new blood supply by the application of a muscle or skin flap, for example, accelerates the secondary development of a malignant tumour because of the tumour's exploitation of the local blood supply.

These procedures are not intended to be curative but rather to provide a window of quality of life that delivers an optimal level of pain management and significantly reduces the need for wound dressings, or intermittent surgery, to address aberrant and spreading odorous wounds.

Whilst it may be difficult to understand that body image and aesthetics may be an issue for a patient in demise, dying in a pain-free environment with a non-fungating, odour-free wound, and in personal dignity, is a human need that never disappears, and should not be forgotten or minimised.

Some aggressive malignant secondary lesions (Figures 6.9 and 6.10) and satellite lesions arising adjacent to malignant melanomas[12] (Figure 6.11) can break down and suppurate and as many are often inoperable, radiotherapy may be considered – but this sometimes leaves weeping, odorous wounds which may be excised and a skin graft, skin flap or dressings applied for temporary relief.

There may be a window of time between the emergence of these obvious lesions and obvious metastatic secondary lesions in the brain, lungs or bones, before death occurs. This requires palliative wound bed management which is important not only for the wound and pain alleviation, but also for body image, an improved sense of aesthetics, and quality of life, even for a short period of time.

The concomitant psychosocial and body image changes which afflict or affect the patient through any periods of remission parallel the potential for recurrence, and fear of death will remain in the patient's mind.

Wounds related to disturbances in the immune system, including AIDS[6], may be longstanding and ultimately life-threatening, and will require continuity of management (Figures 6.2 & 6.3). Modern medications, increasing understanding of the staging of the disease process and the longevity of these patients are significantly improving and wounds are being more adequately managed. Surgery for small lesions can be highly therapeutic for the patient for both wound care and aesthetics.

## Potential for establishing a palliative wound bed management model for non-malignant wounds

Research outlines potential approaches towards establishing models that can be applied within wound care units for palliative wound bed management for non-malignant wounds[10-16]. Utilising an extension of a clinical framework that addresses concepts and principles such as those outlined in Chapter 2 can also be a starting point.

Safety, comfort and independence are as important to the patient who has a wound that will heal, as they are to a patient with a wound that has a chronic or malignant presentation. The emphasis that is placed on particular areas of wound care, pain management, potential for self-care or assisted care, wound aesthetics and psychosocial issues weigh heavily on the individual patient's mind and body.

The principal points to be addressed should include those described within the model proposed in Chapter 2 (Figures 2.1 and 2.2).

**Box 13.2** Proposed case management plan as an objective model for wound bed management (non-malignant).

- Actually assessing and addressing what it is that the patient wishes
- Emphasis on asking the patient what it is that they do not like about their wound and/or treatment
- Providing a range of available options and allowing the patient to determine what the patient considers health professionals can help them with
- Patient, wound and pain assessment
- Psychosocial assessment
- Reviewing clinical risk management
- Addressing the patient's spiritual needs and providing professional assistance wherever possible
- Setting up a multidisciplinary team to address the potential complexity of patient needs
- Setting interim clinical, and patient-achievable goals, through addressing safety, comfort and independence
- Setting preferred and achievable clinical and patient outcomes through addressing safety, comfort and independence
- Auditing preferred clinical and patient outcomes.

**Review**

*Setting goals of care and preferred clinical and patient outcomes*, Chapter 2, Boxes 2.7–2.9. Adapt according to risk management issues and clinical patient needs.

*Auditing preferred clinical and patient outcomes*, Chapter 2, Boxes 2.10–2.12.

## Summary

Rather than being the exclusive province of cancer/oncology, the traditional palliative care model is providing for:

- A disease and chronic wound-focused model of care
- A management pathway co-ordinated to focus on alleviation or amelioration of symptoms, integrated into the individual's overall psychosocial and quality of life needs[5,10–16].

With longer life expectations, increasing levels of chronic wounds associated with diseases such as lower limb vascular syndromes and diabetes mellitus, the 21st Century must retain the concepts and principles of what multidisciplinary professional and humane patient care represents, but within a framework that delivers positive and best practice care outcomes.

As patient care approaches are changing in line with advances in research, medications, technology, and attempts at alternative approaches in the provision of healthcare, wound management must also make similar leaps in parallel with other disciplines[5,10–16].

Current dialogues within reconstructive surgery and wound management forums are ideally placed to take up these challenges.

See recommended websites following the references.

## References

(1) *Mosby's medical, nursing and allied health dictionary*, 4th edn. St Louis: Mosby, 1994.
(2) Bryant R.A. (ed.) *Acute and chronic wounds: nursing management*. St Louis: Mosby Year Book, 1992.
(3) Dealey C. *The care of wounds*, 2nd edn. Oxford, UK: Blackwell Science, 1999.
(4) Naylor W., Laverty D. & Mallett J. *The Royal Marsden Hospital handbook of wound management in cancer care*. Oxford, UK: Blackwell Science, 2001.
(5) Taylor G. & Kurent J. *Clinician's guide to palliative care*. Oxford, UK: Blackwell Publishing, 2003.
(6) O'Connor M. & Aranda S. (eds). *Palliative care nursing, a guide to practice*, 2nd edn. Melbourne Australia: Ausmed Publications, 2004.
(7) Tuthill J. & Garnier S. Prevention of skin breakdown. In: O'Neill J.F., Selwyn P.A.& Schietinger H. (eds) *A clinical guide on supportive and palliative care for people with HIV/AIDS*. Rockville, MD: HRSA, 2003, Chapter 25. http://hab.hrsa.gov/tools/palliative/chap25.html
(8) Mallett J. & Dougherty L. (eds). *The Royal Marsden Hospital manual of clinical nursing procedures*, 5th edn. Oxford, UK: Blackwell Science, 2000.
(9) Smeltzer S.C. & Bare B.G. *Brunner and Suddarth's textbook of medical-surgical nursing*, 9th edn. Philadelphia: Lippincott, Williams & Wilkins, 2000.
(10) Shee C.D. Palliation in chronic respiratory disease. *Palliative Medicine*, 1995 (Jan); 9(1):3–12.
(11) Saphir A. The third way: palliative care gives providers a chance to treat chronic conditions while lowering costs. *Modern Healthcare* 1999 (Apr 12); 29(15):30–3.

(12) Davidson P., Introna K., Daly J., Paull G., Jarvis R., Angus J., Wilds T., Cockburn J., Dunford M. & Dracup K. Cardiorespiratory nurses' perceptions of palliative care in non-malignant diseases: data for the development of clinical practice. *American Journal of Critical Care*, 2003 (Jan); **12**(1):47–53.

(13) Morgan S. Supportive and palliative care for patients with COPD. *Nursing Times*, 2003 (May 20–26); **99**(20):46–7.

(14) Williams A. An overview of non-cancer related chronic edema – a UK perspective. http://www.worldwidewounds.com

(15) Bradley M. When healing is not an option. *Advanced Nurse Practice*, 2004 (Jul 1); **12**(7):50. http://nursepractitioners.advanceweb.com/common/editorial/editorial.aspx?ctiid=613

(16) Center to Advance Palliative Care. *How to establish a palliative care programme for chronic conditions.* http://64.85.16.230/educate/content/rationale/manifestations.html

(17) Ausher B.M., Erikson E. & Wilkins E.G. *Plastic surgery: indications, operations and outcomes.* St Louis: Mosby, 2000.

(18) Hidalgo D.A., Disa J.J., Cordeiro P.G. & Hu Qun-ing. A review of 716 consecutive free flaps for oncologic surgical defects: refinements in donor site selection and technique. *Plastic Reconstructive Surgery*, 1998 (Sept); **102**(3):722–32; discussion 733–34.

(19) Flook D., Webster D.J., Hughes L.E. & Mansel R.W. Salvage surgery for advanced recurrence of breast cancer. *British Journal of Surgery*, 1989 (May); **76**(5):512–14.

(20) Fui A.C., Hong G.S., Ng, E.H. & Soo K.C. Primary reconstruction after extensive chest wall resection. *Australian and New Zealand Journal of Surgery*, 1998 (Sept); **68**(9):655–59.

## Recommended websites

http://www.sbhcs.com/hospitals/hospice/cardiac/

http://www.medicineau.net.au/clinical/palliativecare/palliative

http://www.rnao.org/projects/acpf/topics/cardiac.asp

http://www.nursefriendly.com/nursinglinks/directpatientcare/pain/links/palliativecare.html

http://www.clevelandclinic.org/heartcenter/pub/heartfailure/hf_diseasemanagement.htm

https://www.highmark.com/pdf_file/ger_binder/palliative.pdf

# Principles of Nursing Discharge Management and Community Healthcare Following Reconstructive Plastic Surgery

1. Principles of discharge and ambulatory care following reconstructive plastic surgery
2. Wound management in the home and community healthcare facility following reconstructive surgery

## 1. PRINCIPLES OF DISCHARGE AND AMBULATORY CARE FOLLOWING RECONSTRUCTIVE PLASTIC SURGERY

### Background

Superior outcomes are the result of high quality preparation. With up to 80% of all plastic surgery patients being managed as day surgery and 51% of all cosmetic surgery performed in the office-based setting, an objective and disciplined approach to pre-admission and discharge management are fundamental components of a case management strategy.

In developing a practical discharge plan pathway, a risk screening tool, including an estimated date of discharge, should be completed prior to admission for **every** booked or elective surgical patient. Whilst it is recognised that plans may have to be changed, with an objective process already in place, it is always easier to delay or change a component of care that is in place, than to start from the beginning, as a last-minute exercise[1-5].

For most plastic surgery emergency admissions, it is expected that a discharge plan would be developed for every patient on admission, and certainly within two days of admission. For those patients admitted to critical care or high dependent units, it is expected that the development of a discharge plan will be instigated within two days and reassessed within two days of transfer out of the unit into the surgical or medical unit.

Patients admitted to critical care/high dependency areas may require an increased involvement with the family in the early phases of planning until they are well enough to comprehend the complexity of the situation. These discharge targets will usually be applied to all patients, regardless of the length of stay[1-5].

Day surgery units, office-based surgical centres and many area health services already use their own versions of risk screening tools, with the inclusion of a questionnaire in the pre-admission forms and at triage in the emergency department[1-5]. This is then incorporated in the nursing history.

Health providers have a responsibility for ensuring that risk screening is undertaken for all patients and that the tool is relevant to the needs of different private and public patients, population groups (such as private individuals, people living in residential aged care facilities, drug and alcohol service clients and mental healthcare).

The range of risk screening tools should principally include those administered by medical, nursing staff and interdisciplinary management, in addition to the individual patient questionnaires[1-5].

### Discharge plans in the presence of changing circumstances

The extent of the discharge plan will vary across all patient groups. The majority of patients will require a simple discharge plan that includes:

- Information on the expected date of discharge
- The preferred clinical and patient outcomes of the risk screening tool
- Referrals to other services
- Anticipated requirements for patient discharge care.

It must be also recognised that discharge plans may need to be continually reviewed, and modified, where there is a change in circumstances for the patient. For example, with acutely ill patients following major reconstructive surgery, or where unexpected adverse events occur, it may not be possible to accurately specify the estimated date of discharge. However, a discharge plan should still be developed based on the acknowledged risks associated with the presenting condition and/or proposed surgical procedure(s).

Alterations in the patient's psychosocial needs, and the patient's existing medical condition at the proposed time of discharge, may also significantly require a reappraisal of the whole discharge plan. Poor nutritional status, reduced mobility, an inability of the patient to identify with change, and the new existing circumstances, are also important considerations to address.

Some patients (such as the frail elderly, people with multiple health problems, physical disability, chronic cardiorespiratory diseases, and people who live in residential care facilities or other institutions) will require even more complex discharge planning. Their status should involve dedicated discharge planning staff with the ability to liaise, and make referrals to post-acute and community-based services. This is based on communication and consent from patients and their carers.

Most healthcare facilities aim to keep the GP as the key co-ordinator of all care. It is well recognised that patients get 'lost' in the system. The GP is now considered pivotal in the care plan and so must be included, where possible, in the planning from the beginning. Most referrals to the specialist have come from the GP and, if this is not the case, he or she should always receive copies of any correspondence between specialist and other agencies.

**Box 14.1** Requirements of optimal clinical and patient outcomes.

- Preassessment tools
- Risk screening tools
- Setting clinical and patient goals and outcomes
- A process that allows for auditing patient goals and outcomes.

**Box 14.2** Application of a risk screening tool – clinical and patient benefits.

- Risk screening involves the administration of a questionnaire to ensure that those patients who are at greatest risk of adverse events, receive effective pre-surgery education and problem-specific discharge planning
- A risk screening tool can help identify patients with the greatest needs for post-discharge services, so that they can be referred to necessary services, and receive intensive follow-up
- The use of a risk screening tool can enable early identification of the need for GP involvement in the discharge planning process and should be used to initiate referrals and communication with GPs, community service providers, staff of residential care facilities and other institutions, as necessary
- Hospitals may also use the outcome of risk screening in determining whether patient discharge can be safely managed by ward staff or whether certain patients require the services of a specialised discharge co-ordinator.

**Box 14.3** Identification of patients potentially requiring assistance following discharge.

- Patients with existing healthcare problems who require varying levels of assistance to co-operate with low level prescribed discharge treatments
- Patients who have major surgery and are 'at risk' for postoperative complication
- Patients at nutritional risk
- Patients with low pain threshold
- Patients living alone, at risk of falls, or with failure to comprehend adverse events
- Patients for whom wound dressing self-care is extremely difficult
- Patient likely to have physical self-care problems and for whom rehabilitation is challenging
- Those with caring responsibilities for others
- Patients already using community assistance services prior to admission
- Patients who live long distances from multidisciplinary care centres.

**Box 14.4** Rationale for developing discharge management strategies.

- An important ingredient of total patient care when undertaken in co-ordination with case management
- Places the patient at the centre of the planning process
- Identifies patients for whom timely discharge to less acute care is appropriate, thus freeing up higher care facilities/units for those with greater needs, using healthcare resources appropriately
- Assists the patient in the early procurement of additional or alternative care/resources/aids if required
- Identifying post-discharge needs of patients, particularly patients who are likely to have intensive needs or physical changes made in the home
- Identifies patients who require specialist nurse practitioners for the post-discharge management of, for example, wound care for skin grafts, major flaps and some cosmetic surgery.
- Ensuring that the potential needs of the patient upon discharge can be met:
  - Consultation and communication with the general practitioner
  - Community service providers
  - Staff of residential aged care facilities and other institutions, as necessary.

**Box 14.5** Additional healthcare disciplines required.

- Specialist medical/nursing teams
- Pain management teams
- Nutritional experts
- Occupational therapists
- Mobility and physical balance rehabilitation experts
- Physiotherapists – those involved in early rehabilitation should be advised as directives may be required to be included in specific cases (e.g. post hand surgery, lower limb surgery).

**Box 14.6** Significant patient risk issues following discharge from care unit.

- Inadequate consultation with the patient and significant care providers on discharge as to potential clinical adverse events and measures of patient safety
- Inadequate attention to the maintenance of pain control
- Issues regarding altered mobility and independence, nutrition and wound care dressing supplies
- Inadequate objective planning that includes preferred clinical and patient timeframes and outcomes
- Failure to recognise the individual patient's concerns
- Failure to address the process of projected recovery and wound repair
- Failure to disclose the risks associated with inadequate co-operation/compliance
- Awareness that what the patient hears, understands and carries out, does not always parallel the advice given.

**Box 14.7** Factors that influence patient co-operation on discharge.

- Be as realistic and positive as possible without frightening the patient
- Address the patient directly if appropriate
- Give specific advice and avoid generalisations
- Put all advice in writing
- Stress the importance of the advice
- Use short words and short sentences
- Group the information: these are all the things that are a problem
- Repeat all the information
- Provide written information to the significant care provider and community clinicians
- Request patient or significant care provider to demonstrate any clinical treatments to be undertaken in the home
- Clearly outline the assistance readily available if adverse events occur or progress is not as expected. This means include contact phone numbers and be realistic about who will be available at these phone numbers. It must be someone who knows the case or can access the file otherwise the patient, or whoever is concerned, gets the 'runaround'.

**Box 14.8** The importance of an office-based or surgical outpatient follow-up.

- Ensures the completion of the procedure, allowing for any ongoing specific office-based/outpatient procedures or treatments
- Allows for a review of the needs for the ongoing specific outpatient/community services and supplies, for example:
  - Skilled nursing services including assistance with self care, and wound care
  - Home healthcare including mobility assistance – nutrition
  - Hospice care
  - Durable medical equipment: oxygen, mobility assistance, aids
  - Prosthetics
  - Specialty pharmacy drugs and medicines
  - Allied health – community care.

**Box 14.9** Key issues to be audited and addressed in the outcomes audit.

- Were the key patient issues identified and addressed in a timely and efficient manner?
- Were the services requested provided in a timely and efficient manner?
- Was there adequate and timely consultation and communication with GPs, staff of residential aged care facilities, community providers and other institutions?
- Patient satisfaction
- Carer satisfaction
- Unplanned readmission rates
- Rates of weekday/weekend discharge
- Length of stay (actual versus estimated in the pre-admission discharge plan).

**Box 14.10** Value of outcome audits.

- Identification of other key components for effective discharge planning for incorporation to ensure patient safety, comfort and independence
- Identification of the setting of additional performance targets to ensure patient safety, comfort and independence
- To determine the optimal method for routinely measuring performance against the initial two targets
- Provides a basis for benchmarking clinical practices and outcomes
- Allows for setting in place evidence-based risk management strategies for prevention/minimisation of postoperative adverse events/complications (e.g. haematoma, infection, deep vein thrombosis, pulmonary embolism).

## Audit of discharge practices and measurement of discharge

Healthcare institutions and office-based care facilities will usually undertake outcome audits to meet accreditation criteria and ethico-legal responsibilities, and to evaluate the effectiveness of their practice costs. These audits should include both qualitative and quantitative data on the status of discharge practices through interviews with staff involved in discharge planning and data collection, including review of patient records and consultation with patients, carers, GPs and community service providers[2-5].

**Box 14.11** Expected benefits of objective-based discharge management.

- The development of team-based (interdisciplinary) models of care delivery supported by the availability of specialised discharge planning staff to meet the needs of patients with complex needs
- The active participation of medical officers in development of a discharge plan, including estimated date of discharge, thus using limited resources appropriately
- Input by the GP as part of a team, either as an initial part with the first referral or as the key person within the community
- The involvement of patients, carers and families as appropriate or requested by patient
- Providing a system which can be audited and thus see where management practices can be improved
- Providing for the needs of individuals and groups with special needs, including:
  - Patients following major debilitating surgery
  - The elderly living alone and without significant close carers
  - Patients with additional physical disabilities
  - Patients with mental health problems
  - Patients of non-English speaking background
  - Patients with an intellectual disability
  - Patients who live in residential aged care facilities or other institutions.
- Effective communication between patients, carers (including nursing and significant others) and GPs on medication management and where appropriate, wound dressing care, and specific mobility plans for the patient
- Ensure that hospital staff have a sound knowledge and understanding of the entire healthcare system and the role of general practice and community-based services, supported by systems which provide advice on availability and eligibility of these services
- Regular and timely consultation between all service providers
- Effective timing of discharge meeting patients' transport needs including the special needs of rural patients and patients lacking adequate access to public transport or transport by family and carers
- Ensuring that the patient goals and outcomes are realistically met within the guidelines set down.

## 2. WOUND MANAGEMENT IN THE HOME AND COMMUNITY HEALTHCARE FACILITY FOLLOWING RECONSTRUCTIVE SURGERY

### Background

Ideally, for the greater majority of elective plastic surgery patients/clients, following discharge from hospital, rehabilitation units, short stay or ambulatory care centres, wounds will go on to heal without any adverse events. However there are wounds, surgical or otherwise, which do not always follow exactly the desired and normal sequence of events. These potentially complex wounds can become of great concern to the patient, and to those charged with the responsibility of management in a community setting. For the clinician, this concern must be underpinned with a wide knowledge and understanding of biological disease processes, skill in pain management, mobility/rehabilitation, and empathy that recognises the sometimes overwhelming patient issues that may present due to psychosocial disturbances[1-10].

Although the majority of reconstructive plastic surgery patients will be discharged into the home environment and recover with minimal or no complications, some may not. For example, some patients may have originally been transferred for reconstructive plastic surgery referral, and treatment, from other surgical or medical units, hostels or nursing homes, and some will be discharged to home care, or return to these latter institutions. Follow-up wound care may remain the province of the expert community wound care clinician.

Others, following treated major trauma or disease, may require short, medium or long-term rehabilitation care, but retain the need for wound care in the home, or rehabilitation unit. Community wound care nurse clinicians will often be required to work within a multidisciplinary framework, and this must again reflect the need for patient safety, comfort and independence.

### Responsibility, accountability and clinical governance

The community nurse clinician usually works as a sole practitioner or as an expert within a team environment. This places a major responsibility on clinicians to ensure that adverse clinical events or accidents within their domain of responsibility are prevented or minimised. Addressing clinical risk management, adhering to clinical standards of care, adopting and accepting clinical governance, and setting and auditing goals and outcomes, are essential areas of patient/client care to be addressed[2,3].

## Patient/client time management

With 85% of plastic surgery conducted as day and short-stay surgery, wound care in the home is an expanding role for professional clinicians. Because of the nature of many plastic surgery wounds, the time allocated to each patient/client is increasingly becoming a clinical governance issue. Accurately balancing the available time against the needs of the wound, and the patient's desire for information and reassurance, is an acquired organisational skill.

Original referral sheets, and provision for ongoing treatment notes and treatment rationales that are objectively set out, can provide prior knowledge as to what may be expected both physically and psychosocially. They can also provide guidance when there is a change over of clinicians, reducing repetition, unnecessary treatment changes, and valuable time.

## Establishing a trusting and working relationship

The establishment of a trusting and working relationship is essential with:

- The referring surgeon and general medical practitioner
- The patient and significant others involved in their life.

A change in the way patients/clients are managed has been occurring over the past 40 years. In the past the patient would remain silent, believe everything they were told, and undertake the tasks they were instructed to do, to the best of their ability and resources. Now many patients insist on more. They expect to be:

- Informed of the plan to address their wound and overall physical needs[4]

- Informed of the goals and preferred outcomes of the treatment regime proposed[4]
- Consulted and involved in their care, including financial costs[4]
- Provided with knowledge as to the relevance of the procedures being undertaken
- Informed of ongoing wound status (positive or negative) of the wound care instituted
- Given reasons for any self-care requests and changes in daily activities between visits.

These are fundamental and important aspects of modern community care models. It must also be remembered that a clinician is a 'guest' in the patient's home. This relationship must be respected and nurtured without becoming invasive or intrusive. The patient trusts the nurse who enters their home, and it is within this trust benchmark that care must be delivered.

An excellent working and trusting relationship established with the surgeon and/or GP provides the opportunity to suggest potential changes in medical treatments, dressing/wound care regimes, pain management, and referrals to other disciplines as required. Regular reporting back by phone, letter or email can assist the medical officers in keeping up to date when required to visit or be visited by the patient/client. This is also reinforcing and reassuring to the patient that their interests are considered important and relevant.

## The first encounter

The first encounter with the patient/client and family members is one of relationship building – that old saying of *'first impressions count'* is very true in this setting.

Patients have been known, after the nurse has left, to call the centre responsible for clinician allocation, and request that 'that nurse' not to be allocated to him or her again. Thus it is important to build trust and confidence at this first meeting. Formal provision for dispute resolution must be in place in order that resolvable issues do not escalate and become legal issues.

The nurse will need to demonstrate knowledge of the surgical procedure and the expected wound. The patient may have a strong sense of insecurity having left a hospital or centre, where health professionals were easy to call upon. Returning to an environment where he or she is alone or with others who are also concerned, and wondering what to do, if something goes unexpectedly wrong, can be quite unsettling for all concerned.

## Risk factors affecting healing

If all things were perfect, the patient undergoing reconstructive plastic surgery would be in perfect health. Many risk factors influence the healing process, for example:

- Body build
- Mobility
- Age
- Morbidity
- Nutrition
- Infection
- Potential for desiccation and maceration of wound edges
- Forms of mechanical stress
- Psychosocial status
- Commitment to rehabilitation.

Preoperative risk assessments would have been anticipated to address any existing patient morbidity, and many of the potential adverse events, prior to the hospital admission. Unfortunately, we do not live in an ideal world and some major reconstructive surgery patients are often admitted with significant injuries or with disease-based conditions.

This often results in postoperative acute and chronic wounds being cared for in community settings. Some of these wounds may go on to become increasingly complex requiring palliative-based wound management, often distressing for the patient and consuming vast amounts of health resources.

## Risk management – complications

Complications of surgery and within wounds are especially common amongst patients who are elderly, malnourished, immune compromised, with tumours, and those with varying levels of pain, altered cognition and mobility[6–10].

Patient assessment is vital for planning and no one will argue with this[6–9]. However, in all areas of wound care many clinicians become focused on the wound and fail to see the 'big picture'. This is where educated, skilled and competent community clinicians can come to the forefront.

## Clinician safety

Safety issues relating to lone practitioners entering the homes of patients/clients must also be considered. Maintaining professional attitudes and communication skills and planning of exit strategies are essential for:

- Fending off unwanted overfamiliarity by patient/clients and/or relatives
- Addressing abusive behaviour from angry and grieving patients when progress appears to be slow or regressing
- Addressing issues related to withdrawing care (patient/client dependency) as good progress is made
- Withdrawing in order to move on to the next patient/client.

Contingency/exit plans should be in place that allow the clinician to remove themselves safely from any environment they consider unsafe or to personally feel at risk.

---

**Review**

*Setting goals of care and preferred clinical and patient outcomes*, Chapter 2, Boxes 2.7–2.9. Adapt according to risk management issues and clinical patient needs.

---

## Preparing for the first community visit

When caring for the wound in the home (or community environments) the nurse must first have a referral which provides all the answers to:

- Previous medical and surgical history, including psychosocial status
- Current medications
- Known allergies
- Current surgical procedure and postoperative period of care
- Current wound dressing regime
- Forward date of review by surgeon or GP.

Although no firm assumptions should be made, armed with this information prior to visiting the patient/client, the nurse clinician will already have formed some ideas as to what to expect upon arrival at the residence. The patient/client address will also probably give some indication as to the patient's standing in the community and their socioeconomic status.

### Entering the patient/client home or community healthcare environment

A community nurse, by the very nature of his or her role, will be performing an assessment from the moment their car pulls up outside the patient's home or place of residence.

As the nurse enters the home, he or she is looking at the immediate environment for cleanliness, environmental temperatures, ventilation, possessions, etc. This also helps to form some points of discussion before getting straight into wound care. Many patients will even goes so far as to take the nurse on a tour as they may anticipate a number of visits and the nurse will need to feel familiar with the bathroom, laundry, etc.

This also allows the community nurse to evaluate the need for home environmental assessments by occupational therapists, to assist the patient undertaking activities of daily living, and ease of mobility.

---

**Box 14.12** Basic skills for wound bed assessment, preparation and management.

- Physiology of wound healing, recognising the abnormal
- Diagnosis and management of infection, including current trends for critical colonisation
- Wound care products available:
  - Their cost
  - The funding mechanisms available within various community settings
  - Their best application
  - Usage techniques
- Current wound cleansing techniques within community settings – each area will have standardised protocols of practise
- Knowledge of current thoughts on adjuvant therapies in wound care
- Communication skills, ethical considerations which may be applicable to wound care and psychological and psychosocial assessment skills.

---

## Primary wound bed assessment

There is a wonderful statement used in education for aspiring practitioners in wound care –'look at the *whole* not the *hole*'. The emphasis requires a shift from the wound towards the patient with a wound. This also implies observing the environmental and social factors that may impact on the healing process.

- As previously discussed, normal wounds heal in three distinct phases – inflammation, proliferation and epithelialisation/maturation.
- If seeing an acute wound for the first time within the first three days, it will most probably have some form of redness, therefore the nurse should not panic and cause anxiety to the patient. It would be more appropriate to state to the patient: *'this may be normal and I will review it tomorrow to ensure the inflammation is beginning to subside.'*
- If the wound is on the upper leg, with the surrounding skin being erythematous, and there is an odour of urine within the environment, it may be possible that incontinence is the issue. The erythema may be due to urine causing a 'chemical' burn to the skin around the wound.
- Another common problem is animals (cats, dogs) that may brush past the wound after the patient showers, or sit on the towel while the patient is showering. Animal hair may then be transferred to the wound as the patient dries off.
- Knowing that the wound requires a clean environment, dressing zones and patient clothing must be kept clean. The community nurse should check for this and offer advice on how this may be achieved. Dressings should be stored in a sealed plastic box and placed out of reach
- If the proliferative phase of healing is delayed, the clinician should be concentrating her/his efforts on nutrition, as macrophages, fibroblasts and collagen are nutrient dependant and responsible for most of the work at this stage of healing
- If epithelialisation and maturation are slow, then zinc levels may be studied together with any possibility of repeated trauma. For example, sliding in and out of bed, the nurse may change the patient's bed transfer technique to eliminate trauma on the fresh wound
- Working in co-operation with the surgeon and/or GP is essential as medications and referrals usually are required to come from them

- Digital photos are useful for clinical discussions with medical and nursing colleagues, and to demonstrate positive progress to the patient.

## Diagnosis and management of infection

The community nurse will be assessing the wound at each episode of care. The assessment takes into consideration peri-wound condition[6–9]. Any sign of erythema following acute elective surgery after the first 3–5 days is cause for concern.

The founder of plastic surgery in Australia (Sir Benjamin K. Rank, 1911–2002), was often heard to remark to both medical and nursing students that, if erythema existed, *'on the third day God made pus'*.

If concerned, the nurse should calmly inform the patient that she/he is going to contact the surgeon or reviewing doctor to discuss the current situation and seek advice. It is important at this stage to be calm and reassuring that help will be sought. It is therefore imperative that the first medical point of contact is identified in the discharge letter to the community nurse.

As expected in normal healing wounds, wound exudate levels diminish after several days, but if the levels suddenly begin to rise, and pain is also increasing, it is almost always indicative of impending infection.

## Wound care products available and funding regimes for their procurement

It is not possible to give advice regarding all funding arrangements around the world but it is essential for clinicians to have local knowledge of products available, the actual cost to the patient, and whether the patient can afford the care prescribed.

This is important information, as hospital staff may initiate community care that the patient/client cannot afford to proceed with in the home environment. Some public and private hospitals fund 'hospital in the home' programmes in lieu of hospital bed stays, but many do not. The outcome of this can be that the patient will not be able to co-operate in the designed care pathway, and/or will sacrifice good nutrition in order to pay for dressing products that relieve pain, etc. The community wound care clinician must be creative with these issues in mind, designing wound care programmes that are practical, affordable and have the capacity to realise the preferred wound goals/outcomes.

**Box 14.13** Generic products and their uses.

| | |
|---|---|
| Polyurethane film dressings | protect newly-healed wounds or cover other dressings to water-proof them |
| Polyurethane foam dressings | absorb wound exudate and insulate and protect granulation tissue |
| Hydrocolloid dressings | aid wound debriding, absorb some wound exudate and stimulate angiogenesis |
| Hydrogel dressings | rehydrate dry necrotic eschar and provide some pain relief in certain wound types |
| Alginate dressings | haemostatic properties or for exudate absorption |
| Hydrofibre dressings | exudate management |
| Topical antimicrobial dressings | manage wound bio-burden and colonisation – these include cadexomer iodine, hypertonic salt, silver. |

## Current wound cleansing techniques in the home setting

Once again it is difficult to state outright that most wounds in the community can be cleansed in potable drinking water[6,9]. The nurse must first work within the guidelines set out by her/his employment agency. However, the Joanna Briggs Institute (www.joannabriggs.edu.au) has issued guidelines for clinical practice of wound cleansing in the community.

Wound cleansing helps optimise the healing environment and decreases the potential for infection. It loosens and washes away cellular debris such as bacteria, exudate, purulent material and residual topical agents from previous dressings. Most wounds should be initially cleansed, and at each dressing change, working within the goal of what is trying to be achieved.

## Wound cleansing agents

Wound cleansing agents are solutions that are used to decontaminate wounds following removal of old dressings and prior to the application of a new dressing. As such, they should not be confused with debriding agents that are generally applied and left *in situ* to facilitate the biological removal of slough or necrotic tissue[6,9].

For sheer practicality, accessibility and cost, most wound care clinicians advocate the use of warm, clean (drinkable) tap water or pre-boiled, tepid water for cleansing chronic wounds. There are still some who advocate cleansing acute wounds with warm sterile saline, however there are an equal number of expert clinicians who advocate that acute wounds have less infection rates when cleaned under free flowing warm tap water (*'dilution is the solution to pollution'*[6,9]).

Sterile saline is the preferred cleanser for most wounds because it is physiologic and will always be safe, but the sheer volume required to properly cleanse a wound can be costly to the patient and unnecessary when clean free flowing potable drinking water has been shown to be effective[6,9]. Saline will not clean dirty, necrotic wounds – more aggressive methods are required.

Studies have shown that bacterial growth in saline may be present within 24 hours of opening the container, consequently opened containers should be discarded after initial use[6,9].

Wound care experts do agree that the routine use of antiseptic solutions has little place in wound management. Antiseptics, particularly those which contain cetrimide, have marked cytotoxic properties and therefore should be avoided unless the wound is contaminated or shows clear evidence of infection[6,9].

See recommended websites (wound cleansing and pressure gradients in fluid application) at the end of this chapter.

There continues to be some debate in the use of pressure required to cleanse wounds of superficial debris. It was initially stated that a pressure of 13–18 psi (pounds per square inch) was best – this is now suggested to be 4–15 psi (http://www.fpnotebook.com(s)UR10.htm).

Currently, there are several machine-operated devices available for cleansing wounds, and these employ pressures much higher than this. These devices, however, also employ ultrasound or directional lavage, which does not drive the bacteria deeper into the tissues but rather 'planes' it off in a tangent-like process. Their use is principally confined to specialist wound centres and generally out of the reach of the community nurse. In the hands of the skilled clinician, basic best practice techniques, as described above, provide general practice methods that do not require high costs, transportation and ongoing maintenance. At the end of the day, patients appreciate a warm shower, if possible, or short submersion of a limb in a container, a gentle wash of the wound and surrounding tissues, and moisturisation of dry skin prior to redressing[6,9].

## Current thoughts on adjuvant therapies

There are many non-medical devices available which are suggested to promote rapid wound healing and pain relief. There are few scientific data to support their use. Readers are encouraged to access unbiased clinical reviews of the devices, never believe the person selling the devices, but rather seek independent knowledge, and if at all possible conduct your own research-based clinical trials.

Having said that it is also a well-known fact that if the patient believes the therapy will work then it most probably will – the mind is a powerful organ. There is more and more evidence demonstrating that adjuvant therapies such as touch, music, massage, low-level laser, electrical stimulation, and aromatherapy, may be beneficial when used in conjunction with current medical treatments. Perhaps the old statement *'if it does no harm and the patient is prepared to make the investment'* is worth considering.

## Communication skills, ethical considerations

The community nurse must be able to explain to the patient the overall range of care that is required to promote good wound healing. It is then of value to have the patient repeat this knowledge so that each understands what the other has said or interpreted. The nurse has to be a good listener in order to ensure that both her requests are met as well as those of the patient. Showering is a good example – the nurse may want to keep the dressing dry but the patient wants to shower every day. They must both then come up with a way to achieve this or make compromise and the patient showers every second day when the wound is being taken down for dressing.

It is important that any ethical, religious issues are discussed prior to commencing any procedure. Usually these are discovered in the hospital setting. One expert community wound nurse reported that on first entering the community setting she asked a patient to keep their leg elevated when seated. She then learnt that some religious groups disapprove of the soles of the feet being seen by others, and so her request was not acceptable.

## Patient safety

The assessment of a wound in the community also involves the clinician using all his/her skills of sight, smell, touch, and hearing. It is essential to prevent any additional harm or injury and so a safe environment must be assured. This may mean moving some furniture about for an interim period. Providing fresh air and a clean environment may require 'home help' so a request to other community providers or family may be necessary until the patient can resume an adequate level of mobility and independence.

Nutrition is important, thus the housebound, immobile or ill patient may require community help, or seek assistance from relatives if available. As there can sometimes be internal family feuding, or bad feelings, this request may exacerbate the existing problem. It is better to request assistance outside the family, if this is suspected, and use a community/private agency for regular meals.

## Patient comfort

The assessment and management of any existing physical pain/discomfort, or disturbances to sleep patterns, are also an important component of care[6,9,10]. Pain may not always be physical. One community nurse reported that following a thorough physical and psychosocial assessment she determined that whilst the patient stated the pain was worse at night (despite prescribed regular pain medication and no other obvious physiological cause), the real issue appeared to be loneliness. The TV was moved into the bedroom and was kept on quietly as background noise and the patient slept soundly thereafter.

The issue of patient constipation must be considered when patients are on constant pain-related medications that include an opioid.

## Patient independence

As the wound heals and the nurse visit intervals are extended, the patient can show signs of anxiety. The community nurse must be aware of the bond and dependency the patient has placed on these visits, and it is suggested that before the nurse completely withdraws his/her services, a replacement social programme has been put in place.

The patient must be empowered, wherever they are, with a sense of physical and spiritual wellness, and strength.

Having an holistic understanding of the impact of the wound on the patient's health enables to nurse to assist in planning strategies for ongoing confidence in the return to activities of daily living that include increasing health development, return to work, a daily walk, shopping, maintaining nutrition, and some weekly social outing with other community members.

## Summary

In summary, wound bed assessment requires knowledge of normal versus abnormal, good lighting to perform the assessment, and good record keeping of the wound bed, peri-wound condition, type and volume of exudate, and pain levels.

Wound bed preparation involves the community nurse cleansing and encouraging healthy growth through a clean environment and good diet.

Wound bed maintenance (wound bed management) again implies knowledge of the dietary needs of a healing/remodelling wound, and an environment conducive to good health – clean air, clean surroundings, no stress, happiness and laughter.

See recommended websites (wound management in the home and community healthcare facility following reconstructive surgery) after the References.

---

**Review**

*Auditing preferred clinical and patient outcomes,* Chapter 2, Boxes 2.10–2.12.

---

## References

(1) Parkes J. & Sheppard S. Discharge planning from hospital to home (Cochrane Review). *The Cochrane Library*, 2001(1), Oxford.
(2) National Association for Homecare (USA). *Homecare online – legislation – regulation for patient care*: http://www.nahc.org/NAHC/LegReg/listservcontrib.html
(3) Spath P.L. *Quality management in homecare services* (1999). http://www.brownspath.com/original_articles/qmhome.htm
(4) AORN. *Standard care plan for ambulatory surgery – nursing diagnosis – expected patient outcome – nursing interventions*: http://www.ssmonline.org/ssmonline-media/Documents/25.pdf.

(5) American Society of Plastic Surgeons. *Plastic and reconstructive surgery.* http://www.plasticsurgery.org/

(6) Dealey C. *The care of wounds*, 2nd edn. Oxford, UK: Blackwell Science, 1999.

(7) Flanagan M. A practical framework for wound assessment 1: physiology. *British Journal of Nursing*, 1996; **5**(22):1391–7.

(8) Flanagan M. A practical framework for wound assessment 2: methods. *British Journal of Nursing*, 1997; **6**(1):6,8–11.

(9) Carville K. *Wound care manual*, revised edn. Osbourne Park, Western Australia, Silver Chain Foundation, 1995.

(10) Hampton S. Dressing selection and associated pain. *Journal of Community Nursing*, 2004; **18**(1):14–18.

## Recommended websites

http://www.jcn.co.uk/journal.asp?MonthNum=08&YearNum=2004&ArticleID=713 (Journal of Community Nursing)

http://www.enursescribe.com/wound.htm    (directory/links of websites appropriate to wound care)

http://www.practicenursing.co.uk/forum/    (directory/links of websites appropriate to community wound care)

http://www.nurse-prescriber.co.uk/Journals/MinorAilments2004_skin.htm (directory/links of websites appropriate to community wound care)

http://www.joannabriggs.edu.au/pdf/BPISstpwound.pdf (evidence-based report on wound cleansing and pressure gradients in fluid application)

# Section III

## Perioperative Theatre Management – General Principles of Care

# Chapter 15

# Patient Management in the Operating Theatre

## Background

'Anaesthesia' is derived from the Greek meaning 'without feeling'. 'Analgesia' is also from the Greek meaning 'without pain'. In later descriptions, analgesia has been defined as the loss of **pain** sensation and anaesthesia defined as the loss of **all** sensation. In modern anaesthesia this is described within a triad of events[1,2].

### Box 15.1 Components of the triad of modern anaesthesia.

| | |
|---|---|
| Narcosis | sleep with loss of memory (amnesia) |
| Analgesia | pain relief |
| Relaxation | muscular relaxation. |

Depending on the complexity of the surgical procedures, there may be a requirement for all, or proportions, of each three components. This may be with or without a pre-anaesthetic medication, and commonly with the aid of specific drugs that deliver postoperative retrograde amnesia, and narcotics suited to the individual patient, length of operating time, and the requirement for early/ongoing postoperative pain relief[1–5].

In the much earlier times of anaesthesia, all components of the triad were obtainable only from chloroform or ether. In modern times, the choices are extensive and can be tailored to meet the specific procedure matched to the specific patient's fitness/health/morbidity classification, in particular those who are selected as day or short stay patients.

The American Society of Anesthesiologists has determined risk assessment criteria based on the patient's morbidity, the surgery proposed, and clinical risks associated with the preferred outcome.

### Box 15.2 Assessment for 'fitness for anaesthesia'

- Briefly identify the patient – correct person according to identity bracelet and hospital ID number
- Obtain a medical history, including allergies, existing disease processes and previous anaesthetic experiences
- Perform a brief anaesthesia-directed review
- Conduct a short physical examination
- Review important laboratory results
- Provide an assessment and anaesthesia plan including specific monitoring
- Document the summary, noting that anaesthetic procedures and risks were discussed with the patient (informed consent).

These criteria and the fitness classification have largely been universally adopted (Box 15.2).

See recommended websites (preoperative patient assessment and premedication protocols) at the end of this chapter.

## Fitness for anaesthesia

The overall fitness of the patient may be a difficult issue to resolve in the short space of time available. It must include consideration of all the assessment factors (Box 15.2) as to whether or not the patient is in the best possible state of health, consistent with his or her organic illness, the necessity of the operation, and its urgency.

In the final analysis, the definitive decision can only be made by careful consultation between surgeon, anaesthetist, and the individual patient, wherever possible. Box 15.3 outlines the American

**Box 15.3** Classification of patient fitness (physiological status).

The most common classification is that recommended by the American Society of Anesthesiologists (ASA):

Class I     fit and healthy
Class II    mild systemic illness (such as hypertension)
Class III   severe systemic illness which is not incapacitating
Class IV    incapacitating illness/constant threat to life
Class V     moribund/not expected to live more than 24 hours
'E'         added to above if operation is an emergency

**Box 15.4** Setting clinical and patient anaesthetic goals.

Safety        providing zero or minimal physiological and psychological disturbances
Comfort       optimal anaesthetic and analgesic techniques that allow for intra-operative and primary postoperative pain control
Independence  the early ability for patient mobility that allows the patient to return to perform, for themselves, the functions and activities of daily living[1-5].

**Box 15.5** Addressing principal risk management issues.

- Anticipate possible complications/adverse events and putting in place minimisation/preventative strategies (utilising a risk management assessment)
- Obtain the patient's commitment to co-operation in minimising or reversing those factors (within their control) that may put their life at risk (e.g. smoking)
- Obtain the patient's commitment to a programme of rehabilitation following surgery.

Society of Anesthesiologists guidelines for identifying patient fitness and grades, indicating the level at which patients can be demonstrated to be 'at risk'.

## Anaesthesia in reconstructive plastic surgery

The evolution of short-stay facilities has required a reappraisal of how patients are managed during a minimal timeframe, but with safety and comfort, and to meet the optimal maintenance of the patient's independent status and clinical needs on discharge[1-8].

As a general principle, the selection of the most appropriate anaesthetic approach in reconstructive plastic surgery is based on, for example:

- The procedure proposed to be undertaken
- Assessment of medical and/or surgical morbid risk factors that may lead to adverse events
- The most appropriate techniques that parallel the needs of the procedure, patient safety, pain control and retrograde amnesia.

The value of these techniques/approaches is that:

- They are readily available options
- They can, under controlled conditions, and through interdisciplinary supervised arrangements:
  - Be adapted/modified to meet individual patient requirements in the hospital, home-based environments
  - Meet the needs for most types of redressing needs.

### Examples of specific anaesthetic techniques used in reconstructive plastic surgery

The potential single or combinations or anaesthetic techniques for use in reconstructive plastic surgery are many. The list below outlines and gives examples of the most common techniques used[1-4].

**General anaesthesia**  a state of unconsciousness produced by anaesthetic agents with the absence of pain sensation over the entire body, and a greater or lesser degree of muscle relaxation. The drugs producing this state can be administered by inhalation, intravenously, intramuscularly, rectally or via the gastrointestinal tract. This state is also intended to induce loss of memory.

**Regional block** terms used to describe nerve blocking techniques that anaesthetise one region of the body only. Examples include:

- Brachial plexus nerve block (arm block). Femoral nerve block (one leg) may be by single injection, or catheter for continuous pain management during long procedures and postoperative pain management
- Digital nerve block (a finger or toe). Adrenaline should not be used as this may cause the digital artery to spasm, and not recover, causing irreversible ischaemia
- Spinal and epidural blocks which impede any sensation from the level of injection.

They may be given by single injection or catheter for the period of the procedure or for continuous pain management during long procedures and postoperative pain management. This may be supplemented by a narcotic infusion where there are additional surgical sites, and not covered by the blocks.

**Combined spinal and epidural** with continuous sedation or light general anaesthesia. This combined technique may be used for extended bilateral free vascular breast reconstruction procedures and subsequent postoperative pain management. This may also be supplemented by a narcotic infusion where there are additional surgical sites not covered by the blocks.

**Local skin zone blocks** (e.g. lidocaine (Xylocaine) – short acting – 4–6 hours) which target and block peripheral nerves responsible for sensation in the localised skin zones required for certain procedures (e.g. excision of lesions) may be used alone, or with adrenaline, for vasoconstriction and to enhance the action of the local anaesthetic agent chosen.

Local nerve blocks can be used for major procedures by anaesthetising specific nerves responsible for relatively wide areas of skin, and for example, specific regions such as the mental nerve, to block sensation to the lower lip.

When used correctly, with specific nerves targeted, minimal volumes can attain wide zones of peripheral control of sensory blocking sensations, such as for face lifts procedures, ear correction and breast surgery.

Many surgeons inject local anaesthetic drugs with or without adrenaline, into the surrounding operated tissues as a supplement to oral medications, for postoperative pain management, for example, breast reductions.

All regional and local anaesthetic nerve blocks are commonly used in combination with sedation (usually from the benzodiazepine family) for sleep and retrograde amnesia.

**Topical** e.g. EMLA® applied to the skin surface. Useful for minimal superficial procedures, or prior to insertion of injections, particularly in children. Clinicians wishing to use EMLA® on open wounds for pain management should seek the manufacturer's guidelines for efficacy/safety.

## Monitoring techniques

Best practice and patient safety now require that regardless of the anaesthetic technique chosen, it is now mandatory that full monitoring facilities (i.e. electrocardiogram, oxygen, $CO_2$ levels (capnography), blood pressure, pulse, incorporating and including the five vital signs) are utilised on induction, during the procedure and until all the criteria of postoperative safety are met[1-5].

## Pre- and perioperative nursing care for reconstructive plastic surgery patients

### The preadmission phase

Irrespective of the extent or type of reconstructive plastic surgery procedure there is always the potential for adverse or unpredictable adverse anaesthetic or surgical events to occur. These may result in patient disfigurement, disability, or death[1-5] (review Chapter 14).

As stated previously, during the preoperative assessment session, medical and nursing morbidity and co-morbidity should be identified wherever possible and addressed prior to the patient entering into surgery. Despite this, medical and nursing issues/conditions, due to previously unidentified causes, may remain hidden, and emerge only during the perioperative and/or postoperative phase as complications of the anaesthetic, or surgical event[1-5].

Included in these are the general and specific risk issues related to patients who:

- Are taking medications related to cardio-respiratory conditions, anti-coagulants, aspirin, steroid and anti-inflammatory medications
- Are known 'at risk' for deep vein thrombosis (DVT) related to previous DVT or pulmonary embolism
- Have specific medical conditions such as diabetes mellitus and/or peripheral vascular disease
- Have inherited systemic conditions that have the potential to alter patient cardiovascular safety, and general mobility[9–11].

Increased success of the overall procedure/s occurs if smoking ceases permanently[1–6]. Patients who smoke must be encouraged towards cessation of smoking in all forms for at least 3 weeks both prior to, and following, the surgical procedure. Where possible, and time permits, patients should be directed to smoking cessation clinics for programmes that are under the guidance of professional clinicians.

Short-stay patients also require similar detailed assessments and specific case management protocols to ensure at-risk patients are not disadvantaged particularly by issues relating to some time factors (i.e. long periods of fasting due to unforeseen surgical delays)[12–15].

Pain, hypothermia, hypovolaemia, and deep vein thrombosis will be expanded upon later in this chapter.

## Preoperative psychosocial risk management issues for the surgical patient

**Box 15.6** Psychological risk factors 1.

Anticipatory fear, where the patient has anxiety about the forthcoming surgery or the apprehension may be based on a previous experience. An inhibitory or paralysing sensation, where fear of a previous experience, further injury or death, can significantly cloud the patient's ability to retain information or make objective decisions[1–4,7,8].

Fear of anaesthesia:

- Loss of personal control
- Anxiety about being awake but paralysed during the operation
- Not waking up, dying
- Pain
- Body image (disfigurement)
- Loss of independence.

Despite the patient's desire for particular reconstructive plastic surgical procedures (e.g. an aesthetic/cosmetic procedure), a non-threatening and trusting interdependence between the surgeon, anaesthetist, nurse clinicians, patient and significant carers must exist[3,4,6–8,13–15]. Fear may be a real issue for the patient.

## Psychological risk factors 2 – gaining the patient's confidence

For the patient undergoing anaesthesia, it is often said that the two most important periods are the induction period ('takeoff') and the waking time ('landing'). Gaining the patient's confidence in 'the system' and proposed surgical experience, is basic to achieving the goals and outcomes that are set.

To secure a holistic view of the patient, the nurse clinician must be able to address these and other issues in a quiet professional environment where the patient has the opportunity to ask questions, and the clinician can observe body language and reactions[1–4,7,8]. For some patients who wish to undergo elective surgery but have reservations regarding anaesthesia, pain, etc., additional counselling may be required by the surgeon and the anaesthetist.

The preoperative nursing admission notes should document any fears the patient states verbally or may physically exhibit. Major fears should be communicated to the surgeon immediately. Some patients may change their mind about having elective surgery, often at the last moment, if their early fears are not addressed early, and professionally.

## Physiological risk management

All compromised cells, tissues, and wounds are at risk of increasing morbidity and death due to necrosis when the circulatory system remains under stress for long periods, particularly through reducing blood/fluid volume and pressure[1,2,9–11].

Any alterations in the patient's vascular circulatory and respiratory functions, which are responsible for facilitating the exchange of nutrients and gases at cellular level including the brain, potentially compromises all other major life support systems, and maintaining the integrity of these systems is central[1,2,9–11].

The extent of the surgical procedure, the patient's presenting medical condition, and the postoperative requirements for analgesia largely determine the anaesthetic technique(s) that will be selected.

On induction, and until the completion of the surgical procedure, a range of monitoring techniques will be used. For major procedures, on transfer, the period spent in the post anaesthesia care unit recovery room and surgical unit may require the same degree or intensity of monitoring and care[1,2].

Following major reconstructive plastic surgery, hypovolaemia and hypothermia (leading to adverse vascular events) are stated to be the principal immediate causes for the failure of major wounds to recover early, or for free vascularised flaps, transplants and replants to revascularise[3,4,6]. This is because of the principal effects (red blood cell sludging and vessel rigidity) related to continuing inadequate circulatory volume (dehydration, hypovolaemia), and reduced core temperatures on red blood cells[9,10,12]. This is discussed further later in this chapter in relation to the adverse events that can potentially occur to both the patient and the wound when these issues are not scientifically addressed.

## Dehydration and hypovolaemia

The definitions and identification of dehydration and hypovolaemia in respect of the perioperative phase should not be confused.

**Dehydration** is an excessive loss of water from the body tissues. This may result in disturbances in the balance of essential electrolytes, particularly sodium, potassium and chloride. Dehydration can be mild, moderate or severe.

**Hypovolaemia** occurs when the levels of fluid and/or blood continue to be lost and cannot be compensated by the existing circulatory system.

---

**Box 15.8** Common signs that the circulatory volume is decreasing.

- Headache
- Thirst with dry mouth and lips
- Poor skin turgor
- Flushed dry skin
- Coated tongue
- Oliguria
- Increasing irritability and confusion.

---

**Box 15.9** Dehydration – risk management issues.

Following all forms of surgery, dehydration may be due to:

- Temporary wound oedema
- Preoperative fasting
- Fluid loss during the operative procedure where operating theatre ambient temperatures are required to be high (e.g. up to 30°C during major microvascular surgery)
- Postoperative vomiting
- Minimal oral water intake
- Sweating due to the anxiety of surgery.

These conditions can significantly alter the circulatory volume available, particularly in children and the elderly. In day or short stay surgery patients this may be overlooked, but can be managed by basic intravenous (IV) electrolyte fluid replacement restoring the normal intravascular volume that would have normally been taken in orally by the patient over that period of time[13–15].

---

**Box 15.7** Conditions placing the surgical patient at risk of dehydration and/or hypovolaemia.

- Known previous blood/fluid loss not fully compensated
- Diabetes mellitus
- Burns
- Major reconstructive surgery – multisited wounds including tissue donor sites
- Multisited wounds related to major infections that also require frequent skin grafting
- Chronic wounds that have continuing high levels of exudate
- Multisited major liposuction
- The elderly with anaemia
- Children of all ages.

## Discussion

A recent Cochrane review concluded that the traditional practice of fasting patients for extended periods of time prior to surgery that requires anaesthesia appears to be unnecessary and in fact may place patients at risk of dehydration[12]. It is advocated that 4–6 hours may be adequate for adult patients to fast.

Paediatric anaesthetists will adjust the preoperative fasting period to suit individual children and their needs related to age and food/fluid requirements.

In general, the universality of traditional fasting (food and fluid) periods (e.g. from midnight for morning surgery) continues to come more from rituals than protocols based on evidence, or for convenience to the health institution.

Clinicians working within reconstructive plastic surgery should be conversant with conditions that place the patient at risk for dehydration, or hypovolaemia, that further place both the patient, and the wound, at risk.

- Fasting times
- High patient stress levels
- Observation of the fluid and/or blood loss, short, medium, and long-term, with an accurate fluid loss calculation and replacement programme
- Augmented by vigilance and competent clinical risk assessment, to prevent or minimise potential problems.
- Failure to match fluid loss to replacement can:
- Potentially result in hypovolaemic shock
- Lead to circulatory/cardiac failure
- Potentiate a severe compromise to the structure and movement of red blood cells, further leading to local and general vascular thrombosis[1,2,9–11,15].

## Hypothermia

**Box 15.11** Pathophysiology of hypothermia.

**Normothermia** (normal core body temperature) is generally defined externally as a sublingual temperature of 36°C (96.8°F)[9–11,16–18].

**Hypothermia** (abnormally low body temperature) is essentially defined as a core (internal) body temperature of 35°C (96°F) or below, as a result of exposure to cold.

Some texts set this at 36.6°C (98°F) and further define conditions as:

**Mild** 32–35°C
**Moderate** 30–32°C
**Severe** below 30°C

- Enzyme and biochemical responses are most favourable between 35.6°C and 37.8°C (96–100°F)
- The monitoring, analysis and maintenance of core body temperature is the fourth vital sign in the injured or ill patient (see Chapter 11 – the five vital signs).
- In the person who is mobile, body warmth is generated through the continuity of physical movement, cellular activity, the circulation of warm arterial blood and appropriate warm clothing
- Immobile and/or anaesthetised patients progressively lose body heat unless assisted by warm clothes or adjunct materials (e.g. warming blankets) that retain any heat generated, or more importantly, by ambient room temperatures
- Hypothermia occurs when a physiological core temperature of 35°C (96°F) or below is lowered to a level that progressively alters normal cellular function[1,2,9–11,17,18]

**Box 15.10** Hypovolaemia – definitions and risk management issues.

- Hypovolaemia is stated to exist when the loss of intravascular volume is 15% or greater in a normal adult – mortality from shock ranges from 10 to 31%[9,10]
- With the timing of normalising blood and fluid volume critical to decreasing the significant morbidity or mortality rate, the longer the state of hypovolaemic shock, the greater the risk of adverse events[9–11,16]
- Hypovolaemic shock is an emergency and a life-threatening state which can be avoided by clinicians being alert to conditions that present a danger of hypovolaemia
- Children and the elderly present special problems, as minimal fluid and, particularly blood, loss is highly significant
- In modern anaesthesia this is compensated by medical knowledge of the patient, certain medical conditions:
  - Related to dietary needs (e.g. diabetes mellitus)
  - Extent of the procedure

- Recent recognition of the significant impact of hypothermia on physiological functions following injury and during and after surgical procedures has seen monitoring of the patient's core temperature as an essential component of normal physiological supervision in modern operating rooms[1,2].

## Box 15.12 Primary clinical physiological risk issues – hypothermia.

Hypothermia results from a physiological loss of the ability to maintain an optimal core temperature

- The lower the temperature, the longer it may take to restore normothermia and, with it, adequate respiratory and metabolic functions
- Intrinsic factors include age. Children have an immature hypothalamus, while the elderly have decreasing function of the hypothalamus, causing gradual loss of temperature control mechanisms.
- Rewarming is usually undertaken gradually, but is sometimes required quite rapidly to restore core temperatures for cellular function
- The physiological loss of ability to generate heat because of major injury or surgery affects cellular function or metabolic disturbances
- Use of some vasodilator drugs
- Some anaesthetic drugs may be responsible for the patient having shivering attacks.

Shivering should be brought to the attention of the anaesthetist if the patient's temperature registers at near normal levels. Hypothermia in the operating theatre can result from internal or external factors.

## Box 15.13 Externally imposed factors.

- Extended periods of skin and large wound exposure to cold temperatures
- Overheating, causing sweating (insensitive loss)
- Use of pharmacologically imposed hypotension (for specific procedures to reduce bleeding in plastic surgery, including some free flap reconstructive surgery and craniofacial surgery)
- Administration of cold IV fluids
- Extensive use of cold surgical packs or sponges
- Cold blood/water saturated drapes[1,2].

## Potential clinical risk outcomes in nursing management

The physiological risks of hypothermia to the patient may vary in degree but the potential major complications include those outlined in Box 15.14.

## Box 15.14 Risks to the patient and wound due to hypothermia.

- Physiological changes in all major organ systems, causing alterations in cellular functions as cells function optimally within particular temperature parameters: 35.6°C–37.8°C[1,2,9,10].
- Hypoxaemia leading to patient apathy, confusion, poor judgement, ataxia, dysarthria and potential coma
- Lowered glucose metabolism, which may precipitate acidosis leading to cardiorespiratory arrest, or cardiac rhythmic and electrical disturbances leading to cardiac arrest
- Respiratory disturbances, leading to acidosis and respiratory arrest – this, in addition to an altered fluid balance, may cause major instability in renal function
- There may be disturbances in liver function with an increasing inability to metabolise/detoxify important drugs.

## Box 15.15 Potential clinical risk outcomes in nursing management.

- Normal brain function and reactions are incapacitated when the patient has a general anaesthetic that includes paralysing the muscles of the body
- When normal regulatory response processes by the muscles are unable to respond by, for example, shivering, artificial rewarming responses are required to be instituted to meet the metabolic needs of the body
- The external manifestations of postoperative hypothermia with, for example, varying degrees of shivering and severe discomfort, is most commonly seen early by clinicians in the recovery room or post anaesthesia care unit.
- This may also be as a response to certain inhalation anaesthetic gases used, for example, halothane or similar
- Postoperative shivering can assist in restoring minimum levels of hypothermia but the prolonged

*Continued*

shivering consumes enormous amounts of cellular energy which, in the already perfusion-compromised patient, can lead to acidosis
- The shivering response is suppressed at 32°C (90°F) when the body's rewarming response mechanism becomes ineffective[1,2,9,10,16-18].

## Potential clinical outcomes of hypothermia affecting reconstructive plastic surgery procedures

If hypothermia is not recognised as a potential adverse issue, addressed quickly, and adequately corrected, it may also continue into the clinical unit for up to 72 hours postoperatively. This may have significant effects on vascular outcomes following major reconstructive surgery, particularly free flaps and replants.

Combined with hypovolaemia, this can be an ongoing catastrophic state for reconstructive and microvascular surgical wounds, as during prolonged hypothermia red blood cells carrying the oxygen to the body become increasingly rigid.

As oxygen becomes more strongly attached to the red blood cells during hypothermia, this results in the oxygen-loaded red blood cells having a high degree of difficulty travelling through the capillaries where they are required to release their oxygen and nutrients, in exchange for the by-products of gases ($CO_2$) used to create energy within the cells. Therefore, major systems, including the wound(s) that are in need of oxygen, may now receive little or no oxygen at all from the slow-moving and potentially sludging/clotting red blood cells.

The oxygen-deprived cells must then resort to anaerobic metabolism (to remove the $CO_2$) but that generates only about 10% of normal heat output with increasing levels of lactic acid created as a by-product. For the patient this can be increasingly life-threatening with escalating acidotic respiratory complications. This state, added to circulatory vascular instability, leads to the potential for local and general systemic thrombotic syndromes, finally leading to cardiac arrest[1,2,9,10,16-18].

In reconstructive plastic surgery, nurse clinicians should be on high alert for signs of hypothermia, particularly patients following any major injury and/or surgery combined with procedures longer than two hours, and where the patient has been partially or fully exposed for long periods. Major reconstructive surgery or major liposuction patients, the elderly and children (despite their high metabolic rate) are highly vulnerable[6].

In a major flap and reconstructive surgery, arterial spasm, arterial and venous flow compromise (thrombosis) and subsequent loss of the flap or body part are distinct and high risks. In addition, secondary major complications may result in significant local and systemic infections, as a result of avascular tissue[6].

The increasing recognition of the importance of intra-operative and postoperative hypothermia, including in the surgical unit, is now considered as a serious and potentially life-threatening physiological event that is not uncommon[1,2,17,18].

## Nursing management strategies to prevent hypothermia

### Maintenance of ambient/environmental temperature

The maintenance of ambient/environmental room temperature is considered the key, as under normal environmental and health circumstances, the human homeostatic feedback mechanisms operate to maintain the body's normal core temperature.

It is scientifically acknowledged that maintenance of ambient/environmental room temperature control is the most effective method of sustaining a patient's core temperature at an acceptable level for circulatory and metabolic needs. Because of the variations in ambient room temperatures in operating theatres, recovery rooms post anaesthesia care units and surgical units, the application of the Bair Hugger® should also be undertaken and should accompany the patient back to the clinical surgical unit[1,2,17,18].

Prior to patient entry for major surgery, the operating theatre temperature should be set at 25–26.6°C (78–80°F) and adjusted according to the patient's physiological needs and in response to clinical core temperature monitoring[1,2,17,18].

The application of patient temperature monitoring devices and clinical discretionary judgement are required when there is a potential risk for patient hypothermia, regardless of the extent of surgery or potential body exposure. When the patient is partially or fully exposed for as long as 10–15 minutes after the commencement of anaesthesia, patient positioning, skin prepping and draping, large areas of the skin may be completely exposed and body heat will be lost to the colder environmental temperature. In addition, once surgery begins, internal tissues are exposed, further increasing the potential for hypothermia.

The greater exposure over extended periods of time, the greater the risk of heat loss will be[1,2,17,18]. Wet drapes can also be a source of external cooling. Adjunctive heating should be maintained until the patient is physiologically stable enough to sustain normothermia though increasing physical activity. This may not occur until the patient returns to the surgical unit.

### Administration of IV fluids

Blood and blood products are stored at refrigerated temperatures just above freezing (4°C or 39.2°F) and IV crystalloid solutions are usually stored at room temperatures, consistent with the operating theatre (20°C or 68°F).

For patients already cold, or at risk of increased hypothermia, fluids must be artificially prewarmed (37°–98.6°F) and infused warm, as direct infusion of cold IV fluids into the patient can further decrease the core body temperature dramatically. The patient's body will continue to use valuable energy to warm additional IV fluids. The longer the procedure, the greater the loss of fluid added to the time of internal and external body exposure, the more energy will be generated and utilised which has the potential to lead to metabolic/respiratory acidosis.

### At the completion of the surgical procedure

Prior to completion of the procedure, ambient room temperature should be raised to provide warmth before patient undraping takes place, and patient warmth should be maintained when transferring a patient from theatre to the post anaesthesia care unit, and on transfer to the surgical unit.

As previously discussed, loss of body/skin temperature combined with hypovolaemia also causes significant peripheral vascular shutdown. During and after major plastic surgery this can be disastrous for tissue flap circulation, with infarcts and emboli causing flap loss and unacceptable overall wound outcomes.

Although the effects of progressive hypothermia have only recently been acknowledged in recon-

structive surgery and major cosmetic surgery (major liposuction procedures), recognising and preventing hypothermia and hypovolaemia can make the difference between successful or unsuccessful patient and wound outcomes[1,2,17,18].

### Within the postoperative surgical unit

Following major surgery, the medical and nursing principles and methods of monitoring, documentation and reporting for the five vital signs (including hypothermia prevention) must continue after the patient returns to the clinical surgical unit.

---

**Box 15.16** Addressing hypothermia risk management in the surgical unit.

- The clinical room should have been prewarmed to an ambient temperature of about 25°C and maintained for the first 72 hours, as this is usually the critical period, and longer if deemed necessary
- Continuous core temperature monitoring and maintenance for the initial 72 hours is important, and until the patient and the wound are stable
- When the patient is stable, has some personal mobility and is generating acceptable body heat, the room temperature can be lowered gradually to a more agreeable working level
- This should be assessed based on the patient's ability to sustain an average acceptable core temperature.

---

## Pain management strategies

In addition to the fears already outlined, central to all the concerns that a patient may have prior to surgery, is an intense apprehension related to the potential mismanagement of pain, intra-operatively and post-operatively, and this may perhaps be one of the most significant[1,2,8,11,18–21].

---

**Review**

*Pain management (fifth vital sign)*, Chapter 11.

---

Inadequate objective patient pain assessment, documentation and applied pain management combined with patient demonstrations of anger, fear, and inability to co-operate may become critical issues for nurses to address and to manage effectively.

In some cases where regional or local anaesthetic infiltration has been used and no initial pain may be felt, it remains important that RICE (**R**est, **I**mmobilisation, **C**omfort and **E**levation) is implemented.

The period of a pain-free state may be short lived, and utilising pre-emptive basic RICE principles, with supplementary narcotics or oral analgesics to maintain a therapeutic level, is important for the patient and the wound.

When pain does not exist, the patient can then prioritise and verbalise their issues and concerns, co-operate with requests related to medical and nursing care, and have a sense of personal control and wellbeing.

---

**Box 15.18** Example of surgical interventions requiring applied objective high level pain management strategies.

- Multiple injury
- Burns management
- Major head and neck surgery including craniofacial reconstruction
- Upper and lower limb trauma/surgery
- Reconstructive surgery – free flap vascular transfers
- Major breast surgery
- Abdominal lipectomy with plication of the abdominal wall
- All chest and abdominal procedures that have the potential to compromise normal respiratory function and generate the medical and nursing co-morbidity produced by immobility.

---

**Box 15.17** Critical assessment and evaluation strategies.

- Description of the patient's pain management goals
- What the patient expresses as the pain level documented and analysed, and pain control measures administered accordingly
- The expectation of the potential for the degree and extent of pain in respect of the individual patient's needs
- The type, amount and timing of pain medication required to control the pain
- Specific timing phases to evaluate the degree of pain control attained and reassessment of the patient's wounds and pain control needs as appropriate.

---

Disciplined and planned pre-emptive pain control strategies are essential for all procedures that produce pain or discomfort in the postoperative phase. Specific planning for regional blocks and/or narcotic pain control is essential following many significant reconstructive plastic surgery procedures, and must be explained preoperatively to the patient who demonstrates a fear of pain[19–21].

The principal surgical interventions for consideration are outlined in Box 15.18.

## Maintaining therapeutic control of pain

It is suggested by specialist therapeutic drug advisory groups that as a general rule it is not the actual drug which is important, rather it is the route and frequency of administration[22].

It is also fundamentally important that the selection of the pain-controlling medication is matched to the desired outcome, for example, certain drugs are more suitable for musculoskeletal pain than others. In some cases, a mix of medications (e.g. an opioid, with an oral anti-inflammatory and diazepam) rather than reliance on one (e.g. an opioid) may be appropriate.

For patients remaining in hospital for 24 hours or longer, the use of pain infusions/patient controlled analgesia pumps, including bolus dosages for breakthrough pain substantially contribute to sustained patient comfort, cardiorespiratory compliance, early mobility, early physical and emotional recovery, reduced medical and nursing morbidity, and early discharge.

Adequate selection and dosage of the appropriate oral analgesia (or use of reducing dosages of narcotic intranasal inhalants, or patches (e.g. fentanyl)) should be administered 24–48 hours prior to the complete withdrawal of systemic narcotics to maintain a therapeutic level of pain control and to sustain a sense of safety and comfort in the patient[21,22].

The use of oral, intramuscular and intravenous muscle relaxants (e.g. benzodiazepines) in conjunction with routine pain medications should be considered, for instance as an adjunct to a narcotic or oral medication where muscle spasm is a contributing factor to the pain (e.g. lower limb and facial bone surgery[21,22]).

Pain that is not relieved by narcotics requires a critical reassessment as it often indicates potential problems related to vascular compromise at or surrounding injured tissues, or underlying surgical issues including ischaemia of the tissues and internal wound bleeding or infection[1-3]. Where pain is experienced in relation to tourniquet sites this should be assessed and reported[23]. This is discussed later in this chapter.

### On discharge

On discharge, pain management modalities involving wound targeted medication pre-emptively taken, strictly as directed for the first 48–72 hours, elevation of the part to reduce oedema, and an understanding of what adverse levels of pain may indicate, are important for patient comfort and co-operation.

In addition, circulatory maintenance and fluid balance, regular physical mobility and wearing of anti-embolitic stockings as directed, to prevent/minimise a deep vein thrombosis are important risk management strategies (see Chapter 14).

## Development of haematoma

The development of a haematoma is a risk to a wound following any surgical procedure[3,4,6] and is a potential source of severe pain and subsequent infection if it is not timely treated. Frequent regular inspections and checks should be made for swelling, bleeding, ooze from suture lines, and wound tension in excess of safe or expected normal parameters[3,4,6]. Any adverse signs must be documented and reported immediately.

Gentle gliding touch/movements of the gloved flat surface of the clinician's hand should be used to assess alterations in wound contouring. Clinical observations, visual observations of the patient, the patient's restlessness, sweating, responses to the rising level and type of pain, and examination of increasing size of the wound can provide early indications, alerting staff to problems of internal bleeding.

> **Review**
>
> *Development of wound haematoma*, Chapter 8.

### Internal drainage tubing

Internal drains connected to collecting bottles should be firmly secured to the patient and not to the bedclothes. Tubing should be long enough to allow the patient to move, or to roll over in bed without putting stress on the tubing.

Where several drains exist, each bottle should be individually marked according to its particular wound zone, with drainage levels marked so that individual inputs can be accurately measured against time periods. Surgeons should be asked to provide parameters for reporting drainage in excess to safety limits (i.e. drainage not greater than 20+ ml per hour in the first 24 hours).

## Deep vein thrombosis and venous thrombosis in wounds

Deep vein thrombosis (DVT) is the outcome of the development of a blood clot in the deep venous systemic vessels of the pelvis or lower leg, that remains in an attached and stationary position within the vein, mainly within the femoral, iliac or deep veins of the calf muscle[24-32].

The detachment of a piece of this clot may occur, and travel via the venous system to the lung and, being too large to travel through the vessels in the lung, lead to pulmonary embolism (PE). This has a high potential to cause significant long-term morbidity (if not treated in a timely manner), or untimely death[24-32].

In some patients, PE has been known to occur up to three months post surgery but there is insufficient evidence to link the two events due to the insidious nature and poor aetiological knowledge of the condition. In known at risk patients, preventative measures are imperative at all the preoperative and perioperative stages and on discharge.

There is no known single primary cause of DVT, but some underlying factors that precipitate the condition have been physiologically described[24-32].

A venous thrombosis in large veins blocks the pathway of deoxygenated blood back to the heart and this may set up a permanent local blockage leading to local or regional tissue injury. This is commonly seen in the lower limb and subsequently has the potential to lead to a localised, or multifocal, venous ulceration many years later[9–11].

Whilst it is impossible to identify every potential candidate for DVT, studies have been able to indicate those possibly at low, medium or high risk and as stated these factors should be known by all practising clinicians[9–11,23–31]. The common initiating factor appears to be physical immobility for more than two hours and reduction of blood flow, but even this has not been conclusively proven as a cause and the episode may be a detrimental outcome in an individual already at risk[24–31].

The true incidence of DVT in hospital, and in the community at large, is virtually unknown (suggested to be 1–2 in 1000, mainly women[10,28]. This is because of the nature of the condition, in which silent episodes are thought to occur, not infrequently, and known cases do not require clinical reporting to a central register. With most patients being short stay, most statistical studies have been based on patients presenting to emergency department, and on post mortem figures where pulmonary embolism was the cause of death, and presumed related to an earlier, or previously undetected, DVT.

Many 'silent' episodes do not lead to pulmonary embolism and may go virtually unnoticed and unreported by the individual or patient in hospital or immediately after discharge, but may have the potential to set up adverse events if immobility continues after discharge. The critical period appears to be at or around days 3 to 14–21, but may occur up to 12 weeks later or longer[24–31].

Despite the highly disguised aetiology of this condition and its life-threatening nature, risk management strategies for potential prevention/minimisation are available and should be used in:

- Those patients already identified at risk
- Those who are even slightly suspect
- Patients undergoing specific procedures that may cause periods of complete immobility greater than two hours[28–32].

DVT (silent or recognised) is also a significant precursor to the long-term development of post thrombotic, or post phlebotic syndrome, and venous leg ulcers. These are both insidious in nature and potentially chronic and disabling conditions.

Post thrombotic syndrome is never considered as having been cured, because of the risk of recurrence of DVT related to the chronic nature of the syndrome, and the increased risk of further thrombi developing[28,29]. There may be long periods of remission when disciplined treatment modalities are undertaken.

Such is the life-threatening potential of DVT, the known risk factors should be acknowledged and not underestimated. Nurse clinicians should be advocates for the patient, and practise those prevention strategies that are within their sphere of influence, and alert surgeons and physicians where the pre-existing causes are known or suspected, following the primary nursing patient assessment.

---

**Box 15.19** DVT pathophysiology – the principles.

- Arteries and veins are essentially responsible for life itself and react instinctively to injury and changes in circulatory flow, by clotting or spasm[16].
- Venous thrombosis is the formation of a blood clot within a vein as blood moves from a fluid state to a solid state (a clot)
- Regardless of size or diameter of the vein it is commonly suggested that inadequate arterial pressure and, significantly, immobility are the primary causes in the cessation of venous flow
- Venous flow is principally facilitated by physical activity creating a muscular pumping action and assisted by gravity
- An immobile state assists in creating stasis or pooling of blood that finally coagulates or clots
- The principal physiological causes of venous thrombosis (singly or combined), which are universally accepted, are demonstrated through the three concepts originally described by Virchow in 1846, and known as 'Virchow's triad'[9,10,24–32], as outlined in Box 15.20.

**Box 15.20** Virchow's triad.

| | |
|---|---|
| **Stasis** | low, slow or no flow (hypovolaemia, hypothermia, immobility, gravity – limb below heart level) |
| **Vessel wall injury** | tension (stretching) on the vessel, a vascular laceration, split in, or excess pressure impinging on the internal vessel wall |
| **Coagulation** | blood clotting (predisposing medical factors, or factors responding to stasis and vessel wall injury). |

**Box 15.21** Suggested medium to high risk factors for deep vein thrombosis.

- Prolonged bed rest (i.e. total immobility greater than two hours in the elderly, critically ill, patients with malignancy)
- Long distance travel, because of prolonged immobility. It is unclear if air travel is more risky than other long journeys – for example, by car, train or coach
- Major injuries, immobility or paralysis
- Surgery, especially if it lasts more than 30 minutes to two hours, particularly if it involves the leg joints or pelvis
- Cancer and its treatment modalities, which can cause the blood to clot more easily
- Pregnancy and childbirth – related to hormone changes that make the blood clot more easily and because the foetus puts added pressure on the veins of the pelvis
- There is also risk of injury to veins during delivery or a caesarean
- The risk is at its highest just after childbirth
- Taking a contraceptive pill that contains oestrogen. Most modern pills contain a low dose, which though it increases the risk, is acceptable for most women
- Hormone replacement therapy (HRT) – for many women, the benefits may outweigh the increase in risk
- Other circulation or heart problems[24–28]
- Previous major surgery.

## Clinical diagnosis of DVT

As previously stated, despite the use of a range of minimising/prevention strategies, DVT can, and does, occur unexpectedly. Early recognition and diagnosis of the condition is very important if life-threatening PE is to be avoided and the medium to long-term effects of vascular damage (post thrombotic syndrome) reduced[24–32].

**Box 15.22** Clinical diagnosis of deep vein thrombosis

- Clinical signs may initially be vague but, following surgery, any solicited or unsolicited remark from the patient that they have a cramp or pain in the calf and feel that the leg is swollen must be reported to the surgeon and investigated for a potential DVT if the life-threatening secondary complication of PE is to be avoided/minimised
- The patient should be checked for Homans' sign – calf pain on dorsiflexion of the ankle usually means a positive (+) sign, although a false positive Homans' sign may be present without DVT being present, particularly following knee, hip, pelvic injuries/surgery
- The additional signs of initial calf pain followed by redness, tenderness, slight fever, sweating, and unilateral swelling with calf asymmetry of more that 1 cm, documented by using a tape measure, are also highly important clinical indicators[9–11]
- Patients who report these significant signs and symptoms, and those who are at medium to high risk, with or without chest pain or shortness of breath, should undergo specialist anticoagulant treatment including diagnostic ultrasound, chest X-ray and/or ventilation-perfusion (VQ) scans to rule out PE.

## Clinical risk prevention strategies – patient mobility and discharge

Because it is almost impossible to assess who is endangered, the patient's potential risk, based on existing facts, and the surgery to be undertaken, should be used to determine the risk management strategies. This must be a priority in nursing care in all adult patients undergoing surgery[24,25]. This assessment then allows for prophylactic management to be timely instituted.

There is no single definitive treatment suggested in the literature but in those patients at known risk, a combination of the outlined modalities outlined below, are a 'belt and braces' method of minimising this critical medical complication.

The following outlines suggested modalities for addressing risk prevention/minimising DVT.

**Prophylactic anticoagulant therapy:** (e.g. subcutaneous low molecular weight heparin or new generation anticoagulants as medically ordered). According to the patient's assessed risk, this may be used alone or in combination with the treatments described below.

**Anti-thromboembolic stockings:** for low risk patients, elastic hosiery such as TEDs® are suggested to be effective when the patient is immobile, functioning at a level of compression (17–20 mm Hg) at the ankle.

In immobile patients, the combined application of TEDs®, elevation of the legs on two pillows, further assists in the return of venous blood flow through gravity. This can be further improved by specific and timely leg movements (as directed by physiotherapists) with deep and superficial lymphatic massage therapy techniques applied.

In patients who are awake and can co-operate, appropriate and strict attention to prescribed regular hourly leg movement exercises or, in high-risk patients, the use of mechanical calf pumping devices in the hospital bed prior to, and after surgery, is a very important preventive strategy.

Anti-thromboembolic stockings (elastic hosiery) such as TEDs® are ineffective when the patient is ambulant because of their low level of compression. In the presence of gravity (patient is upright), this requires a greater level of compression over the calf muscles. Thus TEDs® should only be used when the patient is bedbound and TEDs® are, therefore, not advocated for patients on discharge.

**Sequential compression devices:** in the high-risk patient, sequential compression devices (SCD) can increase blood flow velocity up to 250%, to maximise the amount of blood moved by compressing large areas of muscle mass. This increases the fibrolytic activity (removal of material capable of slowing down blood flow), thus increasing the body's ability to protect the vasculature. SCD is highly recommended for use in modern surgical practice.

**Arteriovenous impulse systems:** these can also increase blood flow velocity up to 250%, and maximise the amount of blood moved by stimulating the release of nitric oxide which inhibits platelet aggregation – the principal basis of blood clot formation that produces venous thrombosis and venous obstruction. This technique is highly recommended[25–31].

## Addressing reconstructive plastic surgical patients – DVT

Many patients who undergo major reconstructive surgery and particular types of cosmetic surgery (e.g. breast surgery, abdominal lipectomy, major liposuction) following discharge will go home and stay in bed for a few days, significantly increasing the risk (day 3 – 10+) of DVT, and subsequent pulmonary embolism.

The effects of DVT on reconstructive plastic and related surgical procedures have been reviewed[27,31]. Although the incidence of DVT is stated to be minimal when prophylaxis is practised, the long lasting morbidity of DVT and potential for death should be an enduring signal for a thorough investigation at preoperative assessment time, and all efforts to minimise or prevent its occurrence should be undertaken prior to and post surgery.

The patient who is assessed as medium to high risk should be followed up for long-term prophylactic medical treatment after surgical discharge[27–32].

### *Prophylactic anti-embolic hosiery*

On mobility, and prior to discharge, medium to high-risk patients should have TEDs® replaced with individual custom fitted compression stockings. For the majority of patients, measuring and fitting for postoperative application can be accomplished preoperatively, based on preoperative risk assessment. This should be under the control/supervision of specialist clinicians with accompanying patient education. The following list provides examples of pressures suggested to attain prophylactic management:

| | | |
|---|---|---|
| **Low risk** | pressure producing approximately | 20–30 mm Hg at the ankle |
| **Medium risk** | (post thrombotic oedema) | 30–40 mm Hg at the ankle |
| **High risk** | (post thrombotic oedema) | 40–50 mm Hg at the ankle[31] |

The use of graduated compressing anti-embolitic stockings is highly advocated post surgery and this practice, though uncomfortable at times, may be required to be maintained for up to three months in high risk patients, post discharge.

Stockings should be left off overnight when legs can be elevated on two pillows and TEDs® worn[32]. As previously outlined, all patients to be fitted with compression stockings should be assessed by determining the ankle brachial pulse index[7] to exclude arterial disease, and garments should be fitted by professionals to avoid the risk of arterial vascular damage[32].

Ongoing medical supervision for any ordered medication management of prophylactic anti-thrombolytic regime must be maintained to ensure clotting profiles are at normal levels. In addition, advice regarding continuation or resumption of any previous medications (e.g. aspirin), should be provided. Patients should understand the importance of timely reporting of any signs and symptoms immediately to their medical officer, or the immediate presentation to the closest emergency department.

## Important issues related to venous thrombosis at the surgical site

Venous thrombosis can also manifest itself in the local wound site tissue of patients following procedures such as vascular microsurgery, replant surgery and free flap surgery[6]. This critical complication can result in major negative circulatory outcomes that represent the most common postoperative cause for the loss of the replanted part, or whole or partial loss of a skin/tissue flap.

This is discussed in detail in Section IV – Chapters 18 & 19.

Professional nurses have a large role to play in the minimisation/prevention of local wound thrombosis and DVT, and should be clinically well versed in all aspects of the condition, current strategies to address risk minimisation and prevention management, and advocates for patient safety.

See recommended websites (deep vein thrombosis and pulmonary embolism) at the end of this chapter.

## Postoperative nausea and vomiting

With patients now staying in hospital for shorter periods, postoperative nausea and vomiting (PONV) can be a major and distressing complication of anaesthesia, particularly day case surgery[1,2,5,33]. Many patients find this experience to be the most distressing and often the worst memory of their hospital stay. The consequences have economic implications as well as physical, metabolic, and psychological effects on patients who may find returning to work early, as anticipated, extremely difficult.

---

**Box 15.23** Predisposing factors for postoperative nausea and vomiting.

- Previous history of PONV
- Incidence of gastric disturbances including hiatus hernia
- Low gastric volume with high acidity related to prolonged fasting, narcotics[32]
- Types of procedures (abdominal region)
- Middle ear surgery
- Young females
- Postoperatively, the following are considered the high-risk activities: e.g. excess movement, pain, certain physical postures.

---

### Treatment regimes

Avoidance of general anaesthesia, use of regional techniques wherever possible, maintenance of hydration and circulatory volume, and pharmacologically approved antiemetic drugs are commonly strategies used to avoid PONV.

The use of Zofran® (ondansetron – a selective serotonin antagonist) has been shown to be extremely successful in patients with past history of severe PONV[1,2,33].

## Malignant hyperthermia

This is a rare autosomal dominant trait which gives rise to an unexpected, yet potentially fatal (50%) anaesthetic complication (demonstrated by severe muscle rigidity) arising from an inherited and rare muscle disorder (often unknown prior to surgery) triggered by a reaction to the use of specific hazardous anaesthetic drugs (e.g. halothane) and in particular, neuromuscular blocking agents (i.e. Scoline – succinylcholine – suxamethonium dichloride)[1,2,34–36]. It can occur up to 20 minutes after the induction and up to 24 hours postoperatively.

Treatment includes cessation of anaesthesia, 100% oxygen, dantrolene sodium, a skeletal muscle relaxant, and sodium bicarbonate administered immediately, with correction of acidosis and hyperkalaemia, and cooling procedures. If dantrolene sodium is not accessible within the operating theatre, staff should be able to identify the nearest point of availability (i.e. nearest major teaching/university hospital).

## Preventing intra-operative adverse events – the use of tourniquets

### Tourniquet injuries

A potential region of injury and pain is what is referred to as 'post tourniquet injury'[23]. This is caused by the improper application of a rubber or pneumatic type tourniquet to exclude blood flow to the limb. The pressure should not exceed pulse pressure.

Pressures in excess of those designated for the limbs of children, females and male patients, and failure to follow the protocols set out for their use based on risk management can result in severely damage skin and underlying tissues (muscle, nerves) shear and friction injury. Patients who have had limb tourniquets applied to the skin should be examined following their use for any signs of injury immediately post operatively, and after the regional anaesthetic has worn off.

### Tourniquet pain

A sense of pain not commonly described is one following the removal of a pneumatic tourniquet. This is referred to as 'post tourniquet pain'[22].

- Mediated by unmyelinated, slow conducting C fibres that are normally inhibited by fast pain impulses conducted by myelinated A-delta fibres
- Incidence of tourniquet pain correlates with increasing age and particularly the duration of surgery more common in lower extremity surgery.

## Brachial plexus injury during surgery

Patients undergoing hand surgery will, under normal circumstances, have a brachial plexus block and a tourniquet applied on the upper arm. During the surgical procedure, their arm will commonly be extended at right angles to the body, and placed on an operating hand table.

Extreme care must be taken not to overextend the arm/shoulder backwards, causing stretching and injury to the brachial plexus nerve bundle. This damage may result in temporary or permanent injury to the nerves that are responsible for arm and hand function[1,2]. During normal block recovery, returning sensory function (sensory returns first, and then motor) will occur.

If, following the anticipated return of sensory and motor function, the patient comments on extended numbness time, poor movement, and sharp pain, this must be reported to the surgeon immediately for investigation and appropriate testing.

## Perioperative and postoperative pressure injuries

Extended periods of immobility related to long-term operative procedures (greater than two hours) can include the potential for altered skin integrity and may result in vascular and cellular changes due to the increasing development of dependent oedema in the lower body.

This may be observed on the sacrum, heels or back of the head where procedures are undertaken on the elderly, children, those who are critically ill or injured, or reconstructive procedures of long duration. Protective measures should be instituted to avoid any injury due to these conditions. Non-operated limbs should be protected by padding and supports[1–3,13–15].

## Additional potential adverse events

Risk management strategies to prevent wrong side/site surgery, laser injury, eye injury from prep solutions, burns from diathermy, sharps injury, correct counts of instruments and swabs must also be in place and checked for[1–3,13–15].

# Patient handover responsibilities

Disciplined handover protocols are essential when responsibility for the patient is transferred from one clinician to another[1,2,13-15,37]. Every detail of relevant clinical information must be provided to the nurse who accepts the patient back into the post anaesthesia care unit or the clinical surgical unit area.

## Patient movement following surgery

Whenever possible all patients should be transferred directly to their clinical unit bed, or day surgery trolley, from the operating table (one physical move only) in order to minimise cardiovascular compromises related to postural hypotension in the previously static patient.

It is stated that the most common time for cardiac arrest in the postoperative phase is at the time the patient is transferred from trolley to bed, or bed to trolley. Factors may include repositioning of all abdominal contents, pressure on the diaphragm, fluid movement to the heart, increasing pressure within the left ventricle. With the introduction of the universal patient bed, these episodes are now less likely to occur.

The optimal and safe postoperative resting position of flaps, grafts and reconstructive procedures anywhere on the body may be compromised by multiple bed/trolley patient transfers, so these should be avoided wherever possible.

Following upper abdominal and lower abdominal lipectomy and flap surgery, postoperative instructions should be sought from the surgeon as to the level of leg elevation and parallel sitting position required, to reduce tension on the suture lines, minimise body slippage producing shear and friction over the sacrum, and assist in venous return from the lower limbs[3,4].

## Protecting the surgical site

Following breast reconstruction and lower limb surgery, protective cages should be employed to remove any pressure from wounds, especially skin grafts and skin/soft tissue flaps. This also allows clinical observations to be undertaken without constantly moving covers, etc., which disturbs both the patient and ambient warmth created.

Limbs should be elevated according to the surgeon's orders. It is important not to assume that elevation to assist and increase venous return is automatically desired. Rather, in the early postoperative period, microvascular arterial inflow may be compromised, and lower than normal elevation is required to provide increased arterial perfusion. Competency in neurovascular assessment/observations and analysis of the data collected are essential to respond and provide the correct position for the vascular perfusion and protective needs of the wound. Neurovascular assessment is discussed in Section IV, Chapter 19 and 20.

Tension on suture lines, external pressure on wounds and unintended early movements of the wounded area(s) may initiate bleeding or compromise vascular beds. Pillows, foam support pads and beanbags are useful in resting limbs that are not elevated by formal orthopaedic slings and mechanical supports.

Patients who have had regional arm blocks will lose sensory and motor function until the block ceases to act. Such patients must be protected from unmanageable motor movements that have the potential to cause injury, particularly to the face. Because pain is absent whilst the block is working, neurovascular assessment requires the recognition of other clinical signs such as colour and capillary return.

## Coughing

Previous or current smokers may have severe coughing episodes that compromise the airway by provoking laryngeal or bronchial spasms and compromise the wound[1,2]. Both must be treated immediately and all perioperative nurses should know how to recognise these conditions, be competent in hand ventilation techniques and early management at the onset of an episode, whilst the anaesthetist is arriving. For persistent coughing episodes, if the patient is sufficiently awake, they should be encouraged to place a soft pillow in front of the chest and abdominal wall, supported by folded arms, to reduce any impact on any wounded area.

## Skin care

Because those patients who are required to be bedbound, even for 48 hours, are always at risk of alterations to skin and soft tissue integrity, protocols should be initiated to prevent pressure injury to the sacrum and heels. Two-hourly side-to-side 30° tilts are mandatory, while avoiding pressure on the ischial tuberosities. Physiotherapy or radiology foam wedge appliances are excellent for this purpose as pillows are not of uniform size and may tend to slip. Alternatively, some special patient beds are mechanically able to achieve a 30° tilt.

The heels should also be elevated by raising the bottom of the bed by 15–30° to assist venous return and reduce development of pelvic dependent oedema and venous stasis caused by immobility. The heels should be supported and not touching the bedclothes, to prevent pressure shear and friction on body movement. For patients assessed to be at medium or high risk of pressure injury an appropriate pressure-relieving mattress is essential, especially for critically ill, immobile, obese or elderly, and those patients who are highly dependent on nursing care.

### Surgery in freestanding/ambulatory healthcare units

The American Society of Plastic Surgeons (http://www.plasticsurgery.org/) issued a press release on July 2004 outlining practice advisory recommendations for patient safety strategies for office-based plastic surgery developed since December 12, 2002.

A large number and a wide range of surgery and particularly plastic surgery procedures are practised in freestanding integrated surgical and medical centres[1–4,13–15]. Admission and exit discharge management should be as complete and as safe for the patient as would be expected in any major university teaching healthcare institution, regardless of the extent of the surgery.

Gaining official recognition from appropriate accrediting agencies should be an important goal for the surgical centre. This recognition provides patients with a sense of confidence, which is important in their perception of their encounter with the complex world of healthcare practices.

See Section II, Chapter 14.

## Preferred patient and clinical outcomes

### Box 15.24 Safety.

- The patient was assessed preoperatively for any adverse physiological and psychosocial issues including risk factors that would compromise the preferred patient and clinical outcomes
- Risk factors related to all areas of surgical and nursing management were pre-emptive and effectively addressed
- The procedure was uneventful and conducted within total safety for the patient and staff
- The patient expressed satisfaction with each phase of the entire process.

### Box 15.25 Comfort.

- Assessment of the aetiology of pain and discomfort was an ongoing process and addressed pre-emptively to the complete satisfaction of the patient
- The patient expressed satisfaction with the entire process of pain management at all phases of the surgical procedure and postoperatively.

### Box 15.26 Independence.

- Patient education was ongoing and allowed the patient to be aware of approaching events with the minimum of fear and apprehension
- The patient's level of personal control and independence was considered at all phases of care and addressed to the patient's satisfaction.

## References

(1) Meeker M.H. & Rothrock J.C. *Alexander's care of the patient in surgery*, 11th edn. St Louis: Mosby, 1999.
(2) Fairchild S.S. *Perioperative nursing: principles and practice*, 2nd edn. Boston: Little, Brown, 1996.

(3) Fortunato N. & McCullough S. *Plastic and reconstructive surgery*: Mosby's Perioperative Nursing Series. St Louis: Mosby, 1998.

(4) Goodman T.A. (ed.) *Core curriculum for plastic and reconstructive surgical nursing*, 2nd edn. Pitman, NJ: ASPSN American Society of Plastic Surgery Nurses, 1996. http://www.aspsn.org/

(5) Shields L. & Werder H. *Perioperative nursing*. London: Greenwich Medical Media, 2002.

(6) Ausher B.M., Erikson E. & Wilkins E.G. *Plastic surgery: indications, operations and outcomes*. St Louis: Mosby, 2000.

(7) Spencer K.W. Selection and preoperative preparation of plastic surgery patients. *Nursing Clinics of North America*, 1994 (Dec); **29**(4):697–710.

(8) Moser S. Social service collaboration: meeting the patient's psychosocial needs. *Plastic Surgical Nursing*, 1993 (summer); **13**(2):84–5,119.

(9) Porth C.P. *Pathophysiology: concepts in altered health states*, 5th edn. New York: Lippincott, 2000.

(10) Smeltzer S.C. & Bare B.G. *Brunner and Suddarth's textbook of medical-surgical nursing*, 9th edn. New York: Lippincott, Williams & Wilkins, 2000.

(11) Mallett J. & Dougherty L. (eds). *The Royal Marsden Hospital manual of clinical nursing procedures*, 5th edn. Oxford,UK: Blackwell Science, 2000.

(12) Brady M., Kinn S. & Stewart P. Preoperative fasting for adults to prevent perioperative complications. *Cochrane Database of Systematic Reviews*, 2003;(4): CD004423.

(13) De Fazio Quinn D.M. (ed.). *Ambulatory surgical nursing: core curriculum*. American Society of Perianaesthesia Nursing. London: W.B. Saunders, 1999.

(14) Penn S., Davenport T., Carrington S. & Edmondson M. (eds) *Principles of day surgery nursing*, 1st edn. Oxford, UK: Blackwell Publishing, 1996.

(15) Baker B., Fillion D., Davitt R. & Pinneeotad L. Ambulatory surgical clinical pathway. *Journal of Perianesthesia Nursing*, 1999 (Feb); **14**(1):2–11.

(16) Guyton A.C. & Hall J.E. *Textbook of medical physiology*, 9th edn. London: W.B. Saunders, 1996.

(17) McNeil B. Inadvertent hypothermia in the operating theatre. *Professional Nurse*, 1997 (March); **12**(6):418–21.

(18) Hinojosa R.J. Comparison of three rewarming methods in a post anaesthesia care unit. *Plastic Surgical Nursing*, 1997 (winter); **17**(4):222–5.

(19) Bucknall T., Maniaas E. & Botti M. Acute pain management: Implications of scientific evidence for nursing in the postoperative context. *International Journal of Nursing Practice*, 2001; **7**(4):266.

(20) Hawthorn J. & Redmond K. *Pain: causes and management*. Oxford: Blackwell Publishing, 1998.

(21) Stark P.L., Sherwood G.D. & Adams-McNeill J. Pain management outcomes: issues for advanced practice nurses. *International Journal of Advanced Nursing Practice*, 2000; **4**(1). http://www.icaap.org/

(22) Victorian Drug Usage Advisory Committee. *Therapeutic guidelines: analgesia*, 3rd edn. Melbourne: Victorian Drug Usage Advisory Committee/Interprint Services, March 1997.

(23) Wakai A., Winter D.C., Street J.T. & Redmond P.H. Pneumatic tourniquets in extremity surgery. *Journal of the American Academy Orthopedic Surgery*, 2001 (Sept.–Oct.) **5**(9):345–51.

(24) Autar R. Nursing assessment of clients at risk of deep vein thrombosis: DVT: the Autar DVT scale. *Journal of Advanced Nursing*, 1996; **23**:763–70.

(25) Autar R. Calculating patients risk of deep vein thrombosis. *British Journal of Nursing*, 1998 (Jan 8–21); **7**(1):7–12.

(26) Blondin M.M. Deep vein thrombosis and pulmonary embolism prevention: what role do nurses play? *Medsurg Nursing*, 1996 (June); **5**(3):205–208.

(27) Abs R. Thromboembolism in plastic surgery: review of the literature and proposal of a prophylaxis algorithm. *Annals de Chirurgie Plastique Esthetique*, 2000 (Dec); **45**(6):604–609.

(28) MacLellan D.G. Venous thromboembolism: an insidious hazard. Part 1: incidence, prevalence and sequelae. *Primary intention, the Australian Journal of Wound Management*, 2000 (May) **8**(2):57–61.

(29) MacLellan, D.G. Venous thromboembolism: an insidious hazard. Part 2: prophylaxis and treatment. *Primary Intention, the Australian Journal of Wound Management*, 2000 (August) **8**(3):98–103.

(30) McDevitt N.B. Deep vein thrombosis prophylaxis. American Society of Plastic and Reconstructive Surgeons. *Plastic Reconstructive Surgery*, 1999 (Nov 10); **4**(6):1923–28.

(31) Solomon J.M. & Schow S.R. Potential risk, complications and prevention of deep vein thrombosis in oral and maxillofacial surgery patients. *Journal of Oral and Maxillofacial Surgery*, 1995, (Dec) **53**(12): 1441–47.

(32) Maylor M.E. Accurate selection of compression and anti-embolic hosiery. *British Journal of Nursing*, 2001; **10**(18):1172–84.

(33) Bibby P.F. Postoperative nausea management and patient controlled analgesia. *British Journal of Nursing*, 2001; **10**(12):775–80.

(34) Redmond M.C. Malignant hyperthermia: perianaesthesia recognition, treatment and care. *Journal of Perianesthesia Nursing*, 2001 (Aug); **16**(4):259–70.

(35) Karlet M.C. Malignant hyperthermia: considerations for ambulatory surgery. *Journal of Perianesthesia Nursing*, (USA), 1998 (Oct); **13**(5):304–12.

(36) Fortunato-Phillips N. Malignant hyperthermia. Update 2000. *Critical Care Nursing Clinics of North America*, 2000, (June); **12**(2):199–210.

(37) Anwari J.S. Quality handover to the postanaesthesia care unit nurse. *Anaesthesia*, 2002 (May); **57**(5):484–500.

## Recommended websites

**Preoperative patient assessment and premedication protocols**

http://www.virtual-anaesthesia-textbook.com (Preoperative assessment and premedication

http://www.usyd.edu.au/su/anaes/lectures/Preop_JL.html

http://www.guideline.gov/summary/summary.aspx?doc_id=1854&nbr=1080

**Deep vein thrombosis and pulmonary embolism**

http://www.medscape.com/viewarticle/489427?src=mp (American College of Chest Physicians revised guidelines for prevention of venous thromboembolism – September, 2004)

http://www.rxlist.com/cgi/generic3/arixtra.htm (Risks associated with use of anti-embolitic prophylaxis when epidural or spinal anaesthesia is used – excellent)

http://www.doh.gov.uk/blood/dvt/

http://hcd2.bupa.co.uk/fact_sheets/mosby_factsheets/Deep_Vein_Thrombosis.html

http://www.lifestages.com/health/venous.html

http://health.yahoo.com/health/centers/heart/104.html

http://www.drugs.com/MTM/fondaparinux.html

http://www.pharmacist.com/articles/d_dn_0007.cfm

http://www.fpnotebook.com/HEM174.htm

http://www.medscape.com/viewarticle/463645

**Malignant hyperthermia**

http://www.diagnostic.co.nz/hbook/5ce65a6.htm

# Chapter 16

# Perioperative Paediatric Care in Reconstructive Plastic Surgical Nursing

## Background

Children should not be seen as small adults – physiologically or psychosocially. A child's perception of the world that surrounds them is quite different to the world in which adults live, move, think and function. The care of children at all ages is a highly specialised field with specialised education an essential component of care.

---

**Box 16.1** Examples of knowledge required regarding professional care of the child.

- The expected normal physical and psychological growth milestones
- Congenital or inherited conditions that have the actual or potential to alter the expected normal growth and intellectual development of the child
- Body image – anticipated psychosocial behavioural patterns
- Pathophysiology of common presenting medical conditions within reconstructive plastic surgery
- Pharmacology in respect of the child's types of medication including dosages versus the adult
- Responses to events and timeframes in respect of anticipated anaesthetics, single or multiple surgical procedures, pain/discomfort, and commitments to rehabilitation programmes.

---

Not all children are at the same level of expected social development at the same age, and independent discretionary judgement needs to be practised during the preoperative and perioperative phases of surgery. This can be an extremely stressful time that can be made easier for all if safety, comfort and independence are addressed and adequately managed.

Children need to be engaged within a truthful manner, and forthcoming events should be described to them with care, compassion and in a language they can comprehend. The development and maintaining of trust is fundamentally an important factor in a child's desire for a sense of safety, which must be met before they will comply with any request by the doctor, nurse or parent. In addition, if parents are not engaged in a holistic manner and fully informed of the potential for adverse events, any anxiety felt by the parent will be sensed by the child.

## Psychosocial development

Various parameters have been constructed for describing the basic stages of psychosocial growth, development and behaviour (Box 16.1)[1-6]. Some understanding of this framework assists in addressing the needs of the child and reflecting the child's needs within a particular age structure.

---

**Box 16.2** Basic psychosocial developmental stages of the child.

| | |
| --- | --- |
| From birth to 12 months | development of trust, identity |
| 12 months to 3 years | development of autonomy |
| 3 years to 6 years | development of initiative – desire for increasing autonomy |
| 6 years to 12 years | higher development of both intellectual and motor skills |
| 12 years to 18 years | increasing sense of self-identity. |

---

## Range of paediatric reconstructive plastic surgical procedures

The range of children who can benefit from paediatric reconstructive plastic surgery is extensive and is commonly listed under congenital/inherited, traumatic or aesthetic.

Box 16.3 identifies the diversity of common conditions presenting or referred for corrective, restorative and aesthetic reconstructive surgery. The proposed surgery may require the inclusion of microsurgery and involve a multidisciplinary team who contribute to particular areas of the assessment, reconstruction, nursing and rehabilitation, specific to their area of expertise. Craniofacial surgery is an example of this.

Specialist paediatric units in major teaching institutions associated with universities, additionally provide:

- Diagnostic teams
- Therapeutic care with specific and ongoing information for patients (carers) with a variety of genetic disorders, including:
  - Autism
  - Genetic birth defects
  - Mental retardation
  - Down's syndrome, chromosomal and inherited disorders.

## The hands

Management of birth defects and traumatic injuries of the hand requires the skills of a specialty surgeon as well as a specialist hand therapist or hand rehabilitation unit.

Hand problems managed range from lacerations of tendons and fractured bones, to reconstruction of missing parts by transferring tissue from another area of the body, such as the toe to hand for a missing finger.

## Vascular malformations

Blood vessel malformation may affect the arteries, the veins and the lymphatics. A multidisciplinary vascular anomalies team, consisting of specialists from reconstructive plastic surgery, paediatric dermatology, radiology and paediatric general surgery, meet to evaluate, treat and follow patients with these problems.

## Aesthetic surgery in children

Some young children are teased regarding ear anomalies (e.g. bat ears, large ears) and the child and the parents may desire corrective surgery. This is usually undertaken prior to commencing school to minimise the degree of taunting and potential for psychological effects.

Adolescents may be dissatisfied with the appearance of their nose, ears or lips and seek surgery to make them more pleasing to themselves and their peers. Others may have congenital (e.g. Poland syndrome) breast or chest problems such as asymmetry, underdevelopment or massive breast overgrowth in females, or gynaecomastia in boys (breast overgrowth often due to a hormonal imbalance). Following medical investigations, reconstructive surgery is a viable option for such problems when well thought

**Box 16.3** Example of reconstructive plastic surgical procedures in the child.

- Craniofacial birth defects, including skull deformities, cleft lip and/or palate and other facial clefts, to minor conditions (e.g. tongue tie)
- Ear deformities, congenital or trauma-based
- Facial fractures (usually fractured nose)
- Nasal deformity, congenital or traumatic, and nasal procedures (secondary to craniofacial malformation)
- Facial paralysis (congenital, or acquired following injury)
- Congenital jaw deformities (Pierre Robin syndrome)
- Brachial plexus injury (acquired following trauma)
- Major skin and/or soft tissue defects (commonly benign)
- Tumours of the head and neck (e.g. cystic hygromas, skin lesions including pigmented nevi, hemangiomas, lymphangiomas, baby nevi, congenital hairy nevus, birthmarks
- Cutaneous and subcutaneous tumours of the trunk and extremities (e.g. angiomas, haemangioma)
- Drooling (e.g. related to children with cerebral palsy, Down's syndrome)
- Breast abnormalities (e.g. congenital breast agenesis, Poland syndrome)
- Hand surgery, congenital (e.g. syndactyly, absent digits, extra digits) and acquired repair of tendons, nerves and fractures
- Reconstructive surgery of and acquired conditions (e.g. post trauma, scar revision, keloids, hypertrophic and aesthetically distorting scars, reconstructive surgery of burn deformities)
- Hypospadias (congenital malformation of the urethral opening in the penis)
- Vaginal agenesis/atresia (absence or malformation of the vagina)
- Flap surgery for congenital spinal malformations
- Soft tissue trauma such as dog bites, sporting accidents.

through, and outcome conferences are held with the affected teen, the parents, and the surgeon.

## Anaesthetic risk management issues

**Box 16.4** ASA (American Association of Anesthesiologists) physical status classification.

I   Normal healthy patient
II  A patient with mild systemic disease
III A patient with severe systemic disease limiting activity but not incapacitating
IV  A patient with incapacitating systemic disease that is a constant threat to life
V   Moribund patients

## Preoperative assessment of the child – elective surgery

There remains no evidence-based guideline or system for risk assessment to guide practitioners for determining the best preoperative assessment technique. For simplicity in a complex environment, some anaesthetists have chosen to divide the process into three sections[7] (Box 16.5).

**Box 16.5** Principal areas of preoperative assessment.

- Specific anaesthetic concerns that are rarely an issue outside of anaesthesia
- Patient considerations that may be of importance even for minor surgery
- Issues specific to the proposed surgery.

The parents are advised of this assessment appointment by letter or phone, usually about a week in advance to allow for any special/specific investigations to be undertaken and results returned prior to determining the proposed anaesthetic, surgical and rehabilitation plan. Preoperative assessments will usually last about one hour. Principal components are shown in Box 16.6.

**Box 16.6** Principal components of preoperative assessment.

- The child's general health history, including allergies, history of previous surgery and anaesthetics, and any special medical or psychosocial issues
- Fitness for anaesthetic. This should be ASA-based criteria, for example, Grade I or II to be suitable for day surgery. If there is some concern about the child's level of fitness for elective surgery and an anaesthetic, this should be discussed with the consultant paediatric anaesthetist. Referrals to medical or nurse specialist(s), or allied health personnel may be required to obtain a complete picture of the child's health (e.g. pre-existing medical conditions that require stabilisation)
- Social history, ascertaining who has parental responsibility for purposes of consent, and length of journey time to hospital – this is recommended to be not longer than one hour to reduce anxiety
- Measurement of weight (necessary for drug dosages)
- Baseline pulse oximetry (this is recommended as part of the assessment process)
- Explanation of pre- and postoperative care, including negotiation of level of parental involvement (family centred care) and preoperative phone call (agreeing mutually convenient time for this, and ascertaining contact number)
- Assessment of the levels of child and parental anxiety regarding surgery/admission
- If the child is very anxious, or phobic about hospitals or needles, sedative premedication may be prescribed by the anaesthetist following discussion with the family, if it is agreed that this would be beneficial
- Explanation of fasting times for surgery
- Negotiation of date for surgery with parents, including the possibility of short notice cancellation appointments
- Explanation of what will happen on the day of admission, includes anaesthetic induction and surgery
- Discussion of pain management and demonstration of pain management tool
- Explanation of aftercare at home (e.g. post general anaesthetic care, and specific care and treatment, related to surgery – level of parental competence and commitment to home care)
- Explanation of how long the child will need to be off school, and when able to return to normal activities (e.g. active sports)
- What follow-up appointments will be necessary
- Opportunity for family to ask questions.

All information regarding the anaesthetic, surgery and postoperative care in the home should also be supported in written form for the family to refer to at home. The assessing nurse should provide the parents or primary carer with a contact phone number in order that they may contact him/her with any questions or concerns that may arise after they have left the hospital or pre-assessment office.

A preoperative telephone call should be made the day prior to surgery to check that the child is fit and well for surgery, reinforcing parents' knowledge regarding the fasting and appointment times, and to give the family any additional support necessary.

If the child is unfit for surgery (e.g. has a cold or an infection) the surgeon should be notified, patient checked by the general medical practitioner and a new appointment made when the illness has passed. Parents who may have expressed their availability to come in at short notice if the child recovers quickly should be alerted in time to make arrangements for other responsibilities.

> **Box 16.7** Frequently asked questions from the parents or primary carers.
>
> - Type of anaesthesia to be given
> - How is it given
> - Risks associated
> - Premedication
> - Waking time after anaesthesia
> - Potential to vomit
> - Pain/discomfort
> - Potential lasting effects of the anaesthesia
> - Ability to discuss the anaesthetic with the anaesthetist.

## Preoperative fasting time

It is important to note that the anaesthetic organisations, societies and colleges in most modern countries will have protocols or guidelines regarding fasting for both adults and children (see Chapter 15).

These outline practice guidelines for preoperative fasting, the use of pharmacologic agents to reduce the risk of pulmonary aspiration, and applications to healthy patients undergoing elective procedures. Many children are now allowed clear fluids up to two hours preoperatively to ward off dehydration, particularly on hot days. Despite the guidelines most anaesthetists will assess each patient individually for their needs.

See recommended websites (paediatric preoperative patient assessment and premedication protocols) at the end of this chapter.

## Addressing nursing co-morbidity, clinical nursing risk management and nursing outcomes

As previously stated, children are not small adults and the physiological condition of children in the face of adverse events, especially babies, declines at a much quicker rate than in adults. The five vital signs must be monitored strictly, as the care of children requires not only specialised and specific anatomical and physiological knowledge but also behavioural understanding[1–7].

In respect of behaviour, children do not always act or react in expected ways. Small children cannot describe exactly what they feel, particularly the specifics of their pain. Patience, observation and the ability to interpret verbal and physical signs are essential and any medication prescribed for children must be strictly measured according to ordered dosages and timing.

## Physiological monitoring in children

The anatomical differences (Table 16.1) highlight the specific risks that children present. Children will suffer a cardiorespiratory arrest significantly earlier than adults because of their low rate of reserves. Because of the distinctive needs of children, performance of clinical observations, monitoring, assessment and analysis of data requires special paediatric pathophysiological knowledge and experience in specialist clinical paediatrics, pharmacology and psychosocial sciences.

## Box 16.8 Principal areas of monitoring needs.

- Level of consciousness – alert, awake, drowsy, disorientated, crying, unconscious
- Colour of the skin (blue) is a very early clinical indicator of respiratory embarrassment/compromise
- Pulse – rate rhythm and pulse volume (use stethoscope to calculate apex beat in babies)
- Respiration – rate, depth, freedom from obstruction, good bilateral breath sound on auscultation of anterior and posterior chest (there can be airway obstruction without noise but there cannot be airway noise without obstruction)
- Oxygen saturation of blood measured with pulse oximeter, and if possible, $CO_2$ measurement
- Blood pressure with the proper size of child cuff for accurate readings
- Temperature (monitoring at regular intervals, limiting of body exposure)
- Fluid and blood loss and replacement:
  - Children dehydrate very quickly
  - The circulating volume of children is relative to age, so in babies, for example, small losses can be critical
  - Blood loss must be measured accurately and even minimal amounts of blood must be reported
  - Water and electrolytes are lost in insensible loss and sweating if the child is distressed or in pain
  - Loss of fluid via moderate to excessive, or continuous small amounts of vomiting and loss of fluid via the bowel must also be documented and reported.
- Pain levels estimated by using paediatric pain scales/methods including crying, distress, body language and sweating[8].

**Table 16.1** Paediatric physiological characteristics compared with adults.

| Anatomy/system | Rationale | Suggested response |
|---|---|---|
| **Anatomy** (general)<br>Difference in anatomy responsible for most problems encountered post general anaesthesia. | The smaller the child, the larger the body surface-to-weight ratio. This results in greater potential for heat loss.<br>Babies have relatively large heads, increasing heat loss when exposed. | Maintenance of ambient room temperature rather than use of heavy blankets, as child cannot generate heat at the required level without compromising the metabolic ratio – paediatric Bair Hugger® should be used where possible. |
| **Airway** (specific)<br>Anatomical structure of the paediatric airway predisposes to upper airway hypoventilation. | Head is large with a short neck.<br>Tongue is relatively large in relation to other oral anatomy.<br>Larynx is located at higher level than the adult.<br>Airway is small in diameter, minimal mucosal swelling can critically decrease diameter and increase resistance.<br>Diaphragm is main muscle of respiration. Any increase in intra-abdominal pressure may lead to respiratory embarrassment.<br>Muscle tone is poorly developed. | The child should be maintained on his/her side until completely awake. |
| **Respiratory system**<br>The paediatric patient is predisposed to the ready development of hypoxaemia relative to large body surface-to-weight ratio. | Increased consumption of $O_2$ is required to maintain normal body temperature and increased minute ventilation requirements. | Post-intubation croup and laryngeal obstruction and tracheal retraction should be observed for. |

Table 16.1 *Continued*.

| Anatomy/system | Rationale | Suggested response |
|---|---|---|
| **Cardiovascular system**<br>The cardiovascular system is not fully matured in children:<br>Neonate = 120–140 beats per minute (bpm)<br>Progressive decrease to 80 beats p/mbpm at 12 years.<br>Right ventricle larger than left at birth. Adult right and left ventricular size reached at six months.<br>Blood volume in children generally based on body weight.<br>Heart rate response to hypovolaemia unpredictable.<br>Loss of blood/fluid critical in children. | Cardiac output is rate-dependent.<br>Because of heart-rate dependency of cardiac output, bradycardia more worrisome than tachycardia.<br>Sympathetic innervation is incomplete.<br>Cardiac output twice that of adults because of high-energy demands. | Blood pressure then becomes a guide to adequacy of intravascular volume.<br>Accurate measurement and reporting mechanisms of blood/fluid loss in children is essential. |
| **Temperature regulation**<br>Infants are susceptible to developing hypothermia.<br>(Important to maintain core temperature and skin temperature to avoid metabolic stress.)<br>Decrease in temperature will increase child's oxygen consumption and may result in metabolic acidosis. | Large body surface area relative to body weight.<br>Subcutaneous fat is thin – leads to 400% increase in core conductance.<br>Higher metabolic rate than adults.<br>Hypothalamic temperature control centre is immature.<br>Infants depend on a non-shivering method of heat source, which can only occur in the presence of adequate levels of oxygen, thus hypoxia and metabolic acidosis result in the absence of a natural warming environment. | Maintenance of ambient room temperature rather than use of heavy blankets as child cannot generate heat at the required level without compromising the metabolic ratio – paediatric Bair Hugger® should be used where possible. |
| **Central nervous system**<br>Immature neurological function causes instability of respiration and muscular activity.<br>A higher dosage of drugs required than for an adult to achieve an equal depth of anaesthesia .<br>Brain swelling may occur following major craniofacial surgery.<br>Pain is experienced by children as it is by adults following any form of injury/surgery. | Increased permeability of the blood–brain barrier and lack of myelination leads to accumulation of drugs, e.g. barbiturates, in higher concentration than in adults.<br>Pain can be responsible for the child being unco-operative and distressed, subsequently compromising the reconstructive procedure – especially after free flaps, facial cleft, genital reconstruction and hand surgery.<br>Pain management should not be withheld simply because the nurse fears respiratory complications. Medical or peer advice must be sought. | Narcotic analgesia should not be withheld if the child is distressed and obviously in pain, especially if local or regional blocks have not been used.<br>The use of rectal analgesia is effective immediately post-operatively to establish a therapeutic level to counter the effects of local anaesthesia or regional blocks wearing off in the PACU or in the clinical area.<br>Vascular circulation of the surgical area should be checked to ascertain that the cause of the pain is not vascular compromise caused by tight dressings or inadequate elevation of the limb to allow venous drainage. |

## Risk management issues in intraoperative paediatric management

### Box 16.9 Safety.

- In the perioperative phase, induction of anaesthesia and waking up are critical times
- Children, especially babies, may take longer to recover from anaesthesia depending on the drugs or gases used
- The child should not be forced to wake, in the absence of abnormal observations
- Minimal but safety-based handling will aid easy recovery
- Because most children lack self control when fearful and out of familiar surroundings, their speed and lack of predictability means that staff must never turn their back on a child
- Eyes are always the nurse's best mechanism for clinical observation and clinical monitoring
- It is important to protect the active child from self-injury during the disorientating period of waking
- Clinicians should request additional help at this stage if necessary, to protect the child and the operative site
- Hypoxaemia, hypoventilation, physical coldness or vascular compromise of the operated area must be excluded before pain relieving drugs, or sedation, are administered to an agitated child
- A specific understanding of the pharmacology within anaesthesia is essential as some drugs (e.g. Ketalar® (ketamine)) require that patients are not physically roused, due to psychological effects experienced with provoked awakening (e.g. nightmares, hallucinations)
- Ketamine may be used for short surgical procedures (e.g. removal of sutures) and for burn dressings.

### Box 16.10 Comfort.

- Parents should be encouraged to participate in the recovery process once the child's basic functions are established within normal limits
- Children waking in unfamiliar surroundings and/or in pain, or physically cold, are often inconsolable, even with their parents present
- Local anaesthesia may have been administered prior to the surgery or intra-operatively

- Regional blocks may be administered post surgery for extended pain management
- Paediatric rectal paracetamol administered on completion of a procedure can be very helpful to relieve the child's pain/discomfort and the post anaesthesia care unit staff and parents/carers in providing for postoperative comfort
- Pharmacological guidelines should be strictly adhered to – paracetamol should be strictly administered only under medical orders and not to children who are less than one month of age
- Any form of pre-emptive pain management for children (e.g. narcotics, intramuscular or intravenous, or oral or rectal non-narcotics) should not be withheld if the child is in need and the drugs are administered as prescribed[8]
- Monitoring for adverse effects to narcotics is mandatory, and Narcan® (naloxone hydrochloride) should be available in case it is required to reverse the adverse effects
- In the absence of pain, distressed infants/children are often consoled by a loving hug from parent(s).

### Box 16.11 Independence.

- Most children will move along the dependent to interdependent continuum according to their needs, and demonstrate a sense of growing personal independence
- Older children and adolescents will often be able to demonstrate greater independence, and articulate their needs quite easily
- As previously discussed, whatever their age, a perception of trust established in a pain-free and truly caring environment is essential
- An objective bio-psychosocial preoperative assessment of children provides a holistic view of the child.

## Special issues relating to children in the postoperative phase

Psychosocial issues of physical and mental growth, changing views of the world, the people around the child, personal body image, and family relationships need to be considered as part of the equation when surgery is proposed and undertaken[1–6].

Many children with congenital malformations may require more than one surgical procedure and a mixed range of short, medium or long-term rehabilitation programmes.

In burns management it has been acknowledged that there is an exponential rise in anxiety in relation to the number of anaesthetics the child or young adult has to encounter. Interventions that may precipitate fear, such as injections and needles, anticipation of postoperative pain, and loss of personal control, need to be critically addressed and minimised. Children will quickly demonstrate their fears and every effort should be made to minimise disruption to their daily life and their trepidation in regard to the hospital experience.

Totally restraining children in their bed is extremely difficult in the first few days. In the postoperative phase, physically restraining children in a way that denies them access to toys, games, TV controls, food and so on, should be avoided wherever possible and is gradually falling out of favour. Protocols for specific arm restraints should be not be generalised but the order to do so should be in writing by the specific treating surgeon.

Clinicians should insist on this in order to avoid legal liability should adverse events/outcomes occur (e.g. broken skin, blisters and skin pressure zones). Physical contact and distraction therapy in the form of games or TV are also useful. Without exception, the main factor for continuing co-operation is the absence of pain and discomfort[5].

---

### Review

*Setting goals of care and preferred clinical and patient outcomes*, Chapter 2, Boxes 2.7–2.9. Adapt according to risk management issues and clinical patient needs.

---

## Anaesthesia and primary postoperative dressings in children

In respect of the age of the child and following certain primary procedures, some complex primary dressings or suture removal may need to be performed under light general anaesthesia or sedation.

In children, it is becoming more common for surgeons to use absorbable sutures that do not require removal, but some wounds require the initial use of non-absorbable sutures to ensure wound integrity in areas of potentially active movement.

Assessment of the whole situation and critical discretionary judgement must be exercised to determine whether a short anaesthetic will be needed for removal of dressings, viewing of the wound, removal of sutures, wound cleansing and the degree of redressing and resplinting of the wound required.

Most surgeons will prefer a short/light general anaesthetic for procedures such as removal of tie-over grafts on the hand or near the eye, redressing of large reconstructive flaps, urological and vaginal reconstructions, and suture removal following cleft lip, hand surgery.

For simple suture removal that does not require formal anaesthesia, parents may be requested to give the child oral analgesia or a mild sedative approximately one hour prior to attendance. This is a good practice, particularly before frequent dressing changes in management of superficial and limited area burns.

Many parents have underlying guilt feelings when their children are born with congenital malformations, or are accidentally burnt. The nurse clinician should also observe the behaviour of parents or carers, as an overprotective parent may present particular difficulties that may need to be professionally discussed. It is important to be professional, firm but fair and non-judgemental in assessment and approach to this and, where possible, to include the parent or significant others in the care without compromising on the child's needs.

---

## Summary

Perioperative nursing of children and adults is intense and requires fastidious attention to every minute detail. It must be underpinned with the essential scientific knowledge, exposure to a wide range of acute care clinical experiences, and accurate and disciplined responses to the adverse consequences that may occur.

In the case of short stay patient care, providing a discharge safety net is very important clinically, and in meeting patient quality outcomes. Significant carers may be fearful of potential adverse events and a high level of service satisfaction is anecdotally reported by patients and carers who have received follow-up phone calls four hours after discharge, and on the following day, to check on their status and correct any real or perceived emerging problems.

Excellence in nursing management for both adults and children in the whole perioperative phase, directed towards patient safety, comfort and independence, allows clinical unit and acute care community nurses to provide a high level care where standards are maintained and the special needs of each individual patient can be met.

---

### Box 16.12 Preferred clinical nursing outcomes.

- A trusting and interactive environment was established from initial preassessment stage to exit from the recovery room/post anaesthesia care unit
- There was a physiologically safe and uneventful pathway from admission to final discharge
- The child experienced a pain/discomfort-free surgical and postoperative encounter
- The child was allowed to express his/her views and independent status within a trusting and safe environment
- Parents/primary carers of the child expressed satisfaction with all levels of care of the child.

---

### Review

*Auditing preferred clinical and patient outcomes,* Chapter 2, Boxes 2.10–2.12.

---

### References

(1) Meeker M.H. & Rothrock J.C. *Alexander's care of the patient in surgery*, 11th edn. St Louis: Mosby, 1999.
(2) McCance K.L. & Huether S.E. *Pathophysiology: the biologic basis for disease in adults and children*, 3rd edn. St Louis: Mosby, 1998.
(3) Porth C.P *Pathophysiology: concepts in altered health states*, 5th edn. Philadelphia: Lippincott, 2000.
(4) Smeltzer S.C. & Bare B.G. *Brunner and Suddarth's textbook of medical-surgical nursing*, 9th edn. Philadelphia: Lippincott, Williams & Wilkins, 2000.
(5) Cehaich K. Preparing the paediatric patient for surgery. *Plastic Surgical Nursing*, 1994 (summer); **14**(2):105–107.
(6) Noble R.R., Micheli A.K., Hensley M.A. & McKay N. Perioperative considerations for the paediatric patient: a developmental approach. *Nursing Clinics of North America*, 1997 (March); **32**(1):1–16.
(7) http://www.virtual-anaesthesia-textbook.com/vat/preop.htm#Risk%20Assess
(8) Shin D., Kim C.S. & Kim H.S. Postoperative pain management using intravenous patient controlled analgesia for paediatric patients. *Journal of Craniofacial Surgery*, 2001 (Mar); **12**(2):129–33.

---

### Recommended websites

**Paediatric preoperative patient assessment and premedication protocols**

http://www.umm.edu/plassurg/genrecon.htm
http://www.chw.edu.au/prof/handbook/sect28.htm
http://www.humed.com/plasticreconstructivesurgery/pediatric.shtml
http://www.stlouischildrens.org/articles/kids_parents.asp?ID=237
http://www.med.umich.edu/surg/plastic
http://www.medana.unibas.ch/eng/educ/standard.htm
http://medind.nic.in/iad/t02/i5/iadt02i5p347.pdf
http://www.medana.unibas.ch/eng/educ/standard.htm
http://www.nda.ox.ac.uk/wfsa/html/u12/u1202_01.htm (fasting protocols)

# Section IV
## Applied Reconstructive Plastic Surgical Nursing 1

# Skin Grafts

## Background

### Review

*General wound closure options, including the principal advantages and disadvantages of their application, Chapter 7, Box 7.1, Figure 7.1 & Figure 7.2.*

## 1. TERMINOLOGY

In general biological terms, a **graft** is the transfer or transplanting of human tissue from one region of the body to another, with or without its attached blood vessels[1-8].

**Split thickness skin graft** (STSG) or **free skin graft**, are the terms applied when the blood supply is not attached (e.g. skin is severed and is 'freed' from its blood supply).

**Skin/tissue flaps** is the term applied when the blood vessels remain intact and are transferred with the graft donor tissue[1-7].

In a slightly confusing use of clinical language, the terms **graft** and **transplant** are often applied interchangeably, although the term 'transplant' is now

### Box 17.1 Skin grafting – clinical definitions 1.

| | |
|---|---|
| **Autograft** (autogenic) | from self to self (auto = self) |
| **Isograft** (isogenic) | identical twins (iso = equal) |
| **Allograft/ homograft** | organ transplant between non-identical members of same species |
| **Xenograft** (xenogenic) | from animal, usually pig (or artificial skin) to human |
| **Human tissue culture** | growth of thin epidermis (epidermal grafting) from the patient's own skin via a culture medium[1-7] |
| **Tissue engineering** | bio-engineered or artificially engineered epidermis, dermis or other tissue replacements[9-12]. |

being increasingly used in relation to whole organs from one person to another, whereas 'graft' refers to defined layers of tissue. 'Transplant' may also be the term applied to the free vascular transfer of a big toe to replace an amputated thumb. **Replant** is the term given to restoring a totally severed digit to its original anatomical site[1-7].

## Dermal and fat grafts

Trauma, or the removal of tumours, may leave small contour defects (divots, concavities) in the zone of injury, resulting in a loss of natural form. This may occur in any part of the body, but it is particularly noticeable in the face. Secondary procedures using

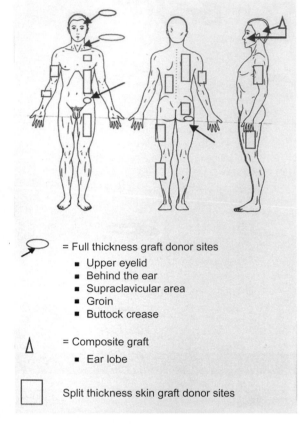

| Box 17.2 Skin grafting – clinical definitions 2. | |
|---|---|
| **Donor sites** | 'donate' harvested tissue |
| **Recipient sites** | 'receive' the donated tissue |
| **Split thickness skin graft** | STSG is defined as the harvesting and transfer of a segment of skin (epidermis and some levels of the dermis are 'split off') by totally separating the donated skin from its blood supply (at the donor site) and transferring the skin to a different part of the body (a recipient site) |
| **Full thickness skin grafts** | FTSG, those where all of the epidermis and dermis are included |
| **Composite grafts** | full thickness skin grafts that are composed of more than one anatomical structure, for example, skin with cartilage (such as a 'V' shaped wedge donated from the ear to the nose)[1–7]. Donor sites here are usually primarily closed and treated as a second wound, expected to heal normally but capable of the same complications as any surgical wound |
| **'Take'** | the term applied when the donor skin is completely adhered to the underlying recipient site bed, regardless of the graft type. The term is also often applied to skin flaps |
| **Open or exposed graft management** | term used when the donor skin is applied and the recipient wound remains exposed as healing takes place |
| **Closed graft management** | term used when contoured dressings are applied to ensure that all areas of the donor skin and recipient site are in direct contact, providing compression to prevent the development of haematoma or seroma, and shear and friction. |

⬯ = Full thickness graft donor sites
- Upper eyelid
- Behind the ear
- Supraclavicular area
- Groin
- Buttock crease

△ = Composite graft
- Ear lobe

▢ Split thickness skin graft donor sites

**Figure 17.1** Donor site examples for skin grafts.

'dermal grafts' shaved free of epidermis, and adipose tissue or fat tissue grafts, may be harvested from appropriate unexposed body regions such as the abdomen.

Dermal and fat grafts are donated to the recipient site(s) by being tunnelled under the epidermis to increase bulk and improve the aesthetic contour in some areas of the face. Outcomes are varied, as these tissues minus their original blood supply often resolve, become smaller or become infected, thus not really achieving what was originally expected or worsening the situation[1–8].

Areas selected for skin graft donation attempt to reflect the colour, efficiency of the blood supply, and depth available for the recipient site. Figure 17.1 shows potential sites of STSG, FTSG and composite grafts, Figures 17.2 and 17.3 show depths/thickness of skin grafts.

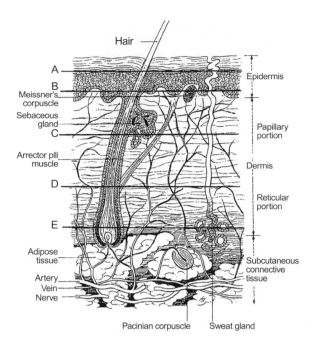

**Figure 17.2** Skin layers and composition.

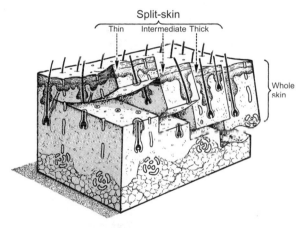

**Figure 17.3** Levels of skin graft donor sites (McGregor I.A. & McGregor A.D., 1995).

## 2. SKIN GRAFTING AS A WOUND CLOSURE OPTION

Not all surgical, trauma or disease-based wounds can be closed primarily. Regardless of the wound's aetiology, alternative methods of skin closure will be considered by surgeons to protect the underlying tissues, and the organism as a whole (the reconstructive ladder)[1–23].

Skin grafting is a specialised and complex method of securing wound closure, and its management requires the entire realm of the clinician's knowledge and understanding of wound repair[1–28]. It is vital that clinicians are able to identify the different types of graft techniques in order that:

- Objective donor and recipient site wound assessments can be undertaken, as wound care is based on the specific needs of both the donor type and recipient site
- Risk management strategies regarding actual and potential adverse events can be put in place
- Preferred clinical and patient need goals and outcomes can be stated and audited.

## 3. SELECTING TEMPORARY OR PERMANENT SPLIT THICKNESS SKIN GRAFTS

Following significant compound tissue trauma, major surgery, major burns, or an increasing loss of skin arising from severe infecting organisms that attack the skin, options must be considered to protect the underlying tissues, and the organism itself[1–16].

For most complex acute wounds, and where adequate skin is not available, STSGs remain a primary surgical option. Skin substitutes may be utilised as temporary cover as a lifesaving measure[1–4,7,9–11]. The primary objective of these procedures is to exclude local and systemic infection, if emergency tissue flaps are not appropriate at the time.

In a large number of specifically selected wounds, this technique is slowly being overtaken by the use of vacuum pressure therapy as wound bed preparation, allowing for any further surgical procedures that may be required, or appropriate, to be planned and undertaken within 5–7 days[2,4,13–17].

STSGs may be permanent or temporary. This decision is made in relation to a range of clinical and morbid factors, state of the presenting wound bed, and whether it is proposed that the graft is to be the principal form of reconstructive wound closure.

This determines:

- The thickness of the donor graft selected
- Specific required quality of the healed skin
- Degree of restored function at the recipient site
- Aesthetic outcome.

## Advantages of temporary STSGs – meshed donor skin

- Temporary thin, or meshed, STSGs may be vital techniques if major skin/tissue flaps are required to permanently close a wound, but are unable to be undertaken within 48 hours of injury time.
- For the optimal results from emergency free vascular flaps, this is suggested to be the most favourable window of time before vessels and oedema in the central wound zone become distorted by excessive oedema and vascular problems.
- Temporary closure also allows reconstructive surgery to be postponed to allow patients to recover from other substantial trauma such as head, chest or abdominal injury. This provides the surgical team time to plan for major reconstructions under significantly improved and relatively stable physiological conditions and particularly the status of the vessels at the site of injury.
- Temporary skin grafts also have an important application in patients with compound wounds which include muscle of questionable vascular status, or exposed bone that has retained some degree of its blood supply from its primary source, the periosteum[1-7].
- Rotation skin flaps to protect potentially injured periosteum or avascular zones of bone, and a thin STSG donor skin acting as temporary closure over the flap donor site, heal quickly. This significantly reduces the opportunity for bacterial invasion and wound infection in the bone to occur in the already medically or traumatically compromised patient[1-7] (Figures 17.4–17.8).
- Where available, negative pressure therapy (VAC®) has become the modern treatment of choice for total wound occlusion in order that the size of the overall wound can be significantly reduced and contamination and infection minimised or prevented[2,4,13-17].
- In smaller wounds, the overall size of some wounds may be decreased sufficiently to allow secondary suturing for closure at a later time. More commonly in larger wounds, the decreased size of the wound (e.g. dermal contraction) significantly reduces the level of reconstruction proposed to be undertaken to improve function and aesthetics.
- To await pathology reports on the type and extent of some tumours (e.g. melanoma, squamous cell carcinoma). Certain skin malignancies may display unusual changes, and it is important that any reconstruction is not compromised by premature use of local skin flaps. These may alter the local blood supply when pathology reports indicate that further local or extensive surgery may need to be undertaken[2-7].
- Some special wounds which are anticipated to contain critical levels of contaminating organisms (e.g. animal or human bites), will often be considered for temporary skin cover to prevent or limit local infection, following debridement, and use of IV (systemic) antibiotics. Secondary reconstruction/repair is then undertaken in a more pristine, uncontaminated environment[7,21].

Thin to intermediate (Figures 17.2–17.10), unmeshed or meshed STSGs are widely used as a temporary or permanent cover in difficult anatomical surfaces, or tissue highly vulnerable to infection, for example, muscle and bone.

- The advantage of meshed skin is that in a range of wound bed conditions, it adheres and conforms effortlessly, and quickly, to the rising and falling raw surfaces and deep crevices within the wound. It is also significantly less vulnerable to haematoma and wound infection[2,4,13-15]
- Its rapidly conforming nature also allows for some movement in important regions (e.g. the chest wall, or in the genital regions) with accelerated healing of the recipient site, and minimal donor site and patient morbidity[15]
- The use of meshed skin is contrasted to the use of unmeshed skin in Figures 17.4–17.10
- The advantages of expanding donor skin reduces the total amount of donor zones required, particularly if there is a plan/need to reuse the donor site at a later date (e.g. major burns)[1-7].

### *Additional advantages of temporary STSGs*

- With the understanding that it is the dermis that contracts and the epidermis is a resurfacing process, some STSGs are used as temporary skin cover[7]
- In the absence of regional and local oedema, the restoration of the biological conditions that promote dermal contraction produces an overall reduction in the wound site area. This then requires proportionally less to be excised and repaired at a later date where the graft is excised and closed, either primarily or in stages. In addition, it may mean that a full thickness graft, skin

flap reconstruction or tissue expansion can be utilised as the permanent reconstruction[1-7]

- Tissue expansion of the adjacent normal skin site may also be considered (Figure 17.11) for secondary or tertiary closure of a healed skin graft site, particularly where function, constant pressure, exposure to the elements, or the cosmetic results, are essential issues[1-7].

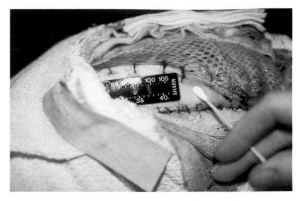

**Figure 17.6** Meshed (STSG) skin applied over groin muscle flap for compound injury to the femur (note observation paddle of skin attached to the muscle).

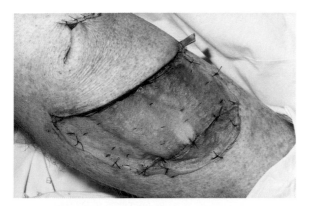

**Figure 17.4** Fasciocutaneous flap rotated to protect avascular bone and temporary split thickness skin graft (STSG) to protect normal bone.

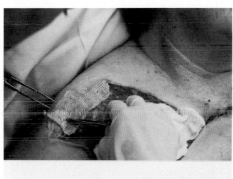

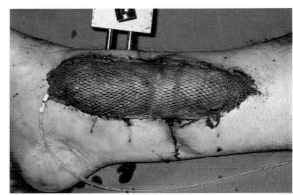

**Figure 17.7** Meshed (STSG) skin applied over muscle flap.

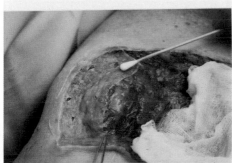

**Figure 17.5** Application of STSG – major breast wound.

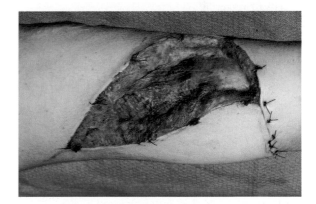

**Figure 17.8** Inadequately managed STSG.

**Table 17.1** Options in wound closure.

| Criteria | Split thickness skin graft | Full thickness skin graft | Skin flap |
|---|---|---|---|
| Blood supply | Needs pink granulating vascular bed. | Needs near-perfect recipient bed. | Carries own blood supply; will cover an avascular, but non-infected wound bed. |
| Availability | Large areas available particularly when meshed. Thin STSG donor sites can be re-harvested after 3 weeks. | Limited – requirement of 'like' tissue recipient site restricts availability. | Limited availability unless free vascular transfer. Surrounding tissue may also be injured. |
| Take | Excellent potential in optimal wound conditions – early timeframe of repair. | Less reliable. Longer to establish. Relies on re-establishment of blood flow in a totally contamination-free environment. Vascular colour initially poor due to slow local vessel fusion. | Healing process is enhanced by the preservation of its own blood supply. |
| Function | Variable: degree of contracture at recipient site may pose a functional difficulty. | Good: reduced/minimal contracture. | Good: minimal contracture allows for the enhanced movement of the repaired area. |
| Aesthetic outcome | Variable: colour and recipient defect may not always be acceptable to patient. Contraction and scarring may be an issue. | Colour and contour usually good quality after scar resolution. | Good: volume, recipient deficit markedly reduced in repair site. |
| Donor defect (the deficiency left after skin/tissue harvest) | Variable: relies on individual's healing process and specific donor site. Contraction and scarring may be an issue. | Surgically marked donor scar – suture line. | Full thickness defect usually produces a noticeable scar – but this will usually flatten out and resolve over time. |

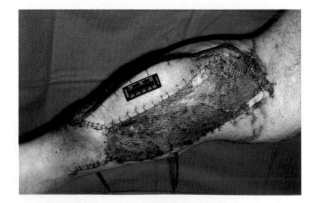

**Figure 17.9** STSG applied over muscle flap allowed to become dry and cracked (often referred to as a 'hamburger flap' because of its bulk).

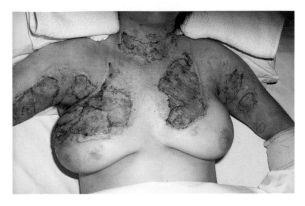

**Figure 17.10** Open STSG to partial thickness burns – chest wall.

- The principal disadvantages of permanent STSGs is that they are often aesthetically unacceptable to the patient (e.g. the face) or subject to hypertrophic or keloid scarring in particular patients
- In certain anatomical fixed skin regions (the lower limb) the healed graft may be subject to secondary injury leading to frequent ulceration
- STSGs used in mobile tissue zones (e.g. some areas of the face in the older patient) will often leave a firm 'wrinkling' effect as the dermis contracts inwards. This is not observed in fixed skin zones, as the dermis is much thinner and dermal contraction is significantly less
- Contraindicated following injures where major skin contraction occurs and/or movement becomes increasingly restricted, such as over joints (e.g. burns or major trauma), surgical options can range from:
  - Z-plasty (Figure 17.12)
  - Thick STSGs for breast or groin (Figure 17.13)
  - Lower limbs (Figure 17.11) – tissue expander in adjacent uninjured region
  - Free flaps to the neck (Figures 17.14 and 17.15) to release the limited function[1–7].

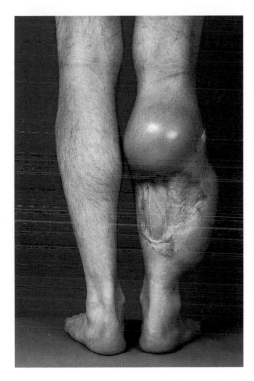

**Figure 17.11** Tissue expander inserted to use local skin for replacement of temporary STSG following severe injury.

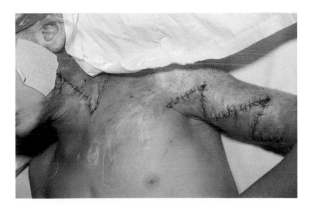

**Figure 17.12** Z-plasty technique used to release contracted skin grafted burn tissue.

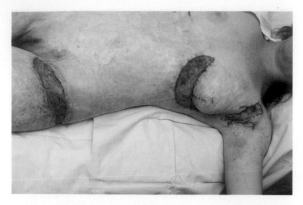

**Figure 17.13** Thick STSG used to release contractures following burns as a child.

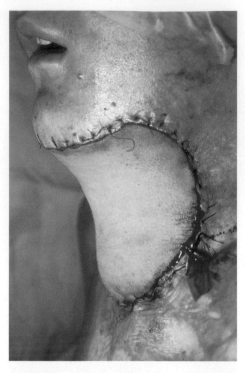

**Figure 17.15** Free flap microvascular transfer from the groin to permanently release scar.

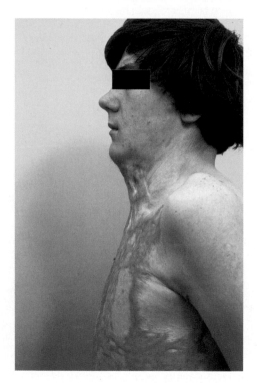

**Figure 17.14** Severe contraction of the neck following burns as a child.

## 4. SKIN GRAFTS – DONOR SITE SELECTION

**Box 17.4** Selecting the donor site to match the needs of the wound.

- Wherever possible, STSGs, full thickness skin grafts (FTSGs) (see later in this chapter) and tissue flap donor sites are selected on the basis of matching the anatomical wound site, restoration of the local function of the skin at the recipient's site, and the aesthetic outcome of the procedure (Figure 17.1)
- In addition, donor site selection is made on minimising the morbidity and associated risk of an additional wound that can significantly alter patient mobility
- The dermis is generally ten times thicker than the epidermis in many locations (e.g. the back), with the skin in equivalent areas in males being thicker than in females
- The depth of the dermis harvested determines the contracting forces in the recipient site as it is stated that in the recipient site it is the living dermis that contracts, and that the donated dermis (in the STSG) takes on the structure and function of the absent dermal layer, so the degree of contraction required is relative[1–7]
- The rule is that the thinner the graft applied to the recipient site, the greater the potential for dermal contraction, and the thicker the graft (which includes a greater depth of the dermis), the less the dermal contraction. FTSGs clearly demonstrate this[1–7].

**Box 17.5** Principal physiological factors influencing donor site selection to parallel wound needs.

- Estimating the size, depth and location/colour of the defect, the type of tissue to be replaced, and donor site delivering the least morbidity and altered patient independence (Figures 17.1–17.3)
- STSGs can be harvested to cover large areas (on the basis of what is readily available, e.g. following burns)
- It must be remembered that the amount of skin harvested creates one or more additional wounds of similar proportion, significantly increasing the patient and nursing wound co-morbidity
- Regardless of the thickness of skin selected, the efficacy of the regional and local blood supply at the donor skin site, and the recipient bed, is directly proportional for the capacity to 'take' and heal, unimpeded[1–7]

- In donor site selection the vascular status (i.e. superior blood flow equals higher quality of the vessels) of the donor skin is extremely important as the potential for take increases if donor skin comes from a well-perfused region
- In all but a minimal number of wounds, the blood supply of the donor site will always be superior to the recipient site
- Any disturbances of vascularity within the wounded area (e.g. secondary injury, avascular zones, critical contamination, previous infection, tumours) (Figure 17.5) will alter the potential for optimal take
- The quality of the vascularity of the surrounding tissue in the recipient site can alter the potential and rate for donor skin graft uptake of a neovascular supply[1,19]
- An understanding of the 'bridging phenomenon' (discussed later in this chapter) is fundamental in assessing the efficacy or merit, in the application of skin in vulnerable wound zones
- Secondary complications, projected healing time rates, functional and aesthetic outcomes of the recipient site, must be considered in the light of this information and these issues largely determine if the skin will be meshed or left intact[1–7].

**Box 17.6** Specific principles guiding selection of skin graft donor sites – practical considerations.

- Skin thickness relative to the age of the patient (see Chapter 6)
- Skin thickness relative to healing potential and potential for complications
- Potential to survive at the recipient site – physiological status of the donor skin and recipient site (i.e. contamination, infection, available blood supply)
- Colour – matching of skin colour for aesthetic compatibility
- Durability – ability to withstand wear and tear relative to the site
- Functional requirements – restoration of function of the part – problems of contractures
- Potential for hair bearing (if required)
- Ability to restore/maintain skin moisture
- Site(s) located in skin zones that are not normally visible when wearing clothing
- Donor sites must be selected in the older person so as not to significantly increase the patient's immobility, degree of self-care and personal independence
- In split thickness skin grafts, the potential to reuse the donor site in approximately three weeks' time if substantial donor skin is required, e.g. burns[1–7].

**Box 17.7** Specific principles guiding selection of skin graft donor sites – aesthetic considerations.

- Following STSGs, skin colour reflecting a totally comparable aesthetic result at both the donor and recipient site is almost impossible to achieve as the donor site may result in a lighter colour (suggested to be due to loss of melanin pigment in the donated skin)[1]
- The recipient site is usually darker than its original colour, and often darker than the surrounding recipient region[1-7]. This can be a source of angst for some patients, but the potential for secondary corrective procedures, or camouflage make-up, are options that can be discussed with the patient[8]
- For skin grafts required on the face, skin is selected from the comparable 'blush zones' of the supraclavicular region, post auricular region, or the scalp
- Selection is also based on suitability in terms of the recipient wound bed's expected short or long-term life needs, potential to withstand secondary injury and immobility
- STSG donor sites are also chosen for their ability to be concealed from normal view, to be free from exposure to UV rays, and from constant irritation from the shear and friction of sharp edges of some clothing[1-8]
- For STSGs used as a permanent replacement for injured or diseased skin, the overall quality of the surgical outcomes will be aesthetically and carefully evaluated by the patient
- For temporary skin cover this has less importance as there is the potential for an improved aesthetic result by further procedures once the primary and timely wound closure objective has been met[1-7].

The final decision in the selection of temporary or permanent STSG, the need for a skin flap, or in some cases the requirement to address the potential for amputation, is made with objective consideration of the immediate needs of the wound, achievable clinical wound outcomes, including detailed discussion, and consent of the patient.

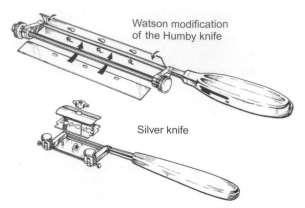

**Figure 17.16** Watson modification of Humby knife and Silvers™ STSG harvesting knives (McGregor I.A. & McGregor A.D., 1995).

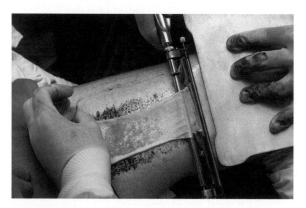

**Figure 17.17** Watson modification of Humby hand-guided skin grafting knife – harvesting of thin STSG.

## 5. STSG HARVESTING TECHNIQUES

Harvesting is the term applied to the technique of removing various layers of skin by hand-held knives (Figures 17.16–17.19), electric or air-driven instruments (Figure 17.20).

See recommended websites (harvesting of split skin graft) at the end of this chapter.

**Box 17.8** Harvested STSGs.

| | |
|---|---|
| **Thin** | epidermis and upper part of the papillary layer of the dermis (Figures 17.17–17.19) |
| **Medium** | epidermis and most of the papillary layer of the dermis (0.012 inch or 0.30 mm) (Figure 17.19) |
| **Thick** | 0.018 inch, or 0.45 mm, of the skin (75–80%), leaving a very thin layer of reticular dermis retaining the skin appendages (Figures 17.24 and 17.25)[1-8,24]. |

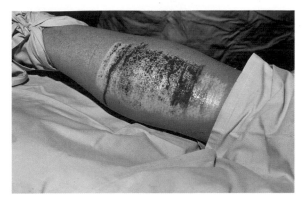

**Figure 17.18** Donor site – thin/medium split thickness skin graft.

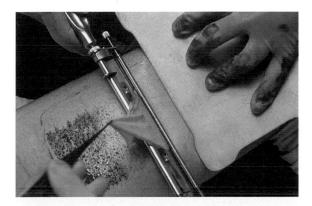

**Figure 17.19** Watson modification of Humby SG knife (harvesting medium depth STSG – most common – easily meshed – excellent take expected).

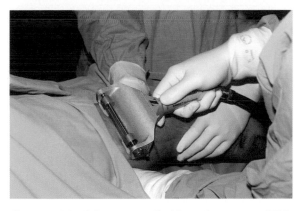

**Figure 17.20** High-pressure air driven dermatome STSG harvesting device – high level of accuracy in depth and width.

**Box 17.9** Braithwaite/Humby handheld knife.

- Handheld skin graft knife, commonly used – degree of accuracy for depth can be average – relies on the skill of the operator (Figures 17.16 & 17.17)
- The use of spreader boards can achieve a more uniform width (Figure 17.17)
- Edges serrated, aesthetic result can be good to average
- Handheld STSG graft harvesting knives require competence in use to obtain a uniform depth and this can often be observed when the donor site dressing is removed and some wound zones remain unhealed (Figures 17.25–17.27)
- There is the potential to convert thick STSG donor sites to full thickness wounds by removing 100% of the dermis, entering the subcutaneous fat layer, particularly in the thin skin of children and older people
- This may result in the donor site itself requiring a thin STSG to facilitate healing or over granulation requiring specific treatment (Figure 17.25)[1–5]
- Thin STSGs can be distinguished from medium/thick STSGs, as thin skin grafts have a translucency that reduces with thickness (Figure 17.17 & 17.24)
- Thin/medium thickness skin has a high potential for optimal take, especially if meshed (Figure 17.7 & Figures 17.21–17.23)
- Thick skin does not mesh well and is usually applied in sheets with holes inserted by sharp pointed scissors or a scalpel blade. This minimises/prevents exudate (haematoma/seroma) collecting beneath the graft (Figure 17.24)
- These perforations allow clinicians to remove exudate and prevent the development of haematoma or seroma when nursed
- Perforations also assist in achieving the same wound bed repair outcomes when grafts are nursed closed
- Problems occur when holes are too narrow and close over with accelerated healing in some wounds.

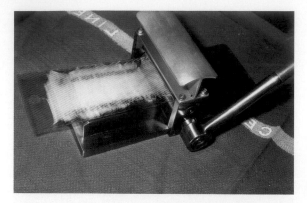

**Figure 17.21** STSG donor skin meshing device.

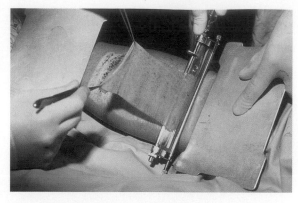

**Figure 17.24** Medium to thick split thickness skin graft – donor skin – meshing ratio minimal to ensure resilient skin cover.

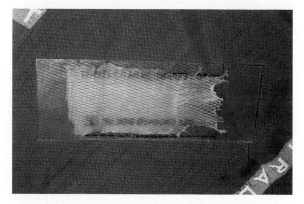

**Figure 17.22** Meshed STSG on plate that determines precise and uniform incisions in the skin (diamond appearance when stretched).

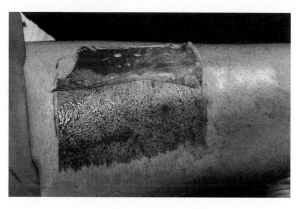

**Figure 17.25** Medium to thick split thickness skin graft – donor site – average harvesting technique – delayed healing may be expected.

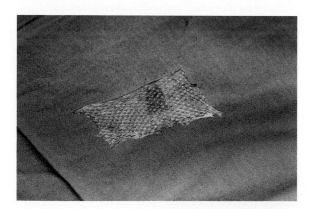

**Figure 17.23** STSG meshed skin ready for application.

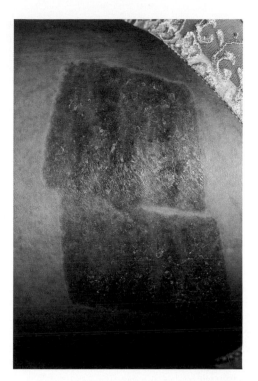

**Figure 17.26** Healing thick donor site – vulnerable to secondary injury – requires protection and wound bed maintenance.

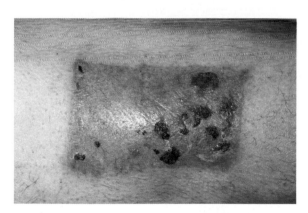

**Figure 17.27** Premature removal of donor site dressing – requires further moist wound healing dressing and wound bed maintenance.

**Box 17.10** Silvers™ skin graft knife technique.

- Small, portable, light and easy to use (Figures 17.16 & 17.19)
- Compare size with Braithwaite/Humby knife (Figure 17.16)
- Allows for harvesting small areas of skin, degree of accuracy quite good
- Useful in hospital and outpatient clinics for small wound defects – provides thin skin, translucent with high potential for accelerated take in optimal recipient site conditions.

**Box 17.11** Electric/air-driven dermatome.

- Demonstrates best practice technique
- Delivers a high degree of accuracy in required depth/width (Figures 17.20–17.23)
- Ability to harvest more skin over smaller available donor zones, due to high degree of width accuracy available
- Serration at edges very minimal and uniformity of depth accuracy provide excellent aesthetic result at donor site
- When meshed (Figures 17.21–17.23) it can be expanded up to 50% and placed on recipient site.

## Pinch skin grafting

With modern analgesia, local anaesthesia, topical local anaesthetic creams (e.g. EMLA®) and the availability of simple STSG harvesting techniques, modern dressings and portable negative pressure therapy, it must also be pointed out that the previous and continued use of 'pinch' grafting is now considered obsolete[7].

Under appropriate conditions, experienced wound care nurse clinicians could be educated to use the small Silvers™ knife (which uses a razor blade) (Figures 17.16 and 17.19), for minimal areas of skin that are required for small wounds in community nursing regions, where medical services are scarce.

**Box 17.12** Disadvantages of pinch grafting technique.

- Take cannot be guaranteed, as the donor skin is usually of full thickness (older patients with thin skin)
- Results of full thickness grafts poor unless the match of donor skin and recipient blood vessels is compatible
- The actual donor graft is the most difficult to ensure take in vascular compromised sites, and sites where oedema is an issue
- Aesthetically, both the donor and recipient sites are generally unsightly and patients are usually unhappy with the checkerboard and peppered divot appearance of donor site outcomes.

## Preparation of harvested skin graft donor skin for temporary storage

When the choice is to delay the application of a STSG to its recipient site, adequate storage preparations must be undertaken to ensure the efficacy of the fragile skin and protect the viability of the cells. Skin may be prepared and stored artificially for up to 21 days immediately following harvesting (see Box 17.13 for storage details).

Application is usually within four hours postoperatively in the surgical unit, or 24–48 hours later when wound bed conditions are more optimal and the patient is feeling more co-operative and settled[1-7].

### *Maintaining stored donor skin viability*

To sustain optimal viability, skin can only be stored in a refrigerator with a constant and uninterrupted temperature of 4°C for up to three weeks (this is usually the same refrigerator used to store pharmaceutical products)[1,7].

Temperature fluctuations within a normal refrigerator can alter the pH of the skin, rendering the cells inactive and subject to toxic changes with elements of the cell beginning to die within 48 hours. Lack of a capillary circulation supporting cellular function contributes to this state.

Stored skin deteriorates exponentially with time (cell death), and faster in the last 10–14 days, and by day 21 the cell nuclei may be irreparably damaged and no longer viable, thus rendering the skin nonviable. The viability of a skin graft can be prolonged when it is stored in 'Hanks' tissue culture solution, which contains plasma and the antibiotic neomycin, but this is rarely used[1,19].

When skin is applied in the surgical unit by the nurse clinicians, any remaining pieces, regardless of size, should be re-stored to avoid subjecting the patient to a further operation if a small piece of skin is required for a slow healing region of the recipient site.

If skin cannot be optimally stored it should be applied immediately it is harvested, or within 4–12 hours for optimal take to occur. As suggested, an alternative, simple and effective method of storing skin is to place it back on the donor bed for up to 24 hours.

The donor skin can be easily removed within 24 hours with minimal injury to the (donor) skin or the recipient wound site, and has a significantly higher rate of take than skin stored within saline gauze at 4°C[1,7].

**Box 17.13** Preparation of STSG skin prior to storage.

- The skin is spread on a piece of Vaseline® gauze with shiny, raw, dermal side upwards, then the skin is folded back onto the raw (shiny) surface of skin, rolled up gently, not folded tightly[5]
- A sterile gauze square (four layers), is prepared with wet normal saline or Ringers solution and the skin is folded and wrapped up gently, not folded tightly, and placed into a large sterile container
- The skin must not be squashed in the jar as this injures the viable cells
- The container should be labelled with the patient's name, hospital number, date of collection, and expected date of expiry (approximately 21 days)
- Labels should be placed on the side of the container, and on the lid, to avoid confusion, particularly if there are two patients with the same or similar names.

**Table 17.2** Donor sites – expected healing timeframes and wound dressing options.

| Expected healing time | | | | |
|---|---|---|---|---|
| Normal wound (primary suture) | Thin split thickness | Intermediate split thickness (most common depth used) | Thick split thickness | Full thickness skin grafts – composite grafts |
| 5–7 days on the face 7–14 days on the limbs and torso 14–21 days on the back – then staged movement to activities of daily living | 7–10 days Epidermis plus part of basal layer of dermis Loss of epithelial appendages minimal | 10–21 days Epidermis plus basal cell layer and most if not all, papillary dermal layer Loss of epithelial appendages minimal | 21–56+ days (should be observed for failure to heal if too thick – may require STSG) Loss of epithelial appendages moderate to high in some sites | 5–7 days (primarily closed – suture line) |
| **Dressing options** | | | | |
| Fixomul®, Mefix®, or Hypafix® dressing/retention tapes Polythene film Silicone based dressing Hydrocolloid thin and/or film, Hypafix®, Mefix®, Fixomul® Thin alginate and/or film or retention tape | | Fixomul®, Mefix®, or Hypafix® dressing/retention tapes Polythene film Silicone based dressing Hydrocolloid thin and/or film, Hypafix®, Mefix®, Fixumul® Thin alginate and/or film or retention tape | | Fixomul®, Mefix®, or Hypafix® dressing/retention tapes Polythene film Silicone based dressing Hydrocolloid thin and/or film, Hypafix®, Mefix®, Fixumul® Thin alginate and/or film or retention tape |
| **Then** | | | | |
| May require temporary compression dressing (gauze, combine and crepe bandage) and elevation for 24–48 hours | | May require temporary compression dressing (gauze, combine and crepe bandage) and elevation for 24–48 hours | | May require temporary compression dressing (gauze, combine and crepe bandage) and elevation for 24–48 hours |
| **Or** | | | | |
| Vacuum pressure therapy (VAC®) for first 48–72 hours then, e.g., moist wound healing retention dressing | | Vacuum pressure therapy (VAC®) for first 48–72 hours then, e.g., moist wound healing retention dressing | | Vacuum pressure therapy (VAC®) for first 48–72 hours then, e.g., moist wound healing retention dressing |

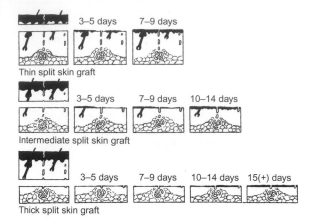

Thin split skin graft

Intermediate split skin graft

Thick split skin graft

**Figure 17.28** Donor-site healing timeframes according to harvested thickness (McGregor I.A. & McGregor A.D., 1995).

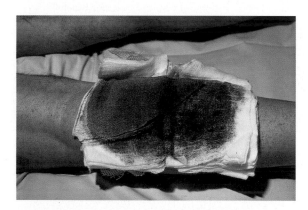

**Figure 17.29** Use of Vaseline® gauze and gauze padding dressing to donor site.

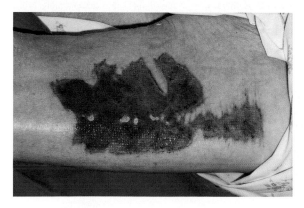

**Figure 17.30** Hypergranulation of donor site wound.

## 6. RISK MANAGEMENT AND THE SKIN GRAFT DONOR SITE

Skin grafts are usually harvested in the operating room with techniques to restrict bleeding in the postoperative phase. Dressings should be selected to match both the depth and expected exudate of the donor site wound – mismatch of wound/dressing selection results in pain and increased wound morbidity. Significant complications and morbidity has been recorded in postharvested skin graft donor sites[1–7,24].

> **Box 17.14** Potential clinical risks following skin graft harvesting.
>
> - Pain
> - Secondary injury
> - Infection
> - Permanent discolouring
> - Hypergranulation (Figure 17.30)
> - Hypertrophic or keloid scarring (Figures 12.7 & 12.8)
> - Skin dryness and potential for secondary bleeding (Figures 17.26 & 17.27).

> **Box 17.15** Principal causes of donor site pain.
>
> - Relegation of the donor site wound to a secondary position in the total care of the patient and their wounds
> - Primary moist wound healing dressing/wound mismatch
> - Engorged new blood vessels may cause pain, especially in the elderly – support bandages or garments are advocated over primary dressings
> - Local shear and friction over the wounded area – where any shear and friction continues to be exerted on the delicate developing epidermal cells, secondary injury is a common feature regardless of the type of dressing applied
> - Thigh anatomy (e.g. sometimes when the bandage is applied to hold all the dressings in place, a 'roll' of flesh is produced above the bandage, so when the patient begins to walk, the bandage pushes the dressings down, causing displacement and further trauma)

- Premature removal of the wound dressings (prior to the anticipated wound bed repair timeframe)
- Failure to address any patient concerns regarding pain and discomfort felt at the site
- Increasing level of wound contamination, leading to infection.

## Selecting STSG donor site dressings

### Review

Chapter 11.

As discussed in Chapter 11, selection of a wound dressing can be science-based, and pristine STSG donor sites provide excellent illustrations of the importance of matching the appropriate dressing to the specific wound depth, exudate and particular wound site.

It must be emphasised that in modern wound care, the previous use of Vaseline®/paraffin or medicated gauze, then plain flat gauze or wool and crepe bandage, is no longer appropriate for the primary dressing of donor site wounds[18] (Figure 17.29). The pain control and healing efficacy of moist wound healing and negative pressure therapy have superseded these dressings[13–19,24].

In addition when Vaseline®/paraffin or medicated gauze or similar is used, external dressings and bandages may become loose with physical movement, causing internal dressings to produce shear and friction across exposed capillaries/arterioles, resulting in sensation comparable to sharp ischaemic pain. This movement occurs as wound bed repair is attempting to take place, the capillaries are injured, and epidermal cells are destroyed, significantly delaying the wound bed repair process.

### *STSG donor site infection*

The local clinical indications of infection are heat, pain, swelling, exudate, odour, loss of function and, in most cases, varying degrees of itchiness. Pain and itchiness are early and significant signs, with cellulitis of the surrounding skin and, on wound inspection, a 'glassy' appearance of the granulation tissue may also be evident[7,24].

A donor site that heals and then breaks down is also probably heavily colonised and hence the new epithelium is 'devoured' by bacteria as soon as it develops[7,21]. Wound bed assessment and preparation, including wound microbiology studies, will be required[21] (see Chapter 8).

## Suggested nursing management options in the presence of donor site infection

**Box 17.16** Suggested treatment options – donor site infection.

- Provide pre-emptive pain management before commencing any dressing removal and wound treatments
- Obtain wound swab for culture and sensitivity prior to any order of antibiotics
- Wash the wound with warm soapy water (plain and non-perfumed soap or medically approved wound detergent) and pat dry with soft non-adherent dressing material (do not use a hairdryer as this will burn the tissues).
- Apply silver sulphadiazine (SSD) cream for 36–48 hours – change dressings four to six-hourly (this procedure would be done for no more than 5–7 days as it is known that SSD cream will delay keratinocytes) or apply a Betadine® pack dressing (1 part Betadine® to 10 parts normal saline) for 5–10 minutes
- For a highly contaminated or infected wound, the use of slow release iodine-based moist wound healing dressings for approximately 48–72 hours is suggested. These are water soluble and the slow release significantly reduces the toxicity of the iodine, but cleans the wound and reduces odour. They should be employed according to the manufacturer's indications for use, including methods and timing of application
- The newer silver-based dressings are also an appropriate choice for these infected donor sites. Either of these dressings can be continued according to manufacturer's instructions until completely healed.

### Additional donor site problems

In a thick split thickness graft, where almost all the dermis was removed, at approximately day 14 the donor wound may demonstrate excessive thickness of the granulation tissue (Figure 17.30) with little or no evidence of epidermal resurfacing.

The patient should be referred for plastic surgical review/consultation as the wound may require a mechanical debridement, hypertonic saline or cell dehydrating-based moist wound healing dressings, a compression dressing and adequate pain management. The patient should be reassured that the situation is readily reversible.

Following this cleansing treatment, a thin split thickness skin graft may be required to facilitate the normal healing process, or the wound may heal secondarily with moist wound healing dressings and continued compression[1-4,19].

### Negative pressure therapy

Although often an expensive option, the application of negative pressure therapy to the donor site for up to 72 hours, followed by a moist wound healing dressing until completely healed, is suggested to be the state of the art method, where available, and where time permits[17].

Evidence-based research has established that excellent, painless and timely clinical wound outcomes for all donor site depths is achieved by negative pressure therapy with (e.g. a non-adherent, non-absorbable dressing) on the surface of the wound itself to prevent the granulation tissue being integrated into the foam dressing, and prevent/minimise pain[17].

It should not be considered absolutely necessary to go to these lengths for all skin graft donor sites, however, those identified as at risk of poor healing outcomes would benefit from this advanced technology.

---

**Review**

*Setting goals of care and preferred clinical and patient outcomes*, Chapter 2, Boxes 2.7–2.9. Adapt as appropriate to the patient's clinical needs.

---

**Box 17.17** Post donor site repair issues.

- Premature removal of donor site wound dressings leave zones of fragile and partially healed wounds
- Retention or silicone interfaced dressings for up to five days will assist further healing, and offer secondary injury protection
- If some areas remain unhealed, then the use of thin hydrocolloids or the antibacterial dressings available will ensure protection and bacterial balance
- A failure to be aware of the varied loss of epidermal appendages that provide the oil and water moisture of normal skin healing will be evident (Figures 17.26 & 17.27)
- The physiological changes related to ageing, disease processes and UV exposure further add to the levels of moisture and oil lost and need to be part of the wound assessment equation with replacement needs maintained until the whole epidermis has resurfaced, and until an acceptable degree of protective normalcy is restored
- A stable wound state may take several months in some patients and in some older patients, and following deep levels of dermis harvested, the need to replace moisture (skin care) and protective measure may continue for a lifetime
- Discharge education should include the ongoing care of the donor site and particularly prevention from secondary injury and sunburn. Wearing soft, non-adhering clothing to cover the donor site, and application of UV protection cream are important to emphasise. Abnormal development of scarring should be referred by the patient to the surgeon for advice and management.

---

## 7. WOUND BED REPAIR IN THE STSG DONOR SITE

---

**Review**

*Wound bed preparation*, Chapter 10.

---

**Box 17.18** Healing in split thickness skin graft donor sites.

- Check with the surgeon as to the donor skin depth and survey the surgical notes to ascertain the type of dressing that has been applied
- This will assist in indicating the level of exudate, discomfort (if any) to be expected, the projected healing timeframe, and accurate timing for primary dressing removal
- Very thin donor sites in reasonably young, well patients heal quickly and sufficiently to be reharvested after approximately 3–4 weeks. In some major surface area burns patients, with minimal donor sites available, this is extremely beneficial[1-7]
- It is recognised that in optimal conditions, complete structural renewal of the epidermis takes approximately 17–19 days, with each epidermal cell taking approximately ten days to migrate to and across the surface[1-7]
- See range of thicknesses and wound outcomes in Figures 17.17–17.27
- See Figure 17.28 and Table 17.2 for suggested donor site healing timeframes in clean wounds, referenced against depth and for suggested moist wound healing dressings
- The general principle is that the thicker/deeper the skin is wounded, or harvested, the greater the loss of epidermal appendages essential in epidermal resurfacing (see Chapter 8)
- As would be expected, this depth is suggested to directly affect the total healing timeframe related to the need for donor site dermal contraction, dermal healing, epidermal resurfacing, and overall wound bed repair[1-7]
- This outline supports the general theory that epidermal resurfacing takes place in both directions, upwards and across, and occurs over a timeframe that reflect the thickness of the donor site wound, patient's age, any morbidity, and blood supply of the donor site[1-7].

**Box 17.19** Thin/intermediate STSG donor wounds heal by re-epithelialisation/resurfacing from:

- Epithelial cells located 1–2 mm from the edges of the wound, migrating towards the centre of the wound
- Mobilised epithelial cells located in the remaining germinal or basal layer of the epidermis, migrating upwards to the injured wound region
- Minimal dermal contraction working in parallel with the resurfacing process[7].

**Review**

*Auditing preferred clinical and patient outcomes,* Chapter 2, Boxes 2.10–2.12.

## 8. PATHOPHYSIOLOGY – SKIN GRAFT 'TAKE' IN THE RECIPIENT SITE

Figure 17.31 demonstrates the physiological pathway of skin graft take in a pristine wound environment. This figure indicates a continuum outlining the initial absence of blood vessels and the values of fibrin as an essential adhering factor, with a gradual uptake of a vascular system to support the donor skin.

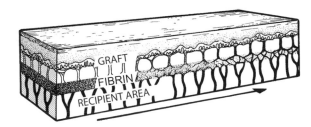

**Figure 17.31** Diagram demonstrating vascular uptake over approximately five days (McGregor I.A. & McGregor, A.D. 1995).

## Principal colours of black, yellow/green, pink/red

| Black<br>No take | Yellow/Green<br>No take | Green/Pink<br>Minimal graft take | Pink<br>Graft take | Red<br>Graft take |
|---|---|---|---|---|
| Wound zone 5 | Wound zone 4 | Wound zone 3 | Wound zone 2 | Wound zone 1 |
| Eschar – potential for development of gross contamination or infection under this lifeless skin | Associated with presence of critical levels of contamination, or infection, e.g. *Pseudomonas aeruginosa* or MRSA | Small to medium islands/zones approximately 30% of granulating tissue and fibroblasts | 95% areas of pink granulation tissue islands/zones (optimal) | Maximum area of granulation tissue 100% (optimal) |
| No blood flow – (avascular necrosis) Wound $O_2$ zero | Limited blood flow – zones of avascular tissue up to 90%. Wound $O_2\downarrow$ | Blood flow variable – $O_2\updownarrow$ | Blood flow excellent – $O_2\uparrow$ | Blood flow excellent – $O_2\uparrow$ |
| Needs WBP including major debridement and MWH dressings | Needs WBP including major debridement and MWH dressings | Needs WBP including basic surgical debridement then STSG $\pm$ meshed skin applied<br><br>Potential for some graft 'bridging' between zones of grafted skin possible | Needs minimal WBP then STSG $\pm$ meshed skin application<br><br>Unmeshed skin should not be placed on non-pink zones | STSG $\pm$ meshed skin application<br><br>Observe for over-granulation of unhealed areas – poor take, needs de-granulating to accept donor skin |

→

*Increasing level of granulation tissue*

## Risk management in skin graft take

Skin graft recipient beds bring clinical risks associated with healing and several principal conditions must be in place for 'take' (adherence to the host/recipient bed) to occur.

> **Box 17.20** Principal requirements to be considered in skin graft take.
>
> - The medical and nursing morbidity of the patient – stabilisation of general medical and nursing issues that inhibit take
> - The physiological status of the recipient wound bed – a granulating wound bed free from contamination and infection[1-7]
> - The physiological condition of the donor skin – skin harvested from a vascular skin zone should have retained a high level of vascular remnants
> - With the graft skin in position – patient co-operation, and immobilisation at the recipient site to match the specific site, healing time required, and the individual patient.

> **Box 17.21** General issues relating to skin graft take.
>
> - In surgical wounds, it is suggested that the deposition of normal fibrin related to the primary inflammatory response to an injury (trauma or surgery) at the recipient site provides the basis of an antibacterial environment and acts as a biological dressings for approximately 48–72 hours and declines thereafter (Figure 17.31)[1-7]
> - In all wounds, the purpose of wound bed assessment and preparation is to ensure that the recipient bed must have an optimal level of quality protein/fibrin exudate present, arising from a normal or restored normal inflammatory process, by removing any biological impediments

- The presence of this exudate is stated to be associated with a healthy vascular wound bed and graft success – its absence is associated with a poorly vascularised wound bed and graft failure[1-7]
- The general theory is that this protein/fibrin substance is attributed with providing the primary adherence of the donor skin to the recipient bed by its sticky 'glue like' consistency. This must not be allowed to accumulate under the graft in any volume, but must simply 'exist' thinly
- It is further suggested that, in this optimal oxygenated and nourishing milieu, a 48-hour window of opportunity exists to facilitate primary donor and recipient vessel anastomosis and allows a circulatory architecture between the donor site vessels and recipient site capillaries to be established
- A reinstatement of the circulatory system (including the lymphatics) is suggested to gradually restore the presence of the physiological negative pressure in the tissues[20]. This aids in restoring the slow but gradual removal of oedema from the wound and cellular growth to increase particularly where gravity may cause the graft to dislodge (Figure 17.33)
- Failure for primary microvascular uptake at this point (48–72 hours) is an indicator of an ineffective wound bed preparation allowing for the potential failure of part or the whole of the graft to take
- It appears that the degree of circulatory efficiency, including the lymphatics, determine the efficacy of both structure and function, and is significantly related to the levels of oedema by days 4–6[1]
- As with all wounds, addressing both the physiological status of the patient, and the regional and local wound condition, provide a clear demonstration of the importance of applying the principles of wound bed preparation for skin graft take to be successful[1-5,7].

Although the precise physiological explanation of the total process of skin graft 'take' remains largely theoretical and no universal consensus has been established, there is general agreement on some areas and this is outlined in Box 17.20[1-7].

**Figure 17.32** Using wound colours (wound bed assessment) to indicate potential for split thickness skin graft take.

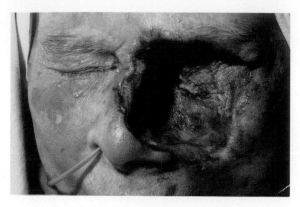

**Figure 17.33** Example of dead space following exenteration of eye for tumour removal and STSG applied.

---

**Box 17.22** Process of initial vascular supply – inosculation.

- When injury occurs, the biological survival instinct is to protect the organism from predatory and opportunistic bacteria by establishing primary and secondary protective responses
- In essence these are the defensive inflammatory responses that initiate the process for restoration of a self regulating vascular response for closed wound repair
- Following injury (surgery or trauma) blood flow is temporarily halted (normal clotting response with concomitant hypoxia) and plasma leaks out of the capillaries into the recipient bed
- This provides an antibacterial environment for approximately 24–48 hours[1–7]
- In a normal closed surgical wound, this action provides a primary protective environment and in the absence of any adverse events healing continues unhindered
- In clean non-contaminated open wounds, the presence of plasma or blood serum exudate arising from the inflammatory process can be observed to have the normal stickiness of plasma. This acts as a form of 'glue', suggested to 'stick' or 'bond' the STSG donor skin to the recipient bed[1–7]
- It is proposed that there is a plasma uptake by donor graft vessels to open the channels but that this does not establish any formal circulation as such (Figure 17.31)[1–7]

---

- It is further suggested that the primary adhesion of the STSG may be partially assisted by a subtle degree of negative tissue pressure (relative to the surrounding venous pumping function) that normally exists within the mobile tissues, and is restored when the open wound is closed off from the external environment[1–7,20]
- No true functioning of lymphatic links is established until approximately days 5–6
- Under normal conditions, empty donor skin vessels have been observed to fill, establishing a nutrient environment
- The graft becomes oedematous and can gain up to 40% in weight as water physiologically follows the plasma
- It is suggested that the occurrence of this action prevents the drying out of the donor graft skin and keeps donor graft vessels open and patent, until vascular connections can be established[1]
- It should be noted that dressings used to secure grafts in fixed skin regions, for example over the pretibial region or the palm of the hand, are assisted by the available bony counter pressures by stabilising the graft in an immobile position
- Excessive external compression (greater than 22–25 mmHg) by wound dressings over any skin graft should be avoided as this can occlude the fragile capillaries at the arterial end, and prevent arterial inflow and normal circulation into and out of the donor skin, resulting in an ischaemic graft[1–7]
- Under normal circulatory conditions, elevation of the limbs to use gravity flow for venous outflow is important to manage risk associated with potential venous congestion, oedema, and microvascular thrombosis, but allow for arterial inflow[1–7].

## Source of continuing graft vascular circulation

As previously stated, researchers vary in their descriptions of how circulation between the donor skin and the recipient bed is established[1]. Some research indicates a replacement of original vessels by a new system established over some days (Figure 17.31). Regardless, for nurse clinicians, Boxes 17.23 and 17.24 reinforce the continued need for immobilisation to prevent shearing forces on establishing vessels, the need for graft protection, and the critical timeframe of immobility.

**Box 17.23** Arterial circulatory uptake process in normal skin grafts.

| | |
|---|---|
| **Day 1** | (24 hours) no connection of collateral vessels in recipient site to donor skin (as above) |
| **Day 2** | (48 hours) initial connection between some vessels of donor skin and recipient site |
| **Day 3** | (72 hours) increasing number of vessels establishing connection – fragile, but functional, and oedema very slowly begins to resolve[1] |
| **Days 4–6** | increasing functional strength and resilience of circulatory system – swelling decreasing – wound bed management requires ongoing protection of the recipient and surrounding site[1–5,7]. |

**Box 17.24** Lymphatic circulation.

- Lymphatic flow of the graft has been demonstrated to return at days 5–6 postoperatively, and essentially parallels the establishment of a reliable, though easily injured, arterial and venous circulation
- Host lymphatics have been shown to link up with pre-existing intrinsic lymphatics within the wound and it is at this stage that oedema and related swelling can be observed beginning to significantly resolve. This is because the 'normal' tissue moist wound healing milieu begins the pathway to restoring its local equilibrium
- In association with the newly established arterial and venous uptake, full circulatory function resumes through a fragile but consistent process, gaining strength, in the absence of secondary injury or development of infection[1–7].

## Wound bed assessment – the recipient site

Objective clinical observation of the regional, surrounding, and local colour of a wound remains one of the universal standards for establishing the vascular status following injury and reconstructive surgery[1–7]. Identification of clinical/physiological risks that prevent or enhance wound repair requires a critical understanding of what these colours can demonstrate in particular wound presentations (Figure 17.32).

Pristine surgical wounds demonstrate the ideal conditions for skin graft take. This ideal situation is unfortunately not always the case. For STSGs, this requires a critical ability for primary wound bed assessment and an understanding of the physiological requirements for graft take. One of the simplest of clinical methods of wound bed assessment has been the use of the local and surrounding wound bed colour to demonstrate differences in wound pathology[18,19]. Although this may appear scientifically simplistic, the experienced observer can accurately predict wound status, aided by scientific testing and data, suitable treatment modalities, and potential healing outcomes.

Within plastic surgery, one of the principal areas in which this technique has been applied is quantifying the degree, or lack of, pink/red granulation tissue, indicating the degree of vascularity and potential for fusion of donor and recipient bed vessels in a wound. This aids in quantifying the level of risk associated with applying donor skin grafts and tissue flaps to wounds[1–8].

Figure 17.32 has been based on recent research to demonstrate the efficacy of the concept of colour and difficulties in affecting skin graft take as universally accepted in plastic surgical practice. A pocket-based guideline has been developed by the authors of this research, reflecting these principles, and may prove extremely useful to the beginning expert both in education and in clinical practice[22].

### Importance of vascular remnants in the donor skin

As donor skin grafts do not bring a blood supply with them, they do bring the vessel remnants remaining in the donor tissue so it is important that the donor skin comes from a highly vascular region[1–7].

Similarly, donor skin requires an optimal blood supply (available via the capillaries in the granulation tissue) to revascularise/fuse with in the recipient bed[1–7,19]. It is stated that regardless of the process of revascularisation, it is not until the fourth day post application (Figure 17.31) that the longevity of vascular efficacy for take can be scientifically demonstrated[1–7]. Clinically, again this sets the timeframe of total immobilisation (usually for 7–10 days) of the wound that ensures optimal graft take.

## Bridging phenomenon – where colour counts

It is suggested that a paradox exits in that it has been observed in some wounds that thin or meshed donor skin, placed over avascular areas, can be demonstrated to receive a blood supply from an adjacent highly vascularised area (see as wound example, Figure 17.32 – zone 3) and its source may be due to a collateral circulation. It has been shown that, if surrounded by richly vascularised tissue, an avascular area of graft as large as 1 cm may still survive. This phenomenon is referred to as 'bridging'[1-7] and is important when attempting to close a poorly vascularised wound bed. Meshed grafts are the choice for these wounds as the skin crosses from zone to zone.

## 9. SKIN GRAFT FAILURE TO TAKE

In the absence of intrinsic medical factors (e.g. the patient is on anticoagulant medication), the principal local causes of a STSG failure to take, following optimal wound bed preparation, are outlined in Boxes 17.25 and 17.26.

The first principle of physiological skin graft 'take' is that nothing must separate the donor skin and the recipient site during the healing (take) phase. The most common causes of graft separation are outlined.

---

**Box 17.25** Principal recipient site conditions preventing skin graft take.

- Separation of the donor skin from the recipient bed (e.g. haematoma or seroma)
- Skin grafts and skin flap donor skin will not adhere to a totally avascular, necrotic, highly contaminated or infected recipient tissue bed[1-8,17-19] (Figure 17.32 – wound zones 5–4), regardless of the quality of the donor skin
- Skin grafts will not 'take' over vital anatomical tissues, such as bone, cartilage or nerve tissue, that have been totally stripped of their blood supply[1-7]
- If some small remnants of a blood supply are available, skin grafts placed over these tissues may adhere but may significantly reduce function due to graft adherence and contraction, especially over tendons[1-7]

---

- The thinness of the grafted skin in these wounds, often being in vulnerable regions, such as the lower limb, have an increased incidence for secondary injury, can be painful, and are often aesthetically unacceptable to the patient[1-5,7]
- In closed graft management, the failure to ensure the securing dressings maintain the donor skin in total apposition with the wound bed allowing haematomas to develop
- Failure to totally immobilise the recipient site to prevent shear and friction
- The development of infection due to unknown causes (e.g. poor donor site preparation or recipient bed preparation)
- In open graft management, failure to immediately remove collections of old blood (haematoma) or serum as they form/appear, from under the graft. These may continue to collect in the first 72 hours
- Failure to elevate the recipient part of the limb resulting in venous congestion
- In open grafted wounds, failure to maintain regular wound bed assessment and wound bed management at the grafted site (Figures 17.4–17.10).

### Issues of take in contaminated/infected tissue zones

In known contaminated wounds, various organisms[1,19,21] may not be immediately obvious, causing grafts to fail by the production of plasmin and proteolytic enzymes which dissolve the important fibrin scaffold to ensure their own survival. For example, beta-haemolytic *Streptococcus*[21] greater than $10^3$, and a glassy/transparent 'film' appearance over the granulation tissue may indicate problems.

Long-term chronic wounds, recurring breakdowns of wounds, and recurring failure of STSGs to take as expected, should be investigated for the normal suspect organisms/bacteria, in particular beta-haemolytic *Streptococcus*, prior to further surgical interventions. Pressure ulcers and recalcitrant non-healing wounds in very ill patients are examples of this.

The presence of abnormal levels of oedema is also a significant contributing factor (e.g. seen in attempts to apply STSGs to highly exuding oedematous venous ulcer wounds), thus the principles of restoring the most favourable healing environment (wound bed assessment and preparation) is as applicable to skin grafts, skin flaps and their donor sites, as to any other wound[1-7].

Overexudating oedematous wounds (usually chronic wounds with vascular disturbances), and overgranulating (proud flesh) wounds accept grafts very poorly. In the latter, wound bed preparation is required and this tissue must be surgically debrided, or the volume reduced by cell dehydrating dressings, compression therapy, and elevation of the part, if possible[1-7].

### Issues of take in irradiated tissue zone

Tissues which have been irradiated, and have lost their intrinsic vascular integrity for angiogenesis (producing new capillaries) or arteriogenesis (producing new arterial vessels from existing arterioles), are also extremely poor candidates for skin grafting[1-7]. It is theorised, though not scientifically proven, that stem cells responsible for the growth factors that initiate angiogenesis, and promote inosculation (vascular fusion between donor vessels and recipient bed vessels), are destroyed by irradiation. Thus, with one of the two factors absent, in a receptive recipient bed, skin graft take is unable to be produced[1-7].

In addition, in post irradiated wounds (breast cancer) or severe burns, the underlying bone or cartilage (particularly in the thoracic or scalp region) may often be avascular, further compromising the proposed recipient wound site.

### Signs of total failure of STSGs to take

> **Box 17.26** Specific principal signs of total failure to take on observation.
>
> - A persistently white graft (no arterial/vascular uptake)
> - A dry, black graft (no vascular uptake, loss of local serum)
> - A persistent bruised appearance (arterial inflow but venous incompetence and inadequate removal of collected haematoma),
> - STSG that is observed moving/mobile across its recipient bed after 72 hours (i.e. critical contamination or infection)
> - An ongoing loss and final absence of any donor graft tissue[1-8].

> **Review**
>
> *Setting goals of care and preferred clinical and patient outcomes*, Chapter 2, Boxes 2.7–2.9. Adapt as appropriate to the patient's clinical needs.
> *Auditing preferred clinical and patient outcomes*, Chapter 2, Boxes 2.10–2.12.

## 10. METHODS OF MANAGING SKIN GRAFTS 1 – CLOSED

As the majority of patients are treated as day or short stay this has accelerated the application of firmly securing dressings such as, tie-over dressings, stapled foam and negative pressure therapy (VAC® system) to attain immobility of the recipient wound site (Figures 17.34–17.41).

> **Box 17.27** Closed STSG graft management techniques.
>
> - Overlay moist wound healing retention dressings may be applied to secure thin STSGs on flat surfaces such as particular regions of the limbs and chest wall
> - Application of compression/contouring and/or tie-over dressings which to exclude dead space, or are on undulating surfaces[1-7] (Figures 17.34–17.41)
> - Figure 17.33 demonstrates a large dead space where the graft was held in place with a tie-over dressing using polythene foam
> - Figure 17.40 demonstrates the research undertaken to determine the optimal placement of staples to gain the maximum efficiency of stapled foam to eliminate dead space, as a modern approach to the tie-over dressing[26]
> - The application of negative pressure therapy/VAC® (Figure 17.41). This can provide the optimal environment for skin graft take absorbing the excess exudate at a regulated and timed compression level particularly in wounds that are concave or have significant dead space[1-7,13-16]
> - The use of non-medically approved negative pressure therapy systems in hospital environments is becoming more common but bed day costs are suggested to be an issue, as is the cost of a portable or non-portable VAC®[13-16]. This may be a case where the cost of not using evidence-based methods is viewed as a cheaper option than the potential for wound breakdown.

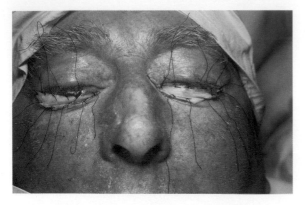

**Figure 17.34** Full thickness skin grafts applied for ectropion (drooping) to the lower eyelids prior to application of tie-over dressing.

**Box 17.28** Immediate aftercare – clinical nursing management issues.

- Where is the wound(s) located?
- Do the surrounding anatomical zones require general nursing care and supportive wound care?
- Consider general hygiene needs, including eye care, oral care, skin care
- Review safety, comfort and independence patient and wound needs on discharge, and ongoing in the community, for a seamless transition.

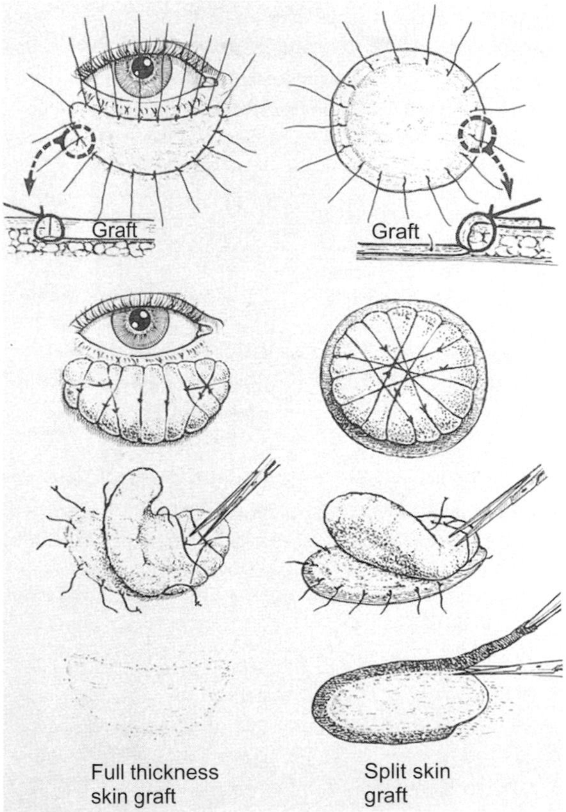

Full thickness
skin graft

Split skin
graft

**Figure 17.35** Tie-over dressing application and removal (McGregor I.A. & McGregor A.D., 1995).

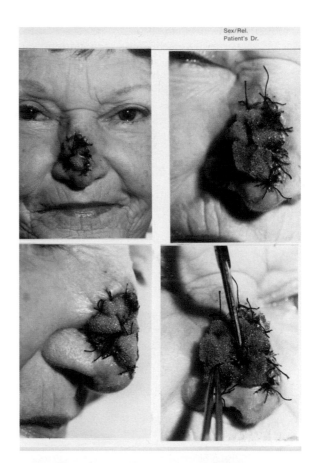

**Figure 17.36** Tie-over dressing to nose (STSG).

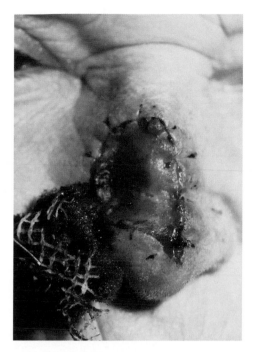

**Figure 17.37** Skin graft to the nose – dressing removal.

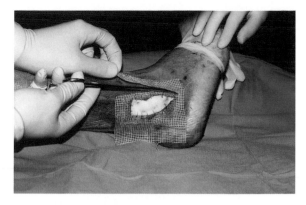

**Figure 17.39** Cutting off excess Vaseline® gauze after STSG stapled into place.

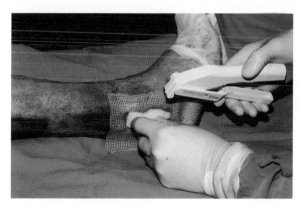

**Figure 17.38** Application of small STSG stapled at the edges used in surgery.

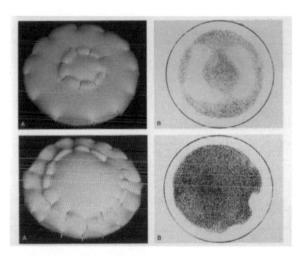

**Figure 17.40** Example of the importance of an evidence-based technique for ensuring uniform compression and optimal opportunity for uniform STSG take. Top (A) Small-circle double-layer dressing. (B) Imprint of the small-circle double-layer dressing. Bottom (A) Large-circle double-layer dressing. (B) Imprint of the large-circle double-layer dressing.

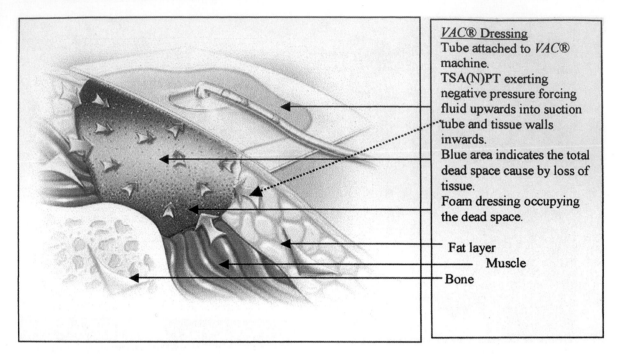

**VAC® Dressing**
Tube attached to *VAC®* machine.
TSA(N)PT exerting negative pressure forcing fluid upwards into suction tube and tissue walls inwards.
Blue area indicates the total dead space cause by loss of tissue.
Foam dressing occupying the dead space.

Fat layer
Muscle
Bone

**Figure 17.41** Using VAC® system to fill dead space over STSG and remove excess exudates. Reproduced with permission, KCI Medical Ltd.

## Closed skin grafts – removal of STSG tie-over dressings

For nurse clinicians, regardless of the dressings used, gentle removal of individual dressing layers is necessary if the graft is not to be disrupted. Tie-over or stapled conforming/contouring type dressings (Figures 17.35–17.37) used to secure STSGs may be removed approximately at days 5–7 after application – day 7 is optimal, allowing for vascular fusing to be secured[5].

Unless there is any evidence or suspicion of infection, open inspections of the graft before this should be strongly resisted to avoid shearing and friction leading to separation of the donor skin from the graft bed. The choice of replacement dressing is based on a wound bed assessment, the healed state of the wound, anatomical site, potential for increased mobility, the surgeon's preference, and the potential degree of patient independence and self-care.

**Box 17.29** Removal of tie-over dressing – clinical nursing practice.

- The process of removal should be discussed fully with the patient
- Prior to dressing management, the patient should be placed in a semi-reclined or reclined position, reassured, and be warm and comfortable
- Pre-emptive analgesia should be considered and discussed with the patient prior to removal of tie-over dressings on the nose, a particularly sensitive region
- Sit comfortably and rest the arms and wrists to reduce normal hand tremor
- As special techniques are required in order that the fragile graft is not inadvertently stripped from its bed, nurses must always request supervision if unsure, particularly when removing such dressings for the first time
- If the dressing appears to be stuck, warm sterile normal saline and a 10 ml syringe should be used to irrigate the dressings initially, and then as required. Some time should be left between irrigating to allow it to be fully absorbed

- First, the outer dressing is carefully removed, minimally disturbing the inner dressing, and sharp pointed scissors are used to cut the black silk sutures over the centre of the tie-over dressing[5] (Figures 17.35–17.37)
- Wool or gauze applied should be removed layer by layer until the paraffin gauze or underlying dressing is exposed over the graft
- It is important not to attempt to collectively remove the paraffin gauze with the outer dressing as this may lift the non-adhered or poorly adhered donor graft skin
- The paraffin gauze or non-adhering dressing must be gently lifted from over the donor skin with any adherence cut free at the precise point of the adherence (Figures 17.35 –17.37)
- The silk sutures surrounding the graft are cut and removed, the status of the graft is inspected, and any blisters are pricked or cut, dabbing with a sterile cotton bud
- The graft should not be rolled as the fluid may lift the adjacent fragile attached skin. Any overlap of dry skin at the wound edges should be trimmed back (Figures 17.35 and 17.36)
- Using normal saline soaked cotton buds, the clinician should gently remove any scabs/eschar and clean away any debris of flaked skin etc, and observe for any dry areas/superficial lifting of skin
- This can be managed by a smear of Vaseline® or topical antibiotic ointment (if prescribed) applied with a cotton bud, leaving the graft exposed or redressed as necessary
- The wound should be inspected by the surgeon and further treatments prescribed based on the status of the take, or any complications within the wound
- A non-adhering contoured dressing and a contoured, conforming polythene foam dressing may be replaced for an additional three to five days to ensure full healing has taken place
- This also aids in maintaining hygiene, protects the wound from secondary injury, and ensures the initial aesthetics of the wound
- It is essential that this dressing has no shear forces, as the graft is still very fragile
- Staples should be removed with extreme care so as not to tear the donor skin.

## General nursing risk management – issues of general patient immobility and special wounds

Regardless of age, there is a consensus that:

- Overall patient morbidity is significantly increased by general and increasing immobility
- Restoration of early patient mobility is a leading factor in avoiding the risks associated with immobility in all age groups, but particularly the older, or normally non-debilitated person.

This knowledge has focused medical and nurse clinicians on reviewing the need for varying degrees of patient immobility following skin grafts in a range of body regions. For example, grafts to the chest and the back require creative methods to allow patient mobility and independence.

For skin tumours on the face, limbs, or the back, and common injuries (e.g. pretibial lacerations) seen in the lower limb, treatment by the application of skin grafts is often the preferred method where direct closure or local skin flaps are not appropriate (usually fixed skin regions and wound dimensions) [1-7].

Following the elective surgical removal of skin lesions, STSGs or very thin FTSGs (e.g. eyelids or nose) are usually applied with tie-over contouring (Figures 17.34–17.37) or retention dressings, and 'splinting' for five to seven days[7]. This allows for a relative degree of mobility, but surrounding eye toiletry or nasal care will be required.

## *Soft tissue and skin tears to the lower limb – issues of immobility*

A large number of skin tumours and soft tissue lower limb injuries are seen in plastic surgery (Figures 17.42 and 17.43) that may compromise or decrease the mobility and independence of the patient for long periods of time. This may result in additional medical and nursing morbidity and significantly alter the patient's independence status.

Assessing the degree of complexity of these wounds and their specific management can best be made by plastic surgeons with their understanding of the blood supply to the skin, and the intrinsic needs for optimal and timely wound repair.

If infection, secondary procedures, and wound ulceration leading to months of dressing care are to

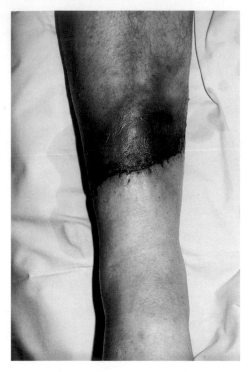

**Figure 17.42** Lower limb injury in the older person – reasonable potential for self-healing.

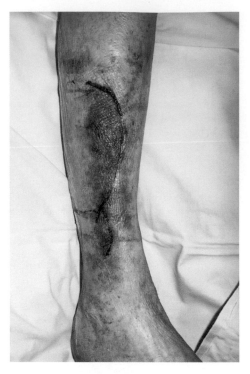

**Figure 17.43** Lower limb injury in the older person – poor potential for healing as demonstrated.

be avoided, critical wound bed assessment by expert clinicians is suggested as important if the optimal treatment is to be applied.

The pretibial region is a fixed skin zone and thus presents the problems of wound tension on the surrounding tissues when the injured skin is reapplied inappropriately (e.g. by the use of tapes or dressings).

In the presence of an inadequate blood supply, non debridement of avascular tissue, early mobility, with continuing shear and friction at the wound site, the wound may breakdown, become infected, leading to ulceration and moving on the pathway towards a chronic wound. Should long-term immobility be instituted patient independence is also at risk.

There appears to be no universal consensus on the correct treatment of these wounds and a number of treatment modalities have been put forward. The following is a case example:

- Assessing the vascular and cellular viability of pretibial traumatised raised skin (Figures 17.42

and 17.43) is particularly difficult. Only expert reconstructive surgeons can truly assess the viability of part or the whole of the damaged skin, its potential survival rate as a viable piece of skin, and its suitability to be replaced as a skin graft.

- If there is any suggestion that the periosteum has been denuded of its blood supply, the potential for graft take is significantly reduced
- Suggested treatment modality based on the evidence:
  - Excision of the avascular raised skin
  - Cleansing of the wound
  - Removing any haematoma or any contaminating material
  - Meshing the skin
  - Reapplication of the meshed skin to the wound has positive wound healing results
  - Potential for take is based on the bridging phenomenon, and revascularisation of the donor skin from the vascular wound edges.

- When expert wound bed assessment is undertaken and appropriate surgical treatment instituted, clinical research by experts in the field reviewing the effects of early mobility in post-surgical or post trauma wounds of the lower limb have confirmed that the controlled mobilisation of the patient after 48 hours of immobilisation, and limb elevation, established no significant risk in the positive healing rate of split skin grafts (88%+)[27,28]
- Splinting where the graft site is close to or over joints produced healing results similar to those for patients confined to bed.
- This practice of early mobilisation where appropriate, appears to significantly reduce the overall morbidity associated with immobilisation observed in all age groups, and significantly enhances the patient's psychological attitude and overall quality of life with little or no risk to graft take[27,28].

## Innervation following successful skin graft take

Following harvesting, the donor skin has no sensation as it is separated from its nerve supply. The return of sensation largely determines the functional usefulness of the graft[1].

**Box 17.30** Process of sensory return following skin graft take.

Degree of return of sensation:

- Skin flaps – complete
- Full thickness grafts – moderate
- Split skin graft – least return.

Degree of rate of return (the process is reversed):

- Skin flaps – slowest
- Full thickness grafts – moderate
- Split skin graft – most rapid.

All types of skin grafts assume the sensation of the recipient site, but innervation can be compromised by complications in wound healing (e.g. scar tissue) within the bed and surrounding tissue. Innervation appears to occur from margins towards the centre and best results appear to come from some regeneration of the previously partly destroyed pathways[1].

Nurse clinicians should be aware of the timing of sensory restoration, as patient education is essential to prevent secondary injury to the wound.

**Review**

*Setting goals of care and preferred clinical and patient outcomes*, Chapter 2, Boxes 2.7–2.9. Adapt as appropriate to the patient's clinical needs.
   *Auditing preferred clinical and patient outcomes*, Chapter 2, Boxes 2.10–2.12.

## 11. METHODS OF MANAGING SKIN GRAFTS 2 – DELAYED APPLICATION

Delaying the application of STSG until the patient has returned to the surgical unit is undertaken for a variety of reasons, and the principal ones are outlined in Box 17.31. The delayed application of the

**Box 17.31** Rationale for delayed application of donor skin to recipient site.

- The wound was contaminated, infected or contained necrotic tissue and has been debrided and wound occlusion following STSG is not clinically appropriate
- When the area requiring grafting is too large for a 'tie-over' type compression dressing or to use a single negative pressure application
- The recipient area is large and in a difficult anatomical position and requires the patient to be awake and co-operative (e.g. the back, chest wall, genitals, buttocks). Again, this may potentially be overcome by applying one or more negative pressure therapy devices at the recipient site to allow for enhanced patient mobility[15]
- Additional skin has been stored in case of breakdown of a skin/tissue/flap, or where the wound has been debrided, bleeding is significant, and/or is considered to continue to be contaminated and not yet suitable for application of skin.

graft may be nursed open or closed, based on surgical decisions[1–7,23–28].

Wet normal saline dressings, occluded with a sealing film dressing, are usually applied in the operating theatre to retain moisture and warmth within the wound. Sterile oxygen catheters, or similar, may be inserted within the dressing material for normal saline to be injected to maintain an optimal moisture level. Alternatively, moist wound healing dressings may be temporarily applied[25].

---

**Box 17.32** Delayed STSG management – open management.

- The open method of STSG is managed through the donor graft being placed on the recipient site and managed exposed to the elements but may be closed at a later time[1–8,23,24]
- On the limbs, this may require forms of immobility such as well padded resting/gutter type splints for a short period, to prevent shear and friction
- Hands and feet should be placed in position of function (check with the surgeon) to prevent foot drop, or flexor tendon contraction in the hand
- The open technique is commonly used in wounds that have doubtful healing properties (e.g. contaminated and chronic wounds), some burns wounds, and extensive compound trauma wounds
- Occlusion of the recipient site is not advocated in the early stages of some specific cases in order to prevent/reduce the incidence of potential infection or compression causing loss of grafted areas
- In open or closed graft management, the graft may be left unsecured to the wound or stabilised with sutures or staples
- Regardless, what can be clinically observed is that ensuring the immobility of the graft on its recipient site, in the first 48–72+ hours, is imperative for primary adherence and overall take
- In some burns, and large relatively well vascularised beds, negative pressure therapy is increasingly replacing the open technique because of potential for infection and the physiological morbidity associated with immobilisation, particularly of the ill and the elderly.

---

**Box 17.33** Addressing clinical nursing risk management prior to application.

- Regardless of the dressings applied in the operating room, appropriate and adequate pain management must be administered prior to commencing any treatments such as dressing removal, dressing changes, or application of the skin
- STSGs should never be applied if haemorrhage occurs when the interim dressing is initially removed postoperatively
- When immediate postoperative bleeding is excessive, the recipient site often requires several hours of compression dressings, elevation or pharmacological intervention[1–8]
- Any applied compression must not exceed the level that would produce ischaemia in the recipient site but must be sufficient to subdue continuing capillary ooze
- Loss of vascular integrity of the granulation tissue would then compromise the capacity of the graft bed to support the donor skin when the skin is applied. Some surgeons may request the use of topical coagulating agents until bleeding has ceased
- Patients who continue to bleed may be on anticoagulant drugs, including aspirin, and should have their coagulation status checked prior to application of skin
- Some post trauma wounds, including thick burns, can pose bleeding problems following extensive surgical debridement – physiological monitoring is essential to ensure fluid balance and general perfusion are maintained
- If moderate bleeding is evident at this point, the clinical nurse should place a calcium alginate dressing on the area, apply a pad and compression bandage, and elevate the area if possible for 1–2 hours
- Some surgeons may prefer to use saline soaked gauze or gauze soaked in, for example, an adrenaline 1 : 200,000 mixture – this can be messy and time consuming, but just as effective
- Excessive absorption may cause cardiac disturbances and patients should be closely observed, particularly those at risk
- Extreme care on removal is required, and gauze should be saturated with normal saline initially and whilst being removed, as the gauze may have lost its moisture and be adhered to the wound bed – this causes bleeding to recommence, leading to extreme pain and discomfort, and patient distress
- Patient medications should be checked again to make certain no aspirin or anti-inflammatory drugs were recently used, or to ensure the patient is not currently taking any anticoagulants, similar medications or natural therapy, and has failed to disclose this fact

- Compression on the wound and elevation may be all that is required but this requires patience and physiological understanding of existing co-morbid factors
- After one to two hours if bleeding continues, moderate compression and a elevating of the recipient area should continue (to utilise the natural law of gravity in reducing arterial flow) and the surgeon should be notified as to the possible medical cause, and this problem addressed
- Once the patient and wound conditions have been satisfied, the choice is then one of open or closed management. The following section provides general guidelines for the care of grafts nursed in an open environment.

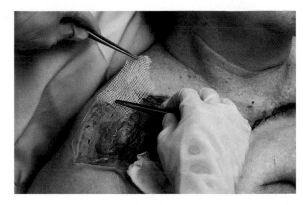

**Figure 17.44** Application of split skin graft – open management.

Table 17.3 Nursing application of delayed split thickness skin grafts. See Box 17.34, Clinical nursing techniques.

| Nursing procedure | Rationale |
|---|---|
| Apply the skin as early in the day as possible. | Allows the intensive time of initial graft care to be done in daylight time and when nursing and medical staff are more readily available if required. |
| Inform the patient and discuss the procedure. | Aids in patient acceptance of the injury or nature of the wound. |
| Allow the patient to inspect the area prior to skin application if they so desire. | Patient should feel he/she is part of the repair process. |
| Always check the name on the skin container and cross-reference with patient. | Skin will only take when the donor and recipient are the same person. |
| Always check expiry date of stored skin. | The longer the storage time the more chance the skin will not take as many cells will have died. |
| Should not be stored for more than 21 days. | |
| Clean recipient bed with normal saline very gently – do not rub. | Graft bed should not be induced to bleed, rather to exhibit a 'healthy' pinkness/redness. |
| Leave wet saline gauze on wound until you are ready to apply skin; remove a little at a time as skin is ready to be applied. | Retains moist cellular wound environment. |
| Unwrap donor skin as near as possible to wound and lay out on flat surface – use bottom of the sterile dressing tray. | Allows for checking skin for size and general thickness. 'Take' time relates to thickness of the donor material so on initial inspection the nurse can assess potential healing time. |
| Inspect donor skin – shiny/smooth side is the underside, dull side is the epidermis or external side. | Important to identify in order that donor (shiny) side is placed onto recipient site. |
| | Dull side with paraffin gauze faces the clinician. |
| | Allows for excess exudate to escape from under the graft. |

**Table 17.3** *Continued.*

| Nursing procedure | Rationale |
|---|---|
| If skin has not been meshed, cut into squares or triangles to fit the wound contour. | Allows for clinician to do early graft care to mechanically remove any exudate. |
| Then cut multiple 'Vs' into the donor skin with sharp-pointed scissors prior to application. *Review Figures 17.44 and 17.45.* | |
| Additional holes may be required after skin application to enable the fluid to escape easily over first 2 days. | Skin that is to be applied in the clinical unit will not be meshed prior to storage. Unless it is placed on a moist granulating surface immediately, loss of moisture from the germinal layer of the epidermis will result and subsequent cellular death will occur quite quickly. |
| In some centres, skin may be meshed in the ward (needs to be done in less than 48 hours of harvest due to skin deterioration) just prior to application to exclude excessive drying of the skin whilst in storage. | |
| Lay skin onto recipient bed shiny side down. | Vaseline gauze helps to stop graft edges from curling on itself. |
| Keep Vaseline®/paraffin gauze on the dull side of the skin until applied to the recipient bed. | Vaseline/paraffin gauze assists in positioning and manoeuvring skin into place. |
| Leave an excess of skin over the normal skin edges and cut remaining excess on day 3 – this skin essentially dries but underneath a collection of moisture may occur and become a focus for infection. | Although it is the dermis that contracts, thick split skin dermal fibres may also contract in the early phase – if excess is not left, the edges closest to the normal skin will be left exposed and may become a focus for infection. |
| Smooth grafts over the bed using swab sticks (using metal or plastic forceps may injure the fragile donor skin) to ensure no air pockets or fluid collections. | Graft will not take if contact/interface with recipient bed is not absolute to allow circulation to be established. |
| Gently remove paraffin gauze from the graft. (Vaseline/paraffin gauze may be left on very small pieces of skin to prevent edge curling and removed after 24 hours). | Allows for observation of development of fluid under the skin. |
| Unless there is an over supply of ooze or a haematoma developing beneath the skin graft, leave applied skin untouched for 2–3 hours or until there is excess exudate which threatens direct contact of skin and bed. | Assists in haemostasis and primary adherence. Allows skin to adhere to the bed by wound fibrin, which has glue-like properties. |
| After 2–3 hours, in the absence of early accumulating fluid, commence half-hourly night and day graft care (usually for first 24 hours) reducing to hourly and 2–4 hourly over the first 48 hours as exudate resolves (more often if drainage is excessive). | Primary take can only occur where the skin and bed are in direct and unopposed contact/interface. |
| Use sterile swab sticks or cotton buds to dab/express fluid from holes and use gentle dabs with swab-sticks between and towards cut holes. | Regular observations ensure no accumulation of fluid as excess fluid prohibits direct contact of donor graft to bed. Direct contact aids imbibition, the uptake of fluids into the donor graft to maintain moisture, and promotes inosculation, the joining of blood vessels from the bed into the donor skin capillaries. |

**Table 17.3** *Continued.*

| Nursing procedure | Rationale |
|---|---|
| With a sufficient supply of holes in the graft, gentle dabbing is the preferred method of removing additional collecting fluid (do not roll the cotton bud across the already adhered skin) Cut more holes if existing holes are insufficient to enable fluid to be expressed out. | Rolling (mechanical shear and friction) the swab sticks over the graft pushes the fluid across areas which may already have primary adherence. |
| Blisters or raised areas of skin indicate collections of fluid or old blood not absorbed. | Fluid or dead space of any sort creates a barrier between the graft and the bed, thus take will not occur and infection will develop in the medium, destroying the entire graft. |
| Snip with sharp-pointed scissors to allow fluid to escape, and dab gently with swab sticks. | |
| Some grafts, following initial take, may be left open during the day and closed at night. | Protects graft from being rubbed off, allows for wound inspections and allows air to circulate and reduce moisture within the graft. |
| Foam/cardboard 'igloos' may be made and placed around the graft site during the night. | Acts as a protection against shear and friction. |
| Specific attention is necessary to the amount of compression exerted by any dressings placed on or around the graft site. | Too much pressure will cause ischaemia to the fragile donor skin and resultant graft death. |
| After 24 hours, some recipient graft sites may need to be wrapped up. Apply a non-adherent dressing, polythene foam pad or acriflavine wool contoured to size of site, then apply gauze and crepe bandage. If on the limb, elevation will be necessary to aid venous return. | Some graft beds may have too much exudate forming under the graft itself due to venous compromise, thus becoming unstable. |
| Negative pressure therapy (VAC®) as the dressing to the skin graft bed is the current state-of-the-art technique. It can be applied following applications of the skin immediately or up to 24+ hours later. | Some patients may become restless or unco-operative and the graft may only be saved by being managed in a closed environment. |
| This can be removed after 48–72 hours and a moist wound healing dressing applied and patient discharged if appropriate. | This technique, used according to the scientific guidelines, assures precise negative pressure that fulfils the uniform physiological requirements of skin graft take/adherence and achieves this uniform level of compression over defined timeframes. |

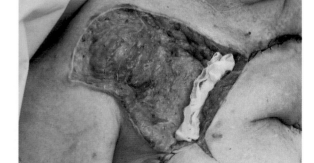

**Figure 17.45** Application of split skin graft – open management – moisture maintenance.

## The application of skin – open STSG management

There are few instances in which the exquisite nature and complexity of biological wound repair is better demonstrated, or aesthetically surpassed, than in the observation of the normal healing processes during the open management of skin grafts[1–7,22–24].

> **Review**
>
> *Setting goals of care and preferred clinical and patient outcomes*, Chapter 2, Boxes 2.7–2.9. Adapt as appropriate to the patient's clinical needs.

---

**Box 17.34** Clinical nursing techniques – preparing the patient and the recipient site.

- Open STSG resurfacing may occur on any part of the body. Some areas are anatomically difficult and present risk to the patient physiologically, and require high levels of care of both patient and wounds by nursing staff (Figures 17.5 & 17.6)
- The patient should be well prepared by discussion of the procedure and reason for undertaking certain procedural actions
- The patient's understanding of what is to occur and their co-operation are essential
- Regardless of where the skin is to be applied, the patient's required physical position should be determined and potential physical safety issues assessed:
  - Does the patient need to be placed on his/her face or side for 3–4 days?
  - Does the patient require a pressure relieving bed for long-term immobility?
  - What will be the toileting and feeding protocols?
  - Does the patient require physiotherapy to manage alterations in mobility (e.g. physical exercises to maintain body strength)?
  - Does the patient require massage therapy to ensure venous and lymphatic drainage?
- For limbs, resting splint material may be required such as plaster of Paris or a custom made thermoplastic mould. This should be prepared prior to laying the skin, to avoid disruption by shear and friction of the laid skin
- It is important to ensure, in the lower limb, that the risk of 'foot drop' is prevented through splinting the foot in its anatomical position of function
- The splints must be well padded to exclude incidence of pressure ulcer development, especially on the heel
- The limb should be placed in the splint, elevated on a pillow, and the patient made comfortable prior to skin application
- Ongoing assessment of potential pressure points is essential – any reports of a burning feeling, or pain should be addressed immediately.

## 12. DISCHARGE INFORMATION AND EDUCATION

**Box 17.35** Patient information for the long-term protection of the donor and recipient site.

- STSGs that have been meshed will retain a lattice or diamond-shaped appearance (Figures 17.6 and 17.7)
- For most, this may last a lifetime, for a few the unevenness of the skin may resolve with varying degrees, but rarely, fully. The patient must understand this. Some attempts to reduce the effect have been attempted by the use of dermabrasion, laser therapy or compression pad and bandage techniques, but with limited success
- Skin care through wound bed management is important
- For a couple of months skin will have some numbness – it will take time to fade to a pale colour and for epidermis/dermis to strengthen and toughen
- The donor and grafted site should be protected from any secondary injury by avoiding rubbing, hot showers, heaters, sunlight (using factor 15+ UV protective cream) and cold extremes
- As instructed, the site should be washed daily with non-fragranced soap and warm (not hot) water and patted dry with a soft towel
- A hairdryer must not be used to dry the wound as this may cause fragile skin to burn
- Use simple non-fragranced moisturising creams frequently (e.g. Sorbolene, glycerin, aloe vera, vitamin E oil or cream) gently massaged (not rubbed) into grafted and donor sites (at least three times daily) and as necessary, if the skin is drying out easily
- Any sign of skin breakdown, particularly vesicles or blistering, should be reported immediately to reduce the development of ulceration and infection, particularly in the lower limb
- Wearing contoured foam support pads (shin protectors) during the day over any lower limb sites can protect against accidental bumping or abrasions

- Support bandages and stockings should be applied only as instructed by nursing staff or those charged with their application
- On the lower limb, support stockings must not be put on an affected limb unless an ankle brachial pressure index is first undertaken to assess arterial perfusion
- Inappropriate application of pressure garments may cause further vascular compromise in patients with doubtful circulation, leading to ischaemia, and potential for loss of a limb. Diabetes mellitus patients also fall into this category
- Support stockings must be removed at night on retiring to bed to allow for optimal arterial inflow and venous outflow in the recumbent position unless the patient is up regularly overnight
- In the presence of excessive scar development, the patient should seek plastic surgical advice as to the diagnosis and appropriate treatment
- The development of hypertrophic or keloid scars should not be considered normal unless proper medical advice is obtained and the condition confirmed as 'normal' for that individual patient.

---

**Review**

*Auditing preferred clinical and patient outcomes,* Chapter 2, Boxes 2.10–2.12.

---

## 13. FULL THICKNESS SKIN GRAFTS

Full thickness skin grafts (FTSGs) are composed of the epidermis and dermal layers that constitute the organ of the skin[1-7] (Figure 17.34).

They differ from 'composite' grafts, which consist of a tissue layer in addition to the skin. (Figures 17.46–17.48).

The donor skin is excised as a surgical procedure, with a surgical scalpel, and so they do not require specialised instruments for their harvesting and can be closed by primary suturing. Figure 17.1 shows the potential and common sites used.

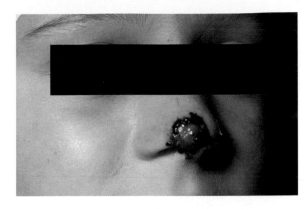

Figure 17.46 Composite graft 1 – day 2.

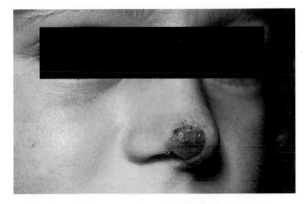

Figure 17.47 Composite graft 2 – day 5.

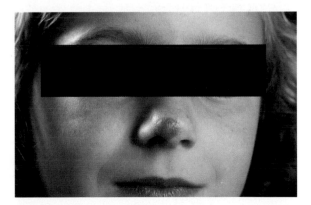

Figure 17.48 Composite graft 3 – day 24.

**Box 17.36** Basis on which the choice of donor sites for full thickness skin replacements is selected.

- Skin colour, tissue resemblance, or thickness that is required to be reflected at the recipient site (e.g. upper eye lid donor tissue for lower eyelid)
- Selecting a donor site that can be disguised by wearing of clothes, or behind, for example, the ear or in the groin
- The mobility of the donor site skin in order that primary closure of the donor site can be undertaken
- Eyebrows may be reconstructed by donor sites located in the scalp hairline, or by a tunnelled vascularised island flap based on the temporal vessels[2-5].

**Box 17.37** Function of FTSGs.

- FTSGs make excellent long-term grafts, as they contract the least of all skin grafts
- In children they will usually continue to grow with a child and they have excellent texture and pigment (skin colour) appearance
- FTSGs simulate normal skin that has not been injured, making them the ideal choice for skin replacement following burns scar contractures at the eyelids or the nose. However, because large areas often require grafting (e.g. the neck), they are unfortunately not always a practical solution (issues of re-establishing a viable blood supply)[1-7] and have largely been replaced by free flaps (Figure 17.15)
- FTSGs are harvested from sites according to the thickness required at the recipient site. An example is use of thin FTSG of the upper eyelid as a donor site to fill defects on lower eyelid (Figure 17.34)
- These defects maybe the result of congenital disorders, skin tumours, burns, or to correct drooping of the lower eyelid (e.g. ectropion, Figure 17.34), due to gravity of the ageing skin[1-7]
- Thick FTSGs are useful for restoring function and form to the nasal tip where cartilage is not missing and contraction from thinner STSGs may interfere with nasal function and particularly aesthetics. For example, the supraclavicular area of the neck with contains the 'blush' effect common to the face. This area is an excellent donor site for the face, particularly the nose, as the donor skin will blush in parallel with the face[1-7]

- Some surgeons use the crease of the wrist for a donor site to repair a defect on the hand following skin loss injury to a finger. This may have social implications as it may be wrongly assumed at some later stage that the person has attempted suicide
- The mobile skin on the lateral surface of the hand below the fifth finger and the elbow crease may also be used
- FTSGs may be used in severe cases of Dupuytren's contracture of the hand where Z-plasty is not possible and amputation of a finger/s may be considered
- FTSGs for this hand surgery are usually harvested from the groin or upper inner arm
- Immobilising hand splints are removed four to five days postoperatively and sutures left in for up to ten days
- Some surgeons will redress the hand 24 hours post surgery and apply flexible silicone or fixation sheet dressings and institute passive hand therapy immediately to reduce joint stiffness
- Flexible fixation sheet/retention dressings are usually applied after the splint is removed and hand therapists engaged to commence early rehabilitation, reducing the contraction
- FTSGs may also be used on the foot and usually combined with the use of local axial skin flaps
- The foot is an area with zones of constant shear and friction and varying degrees of shifting pressures. Nurse clinicians should educate the patient regarding protection of the flap and grafted zones
- Healing is a slow and fragile process because of the specialised blood supply
- Success may not be obvious for up to two weeks with desiccation of the thick epidermis occurring more than once
- Remobilisation is slow and the wound needs continuing protective covering and a programme of independence should be supervised by a physiotherapist.

# Wound bed repair and maintenance

## Box 17.38 Wound safety issues – FTSGs re-establishment of vascular pathway.

- The fundamental principles for skin graft take in FTSGs and composite grafts parallels STSGs and the absence of these is the main reason for failure of grafts to take[1-7]
- As with thin STSGs (in optimal conditions) the closer the proximity/interfacing of the FTSG donor skin vessels to the recipient bed vessels, the more reliable and quicker the potential for early revascularisation and take
- The potential for thick FTSG to take is high when the hypodermal fat has been completely excised from the dermal base, reducing the distance between donor and recipient site vessels
- Avascular fat cells can be a source of contamination and potential infection
- Nurse clinicians should exercise caution when removing primary dressings (usually tie-over), as revascularisation may be slow and the graft fragile
- Open wounds require daily hygiene care with normal saline and cotton buds, and Vaseline® regularly applied to wound edges to maintain suppleness.

## Box 17.39 Donor site wound bed repair and management.

- FTSG donor sites are usually closed by primary continuous sutures (e.g. absorbable or non-absorbable monofilament nylon) and heal as normal primary intention wounds[1-7]
- If donor sites are around the face (e.g. upper eyelid, behind the ear, side of the neck, joint creases) they will often be superficially healed in five to seven days but require longer for restoration of dermal strength
- The choice of a wound dressing for the donor site is based on the anatomical site, the age of the patient, size and site of the donor site, and any mobility required can be designed to meet the individual patient needs.

## Box 17.40 Wound comfort issues – pain.

- In the first 24 hours any expression of undue pain will potentially be due to haematoma or undue dressing compression within the wound causing ischaemia to underlying tissue[1-7] – this may result in loss of the graft
- Pain should be reported to the surgeon immediately as sutures may need to be removed
- After 48–72+ hours any ongoing pain is usually related to the early development of infection with the traditional clinical signs becoming evident.

## Box 17.41 General wound care.

- In addition to the donor and recipient site wounds, general nursing care issues of safety, comfort and independence, as discussed in Chapter 4, must be addressed
- Regardless of the wound site, basic general and local hygiene care of adjacent regions is extremely important
- Wounds on the face may require regular eye, nasal or oral care not only for the prevention of infection and hygiene, but to provide the patient with a sense of comfort, wellbeing, and professional attention to detail
- It also provides an opportunity to closely observe the wound's healing progress, or to identify early signs of potential adverse outcomes.

### Review

*Setting goals of care and preferred clinical and patient outcomes*, Chapter 2, Boxes 2.7–2.9. Adapt as appropriate to the patient's clinical needs.

*Auditing preferred clinical and patient outcomes*, Chapter 2, Boxes 2.10–2.12.

**Box 17.42** Vascular uptake of composite grafts.

- Composite grafts are so called because they are 'composed' of full thickness skin and cartilage[1-7]. These combine to restore both function and form in specific anatomical region, mainly on the face
- Composite grafts may also be harvested from the ear and used to replace lost skin and cartilage of the nose, to restore the structural form, function, contour and normal aesthetic appearance. In composite wounds on the nose, these are normally left exposed so as not to exert any pressure and for vascular observation
- The process of vascular uptake in these wounds is not well understood.

  Figure 17.46 = day 2, Figure 17.47 = day 5, Figure 17.48 = day 24.

- The complexity of the linkages and re-establishment of a normal blood flow remains largely theoretical, but it is suggested that the 'bridging' phenomenon is perhaps at work, with overall revascularisation being assisted by vessels at the edges of the donor wound joining up with vessels at the edge of the recipient wound
- Normal composite graft revascularisation is less reliable than STSGs, as the donor vessels and the recipient vessels may be 5–10mm apart, because of the thickness of the dermis, and uptake determined by the vascular status of the previously injured recipient vessels
- The first 48–72 hours appear to be critical, and with oedema present as in any other wound, this potentially increases the distance between donor and recipient vessels
- The external demonstrations of the haemodynamics of establishing a circulation in these wounds is likely to lead the nurse clinician charged with vascular observations to believe that failure to take is occurring, as areas of whiteness and blueness are evident up to 4–5+ days
- In the early phase the cyanotic discoloration may be also be observed in the graft due to thrombi within some of the microcirculation
- In the first 7–10 days, it is difficult to predict 'take' following composite grafts and it is often said that they look worse before they look better[1-7] (Figure 17.46 versus Figure 17.48)
- This phenomenon relates to the vascular uptake which is slower and various changes of colour are exhibited that move from a pale white to a blueness, before exhibiting the pinkness from within the new skin as desiccation of the avascular outer layers of epidermis and superficial dermis takes place.

## 14. COMPOSITE GRAFTS

The loss of composite tissue from, for example, the nose or the ear due to skin cancers, or trauma caused by burns, bites from dogs or humans, can be functionally and aesthetically unacceptable to the patient.

Reconstruction is frequently undertaken as a secondary procedure (elective) to avoid the problems of initial high levels of critical contamination and almost inevitable infection, associated with loss of blood supply and the high levels of bacteria living within the human and animal oral cavities[1-7].

The loss of cartilage at the nasal tip results in collapse of the columella, giving the appearance of a flat unaesthetic tip.

### *Clinical nursing management – composite grafts*

**Box 17.43** Clinical vascular observation.

- Postoperative nursing observation is as for normal vascular observations, and accurate descriptions and charting of colour and pain are important to predict progress
- In composite grafts, the thickness of the donor skin may obscure early blood supply establishment; arterial supply comes first, and venous second, explaining the early phenomena of blueness and swelling[1-7]
- If these wounds continue to remain white for more than four days, arterial compromise must be expected and regular progress reported to the surgeon
- If the graft remains blue and swollen, venous compromise must be suspected[1-7]
- No absolute judgement should be made about the viability of the graft until the first five to seven days have passed
- Connection of the blood vessels is often slow, unpredictable and obscured by the outer layers of normally avascular epidermal layers of the skin
- The failure to demonstrate any form of revascularisation by day 7 will mean the graft is usually lost but this may not be visually evident in the first instance and the waiting game is played out until take becomes evident or, conversely, the graft simply dislodges[1-7].

**Box 17.44** Composite grafting – wound bed management and repair – nursing management.

- Vaseline® or neomycin ointment should be reapplied regularly. This can be accomplished with a cotton bud as frequently as required, preventing dryness and the cracking of the donor graft and surrounding skin
- Desiccated tissue then collects around the circumference of the wound, is loose and may be gently removed
- By days 5–7, the outer epidermal layer may form a blister and desiccate (peel off) to reveal pink areas of new epidermis
- A failure of the graft to take will be demonstrated by an overall dry/dehydrated scab and will simply self-dislodge[1–7].

**Box 17.45** General nursing care.

- Nursing care of grafts to the nose also includes four-hourly gentle internal nasal toilets to maintain normal hygiene
- A nasal bolus to collect any exudate should be employed as long as any drip continues
- The nose is an extremely sensitive organ and the desire to touch, blow, sneeze, etc. is almost irresistible
- Clinicians must institute measures to protect the wound from pressure, shear and friction, day and night, and the patient or home carer can be guided in this process prior to discharge
- Donor sites, often from the ear lobe, are repaired by primary suture and usually dressed with a protective retention tape, or contouring acriflavine wool and crepe bandage – this is removed after 48 hours
- The patient should be educated not to lie on the donor ear compromising the blood supply to the donor site
- Healing of the donor site is in about five to seven days depending on the age of the patient
- Maintenance of moisturisation, post-suture removal and use of UV protective creams should be frequent and ongoing.

**Review**

*Setting goals of care and preferred clinical and patient outcomes*, Chapter 2, Boxes 2.7–2.9. Adapt as appropriate to the patient's clinical needs.
*Auditing preferred clinical and patient outcomes*, Chapter 2, Boxes 2.10–2.12.

**Box 17.46** Discharge management.

- Hot shower water running over the wound, or rubbing of the wounds after showering or bathing should be avoided to prevent secondary injury to the fragile tissue
- The application of Vaseline® should continue until the normal moisture returns to the wound and surrounding skin
- Wearing a hat, and applying UV protective creams whenever entering the outside environment are additional protective measures
- The use of hairdryers close to the wound must be avoided to prevent the new skin burning and drying out.

## 15. ENGINEERING SKIN TISSUE FOR WOUND BED REPAIR

Engineered skin tissues are of two principal types, those for temporary use and those for permanent application[1–7,9–12].

### Cultured human keratinocytes

This is non-bio-engineered epidermis that is grown in a scientifically devised culture medium that may take up to three weeks. Cultured epithelial grafts grown from the patient's own skin are only suitable for superficial and superficial partial thickness burn wounds and although their success rate is limited, they may save the patient's life by preventing recurring infection until more permanent measures can be instituted.

It is suggested that the lack of success of take may be due to lack of viable dermal structure and basement membrane zone for anchoring purposes. These grafts are only a few cells thick, and as such have very limited use for chronic wounds. They are easily damaged, so secondary injury and the development of wound ulcers are common.

In another area of research, the development of spray-on (aerosol) cultured keratinocytes has been used with excellent results in superficial/partial thickness scald burns on children, at the Burns Unit at Royal Perth Hospital, Western Australia (see http://www.clinicalcellculture.com/one/01_03_board.asp, for further information).

## Human allograft derived product

Bio-engineered (e.g. Alloderm® is processed allograft dermis). These products are engineered from human cadaver skin intended for permanent dermal transplanting. They undergo a special process to remove fibroblasts, endothelial cells and epidermis to exclude immune response. The resulting product is a cellular dermal collagen matrix which is immunologically inert, retains elastin, and has a basement membrane complex enabling it to sustain a STSG. The STSG is applied about three weeks or more after the primary procedure, when granulation tissue has grown into the dermal transplant and can support the STSG.

The Alloderm® product is freeze dried and reconstituted in the operating room prior to application. Some benefits have been demonstrated in post burn reconstructive surgery for severe burn scar contracture in the neck region, and it may be used instead of free flap reconstructive surgery in selected patients.

No benefits have been established in chronic wounds as no stimulation of the wound environment has been demonstrated that would provide/initiate tissue strength to assist in preventing against secondary injury.

## Human dermal replacement

Bio-engineered (e.g. Dermagraft-TC® – Apligraft® – TransCyte™). These are permanent dermal replacements cultivated from human diploid fibroblast cells on a three-dimensional polymer scaffold with fibroblast cells derived from foreskin following circumcision. Fibroblasts are important in the secretion of growth factors and matrix proteins for enabling STSG resurfacing and ultimately wound closure.

## Risk management in human tissue engineering

In the science of tissue engineering, one of the goals is to discover ways for humans to recreate the embryonic capacity for authentic tissue regeneration that exists in the unborn but ceases after birth, with the exception of, for example, the liver. No explanation has been forthcoming for this phenomenon, but some progress is being made in laboratories in relation to stem cell research.

The need to ensure patient safety and restore function that is combined with acceptable aesthetic results drives the research for tissue replacement products where the patient cannot be the donor[1–7,9–12]. Stem cell research holds some promise but is in its infancy. The distance between hypothesis and applied ethical practice remains very wide in most instances. In addition, immunological difficulties related to transplant remain largely unsolved but are increasingly better understood.

The current research into tissue engineering covers almost every tissue in the body, particularly skin, cartilage, tendon, vascular tissue and bone, towards the growth for replacement of whole organs.

Gene-based research is costly, complex and often very controversial, but in many instances may hold promise for extraordinary discoveries in tissue formation[1–7,9–12].

In modern science, the most significant issues in contemporary grafting from human to human or between human and animal species is that of rejection and the inheriting of conditions such as AIDS, hepatitis B,C, or D, autoimmune syndromes, or any unknown or atypical diseases or viruses that the donor may be carrying[1–8].

The search for scientifically developed tissue replacement (tissue engineering) free from any biological contamination, rejection or re-absorption problems, is one of the 21st Century's challenges in wound management[1–7,9–12].

## Contemporary progress in tissue engineering and application to patient care

As a replacement for severely damaged or irretrievably injured skin, there is no substitute for the patient's own skin, but in some instances, such is the extent of the overall injury (e.g. burns), that temporary or permanent substitutes are sought.

Historically, research into skin substitutes has focused on burns and lower limb ulcers and has been seen as useful to replace split skin grafts (which can present morbidity and problems of pain, infection, delayed healing, severe contractures, and poor aesthetic results)[1–7,9–12].

In plastic surgery, the treatment of burns victims has combined modern resuscitation measures with attempts to temporarily or permanently replace lost skin. This has led to limiting the degree and rate of infection, the main cause of extensive patient morbidity or death, and increasing the survival rate of extensively burnt patients[1–7,9–12]. It has also generated a continuing search for better substitute products to protect against infection but with lasting protective, functional and aesthetic properties.

The use of any skin other than that of the individual patient presents important ethical and immunological issues, for reasons previously mentioned. Cost is also a principal factor, limiting the use of many of these products and, in many institutions, a specific criterion for their use (e.g. no contemporary alternative) must be met before purchase is permitted. Nursing management parallels the care of skin graft recipient sites and the specific recommendations outlined by the manufacturers of each specialised product.

## The future

The contemporary science of skin tissue engineering is multifaceted, ranging from using the patient's own skin to grow sheets of epidermal layer skin replacement through to the development of dermal matrix or scaffolds to support epidermal cells, and to the areas of stem cell stimulation for the growth of new blood vessels that will assist in the epidermal resurfacing. The artificial growth of a dermal scaffold with attached epidermis that will integrate ('take') into the subcutaneous tissue of all patients, unhindered at all stages of repair, is one of the 'Holy Grails' of reconstructive plastic surgery[1–7,9–12].

See recommended websites (skin substitutes) following the references.

## References

(1) Kelton P.L. Skin grafts and skin substitutes. *Selected Readings in Plastic Surgery*, 1999; **9**(1):1–24.

(2) Aston S.J., Beasley R.W., Thorne C.N.M. *Grabb and Smith's plastic surgery*, 5th edn. New York: Lippincott & Raven Publishers, 1997.

(3) McCarthy J.G. (ed.) *Plastic surgery, volumes 1–8*. Philadelphia: W.B. Saunders, Harcourt Brace, 1990.

(4) Ausher B.M., Erikson E. & Wilkins E.G. *Plastic surgery: indications, operations and outcomes*. St Louis: Mosby, 2000.

(5) McGregor I.A. & McGregor A.D. *Fundamental techniques of plastic surgery and their surgical applications*, 9th edn. Edinburgh: Churchill Livingstone, 1995.

(6) Morris A. McG., Stevenson J.H. & Watson A.C.H. *Complications of plastic surgery*. London: Baillière Tindall, 1989.

(7) Peacock E.E. Jnr. *Wound repair*, 3rd edn. Philadelphia: W.B. Saunders, Harcourt Brace & Company, 1984.

(8) Goodman T.A. (ed.) *Core curriculum for plastic and reconstructive surgical nursing*, 2nd edn. Pitman N.J.: ASPSN, American Society of Plastic Surgery Nurses, 1996. http://www.aspsn.org/

(9) Hansen S.L., Voight D.W., Wiebelhaus P. & Paul C. Using skin replacement products to treat burns and wounds. CE Article, Advances in skin and wound care. *The Journal for Prevention and Healing*. 2001 (Jan/Feb); **14**(1):1–18.

(10) Miller M.J. & Patrick C.W. Tissue engineering. *Clinical Plastic Surgery, (USA)*, 2003 (Jan); **6**(1).131–4.

(11) Lindblad W.J. Wound healing, regenerative medicine and tissue engineering: a continuum. *Wound Repair and Regeneration*, 2002 (Nov–Dec); **10**(6):345.

(12) Patrick C.W. Tissue engineering strategies for adipose tissue repair. *Anatomical Record*, 2001 (Aug); **263**(4):361–6.

(13) Banwell P., Withey S. & Holten I. The use of negative pressure to promote healing. *British Journal of Plastic Surgery*, 1998; **51**(1):79–81.

(14) Thomas S. An introduction to vacuum assisted closure. 2001.http://www.worldwidewounds.com/2001/may/Thomas/Vacuum-Assisted-Closure.html

(15) Greer S.E., Duthie E. & Cartolino B. Techniques for applying subatmospheric pressure in wounds in difficult regions of the anatomy. *Journal of Wound Ostomy*, 1999 (Sept); **26**(5):250–3.

(16) Mullner T., Mrkonjic L., Kwasny O. & Vecsei V. The use of negative pressure to promote the healing of tissue defects: a clinical trial using the vacuum sealing technique. *British Journal of Plastic Surgery*, 1997; **50**(3):194–9.

(17) Genecov D.G., Schneider A.M., Morykwas M.J., Parker D., White A.L. & Argenta L.C. A controlled subatmospheric pressure dressing increases the rate of donor site

re-epithelialisation. *Annals of Plastic Surgery*, 1998 (March); **40**(3):219–25.

(18) Flanagan M. *Wound management*. New York: Churchill Livingstone, 1997.

(19) Dealey C. *The care of wounds*, 2nd edn. Oxford, UK: Blackwell Science, 1999.

(20) Guyton A.C. & Hall J.E. *Textbook of medical physiology*, 9th edn. London: W.B. Saunders, 1996.

(21) Bowler P.G., Duerden B.I. & Armstrong D.G. Wound microbiology and associated approaches to wound management. *Clinical Microbiology Reviews*, 2001 (Apr): 244–69.

(22) Cohen M., Giladi M., Mayo A. & Shafir R. The granu-lometer – a pocket scale for the assessment of wound healing. *Annals of Plastic Surgery*, 1998 (Jun); **40**(6):64[1–5].

(23) Snyder R.J., Doyle H. & Delbridge T. Applying split thickness skin grafts: a step by step clinical guide and nursing implications. *Ostomy Wound Management*, 2001 (Nov); **47**(11):20–6.

(24) Fowler A. Split thickness skin donor sites. *Journal of Wound Care*, 1998 (Sept); **7**(8):399–402.

(25) Dahlstrom K.K. A new silicone rubber dressing used as a temporary dressing before delayed split skin graft-ing. *Scandinavian Journal of Plastic and Reconstructive Hand Surgery*, 1995; **29**:543–5.

(26) Wolf Y., Kalsih E., Badani E., Friedman N. & Hauben D.J. Rubber foam and staples: do they secure skin grafts? A model analysis and proposal of pressure enhancement techniques. *Annals of Plastic Surgery*, 1998 (Feb); **40**(2):149–55.

(27) Bodenham D.C. & Watson R. The early ambulation of patients with lower limb grafts. *British Journal of Plastic Surgery*, 1971; **24**(1):20–2.

(28) Wallenberg L. Effect of early mobilisation after skin grafting to lower limbs. *Scandinavian Journal of Plastic and Reconstructive Surgery and Hand Surgery*, 1999 (Dec); **33**(4):411–13.

## Recommended websites

**Harvesting of split skin graft**

http://www.surgical-tutor.org.uk/default-home. htm?core/trauma/skin_grafts.htm~right

**Skin substitutes information**

http://www.burnsurvivor.com/skin_substitutes.html

http://www.burnsurvivor.com/resources_articles_ culturedskin.html

http://www.clinicaltrials.gov/ct/gui/show/ NCT00004413

# Chapter 18

# Microsurgery

## Background

The term **microsurgery** defines a surgical technique that involves micro dissection and micro manipulation of particular body tissues. Microsurgery is undertaken using a high-powered electronic microscope. This provides greater levels of magnification, or enlargement, than the naked eye can see (Figure 1.6). With this level of magnification, specialised instrumentation is required to accommodate the type of microsurgery being undertaken. The origins of these instruments are based on traditional jewellers' forceps, used to repair fine watches.

Microsurgery is an essential part of almost every branch of modern surgery. For instance, most areas of reconstructive plastic surgery, vascular surgery, neurosurgery, surgery to the inner ear, eye surgery, and some areas of gynaecological surgery could not be undertaken without the use of a microscope to magnify blood vessels, nerves and microscopic tubular tissues[1-6].

The term microsurgery may also be used to describe the surgical repair of both larger nerves and blood vessels, using custom designed surgical loupes. These are reading-type glasses fitted with special 2–8 times normal magnified lens. Many plastic surgeons wear loupes as a routine for most delicate surgical, and particularly paediatric reconstructive procedures.

In reconstructive plastic surgery, microsurgery may be undertaken to repair injured nerves (post trauma) and/or blood vessels, or as part of an elective reconstructive procedure[1-6].

## Microsurgery – clinical applications

Although the term **microvascular** strictly refers to the portion of the vascular system that is composed of the capillary network, it is applied to surgery of small arterial and venous vessels.

Some areas of reconstructive surgery require a complex approach with microsurgery as a method that:

- Facilitates the transfer of skin and other tissues from one region to another with vessels attached (free flaps)
- Facilitates an approach that allows injured tissue to be repaired using existing and remaining viable tissue at the site of the injury (cut vessels and nerves).

Any surgical situation that requires movement or repair of nerves and vessels may potentially require magnification in order that these anatomical components may be seen in their injured/uninjured true state[1-7].

Some variations on the theme of microsurgery are used. Whilst microsurgery as reconstructive surgery may be concerned with both nerves and blood vessels, 'reconstruction' may not always contain both. For example, free flap breast reconstruction may be described as microvascular. That is, it is concerned with a reconstructive procedure where blood vessels only are joined using a microscope.

Microsurgical techniques can provide other advantages. Neurovascular surgery island flaps are common forms of surgery in the hand to replace lost sensory skin to vital fingertips such as the index and thumb (Figure 19.9).

The flap is transferred from one side of an adjacent finger intact, that is, not separated from its neurovascular base, and tunnelled under the hand skin to its new destination. Perhaps not truly microsurgery, nonetheless micro-dissection and micro-manipulation of the tissues is often undertaken using a microscope to ensure that vital structures are not injured during the dissection.

Muscle (containing vessels and associated nerve) or single nerves may be harvested and used as a free flap muscle transfer to reconstruct the face following disease (parotid tumours, acoustic neuroma or severe facial trauma), where the facial nerve has been injured or removed. Innervated muscle can provide a degree of contour restoration, but results can vary greatly. This procedure is more commonly done in units that specialise in this type of reconstructive surgery.

Depending on the size and length of nerve required, nerves (micro nerve grafts) may be harvested from particular sites in the body which are minimally exposed to direct injury, or sight, for example the back of the leg (sural) or anterior forearm. These nerves are then used, for example, to repair a major nerve in the face, arm or hand where

injury or disease has resulted in loss of some part of the nerve itself.

As nerves are stated to restore their function at the rate of approximately 1 mm per day, the outcomes can be quite unrewarding. For example, if all the nerves are cut at the wrist, the chance of having a

---

**Box 18.1** Risk management issues in microsurgery.

- Microsurgery related to small vessels is not without risk and problems (Virchow's Triad)
- Injury to blood vessels whether intentional or unintentional may lead to:
  - Infarcts or thrombosis
  - Vessel 'spasm' (causing the cessation of blood flow). This is a reaction that may occur when the wall of an arterial vessel is 'injured' during the normal process of surgery, as a result of trauma, undue pressure, or degrees of accidental vessel kinking[1-7]
- These responses are all well recognised in circulatory physiology. How to avoid their occurrence, or restore normal and continuing flow, is a challenge for all microvascular surgeons undertaking reconstructive procedures
- Surgeons agree that the greater the level of tissue manipulation, the smaller the vessel, and the greater the tension at the suture line of the blood vessel, the greater the risk of thrombus formation and arterial spasm
- The use of anticoagulation therapy (e.g. Dextran, heparin, aspirin, fibrinolytic agents) in the prevention of thrombus formation remains controversial, but continues to be used prophylactically
- Multiple reports confirm the use of medicinal leeches in attempting to salvage a failing flap that has venous compromise
- Microsurgery for nerve repair may result in a highly sensitive and painful neuroma at the site of anastomosis
- Further surgery may be required, or nerve desensitising programmes by hand therapists to assist in correcting the problem.

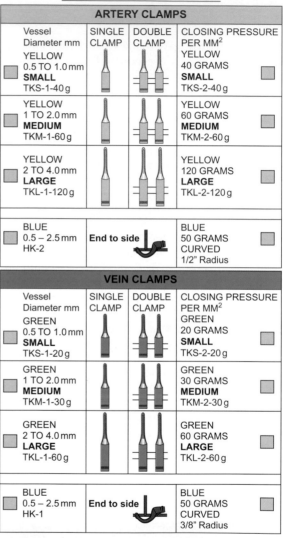

**Single use Bear vessel clamps**

| ARTERY CLAMPS | | | |
|---|---|---|---|
| Vessel Diameter mm | SINGLE CLAMP | DOUBLE CLAMP | CLOSING PRESSURE PER MM² |
| YELLOW 0.5 TO 1.0 mm **SMALL** TKS-1-40 g | | | YELLOW 40 GRAMS **SMALL** TKS-2-40 g |
| YELLOW 1 TO 2.0 mm **MEDIUM** TKM-1-60 g | | | YELLOW 60 GRAMS **MEDIUM** TKM-2-60 g |
| YELLOW 2 TO 4.0 mm **LARGE** TKL-1-120 g | | | YELLOW 120 GRAMS **LARGE** TKL-2-120 g |
| BLUE 0.5 – 2.5 mm HK-2 | **End to side** | | BLUE 50 GRAMS CURVED 1/2" Radius |

| VEIN CLAMPS | | | |
|---|---|---|---|
| Vessel Diameter mm | SINGLE CLAMP | DOUBLE CLAMP | CLOSING PRESSURE PER MM² |
| GREEN 0.5 TO 1.0 mm **SMALL** TKS-1-20 g | | | GREEN 20 GRAMS **SMALL** TKS-2-20 g |
| GREEN 1 TO 2.0 mm **MEDIUM** TKM-1-30 g | | | GREEN 30 GRAMS **MEDIUM** TKM-2-30 g |
| GREEN 2 TO 4.0 mm **LARGE** TKL-1-60 g | | | GREEN 60 GRAMS **LARGE** TKL-2-60 g |
| BLUE 0.5 – 2.5 mm HK-1 | **End to side** | | BLUE 50 GRAMS CURVED 3/8" Radius |

**Figure 18.1** Microvascular clips for anastomosis of vessels; end to end; end to side (AROSurgical® Bear™ vessel clamps) – see full range of specialised instrumentation (website: http://arosurgical.com/products.htm).

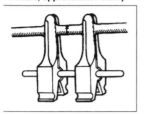
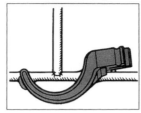

**End to end anastomosis with a double, approximator clamp**

**End to side anastomosis with an end to side clamp**

**Figure 18.2** Macro demonstration of end to end, and end to side anastomosis.

viable functioning hand is almost zero as the flexor tendons and blood vessels will also certainly be involved. As stated previously, the blood supply to the body is circulatory with a collateral backup system, the nervous system is not circulatory and as such lacks this structural/functional advantage.

## General principles of microsurgery and microvascular surgery

As previously stated, specialised instruments based on those used by jewellers for fine work in watch repairs, have been designed, and are essential to manipulate and minimise injury to fine tissues.

This also allows for the use of specialised sutures in sizes that range in size from 7–12 microns that are required to match the range of vessels and nerve sizes for repair. The use of these sutures requires various levels of magnification for accurate manipulation. The size of the sutures and instrumentation available is proportional to the size of the fine vessels

that can be repaired, such as the microscopic repair of very small arteries, and fine capillary vessels[1-7].

Specialised microvascular clips with specific pressures are designed to 'clamp' off vessels of various sizes. This provides the least injury to the vessel when it is clamped and whilst anastomosis is being undertaken. The two techniques of vessel anastomosis are end to end and end to side. It is suggested that end to side anastomosis presents the least risk of complications[1-7] (Figures 18.1 and 18.2).

## References

(1) Tittle B.J., English J.M. & Hodges P.L. Microsurgery: free tissue transfer and replantation. *Selected Readings in Plastic Surgery*, 1993 (Jan); **7**(11):1–31.
(2) Kayser M.R. Surgical flaps. *Selected Readings in Plastic Surgery*, 1999; **9**(2):1–63.
(3) Aston S.J., Beasley R.W. & Thorne C.N.M. *Grabb and Smith's plastic surgery*, 5th edn. New York: Lippincott & Raven Publishers, 1997.
(4) McCarthy J.G. (ed.) *Plastic surgery, volumes 1–8*. Philadelphia: W.B. Saunders, Harcourt Brace, 1990.
(5) Ausher B.M., Erikson E. & Wilkins E.G. *Plastic surgery: indications, operations and outcomes*. St Louis: Mosby, 2000.
(6) Ruberg R.L. & Smith D.J. *Plastic surgery: a core curriculum*. St. Louis: Mosby. 1994.
(7) Morris A. McG. Stevenson J.H. & Watson A.C.H. *Complications of plastic surgery*. London: Baillière Tindall, 1989.

## Recommended website

**Demonstration of microsurgical clamps, instrumentation, sutures and anastomotic repair**
http://www.arosurgical.com/products.htm

# Chapter 19

# Reconstructive Skin and Soft Tissue Flaps

**Review**

Chapter 5, Chapter 7, including: Figure 7.1, *principal wound closure options* and Figure 7.2, *general advantages and disadvantages of principal wound closure options*, Chapter 15.

The survival of any flap is largely predetermined by three factors, excluding patient health status:

- The planning process
- The vascular and mechanical capacity of the donor tissue to remain viable
- The efficiency of the early monitoring process that alerts the team to adverse vascular events.

Flaps have principally been defined as local or distant, but such is the scientific advancement in the understanding of the functional microcirculation of the blood supply to the skin, these terms have been further classified (Figure 19.1).

## Background

Tissues (e.g. skin, fascia, muscle, bone) that are congenitally malformed, traumatised, or have a benign or malignant tumour that cannot be corrected with simple forms of treatment modalities, may be considered for surgery that requires the movement of other suitable tissues as a replacement[1–11].

Ongoing research into the micro blood supply to the skin, and its primary and secondary sources, has provided a greater understanding of blood flow structure and flow throughout the whole skin architecture. This research, based on functional anatomy and identification of vascular patterns has allowed an increasing diversity of single tissues, and combinations of tissues to be transferred, to provide a wide range of options for reconstructive purposes.

## Flap definitions

A **flap**, as distinct from a **skin graft**, is defined as any form of tissue that can be successfully transplanted or transferred to a local of distant site of the body whilst retaining its own blood supply (arterial, venous and capillary) at all stages of its transfer. It may, or may not, have a scientifically identifiable source of its blood supply[1–8].

**Box 19.1** Classification of flaps.

Flaps can be classified according to:

**Method of movement**

- Local, within close approximation to the recipient site
- Distant, the donor flap is placed on a distant recipient site:
  - Donor flap raised and located on a distant recipient site – relies on vascular uptake at the recipient site (Figures 1.5 & 19.8)
  - Remains attached to the donor site with vessels intact – axial pattern
  - Is cut free from its blood supply, transferred to a distant site and attached to recipient vessels – a free flap.

**Blood supply**[1–8]

- Random, undefined blood supply
- Axial, designed on a pre-existing known arterial or venous source
- Free, is cut free from its blood supply, transferred to a distant site and attached to recipient vessels.

**Composition** (skin, fasciocutaneous, skin and fascia, muscle, myocutaneous, muscle and skin, free flaps).

No classification is totally adequate and there may be an overlap, so combinations are often used.

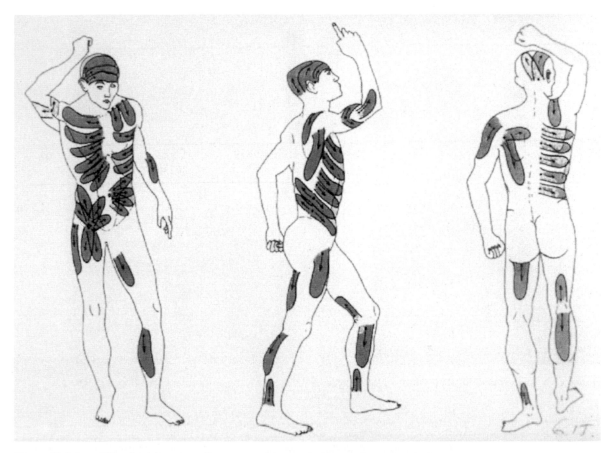

**Figure 19.1** Example of axial pattern flap sites. With permission: Professor G.I. Taylor.

## Method of movement

**Box 19.2** Method of movement – local skin flaps.

Elevated from the tissues in the immediate vicinity of the primary defect

- Random flaps may be used on most parts of the body but with major dimensional restrictions (breadth : length ratio), related to the random nature of their blood supply
- Local flaps are described as 'rotation', 'transposition' or 'advancement', relating to the manner the flap is required to be moved into the (defect) recipient site
  - Advancement flap – moves directly into the defect without lateral movement (Figures 19.2 & 19.3)
  - Transposition flap – moves laterally into the defect creating a secondary defect – primarily repaired (Figures 19.4–19.6).
  - Rotation flap – moves in a circular direction directly into the defect – secondary defect may require skin graft (Figure 17.4).

The above three local flap types are commonly seen on the face, but may be used to cover defects (for example) on the hand, foot, anterior surface of the tibia, or sacrum.

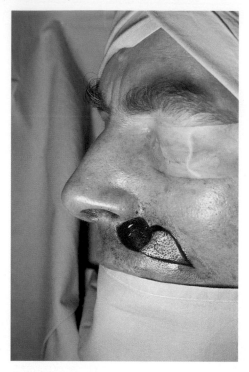

**Figure 19.2** Post removal of skin lesion.

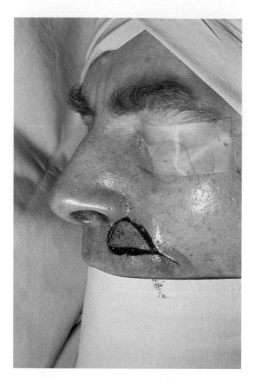

**Figure 19.3** Advancement skin flap for closure.

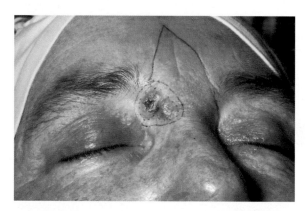

**Figure 19.4** Basal cell carcinoma in the glabella region with flap closure design.

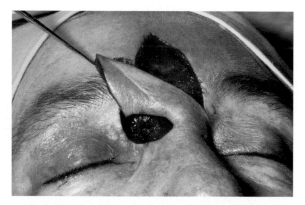

**Figure 19.5** Excision of lesion and rotation of flap.

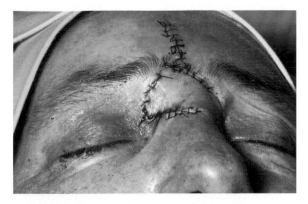

**Figure 19.6** Flap and direct donor site closure.

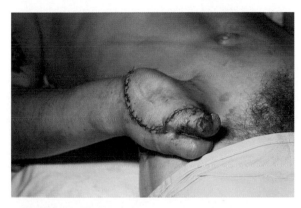

**Figure 19.7** Abdominal flap to the hand (blood supply remains in the donor flap until uptake at approximately 21 days – staged procedure) – donor site skin grafted.

**Box 19.3** Method of movement – distant flaps – axial pattern.

A **distant flap** remains attached to the donor site. It is disconnected when vascular connection is deemed to have been established at approximately 2–3 weeks
Examples:

- A skin-based groin flap elevated attached to the hand (Figure 19.7)
- A flap raised from one leg and placed on the opposite to protect the tibia – cross-leg flap (Figure 19.8) (Skin grafts are required to replace elevated skin). These procedures are less common since the evolution of, for example, axial pattern and free flaps, but they still have a place in some cases or societies where microvascular surgery is difficult to undertake
- May also be used for example, forehead to nose (forehead rhinoplasty – see Chapter 30)
- Deltopectoral tissue flap to the jaw
- Small tube pedicles made from surrounding local skin, including tissue expansion, are used in ear reconstruction to create the rim of the ear (Figure 19.10). These require division and setting into recipient site at approximately 2–3 weeks after initial movement – any excess skin is discarded.

**Axial pattern flap** – for example, skin raised on its vascular territory (identifiable artery and vein) left attached at the donor site, and located intact to an adjacent region.
**Special flaps**, e.g. neurovascular island flap (Figure 19.9).

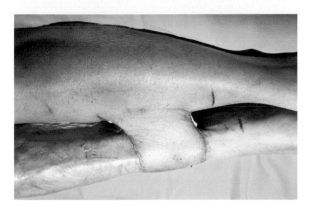

**Figure 19.8** Cross leg flap (blood supply remains in the donor flap until uptake at approximately 21 days – staged procedure) – donor skin raised from undersurface of opposite leg to protect compound injury of the tibia – donor site skin grafted.

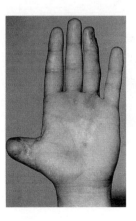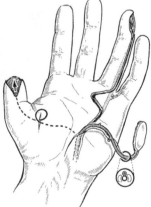

**Figure 19.9** Neurovascular island flap – ring finger to thumb providing reconstruction and innervation for protection from injury – donor site skin grafted.

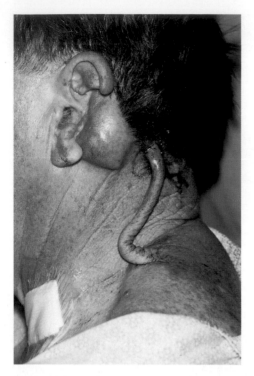

**Figure 19.10** Ear reconstruction using tissue expander and local tissue tubed pedicle for rim contour.

**Box 19.4** – Method of movement – distant flaps – free flaps.

- Free flaps are skin/tissues harvested with donor vessels remaining attached to the donor tissue but are cut or 'freed' from their original site
- The vessels that support the donor tissue mean blood flow is temporarily interrupted, and re-established by joining the donor vessels through microsurgical techniques to appropriately selected vessels, at a wound defect site, distant from the original harvested region (see Chapter 18).
  - A radial forearm flap transferred to the lower limb (Figure 19.13)
  - Groin flap to the lower leg (Figure 19.14)
  - Groin flap to severe hand injury (Figure 19.20)
  - Breast reconstruction following malignancy (Figure 19.21)
  - Muscle flap with areas of skin, but requiring STSG to remaining muscle, as muscle size was too larger for the source vessels to support an equal amount of skin
  - Specialised compound tissue flaps for the treatment of lymphoedema (Figure 1.7)[1–8].

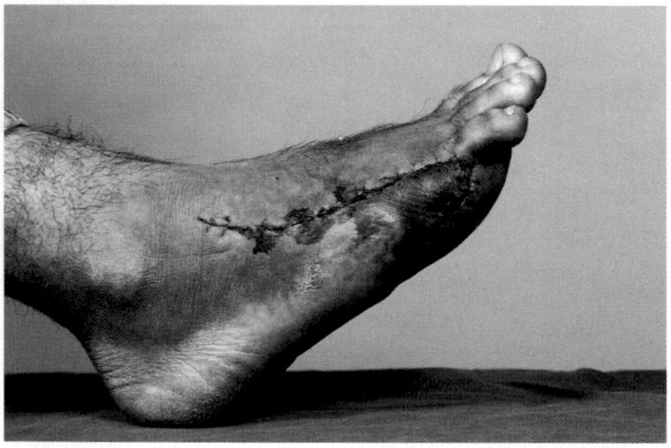

**Figure 19.11** Shearing injury to the lateral side of the right foot – loss of distal zone due to inadequate understanding of the angiosome concept relating to specific vascular territories of the body's skin.

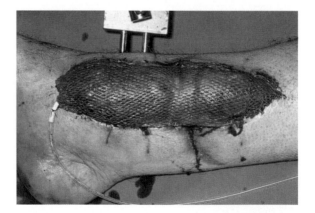

**Figure 19.12** Compound fracture of tibia – gastrocnemius muscle rotated to protect bone – meshed STSG for muscle protection – temporary internal negative pressure drainage system to drain dead space left by muscle transfer.

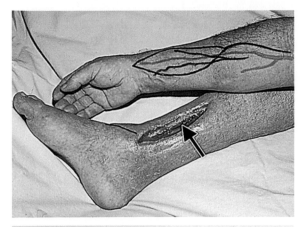

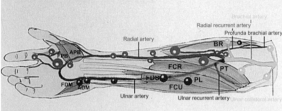

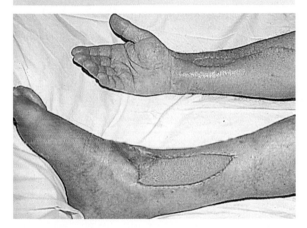

**Figure 19.13** Free vascularised radial forearm flap to foot – demonstrating vascular anatomy – state-of-the-art technique – eliminates staging. With permission: Professor G.I. Taylor.

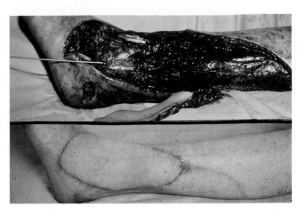

**Figure 19.14** Latissimus dorsi muscle with attached skin to reconstruct compound injury of the foot.

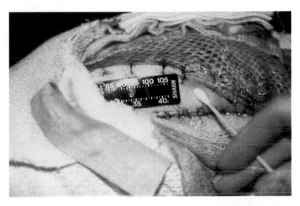

**Figure 19.15** Compound free vascularised groin muscle flap to compound fracture of the femur – skin paddle for monitoring techniques.

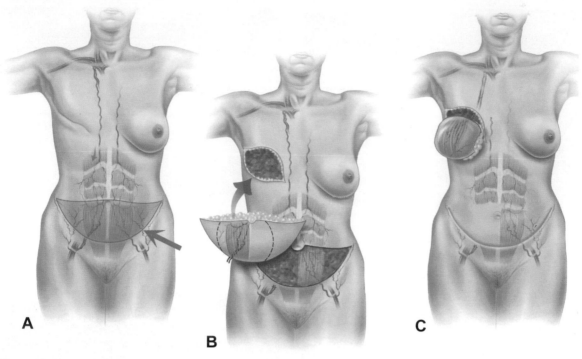

**A**

**B**

**C**

**Figure 19.16** Illustrative representation – TRAM flap. With permission: Professor G.I. Taylor.

## Classification according to blood supply

**Box 19.5** Defining flaps by the source of their blood supply.

- 'Random' pattern skin flaps are so called because the small blood vessels are not specifically identified[1-7]
  - As such, blood vessels are stated to be 'randomly' distributed within the skin or so small as to be unidentifiable
  - With modern research and better understanding of the micro blood supply to the skin, and identifiable patterns of distribution, major surgery such cross leg flaps, abdominal flaps to the hand, and tubed pedicles are less frequently used (Figures 1.3, 1.5 and 19.7–19.10).
- Figure 19.11 demonstrates a lack of understanding of the random nature of the blood supply to the lateral side of the foot. The shearing type laceration has stripped the cutaneous blood vessels from the fascia and the distal portion has died. This required debridement, skin graft and a substantial time in hospital
- 'Axial' pattern flaps are so called because their specific blood supply (artery, vein, lymphatics) can be identified, remain attached to their source, and are moved on an arc or an axis, to an adjacent site (e.g. latissimus dorsi muscle flap rotated/tunnelled under the skin of the axilla for use in breast reconstruction)
- Research has allowed both axial and free flaps to be developed with greater flexibility in width and length, with increased ability for flaps to survive[1-7] (Figures 5.5, 19.1 & 19.12 – gastrocnemius muscle split and one half rotated to cover compound fracture of the tibia and fibula – skin graft to muscle)
- Free flap transfer is a specialised technique where the vascular pedicle is cut (freed) from its host vessels and the skin/tissue and vessels are relocated and attached by microsurgical techniques to the pre-identified recipient bed host vessels.
  - May be a single tissue (skin) or composed of more than one – see Box 19.6
  - 'Free' flap transfer is based on the axial flap concept – source vessel and anatomical/vascular territory is responsible for is identified and the extent of the distribution understood allowing for larger sized tissue flaps to be used – (e.g. radial (artery) forearm flap, Figure 19.13).

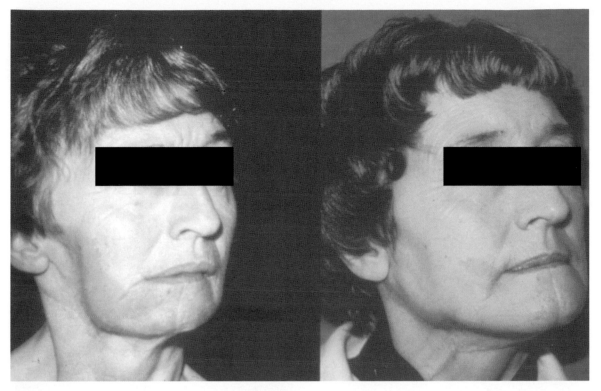

**Figure 19.17** Free vascularised bone graft (fibula) for jaw reconstruction – before and after surgery for tumour removal.

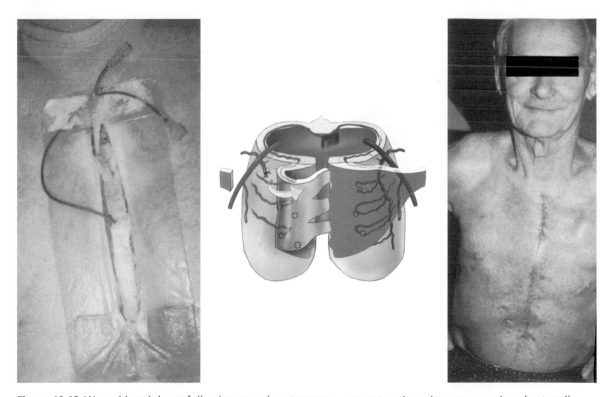

**Figure 19.18** Wound breakdown following open heart surgery – reconstructive microsurgery using chest wall muscle flaps allowing primary skin closure to protect the chest contents.

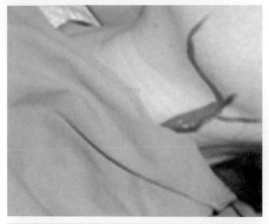

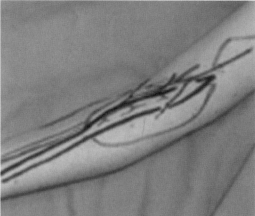

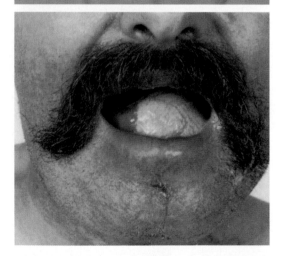

**Figure 19.19** Innervated radial forearm flap used to reconstruct the tongue following partial glossectomy for removal of malignancy.

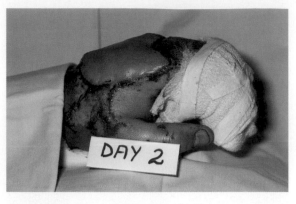

**Figure 19.20** Free vascularised groin flap to compound injury of the hand – demonstrates excellent vascular perfusion at day 2 post surgery.

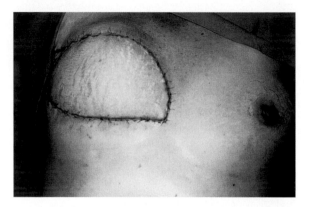

**Figure 19.21** Immediate trans rectus abdominis muscle (TRAM) flap to the breast with prosthesis inserted for volume – (post mastectomy reconstruction – nipple reconstruction undertaken as a secondary procedure).

## Classification according to composition

### Box 19.6 Tissue composition of flaps.

**Single tissue flaps** – examples:

- Cutaneous (skin) flap – composed of full thickness skin and the superficial fascia (e.g. forehead flap to the nose (Figures 19.4–19.6))
- Muscle – transfer of muscle for bulk without skin (e.g. to the breast, or used to bring a blood supply to bone with compromised blood supply and loss of soft tissue and skin such as observed in major compound fractures in the limbs (Figure 19.12)).

**Composite flaps** – free flaps are composed of more than one layer of tissue, for example:

- Fasciocutaneous – skin, superficial and deep fascia – radial forearm flap to lower leg (Figure 19.13)
- Myocutaneous = muscle including deep and superficial fascial layers to skin layer – examples:
  - Latissimus dorsi muscle including skin, transfer to the lower limb (Figure 19.14)
  - Transverse rectus abdominis muscle (TRAM) used for major compound injury to lower limb – small zone of skin remains for skin and temperature flap monitoring (Figure 19.15)
  - Transverse rectus abdominis muscle (TRAM), used for breast reconstruction – all skin used – (Figure 19.16).
- Osseocutaneous – bone, muscle and fascial layers to skin layer
- Osseous – bone with pedicle blood supply via muscle (e.g. contoured bone replacement to reconstruct the jaw – free fibula transfer (Figure 19.17), other donor sites (e.g. the hip, rib, ulnar or fibula).

**Free flaps designed to meet specialised wound needs:**

- Figure 1.10 – latissimus dorsi muscle transfer to close dehisced chest wall
- Figure 19.18 – pectoral muscles transferred to close dehisced chest wall
- Figure 19.19 – radial forearm flap to reconstruct a defect left following excision of cancer of the tongue.

**Specialised composite tissue** – sensory = skin with nerve and vessels (e.g. neurovascular island flap transferred from the inside of one finger to a defect in another – to the areas of critical need for sensory perception, for example, the finger tips – Figure 19.9)[1–7].

### Box 19.7 Clinical operational definitions.

- The wound zone to be reconstructed is called the primary defect
- The wound zone from which the flap is harvested is called the secondary defect
- Reconstructing the primary defect with a harvested flap is called insetting
- The pedicle is the vessels which are attached to the donor flap – may be described for either local or distant flaps
- The proximal end of any flap is at its base where vessels enter and are at their largest
- The distal end is the furthermost point from the base or proximal end of the flap where the vessels are at their smallest
- The central portion/point between the distal and proximal ends meet is called the 'bridge' segment, an important region where vascular problems may occur as vessels begin to branch off in various directions, and decrease in size[1–7].

### Box 19.8 Principal risk issues to be addressed that may affect outcomes.

- As for any form of medical/surgical intervention, major flap surgery will require an intensive, well organised, interdisciplinary approach, and a model of care which all team members (i.e. surgeon/s, nurse clinicians, dietician, physiotherapist, occupational therapist, counsellors) can call upon as appropriate to provide specific input, have a stated role, and a collective responsibility[1–29]
- Excellence in planning, as a process, has been clearly demonstrated to influence optimal interim clinical and patient goals, and preferred clinical and patient outcomes
- Any failure to address actual or potential clinical/patient risk factors pre-, peri-, and postoperatively, or to set nursing observation and wound goals and outcomes, can lead to loss of part or the whole of the flap
- Regardless of the size or perceived simplicity of a flap, best practice vascular observation and reporting practices are essential to identify any complications of the specific flap

*Continued*

- Detailed wound care planning from the preoperative to rehabilitation phase is critical to ensure that immediate and surrounding tissues are protected[1-29]
- A donor flap may create an additional wound, both donor and recipient sites have the same potential for failure as any wound for the same principal reasons (already discussed in Chapter 8).

See recommended websites (tissue flaps) at the end of this chapter.

# Surgical selection of reconstructive procedures

**Box 19.9** Principal rationale for the selection and application of a flap type.

| | |
|---|---|
| **Protective** | protecting exposed tissues from further trauma and opportunistic organisms |
| **Corrective** | correcting tissue defects and contour abnormalities |
| **Restorative** | restoring functional requirements and overall aesthetics |
| **Palliative** | providing a tissue and/or skin cover that offers comfort and aesthetics. |

For all wound defects, in deciding the reconstructive procedure to be undertaken, the regional extent, depth, and degree of anatomical and functional injury, disease or congenital malformation will be considered. The available anatomical and functional tissue options will be reviewed to determine how the best protective, functional, and aesthetic outcomes can be achieved.

When faced with complex trauma-based tissue defects, reconstructive plastic surgeons may use temporary methods (e.g. skin grafts, vacuum pressure therapy for wound protection/healing, or choose from a range of reconstructive flap options to parallel the particular needs of the wound at the specific time of presentation. These surgical options are referred to as the 'reconstructive ladder'[1-5] (Figure 7.1). This is a dynamic tool that provides step-by-step wound repair options. More than one step, or procedure, may be combined with another to achieve

wound closure. Figure 19.15 shows muscle flap with skin paddle for vascular observation, plus skin graft to protect the muscle.

**Box 19.10** Principal questions asked to determine surgical procedure.

- The medical status of the patient
- Is this a lifesaving procedure, limb salvage surgery, elective surgery, or palliative management?
- Potential for long-term survival of the patient
- What tissues are/will be missing (e.g. skin, fascia and muscle, muscle and bone)?
- What tissues are available?
- What clinical medical and nursing morbidity and co-morbidity would be created in moving the desired tissues for wound coverage?
- What secondary or tertiary procedures will be required at a later date, if any?

**Box 19.11** Flap success – principal events.

**The presence of:**

- Wound bed assessment – the identification of the most appropriate procedure for the specific wound
- Wound bed preparation – removal of the physiological and psychosocial impediments that may lead to adverse events and outcomes
- The overall surgical planning process (use of risk management process from assessment to rehabilitation) – a multidisciplinary approach considered to be essential for optimal clinical and patient outcomes
- Pre-emptive risk assessment, application of processes that address timely recognition of correction of potential adverse physiological and psychological events
- The timely recognition and correction of adverse episodes
- A team approach, including specialist nursing
- A high quality of nursing care provided to the patient and the wounds
- The ability for the patient to co-operate wherever possible, at all stages from pre-operative to rehabilitation.

**The absence of:**

- Adverse internal clinical factors (e.g. hypovolaemia, hypothermia, haematoma, wound tension – kinking of the pedicle particularly at the proximal end, pres-

sure from within the wound tissue such as oedema or haematoma, exertion of pressure on the vascular pedicle)
- Adverse external clinical factors (e.g. pressure on the wound causing exertion of pressure on the vascular pedicle) that may lead immediate flap failure[1-8]
- Known issues of potential sleep deprivation, anxiety, depression.

---

**Box 19.12** Flap failure – principal surgical events.

- Inadequate preoperative patient assessment, including identification of congenital vascular anomalies, blood clotting problems
- Failure to address primary clinical and patient risk management issues (e.g. smoking, nutrition)
- Poor patient selection by the surgeon (e.g. high incidence of failure in patients with previous injury at the recipient site (scar tissue and vascular rearrangements), those who smoke, patients with poor commitment to success including rehabilitation)
- Poor specific planning of the procedure
- Inadequate technical competence.

---

**Review**

*Perioperative management of adults and children,* Chapters 15 and 16.

---

**Box 19.13** Principal immediate postoperative physiological reasons stated for flap failure.

- **Physiological**
  - Hypovolaemia – inadequately controlled management of circulatory fluid balance in the operating theatre and clinical surgical unit
  - Hypothermia – inadequately controlled management of normothermia in the operating theatre and clinical surgical unit

- Failure of early identification of adverse vascular events that allows timely correction
- Failure to maintain ongoing pain control.
- **Mechanical** disturbances:
  - Vessel kinking due to swelling or position of patient/flap
  - Vessel spasm
  - Arterial or venous obstructions
  - Vessel and/or flap tension (due to flap too small for the site, oedema, haematoma).
- Inadequate set parameters for monitoring and reporting protocols that reflect best practice available
- Lack of specialist nurses competent in advanced nursing practices that include a high level of vascular observation, analytic and reporting skills
- Unresolved haematoma leading to wound infection[1-8].

---

# Clinical nursing risk management and setting clinical nursing outcomes

**Box 19.14** Principal preoperative clinical and patient needs – nursing.

- Preoperative assessment
- Addressing nursing morbidity and co-morbidity identifying core clinical issues
- Addressing clinical nursing risk management
- Developing clinical and patient goals for stages of management
- Establishing best practice monitoring and reporting tools
- Developing and auditing clinical nursing outcomes.

---

## Patient handover – post anaesthesia care unit to surgical unit

A full patient and procedural handover by the surgeon, anaesthetist and post anaesthesia care unit staff is indispensable if nurse clinicians in the surgical unit are to understand the nature, extent, and degree of patient care that may be needed for basic or complex procedures, including highly dependent acute care patients, and critically ill patients.

Wherever possible it is helpful for the surgical unit staff can actually see part of the surgical procedure, in order to appreciate the postoperative requirements.

---

**Box 19.15** Principal postoperative information required – post anaesthesia care unit to surgical unit.

- Full explanation of the procedure, including any adverse events intra-operatively
- Information regarding the procedure that includes a check with the surgical and nursing team regarding the potential for complications, to determine whether specific or additional observations and reporting mechanisms are required[10–19]
- Description of any anticipated adverse events related to the procedure
- An audit of any respiratory assistance (tracheostomy), nasogastric tubes, percutaneous endoscopic gastrostomy (PEG), and urinary catheter[20–23]
- An audit of all 'invasive' lines providing perfusion monitoring status, pain management, thermal monitoring, adjunctive flap monitoring
- Review of the documented objective and clinical observations, overall physiological status of the patient and flap and monitoring devices in place, particularly those applied to measure flap perfusion, flap and patient hypothermia, patients circulatory status and hypovolaemia[10–19]
- A check of the operation notes to establish what type of anastomosis has been undertaken and the number of veins used and which part of the flap is the proximal end and which is the distal end
- The pain management protocols which have been arranged to provide patient safety, comfort and independence
- Antibiotic therapy, antiembolic therapy
- The number and location of wounds[28]
- A final critical and complete assessment of the patient, and completeness of medical guidelines by the receiving clinician, in order to be satisfied that a safe transfer of the patient to the receiving unit is not at risk.

---

# Clinical nursing management – the surgical unit

**Box 19.16** Patient and flap safety.

- Pressure relieving beds should be considered essential following major reconstructive surgery until the patient is mobile
- Preparation of the receiving environment, including ambient room temperature control
- Temporary postoperative placement in the high dependence unit or intensive care unit (ICU)
- For patients with multiple major wounds (for example, combined chest wall and abdomen, upper and lower limbs), prolonged procedures, or unavailability of appropriate specialist nursing care in the surgical unit, the range of patient risks and physiological dependency may be better addressed by placement of the patient in the ICU for the first 48 hours[1–7,9 29]
- This may be necessary following reconstructive procedures for major trauma, and major head and neck reconstruction, where tracheostomy is used, and the patient's general condition is unstable
- With the complexity of the procedure, multitude of surgical sites, length of the time for the operative procedure, and general surgical 'assault', the patient's cardiorespiratory, renal perfusion or pain status must not be compromised, as any disturbances of the major life support systems will ultimately compromise the flap
- For the first 48–72 hours, regular and objective vascular inspection of the flap by specialist nurses with expertise in flap monitoring and reconstructive surgical wound management may be required. This may necessitate the presence of a specialist nurse coming from the plastic surgery unit to undertake such observations
- Protective frames must be used to protect the flap from wound pressure related to potential blanket loading attempting to restore/maintain body temperature
- In nursing care of major flaps, one of the most complicating factors in general patient care is the issue of sleep deprivation suffered by patients in the first 72–96 hours, where life support systems, pain management, vascular observation, wound care, and general patient care are constantly in progress
- This results in psychological anxiety, mental confusion, and an inability to co-operate in nursing and physiotherapy activities that protect the patient from life-threatening complications such as deep vein thrombosis (leading to pulmonary embolism), chest

infections, nutritional deficits, a range of wound complications, and development of pressure ulcers that can lead to local and systemic infections

- In the first 72–96 hours, it is critical that unless adverse events are occurring, observations and treatments should be undertaken as a collective set of tasks at the same time
- Constant prodding, probing, touching, dressing inspections, and unnecessary noise around the patient are to be avoided
- The patient must be cared for separately to other patients to ensure that general environmental disturbances are limited
- Where possible, strictly prescribed periods of rest for the patient should be part of the overall plan of postoperative recovery in the first few days, and longer if required
- Some patients respond well to low-dose (i.e. 2.5–5 mg) diazepam three times daily, or similar, for the first 72 96 hours to reduce anxiety and general muscle tension, and this also allows for some prescribed periods of rest
- Night sedation should also be considered. Pharmacologically titrated, this can also assist in reducing the amount of narcotics required.

---

**Box 19.17** Patient comfort.

- Whilst pain management is an essential component of patient management, signs of overdose of narcotics should be observed for
- Respiratory difficulties, low oxygen saturation, remarks such as 'ants crawling on the skin', and constant scratching of the skin, are usually an indication that excessive narcotic particularly morphine, is being administered
- As stated previously, in the essential need for optimal pain management, adjunctive medications or alternative therapies may need to be administered/applied, and the use of medications such as diazepam may significantly reduce the amount of narcotics required.

---

**Box 19.18** Patient independence.

- When the patient's general condition and flap have stabilised, the planned rehabilitation phase should be reappraised and instituted as appropriate
- Social integration into multiple patient units can be an important transition from the isolation of a single room, and psychologically indicate a positive step upwards towards recovery
- Psychosocial care must remain paramount throughout the recovery process, and patients should be given every opportunity to discuss all areas of their care, their feelings about any complications, and impediments to overall recovery
- Where the recovery is unimpeded, the patient will respond to positive reinforcement by staff, for their commitment to co-operation throughout the experience
- Psychologists may be required in counselling sessions where patients and/or carers express anger, grief or despair at any adverse events that:
  - Reflect congenital, traumatic or disease-based conditions that are potentially life threatening
  - Significantly alter body image
  - Diminish the patient's quality of life
- Patients and significant carers ought be offered appropriate counselling, and alerted to community assistance that may be available.

---

## Monitoring and observing flaps

As outlined in Boxes 19.1–19.6, it is clear that all tissue flaps are not the same, because flaps present for nursing care in many various forms. This may present issues in monitoring protocols, although principally there are more similarities than differences. These are discussed in this section.

For specialist nurse clinicians the three fundamental practice principles are:

- A basic understanding of the principal source and pathway of the blood supply to the skin
- An understanding of how this knowledge influences monitoring principles
- A basic understanding of the physiological and mechanical reasons for interruption of, or total obstruction of, blood flow.

## Non-buried and buried flaps

For further ease in describing and monitoring, random, axial and free flaps can also be:

- Non-buried flaps – exposed primary tissue layer (e.g. fasciocutaneous – skin, and some axial-based muscle flaps – muscle)
- Muscle partially buried but has skin paddle for monitoring (e.g. musculocutaneous)
- Buried flaps (e.g. some muscle flaps).

## Best practice monitoring practices

Best practice vascular assessment is based on:

- Current accepted objective monitoring techniques
- Skilled methods of interpretation to flag early adverse events
- Timely reporting procedures
- Interventions that reverse or minimise adverse events.

Unfortunately, there are often ambiguous and mixed signs presented by a flap. This can pose interpreting difficulties for the nurse clinician in deciding whether what is observed is indeed a problem, and more importantly, worthy of reporting.

At present there are no stated empirical (exact scientific/objective) guidelines on which clinical monitoring can be based to provide an independent response to the status of a flap, at a given time[1–7,10,11,14–19]. What is available is essentially skilled discretionary judgement (an inexact scientific conclusion) assisted by technical aids. For example, dermal pricking with an 18 or 23G hypodermic needle remains the gold standard for determining the vascular status of a flap with a skin paddle[1–7,10,11,14–19].

The salvage of a failing non-buried (i.e. fasciocutaneous) or a buried flap (e.g. muscle), although primarily difficult with the naked eye, is stated to directly relate to the early identification of an emerging microvascular problem. This intense relationship between an arising vascular problem, and timing of a salvage procedure, has accelerated the search for methods that can alert clinicians at the earliest point to any emerging microvascular complication[1–7,10,11,14–19].

Nonetheless, the range of traditional monitoring techniques, outlined in this section, remain as sup-porting guiding principles and modalities to provide assistance in the difficult analytical decisions that need to be made. These decisions are made in relation to the timing of attempts to salvage inadequately functioning flaps by removal of sutures, re-exploration of the anastomosis and vessels, or removal of thrombotic plugs blocking circulatory flow.

### Non-buried flaps – monitoring

In non-buried flaps, plastic surgeons may vary in their choices by single or collective methods including adjunctive (probes) flap monitoring (see Boxes 19.19–19.34).

### Buried flaps – monitoring

Buried flaps (e.g. muscle) that do not have an external skin paddle for monitoring purposes present major problems for early recognition of vascular compromise. This is because there are two layers of tissue for the microvasculature to pass through, and exposed muscle dies slowly (Figure 5.7).

#### Flap salvage issues

It has been demonstrated that flap salvage rate can be as low as zero, particularly where a 'skin paddle' (attached to the muscle, as in a myocutaneous flap (Figure 19.15)) is not available for observation.

Alternatively, with skin paddles available, an inadequate blood flow (to the skin paddle) may see the skin alone begin to necrose and some dryness of the surrounding muscle. This usually requires debridement of the necrosed skin and the exposed muscle to be skin grafted, to avoid infection.

One research group has indicated that the use of an implantable Doppler probe can provide a salvage rate of significantly higher levels[19].

#### Adjunctive vascular monitoring

Some units have demonstrated the advantages of, for example, advanced laser Doppler flow monitoring meters/probes, or transcutaneous oxygen monitoring, as basic observation tools, but there is no scientific consensus on their use, with other units suggesting the use of a combination of observation tools.

It is suggested that the use of Doppler probes must be tempered with the knowledge that the image provided is a reflection of larger vessel perfusion and not micro perfusion, and may give a false positive at tissue level. Nonetheless, research has indicated that, with combined techniques and highly competent clinicians assessing the data, salvage rates can be high.

Substantial research has been, and continues to be, undertaken to find a cost effective objective process that meets the criteria of reliable and repeatable research processes, and methods that provide early warning systems are emerging as technically assisted monitoring of the microvascular system becomes more refined[1–7,14–19].

It has also heightened the level of research to eliminate or minimise, wherever possible, the mechanical reasons for vessel reactions to injury that include increasing tension on the vessels, regardless of the cause (e.g. venous thrombosis, vessel spasm).

---

**Box 19.19** Flap monitoring techniques – requirements.

- Safe and simple to undertake
- Not cause secondary injury to the flap
- Represent results that are reproducible by each person undertaking the monitoring procedure, using the same techniques
- The results must be able to produce outcomes that confirm the reliability of the analysis
- Should only be conducted by clinicians who have been educated in advanced nursing practice, the specifics of the monitoring procedures, rationales for use, and independent discretionary judgement and interpretation of results.

---

**Box 19.20** General principles of flap monitoring.

- Adoption of an objective monitoring process
- The earlier the problems are identified, the better the outcomes[1–7,14–19]
- Primary flap observation goals must be criterion referenced for early identification of adverse event/potential complications, if optimal outcomes are to be realised
- Consider adopting a common unit-based strategic plan, based on a 3–4 tiered assessment protocol, and supported by criterion referenced numerical scales, similar to pain management documentation
- Collected data would be analysed and utilised as a primary or secondary reporting system
- Colour coding of, for example, red, blue and black to identify the concerns of the nurse clinician, may then be applied
- Any doubt in the nurse clinician's mind can be solved by collecting the documentation on the overall physiological patient status, including the flap, and phoning the surgeon for advice and directives, whatever the hour
- Mechanical aids should only be applied as an adjunct to the critical observations of wound pain, tissue colour, capillary refill (where possible), wound swelling, dermal bleeding
- Set timing for monitoring
- An agreed timing of monitoring should be established based on the existing research regarding flap survival times
- In the initial stages, some important applied clinical research has demonstrated hourly monitoring for the first 72 hours as preferable with a downgrading of the timing in optimal conditions[17]:
  - Half to one-hourly for the first 72 hours
  - Then two-hourly for the following 12 hours (84 hours post surgery)
  - Then three to four-hourly for following 12 hours (96 hours post surgery)
  - Then as surgically stipulated.
- Documentation should be via a graph/chart to clearly demonstrate an impending adverse incident, or a changing pattern of flap perfusion that may lead to an adverse event
- Subjective language that may allow for ambiguity of interpretation (e.g. such terms as 'good', 'poor' or 'inadequate') should be avoided
- Reporting parameters can be set to provide an early warning system for addressing a flap in potential eminent danger of failure
- Monitoring process must reflect the evidence that suggests that the earlier the identification of problems of vascular perfusion, the better the results of flap salvage.

**Box 19.21** Flap monitoring 1 – available techniques.

Vascular monitoring techniques can generally be divided into three pathways[1–7,14–19].

| | |
|---|---|
| **Objective** | invasive – internal monitor probes, dermal pricking |
| **Semi-objective** | non-invasive – observation, increasing flap tension, pain, colour and temperature – may include dermal pricking |
| **Combination** | utilising subjective and a selected invasive probe |

- Semi-invasive dermal bleeding is the single most accurate and reliable[1]
- Colour, capillary blanching, and flap temperature only, is the least reliable[1]
- Because of cost and lack of universal availability of technical adjuncts, clinical observational evidence plus dermal pricking remains the gold standard.

**Box 19.22** Flap monitoring 2 – technical – adjunctive.

| | |
|---|---|
| **Instrument-based methods** | (objective): temperature probes, transcutaneous gas, pH probe, laser Doppler with an intermittent or continuous readout, pulse oximeter, photoplethysmography. For many surgical units the initial costs, recurring/replacement costs of probes, and maintenance of some specialised equipment, are prohibitive, and their efficacy not adequately proven to justify the expense |
| **Chemical tests** | IV fluorescein (objective) – look for viable tissue under ultraviolet light, dye persists for 48 hours, not easily repeatable |
| **Radioisotope clearance** | (objective) – expensive, invasive and non repeatable. |

**Box 19.23** Essential clinical equipment to achieve positive monitoring.

- Good lighting is essential (same type each time)
- Lighting should not deliver heat as this may burn the flap skin
- Objective total management patient/flap-based monitoring chart (i.e. for free flap, use critical care type charting that includes general patient perfusion, respiratory measurements, renal function, pain status, flap vascular perfusion, and nutritional intake)
- Sterile swab sticks or cotton buds to exert gentle pressure on the flap to test for capillary return (Figure 19.15)
- Number 18 or 23-gauge sterile hypodermic needles for dermal pinpricking to assess the colour of the blood exudate indicating perfusion status
- Skin temperature probe, optional (Figure 19.15) – adhesive type – useful but not reliable
- Dressing tray with suture removing scissors in case sutures require immediate/emergency removal.

**Box 19.24** Principal colour definitions utilised in flap monitoring.

Surface skin colour

| | |
|---|---|
| **Pink** | normal (Figures 19.15, 19.21 & 19.24) |
| **Red** | normal – some early degree of venous congestion – early sign – (Figures 19.20 & 19.24) |
| **White, pallor** | arterial insufficiency (Figures 19.22 & 19.23) |
| **Blue, purple, mottled** | venous insufficiency (Figures 19.22 & 19.23) |
| **Black** | necrosis – zones of flap demise (Figures 19.22 & 19.23) |

Capillary refill = time taken for capillaries to refill following pressure being exerted on the skin – pressure should be soft – firm pressure takes longer giving false positive result.

| | |
|---|---|
| **Arterial** | normal = 1–3 seconds |
| **Venous** | normal = 3–5 seconds (unreliable tests) |

- Flap temperature – surface temperature of skin at flap site – (normally 36–36.4°C) usually described as warm or cool to cold – unreliable test

- Tenseness of the flap tissue, on a continuum from soft to firm to very firm
- Dermal bleeding – colour of blood exuding following pricking of skin with sterile 18 or 23 G needle, for example:
  - Red/pink blood indicates arterial efficacy
  - Dark blue blood (loss of oxygen) venous congestion, particularly in the presence of increasing swelling.

Only a surgeon should undertake the dermal pricking technique, unless the nurse is clinically instructed to do so, and understands the implications of the exuding blood colour.

---

**Box 19.25** Random pattern flaps – principal causes of failure.

---

- The risk of arterial complications is minimal when local random flaps are used, the principal vessels are not cut, tissues are gently handled, and the flap is sutured into place without tension
- Arterial complications that occur may be due to increasing tension within the wound caused by haematoma, oedema, or the tension placed during insetting
- Spontaneous arterial infarcts or spasm[1-7]
- Principal causes of random flap failure are:
  - Mechanical tension on the flap (flap too tight – no margin for error in planning – inflammatory oedema further adding to flap tightness)
  - Kinking of the flap[1-7].

Flap rescue – the removal of sutures will usually resolve the problem, but leave a defect. This may require:

- Four-hourly normal saline dressings covered with an occlusive film dressing
- Moist wound therapy dressings
- Potential debridement, secondary suture, or a skin graft, if the defect does not close as the swelling resolves.

---

**Box 19.26** Clinical monitoring process.

---

**Arterial perfusion:**

- Use a cotton bud to test vascular response in normal surrounding skin

- Use a sterile cotton bud to test vascular response in the flap
- Emerging flap failure is demonstrated by an acute phase (within 48 hours)
- Viability or failure of the flap determined within 1–2 days.

**A healthy random pattern flap:**

- Pink
- Blanches on gentle pressure
- Returns to pink colour as quickly as in the surrounding skin – 1–3 seconds (arterial sufficiency)
- Warm to touch
- Soft texture
- No tension (tension is a common cause of flap failure, particularly at the distal end)
- Swelling is within normal limits expected as for inflammatory response (venous efficiency).

**Arterial insufficiency:**

- Pain usually sharp
- Capillary return greater than five seconds, signifies arterial insufficiency
- Colour pale and becomes white
- Flap feels cool – loss of warm arterial blood
- Blanching becoming increasingly less distinct – increasing loss of arterial flow
- Finally, flap becomes dehydrated – flat – colour black[1-7].

**Venous perfusion:**

- Normal venous return is approximately 1 second – referred to as brisk.

**Venous insufficiency:**

- Flap skin acutely swollen, congested, cyanosed with increasing tension (venous congestion suggested by mottled purple/blue colour, plus oedema related to the inflammatory process) increasing dull and throbbing pain
- Dermal pricking indicates dark blue (deoxygenated) blood
- Tissue becomes shiny due to swelling and tension – blistering may appear
- Demarcation line (point at which circulation begins and ends) of vascular insufficiency becomes clearer
- Flap may be warm or cool – loss of warm arterial blood
- Pain reduced as swelling resolves
- Signs of necrosis become evident – colour moves from mottled purple/blue to black, indicating necrosis and flap demise[1-7].

**Box 19.27** Axial pattern flaps – monitoring process.

Differences in vascular response from random pattern flaps:

- The difference in the circulatory dynamics of random and axial pattern flap types is different and strikingly shown in the skin colour of each[5]
- The healthy axial pattern flap shows extreme pallor for several days with virtually no circulation apparent/demonstrated in the skin
- Difficult to distinguish vascular viability in this time by use of cotton bud pressure but monitoring should not cease – all clinical indicators of vascularity require documentation for up to five days
- Circulatory compromise often caused by kinking of the vessels and pressure of internal oedema caused by normal inflammatory process – suture removal may be required
- Elevation of the part for venous return important
- Area of concern is where circulation appears sluggish – usually in the centre of the flap
- Main area of potential necrosis is the central zone clinically demonstrated by an early cyanotic island emerging
- Circulation to other areas of the flap may be assisted by revascularisation from the surrounding tissues at the flap margins
- The first 72 hours are the critical period of potential vascular compromise – flaps that survive the first 48 hours will usually do well but monitoring should not lapse
- Axial pattern flaps that require re-exploration due to vascular compromise demonstrate mixed recovery[1-7].

**Box 19.28** Exposed muscle flaps axial pattern and free vascular transfer – monitoring process.

- Avascular muscle flaps
- Exposed muscle flaps (axial or free vascular transfer) die slowly due to their complex circulatory distribution
- Indicators include increasing dryness of the muscle and darkening of the muscle colour
- Applied skin grafts also become dry and do not take
- There is an increasing darkness in the colour blue, and signs of dehydrating tissue and finally, muscle death[1-7].

## Free vascularised flap transfer

The accepted statistical average of free flap failure is approximately 5–10%[1-7,10,11,14-19]. The percentage is suggested to be lower if the flap is 'delayed' prior to the main procedure.

Figures 19.17–19.19 demonstrate how buried flaps can be successful, despite the inability to monitor ongoing vascular status. Figures 19.20 and 19.21 display blood flow that is excellent, adequate at dermal level. Figures 19.22 and 19.23 are basic diagrammatic representations to assist in understanding how non-buried free flaps can, and do, fail. These

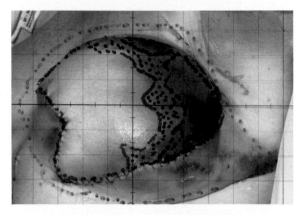

**Figure 19.22** Diagrammatic representation – increasing potential problems of blood flow in flap as it reaches the distal zone. From Teaching Notes, Jill E. Storch.

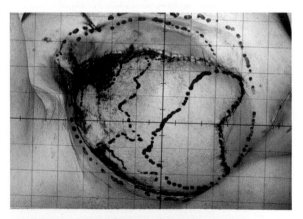

**Figure 19.23** Free TRAM flap demonstrating recovered zones of vascular perfusion in relation to Figure 19.22. Adapted from Teaching Notes, Jill E. Storch.

figures utilise colour to demonstrate how blood supply that is initially sufficient and slowly compromised is externally displayed in the skin at both the proximal and distal zones of the flap.

See markings over the tissue zones in a non-buried flap (Figures 19.22 & 19.23) outlining the viable zones versus the compromised zones at a particular given time. The black point is the distal end of the flap.

The message here is that in flaps that have exposed skin, firstly dermal bleeding and secondly skin colour are the primary clinical indicators of the tissues blood flow at the superficial or deep facial source levels (Figures 5.6–5.8).

See recommended websites (free flaps and flap monitoring) at the end of this chapter.

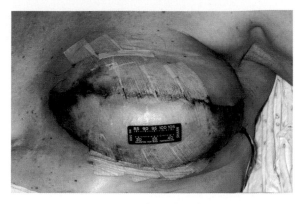

**Figure 19.24** Free TRAM flap to breast demonstrating avascular zones at both lateral zones.

---

**Box 19.29** Free flaps – physiological issues – arterial flow 1.

Based on the concept and principles of Virchow's Triad

- Despite all attempts to prepare the patient and the modern understanding of the blood supply to the skin, flaps can still fail[1–9,14–19]
- Arteries are high flow vessels and the organism's survival depends on the continuity of circulatory flow
- Continuing arterial pressure and flow problems do not bode well for the survival of the flap cells, which need oxygen to function any blood stored in the veins will thrombose
- Small bleeding arteries/arterioles, attempt, where possible, to clot, reduce blood loss and redirect the flow
- If the vessel is medium to large in size, and the normal intrinsic measures to halt the bleeding are inadequate, the patient will either continue to bleed (a haematoma will develop) or exsanguinate
- In general, arterial complications, particularly in free flaps, frequently occur directly following the anastomosis in the operating room, or the postoperative recovery room, and are dealt with immediately
- 'Vasospasm' is the term given to the reaction of vessel walls to injury (especially arteries) where the spasm (an involuntary muscle contraction (safety response) resulting in collapse of the vessel) causing blood flow to cease, may be the major issue
- This may result in the development of multiple emboli develop in smaller vessels, temporarily or permanently.

---

**Box 19.30** Free flaps – physiological issues – arterial flow 2.

- Postoperatively, disturbances in arterial flow are related to, for example, vessel kinking, or problems such as disturbances within clotting mechanisms, general hypovolaemia causing insufficient arterial volume, pressure and flow or hypothermia causing peripheral vasoconstriction[1–7]
- With the potential for increased blood viscosity due to hypovolaemia, a decrease is desirable to minimise thrombosis – some units accept maintenance of a haemoglobin level of 10 g or haematocrit of 30, as optimal to reduce the potential for thrombosis, but this is only acceptable in the presence of normovolaemia[1–7]
- In free flap transfer of tissue, the division of an artery and its subsequent microsurgical anastomosis to a distant artery can initiate the normal vascular injury response, and cause clotting complications that can often determine the success or failure of the flap[1–7]
- In reattaching arterial vessels, many surgeons often undertake 'end to side' arterial anastomosis of vessels (like a 'T' rather than vessel 'end to end') (Figure 18.2)[1–7]
- This type of anastomosis is suggested to reduce the risk of vessel leakage, arterial spasm or clotting problems, which are commonly seen to occur with the end to end technique

*Continued*

- The numbers of arterial complications that occur in the postoperative surgical unit are stated to be minimal[1-7]
- Any technical difficulty encountered intra-operatively, or in the first four to six hours postoperatively, is usually arterial, and can often be corrected immediately as the patient may not have left the surgical suite[1-7]. This should not discount the fact that venous problems may also occur, as the most critical time for a vascular crisis is in the first six to eight hours postoperatively[1-7,14-19]
- The minimisation/prevention of vessel injury is very important, as arteries are extremely susceptible to emboli and vessel spasm, when even minimal injury is inflicted
- Any vascular issues that occur prior to discharge from the operating suite must be considered fundamental to flap survival, and prior knowledge of this by nurse clinicians in the surgical unit can heighten sensitivity to the importance of specific postoperative vascular monitoring needs
- Pre-emptive use of, for example, IV Dextran, or unforeseen disturbances in arterial and venous flow, may require pharmacological control with use of anti-clotting agents to dissolve the clot, or surgical intervention to remove it
- Bleeding within the wound tissues (arterioles or capillaries) caused by, for example, increases in postoperative blood pressure, leaking from the anastomoses, or inappropriate elevation of the operation site, can create a haematoma and/or oedema and swelling under the flap. This will cause wound tension and increasing pressure on the important micro vessels and peripheral nerves.

---

**Box 19.31** Free flaps – arterial compromise – clinical assessment.

**Arterial compromise:**

- Arterial obstruction is initially demonstrated by a white/pale colour (absence of oxygenated blood) of the wound/wound edges, and particularly the distal portion
- Pain is sharp, unrelieved by narcotic analgesia and unresponsive to lowering of the part below the level of the heart (where possible) to increase arterial blood flow[1-9,17-22]
- Normal parameters for capillary return is within two to three seconds. If capillary return is more than three seconds (5+), this indicates inadequate arterial flow
- Brief compression to assess capillary return should be consistent in its application and the instrument used (e.g. a cotton bud), as the instrument and degree of compression exerted can produce different results
- In darkly pigmented skinned people this test is of little value, except pink zones of the toe and fingernails
- Wound may feel cool due to lack of warm arterial inflow – not a reliable indicator
- Flap temperature, + or – is the threshold set by surgeon for reporting (normally 36°C–36.4°C). Coolness of the flap can suggest potentially poor arterial perfusion and increased temperature, implies potential venous compromise, but these are not considered reliable indicators
- The reporting timeframe here is exceedingly vital in rescuing a flap from avascular necrosis, and tissue death, as the maximum ischaemia time allowed is usually not in excess of six hours
- Time is of the essence, as after 12 hours (following anastomosis) of ischaemia, the rescue of a failing flap is, more often than not, irreversible[1-7,10,11,14-19].

---

**Box 19.32** Reperfusion injury.

Stated to be the result of restored arterial pressure and volume following cessation for short or intermittent periods of time:

- When blood flow is inadequate cell function is slowed, or stopped, and waste products accumulate
- This material is catapulted into the partially injured and normal tissues, causing cellular metabolic disturbances and the potential for death of tissues and ultimately part of, or the entire, flap
- With multiple injury reperfusion, cytotoxic material is also released into the circulation
- Large amounts of circulating lactic acid can be detrimental to cardiac rhythms[1-7].

**Box 19.33** Free flaps – physiological issues – venous flow.

**Venous compromise:**

- Principally, most postoperative flap complications are said to be venous and the common cause is thrombosis (particularly in free flaps)[1–7,10,11,14–19]
- These mainly occur in the postoperative phase, late in the recovery room, or back in the surgical unit
- As most vascular problems are venous, in some selected flaps the practice of using two veins as a backup precaution may be undertaken in some
- This is a surgical choice and will relate to individual flap procedures, and specific risks associated with the perceived survival of the flap
- Internal pressure on the anastomosis, or inappropriate positioning of the flap, may cause kinking of the vascular pedicle, leading to spasm and inadequate arterial inflow and/or venous outflow
- Venous complications frequently require the patient to return to the operating theatre for removal of the obstructing thrombosis/clot
- Flaps that require re-exploration due to vascular compromise demonstrate mixed recovery
- Patients who require repeated major surgery may become increasingly physiologically compromised (hypovolaemia, hypothermic) nutritionally deficient, sleep deprived, anxious/depressed and, as a result, less co-operative or self-caring
- Psychological reinforcement and reassurance is important at all stages of nursing care and this is heightened when the potential for flap failure becomes evident to the patient[1,7].

**Box 19.34** Venous compromise – clinical assessment.

- Wound/wound edges are dark blue (loss of haemoglobin in the blood)
- Wound is swollen
- Pain dull and throbbing, which may be temporarily relieved by narcotic analgesia (but this is short term)
- Colour remains unchanged by elevating the limb (fails to respond to gravitational assistance) and swelling may further increase if there is arterial inflow, but venous thrombosis is total
- The wound may feel warm as there is some arterial flow in, but again no venous escape is possible

- Capillary return is less than three seconds (–1) and is referred to as 'brisk' = venous obstruction
- Brief compression over a small zone of the wound, to assess capillary return, should be consistent in its application, including the instrument used, as the degree of pressure exerted can produce different results (in dark-skinned people this test is of little value)
- Engorged flaps due to venous obstruction demonstrate little or no blanching due to inability to compress vessels, which may be deep within the wound structure[1–9]
- Blistering usually occurs as fluid leaks out into the germinal epidermal layer due to underlying pressure
- The use of medical leeches in venous compromise is often seen as a last resort to salvage at least part of the flap, but success is very limited
- Use of medical leeches could be instituted early, or as a first resort in free flaps that have the potential for, or demonstrate early venous difficulties (see Chapter 21, Bitten ear, Case Study and Figure 21.10)[8]
- Figures 19.22 and 19.23 demonstrate complex vascular problems in a free TRAM flap to the breast, as opposed to Figure 19.21.

## Comfort

**Box 19.35** Pain management – effects on vascular monitoring.

- Following major flap surgery, the patient will require an IV narcotic infusion for the first three to four days at least, or until comfort is controlled by oral analgesia, and pain-free mobility is established
- Continuous epidural/spinal anaesthesia is extremely desirable and highly recommended where possible in chest wall and lower body/limb reconstruction, but requires specialist nurse accredited observations because of circulatory changes that may occur
- Continuous regional arm blocks provide excellent pain management for major reconstruction on the upper limbs. These techniques allow for the patient to be returned to the operating theatre, if necessary, with minimal disruption to the patient's overall condition
- It should be noted that direct pain assessment may be difficult to utilise as an indicator for vascular compromise, if the patient has a regional block (e.g. arm block or epidural) as pain signals are obscured.

## Withdrawing pain management

The patient should sit up wherever possible (about 30°–45°) to assist ventilation by expansion of the chest wall and diaphragm. This also significantly assists in venous return as the diaphragm and abdominal muscles force the lower body venous blood into the right ventricle. Following major surgery to the chest and/or abdomen, this can be painful and lead to adverse events if optimal pain

---

**Box 19.36** Wound bed management.

- Where possible the patient should sit up to ensure respiratory and circulatory integrity
- Elevation of the body part or limb should be undertaken as directed
- Major skin flaps are managed open to the environment with minimal dressings applied to facilitate positive perfusion at arterial entry, and venous exit, and allow for clinical monitoring/observation of the flap
- Vacuum pressure therapy has been advocated for dressing management to facilitate the removal of excess oedema but is not widely used
- Dressings used on or around a flap must not deliver any degree of compression or pressure on the wound
- Warmed saline packs may be applied to zones of exposed muscle not protected by meshed skin grafts
- Wound hygiene is essential and surrounding dressings should not be allowed to collect large amount of exudate and become saturated
- Only loose bandages over or around flap zones are recommended as any firmness may easily cause a problem in a fragile flap wound, particularly causing capillary perfusion injury
- If a muscle flap is carried out, for example on the lower limb, skin grafts (meshed) will be used and may be primarily nursed open (Figures 19.12 and 19.15) or closed with tie-over dressing
- Skin graft management (see Chapter 17)
- It is essential to check for the presence of multiple wound sites, for example vein graft, skin graft donor sites, and wound drains, as multiple wound sites significantly increase the potential for complications and patient morbidity
- The multiplicity of different wounds requires the ability to manage each wound individually, be aware of the potential complications and maintain a constant vigilance for adverse events that may compromise the entire procedure, such as the emergence of wound infection at a distant site.

---

**Box 19.37** Wound bed management – special issues with free vascularised muscle flaps – open management.

- Avascular or a compromised circulation causes muscle to expire slowly for various complex physiological reasons
- The use of a free vascularised muscle flap to cover, for example, compound fractures and exposed bone without a small area of skin 'paddle' that can be used as a vascular monitor or the use of an implanted Doppler probe, can present problems of blood flow assessment
- In the initial 72 hours, it can be very difficult for nurses monitoring these flaps to detect changes, with or without meshed skin grafts having been applied, but some external signs are available for clinicians
- In the absence of an implanted Doppler probe, the principal signs are:
  - The significant absence of serous/protein exudate expected in the first 72 hours as part of the normal inflammatory process
  - Progressive dryness of the surface of the muscle, dryness of the graft tissue and subsequent failure of skin grafts to adhere
  - STSGs will not adhere to devascularised muscle because of the absence of the 'sticky' protein exudate to assist in adherence and neovascularisation
  - Continuous darkening of the usually red/pink muscle, and a shrinking of the muscle bulk can be gradually observed with an obvious drying of the skin graft
  - If the muscle is viable and application of the donor skin is delayed (i.e. 12–24 hours), normal saline packs are applied four-hourly, or may be applied with an irrigating catheter inserted between the gauze layers and an occlusive plastic film to maintain wound moisture and wound warmth
- Because of the problems of meshing skin after 24 hours (see Chapter 17), and the potential for poor take of the graft, the donor skin is usually applied directly to the exposed muscle in the operating room or unmeshed stored skin applied
- Non-meshed skin can be applied at a time according to the surgeon's wishes, but as muscle is very prone to drying and infection, this is usually within 8–12 hours postoperatively, as described in Chapter 17.

management is withdrawn without an objective programme in place for opioid cessation.

As the patient recovers, their narcotic dosage should be reduced gradually. When the patient is taking oral fluids, oral analgesia can be provided four-hourly strictly for 72+ hours to maintain a therapeutic level as mobilisation is introduced, and narcotics are titrated downwards.

Some mobilising patients may benefit from therapeutic manual lymphatic drainage to unhindered limbs and body parts to increase lymphatic flow, mobilise the immune system, and for its therapeutic relaxation.

**Box 19.38** Flap suture lines and areas following dermal pricks.

- Wound care to the suture lines should be two-hourly or as necessary – any sutures or staples should be individually and gently cleaned with warm normal saline, or a non-alcoholic solution using a sterile cotton bud, or gauze swab with a gloved hand
- A thin smear of Vaseline® or topical antibiotic ointment (as prescribed) should be frequently applied over the suture line and the surrounding skin to prevent any primary cracking of the skin due to dryness and tightness of the skin due to swelling
- Until healed over, a thin smear of Vaseline® or antibiotic ointment (as prescribed) should be frequently applied over the wounds imposed by dermal pricks, to prevent the introduction of bacteria
- The use of antibiotic ointment is discouraged if the skin pH, etc., is restored, as it should be able to defend off opportunistic bacteria

## General nursing care

**Box 19.39** Independence – the rehabilitating phase.

- Patients may be acutely ill for several days, be completely dependent on nurse clinicians, and will require strict 24-hour attention to detail in every area of nursing care[10–15]
- Patient needs may be increasingly accentuated by repeated need to be returned to the operating theatre for flap salvage procedures
- Multidisciplinary care is essential and the physiotherapist is an important team member to ensure maintenance of cardiorespiratory integrity and for providing muscle strengthening exercises that assist the recovery and rehabilitation phase.

**Box 19.40** General nursing care.

- The nurse should observe for emerging nutritional deficits in critically/seriously ill patients or patients who had a nutritional deficit pre-operatively[20–23]
- Patients with tracheostomy tubes and *in situ*, nasogastric tubes or percutaneous endoscopic gastrostomy (PEG), require specialist nutritional monitoring, and should not be allowed to enter into negative nitrogen status[20–23]
- Wound care related to PEGs to ensure against inflammation, hypergranulation[23] and discomfort, and safe positioning of nasogastric tubes to prevent pressure ulceration on the nasal rim should be included in the patient risk checks undertaken at each treatment episode
- Patients with compromised mobility, severely ill patients, patients at nutritional risk, and those with cancer, are at a very high risk for pressure ulcers, particularly on the heels, and because of this reduced mobility should be nursed on special pressure relieving beds and the heels elevated at 30° off the bed
- Evidence suggests that patients with cancer are at high risk (e.g. in plastic surgery, head and neck cancer) and, as discussed in Chapter 15, pulmonary embolism (PE) is often only diagnosed at post mortem, and data as to previous aetiology is not recorded[21,22,24–27] (see Chapter 15 – recommended websites)

*Continued*

- Following upper body surgery, two pillows should be placed lengthways under the legs to assist in venous return, and elevation of heels
- Reports suggest that following plastic surgical procedures, the incidence of deep vein thrombosis and PE is minimal[24,25]
- Anecdotally, there have been reports of deep vein thrombosis in patients (following discharge) who fail to observe mobility requirements, and use antiembolic stockings following, for example, major lipectomy, breast surgery, or substantial liposuction
- Discharge education should cover the need for regular mobility, and the means to identify important signs and symptoms of deep vein thrombosis or PE, seeking medical attention immediately if there are any concerns
- Patients who have had major reconstructive surgical procedures may undergo a sense of grief and loss, become depressed due to altered hormonal balance, boredom or negative perception of their condition – this component of care should not be forgotten
- When the reconstructive surgery is on the face, regular oral, eye and nasal toilets should be instituted to maintain regional wound hygiene[11,21,22]
- General basic patient hygiene (e.g. shaving for males, oral and denture care, hair care) is important for self-esteem and a sense of wellbeing in the patient
- The provision of psychosocial care and reassurance is an important area of nursing care in the primary phase as safety, anxiety and a sense of disorientation may occur
- For younger patients, occupational/play therapy is important to relieve boredom in the recovery and rehabilitation period
- Constipation, related to opiate-based analgesic medication, should be avoided by good dietary or medicated prevention strategies, to exclude physical straining, particularly following TRAM flaps[21,22]
- For patients who have had reconstructive surgery that includes surgery to the abdomen, it is important to ensure that the gastrointestinal system is functioning appropriately by checking bowel sounds, to exclude paralytic ileus, particularly following bilateral free TRAM flaps
- Staff may be required to manage patient anger and distress over the potential loss of life due to cancer, loss of a limb, loss of independence, or altered body image
- Calmness, professionalism and the use of professional counsellors are important. Initially, staff subjected to 'difficulties' with patients should elicit an experienced senior colleague for support, and the surgeon should be alerted.

**Box 19.41** Special risk management issues related to free flaps to the head and neck.

- Major reconstructive surgery to the head and neck can initially result in the patient being totally dependent and requiring critical care (ICU) nursing[17]
- ICU to step-down unit stay may be for as long as it takes for the patient to become physiologically stable, for the patient to feel comfortable with his/her airway management (tracheostomy), and for the flap to achieve vascular competence
- Vascular assessment of radial forearm free flaps to reconstruct oral defects may present particular difficulties in vascular assessment, when invasive adjunctive instrument-based methods are not available
- Assessment of the flap inside the mouth can be clinically difficult when the mouth and wound is swollen and painful
- Buried free vascularised bone grafts (Figure 19.19) provide even more difficulties, especially when monitoring is compromised by external frames, or immobilising wires – the use of internal Doppler probes are extremely valuable in these cases
- Clinicians should request from the surgeon the specific monitoring sites and parameters that can be observed and reported
- Potential complications can be extremely high in these complex procedures as the tumours are often advanced, the patient is nutritionally compromised, depressed, and has a sense of impending death
- The knowledge that surgery is only one part of a proposed triad of surgery, chemotherapy and/or radiotherapy, may contribute to a sense of apprehension and fear.
- Observe for:
  - Flap compromise/failure
  - Infection
  - Permanent airway changes
  - Healing problems related to multiple wounds
  - Development of pressure ulcers related to severe illness[21,22].
- Preoperative risk management can reduce the nursing morbid and co-morbid factors and provide assistance to the immediate surgical outcomes
- Family or significant carers may be shocked at the unexpected sight of the patient undergoing critical medical/nursing management
- Preoperative professional psychological counselling for the patient and significant carers should be considered an essential part of the preoperative wound bed preparation and patient outcomes. Issues of specialist nutritional risks[20] are also discussed in Chapter 9.

**Review**

*Setting goals of care and preferred clinical and patient outcomes*, Chapter 2, Boxes 2.7–2.9. Adapt as appropriate to the patient's clinical needs.

---

**Box 19.42** General discharge principles.

- Clinicians should undertake discharge risk management and address patient and wound needs in the home environment
- Provide the patient with any special discharge education two to three days prior to discharge and reinforce with written notes
- Undertake the mobilisation programme as directed, reinforcing any special instructions and enlisting professional allied health assistance as appropriate
- Educate the patient in the principles of general hygiene in respect of wound site/s and report any wound disturbances
- Educate the patient to report any increasing or unusual swelling, or persistent pain not relieved by oral pain medication, regardless of the site
- Only apply compression dressings or elastic support garments over or around the flap wound as instructed
- Encourage the patient to avoid pressure or rubbing on wound when wound hygiene is undertaken, and to apply ointments or moisturising creams as instructed to maintain soft skin environment and prevent cracking and potential for infection
- Encourage protection of the wound from the sun – use UV protective cream
- Clinicians should audit preferred patient outcomes and reassess of any specific areas of patient care needs.

---

**Review**

*Auditing clinical nursing goals and outcomes*, Chapter 2, Boxes 2.7–2.12.

**References**

(1) Kayser M.R. Surgical flaps. *Selected Readings in Plastic Surgery* 1999; **9**(2):1–63.
(2) Aston S.J., Beasley R.W. & Thorne C.N.M. *Grabb and Smith's plastic surgery*, 5th edn. Philadelphia: Lippincott & Raven Publishers, 1997.
(3) Daniel R.K., Kerrigan C.L. Principles and physiology of skin flaps. McCarthy J.G (ed.). *Plastic surgery, Vol. 1*. Philadelphia: W.B. Saunders Co., 1990: 275–328.
(4) Ausher B.M., Erikson E. & Wilkins E.G. *Plastic surgery: indications, operations and outcomes*. St Louis: Mosby, 2000.
(5) McGregor I.A. & McGregor A.D. *Fundamental techniques of plastic surgery and their surgical applications*, 9th edn. Edinburgh: Churchill Livingstone, 1995.
(6) Tittle B.J., English J.M. & Hodges P.L. Microsurgery: free tissue transfer and replantation. *Selected Readings in Plastic Surgery*. 1993; **7**(11):1–31.
(7) Ruberg R.L. & Smith D.J. *Plastic surgery: a core curriculum*. St. Louis: Mosby, 1994.
(8) Taylor G.I. *Research report of current clinical investigation*. The Reconstructive Surgery Research Unit, University of Melbourne Australia 2001–2003.
(9) Morris A. McG., Stevenson J.H. & Watson A.C.H. *Complications of plastic surgery*. London: Baillière Tindall, 1989.
(10) Fortunato N. & McCullough S. *Plastic and reconstructive surgery*. Mosbys Perioperative Nursing Series. St Louis: Mosby, 1998.
(11) Goodman T. *Core curriculum for plastic and reconstructive surgical nurses*, 2nd edn Pitman N.J: American Society of Plastic Surgical Nurses Inc., 1996. http://www.aspn.org
(12) Hudson G., Scott J. & Beaver M. Warming up to better surgical outcomes. *AORN Journal* (USA), 1999 (Jan); **69**(1):247–8, 251–3.
(13) Mathias J.M. Warmer patients, better outcomes. *OR Manager* (USA), 1999 (Oct); **15**(10):39.
(14) Dinman S. & Giovannone P.A. The care and feeding of microvascular flaps: how nurses can help prevent flap loss. *Plastic Surgical Nursing*, 1994 (autumn); **14**(3):154–64.
(15) Haskins N. Intensive nursing care of patients with microvascular free flaps after maxillofacial surgery. *Intensive Critical Care Nursing*, 1998 (Oct); **14**(5):225–30.
(16) Bornmyr S., Martensson A., Svensson H., Nilsson K.G. & Wollmer P. A new device combining laser Doppler perfusion imaging and digital photography. *Clinical Physiology*, 1996 (Sept); **16**(5):535–41.
(17) Devine J.C., Potter L.A., Magennis P., Brown J.S. & Vaughan E.D. Flap monitoring after head and neck reconstruction: evaluating an observation protocol. *Journal of Wound Care*, 2001; **10**(1):525–30.

(18) Heller L., Levin S. & Klitzman B. Laser Doppler flowmeter monitoring of free tissue transfers: blood flow in normal and complicated cases. *Plastic and Reconstructive Surgery*, 2001 (June); **107**(7):1739–45.

(19) Disa J.J., Cordeiro P.G. & Hidalgo D.A. Efficacy of conventional monitoring techniques in free tissue transfer: an 11-year experience in 750 consecutive cases. *Plastic and Reconstructive Surgery*, 1999 (July); **104**(1):99–101.

(20) Kinn S. & Scott J. Nutritional awareness of critically ill surgical high dependency patients. *British Journal of Nursing*, 2001; **10**(11):704–709.

(21) Mallett J. & Dougherty L. (eds) *The Royal Marsden Hospital manual of clinical nursing procedures*, 5th edn. Oxford, UK: Blackwell Science, 2000.

(22) Smeltzer S.C. & Bare B.G. *Brunner and Suddarth's textbook of medical-surgical nursing*, 9th edn. Philadelphia: Lippincott, Williams & Wilkins, 2000.

(23) Rollins H. Discussion: hypergranulation tissue at gastrostomy sites. *Journal of Wound Care*, 2000 (March); **9**(3):127.

(24) McDevitt N.B. Deep vein thrombosis prophylaxis. American Society of Plastic and Reconstructive Surgeons. *Plastic Reconstructive Surgery*, 1999 (Nov); **104**(6):1923–8.

(25) Moreano E.H., Hutchison T.M., Graham S.M., Funk G.F. & Hoffman H.T. Incidence of deep vein thrombosis and pulmonary embolism in otolaryngology – head and neck surgery. *Otolaryngology – Head and Neck Surgery* 1998 (June); **118**(6):774–84.

(26) Maylor M.E. Accurate selection of compression and antiembolic hosiery. *British Journal of Nursing*, 2001; **10**(18):1172–84.

(27) Brevet T. Antiembolism stockings for prevention of and treatment of deep vein thrombosis. *British Journal of Nursing*, 1999 (Jan 14–27) **8**(1):44–9.

(28) Sidebottom A.J., Stevens L., Moore M., Magennis P., Devine J.C., Brown J.S. & Vaughan E.D. Repair of the radial forearm flap with full or partial thickness skin grafts. *International Journal of Oral and Maxillogacial Surgery*, 2000 (June); **29**(3):194–7.

(29) Morton R.P. The need for ICU admission after major head and neck surgery. *Austraila and New Zealand Journal of Surgery*, 2002; **72**(1):3–4.

## Recommended websites

**Tissue flaps**

http://www.emedicine.com/plastic/topic242.htm#section~author_information (flaps, random skin flaps (excellent)

http://www.centerforrestoration.com/breastrecon/beforeafter.html (breast reconstruction before and after photos – excellent)

http://www.raft.ac.uk/plastics/patient/head_and_neck_cancer.html

**Free flaps and flap monitoring**

http://www.plasticsurgery.com/gallery/list.asp?procID=30 (before and after photos – breast reconstruction post mastectomy)

http://www.sma.org/smj/96abplas.htm (information on free flaps)

http://www.plasticsurgery.org/search-results.cfm?SRCHSTRING=flaps (before and after photos – breast reconstruction post mastectomy)

http://www.moor.co.uk/app_flap_monitor.htm (information about Doppler probes)

http://www.ibd.nrc-cnrc.gc.ca/english/spec_e_skin.htm (using optical spectroscopy and imaging to predict skin flap survival)

# Chapter 20

# The Hand

## Introduction

*'The hand, more than any other body part, enables man to control and manipulate the surroundings. Hands are used in activities of daily living, employment, play, combat, and when disabled, the patient loses much of his quality of life. The repair of hand injuries or reconstruction of congenital defects requires precise surgical technique. Nursing care must be equally precise since the patient's quality of life depends on it.'*[1]

In all cultures the hand is a significant physical feature and important in everyday survival. It is instrumental in providing art, culture, and industry in our community. In many societies, it has such significant cultural and psychological meaning, that amputation is undertaken as retribution for certain criminal, religious or anti-social behaviours.

As any part of the human anatomy, the hand is subject to similar congenital, traumatic or disease-based conditions that can render it partly or fully dysfunctional[2 6]. Loss of the functional properties of the hand can represent a significant loss of livelihood for the individual and a substantial cost to the community.

As with all areas of complex injury and/or elective surgery, clinical case management that includes risk management, stating realistic and achievable outcomes, can significantly reduce the potential for adverse events, clinical management, and difficulties in patient co-operation.

Table 20.1 outlines the common conditions that present for hand surgery[3–6]. Table 20.2 outlines the stated statistical figures for hand surgery in the USA[3–6].

## Structural anatomy of the hand

### Box 20.1 Definitions relating to anatomy of the hand.

| | |
|---|---|
| **Dorsal** | back of the hand |
| **Palmar** | front of the hand |
| **Proximal** | nearest the forearm (wrist) |
| **Distal** | farthest from the forearm (fingertips) |
| **Medial** | in the middle[2–6]. |

### Box 20.2 Outline of structural anatomy of the hand 1.

**Bones of the hand:**

- See Figure 20.1 for general view
- Figure 20.2 – structure of the distal end of the finger and fingernail.

**Muscles and tendons of the upper limb:**

- Tendons arise from muscles in the forearm
- Figure 20.3 displays the extensor tendons on the back of the hand – weak – allows hand to extend backwards – required to balance the flexor tendons
- Figure 20.4 displays the flexor tendons of the palmar surface – very strong – required for physical power and strong grip.

**Nerves of the upper limb:**

- Figure 20.5 displays the distribution of the nerves of the upper limb that arise from C5–T1 (source of all motor and sensory function of the upper limb)
- Figure 20.6 displays the important source, and distribution, of cutaneous nerves of the hand.

**Table 20.1** Common conditions that present for hand surgery. Examples only[2–5].

| Elective | Trauma | Congenital |
|---|---|---|
| Rheumatoid arthritis<br>Joint replacement procedures following disease or trauma | De-gloving injury<br>Compound injuries (bone, soft tissue, and sometimes nerves, vessels, tendons)<br>Closed fractures<br>Rupture of tendons<br>Direct tendon and or nerve injury – sharp injury | Congenital absence of digits<br>Accessory digits (commonly thumb or little finger)<br>Bone deformities (absence of and/or malformation of the bone) |
| Dupuytren's contracture | Laceration and stab injury<br>Crush injury<br>Infections<br>Animal and insect bites<br>Human bites | Congenital malformation seen in association with particular syndromes<br>Vascular malformations<br>Syndactyly (partial or full webbing of digits – may include bone) |
| Trigger finger | Thermal injury (heat or cold)<br>Electrical burn injury | Soft tissue benign lesions including vascular lesions |
| Soft tissue tumours – cysts<br>Carpal tunnel syndrome<br>Ganglion | Vascular injury<br>Tendon injury<br>Nerve injury<br>Brachial plexus injury (adult – usually sporting related)<br>Brachial plexus injury (child – usually birth injury) | |

---

**Box 20.3** Outline of structural anatomy of the hand 2 – the thumb.

- Humans are the only animals that can oppose all fingers to the thumb, thus the thumb is considered to represent 50% of the hand
- Without the thumb the ability for fine pincer function is not possible
- When the thumb has been amputated, under the right conditions, replant is considered, alternatively large toe transfer may be considered to recreate the thumb
- Compensation following accidents is based on the worth of each finger to perform certain functions in descending order, after the thumb[2–6].

**Box 20.4** Outline of arterial blood supply to the palm of the hand.

- Vascular malformations are not unusual in the human body, some of them can be life-threatening while others remain unknown/unseen for the patient's lifetime
- The unique arterial/venous structures in the hand have a specific architectural pattern but a range of malformations/variances may be observed
- The normal blood supply to the hand is constructed in an arch (Figure 20.7, on the left = normal)
- Branches move off this primary arch, proceed up the sides of each finger and form smaller arches at the distal end of each finger
- Figure 20.7, on the right = abnormal, where the radial and ulnar vessels fail to join but radial artery is patent, supplying the digits
- The hand can function on one patent single ulna or radial artery[2–6].

**Table 20.2** Scope and statistics for hand surgery in the USA[2–5]

| Hand surgery – the scope | Hand trauma – types of wounds | |
|---|---|---|
| Incidence in the USA 15 million per year | Opens | 65% |
| Congenital malformations | Crush | 22% |
| Trauma | Burns | 3.0% |
| Implants | Fractures | 2.5% |
| Reconstructive | Other | 7.5% |
| Burns | | |
| Degenerative | | |
| Tumours – benign or malignant | | |
| Cosmetic | | |

| Mechanism of injury – the scope | Parts of hands injured | |
|---|---|---|
| Laceration | Fingers | 66% |
| Crush | Metacarpal region | 27% |
| Avulsion | Wrist | 4% |
| High pressure injection | Multiple zones | 3% |
| Burns/freeze | | |
| Chemical | | |
| Assault | | |

| Occupation of the patient | | Principal causes of accidents | |
|---|---|---|---|
| Unskilled worker | 90% | Inadequate use of equipment | 35% |
| Transport workers | 2.5% | Lack of attention or no prevention during work | 21% |
| Service workers | 35% | Incorrect position of hands | 11% |
| Other | 4.5% | Machinery not turned off | 11% |
| | | Bypass security measures | 8% |
| | | Other | 17% |

| US statistics | Hand injury/surgery key word |
|---|---|
| 7 903 850 workdays lost through hand injury in 1 year | ELEVATE |
| Average of 23 days lost per injury | |

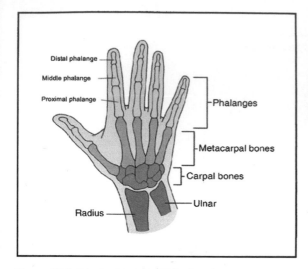

**Figure 20.1** Principal bones of the hand.

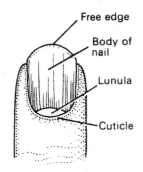

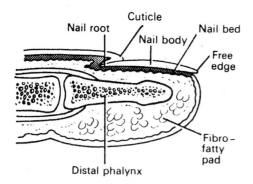

**Figure 20.2** Anatomy of the distal phalanx and nail bed.

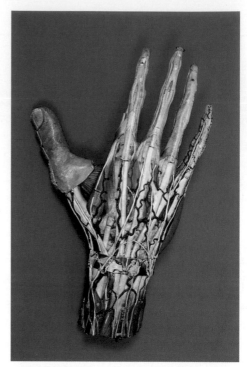

**Figure 20.3** Anatomy of the back (extensor) of the hand.

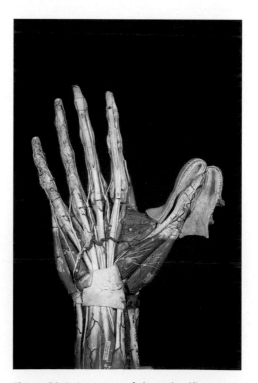

**Figure 20.4** Anatomy of the palm (flexor) of the hand.

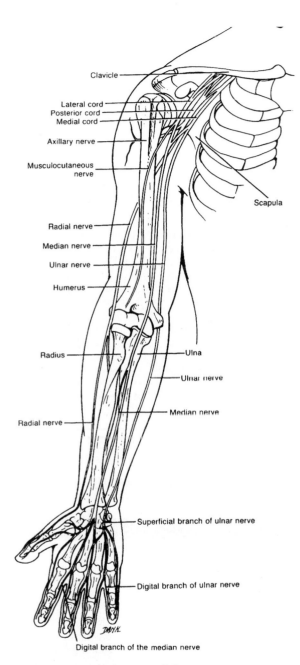

Figure 20.5 Principal nerves of the arm.

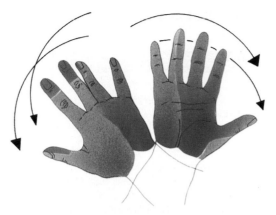

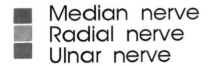

# CUTANEOUS NERVES

Median nerve
Radial nerve
Ulnar nerve

**Figure 20.6** Distribution of cutaneous nerves in the hand.

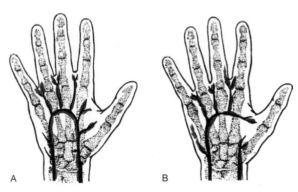

**Figure 20.7** Normal (A) and abnormal (B), vascular arch in the palm of the hand.

## Testing for the integrity of the vascularity of the hand

**Box 20.5** Allen's test.

- Allen's test is an examination used to determine the patency of the radial and ulnar arteries[7]
- In some individuals the blood supply from one of these may be negligible, injured or congenitally absent
- It is important for clinicians to check for both pulses prior to performing procedures that might interrupt supply from one of the arteries, such as an arterial 'stab' to obtain blood to measure arterial blood gases, or the insertion of an arterial line for continuous perfusion monitoring
- Surgeons will always undertake this test on a patient when seeking to harvest a radial forearm flap based on the radial or ulnar artery.

**Box 20.6** Undertaking Allen's test.

- With the patient's hand facing towards the examiner, the patient is asked to make a fist to force the blood from the hand
- It is suggested that if the patient cannot make a fist, the efficacy of the test may be in doubt as the blood remains in the hand
- The index and middle fingers of the examiner's hand are placed upon both the ulnar and the radial arteries and are pressed upon by the clinician, using the fingertips of both hands to occlude flow for approximately one minute
- This leads to blanching, the hand goes white
- Then one of the arteries is released and, in the normal case, the blanching disappears (red/pink colour recovers in about five seconds) over the whole of the hand
- This is repeated with both arteries. In theory, a whole normal blood supply of the hand can come from an artery but the hand cannot survive on the ulnar artery alone, as it can on the radial artery
- In anatomical congenital malformations, a collateral circulation appears to have taken up the role of the radial vessel
- Accidental loss of integrity of the normal radial artery, or both vessels, means loss of blood supply to the hand

- Ischaemia results, with potential amputation of the hand required[7]
- Following injuries to the wrist, surgeons will explore the wound to assess the patency of the radial artery and repair any division or laceration of the vessel by microsurgical techniques.

**Box 20.7** Aetiology of hand injury.

- Hand injuries make up a substantial number of all injuries that present to the emergency room (suggested to be 5–10% of all presentations – 30% in some demographics – for example, in large industrial zones[5,6]). See Tables 20.1 and 20.2 for common conditions and statistics on hand trauma and types of injury
- Injuries to the fingertips and fingernails are the most common[6] (Figure 20.8 shows a crush injury to the thumb pulp with fracture of the distal phalanx, and a Kirschner wire inserted)
- Most hand injuries are due to knife accidents during use in the home, workplace accidents, or may be as a result of fights or assaults[5,6].

## Risk management and clinical outcome issues

**Box 20.8** Safety.

| | |
|---|---|
| Haematoma | (early): unresolved, leading to acute compartment syndrome |
| | (long-term): tissue fibrosis and loss of function |
| Oedema | (early): unresolved swelling leading to acute compartment syndrome |
| | (long-term): tissue fibrosis and loss of function |
| Infection | leading to chronic stiffness and loss of function. |

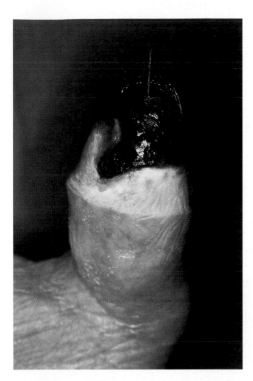

**Figure 20.8** Avascular necrosis of the distal portion of the finger following crush injury.

## Wound repair and closure – risk management issues in the hand

Skin closure following any form of surgery or injury to the hand is not simple, and where possible needs to follow the skin lines that prohibit tension, and the development of postoperative skin contractures[2–6].

With the 'fixed' nature of the skin on the palm of the hand (the flexor surface), and fingers, and their specialised blood supply, the normal use of Z-plasty or 'zigzag' (Figures 20.9 & 20.10) incisions made within the skin's lines of tension may not be entirely possible following trauma, and for the removal of some tumours[3–6].

To prevent severe skin tension, or replace important lost skin cover, particularly in severely injured hands, full thickness skin grafting, local, or free vascular skin flap surgery, will often be required[3–6].

On the back of the hand (extensor surface) the skin is essentially mobile, allowing for direct wound closure to be undertaken when only minimal skin needs to be excised. A thick split skin graft may be required to 'resurface' and protect the extensor surface when wider surface skin tumours are removed. This provides free movement of the tendons and allows the hand to open and close, with minimal restriction (Figures 20.11–20.13).

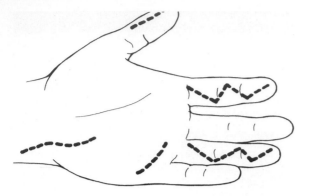

**Figure 20.9** Elective surgical incision marking of the finger to prevent skin contraction.

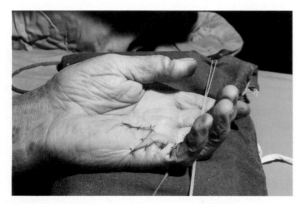

**Figure 20.10** Surgical incision marking of the hand preoperatively for Dupuytren's contracture of the fifth finger.

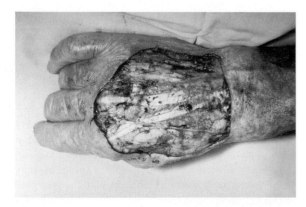

**Figure 20.11** Excision of multiple skin tumours from the back of the hand (bloodless field using tourniquet).

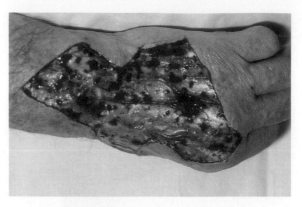

**Figure 20.12** Excision of multiple skin tumours from the back of the hand (removal of tourniquet – clear view of veins).

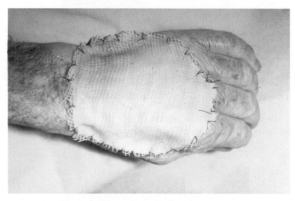

**Figure 20.13** Thick split thickness skin graft to back of the hand as a resurfacing technique.

## Skin tension due to trauma, postoperative haematoma or excess oedema

### *Case examples*

#### *Electrical burns*

In some instances following trauma or surgery, the potential development for haematoma, increasing oedema or muscle damage may be a risk to the overall structure of the hand[3–6].

The hand will usually be placed in a 'resting' splint as this allows for wound oedema to develop that can be observed, any skin damage to emerge, and permits interim dressing management (Figure 20.14). It also allows for potential surviving tissues to be identified and surgical planning to address the issue of restoring tissue viability where possible.

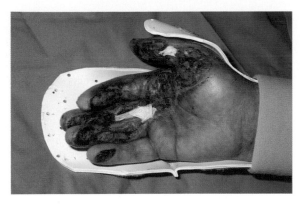

**Figure 20.14** Injured hand managed open with resting splint – electrical burns – injury extent to skin and underlying tissues may remain unknown for up to 21 days.

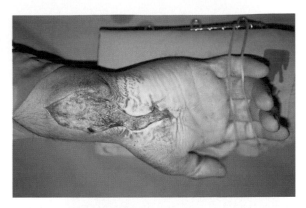

**Figure 20.16** Relieving incisions for compartment syndrome of the hand following crush injury – palmer side.

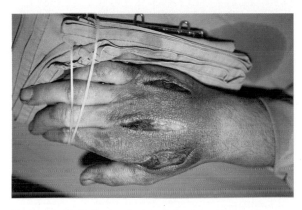

**Figure 20.15** Relieving incisions for compartment syndrome of the hand following crush injury – dorsal side.

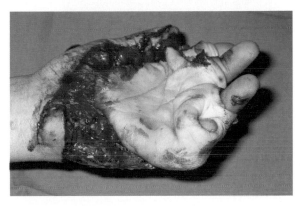

**Figure 20.17** De-gloving injury of the hand due to hot industrial roller – on presentation (required amputation).

## Compartment syndrome

Compartment syndrome (Figures 20.15 & 20.16) can occur when swelling is greater than the skin can contain, and relieving incisions will need to be made to salvage the hand[3–6].

## De-gloving injury

Figures 20.17–20.19 display severe hand trauma following accidental compression in a mechanised hot roller, experienced by a factory worker. A de-gloving injury occurred as an attempt was made to pull the hand out.

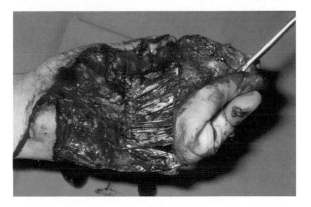

**Figure 20.18** De-gloving injury of the hand due to hot industrial roller – dorsal surface.

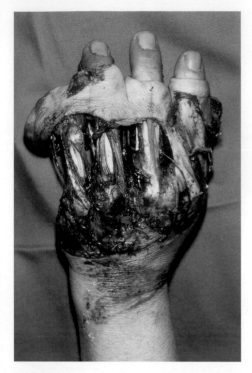

**Figure 20.19** De-gloving injury of the hand due to hot industrial roller – palmar surface.

Burning of the intrinsic hand tissues also occurred, destroying the neurovascular anatomy and tendons. The hand required amputation.

### Finger avulsion injuries

Figures 20.20 and 20.21 display why rings should be removed when working in certain environments. This patient required an amputation of the finger due to ring avulsion injury, where the vessels and nerves on both sides of the finger were torn and crushed when the ring was caught on a moving hook.

### Tendon injuries

Extensor tendon or flexor tendon injuries (Figure 20.22).

### Nerve injury

Figure 20.23.

### Superficial partial thickness hot water burns

Figure 20.24.

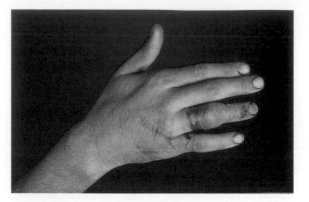

**Figure 20.20** Ring avulsion injury day 1.

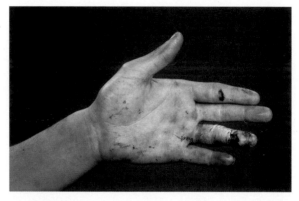

**Figure 20.21** Ring avulsion injury day 2 (required amputation).

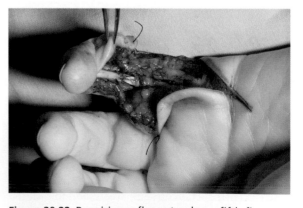

**Figure 20.22** Repairing a flexor tendon – fifth finger.

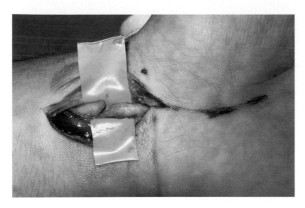

**Figure 20.23** Microsurgical median nerve repair at the wrist.

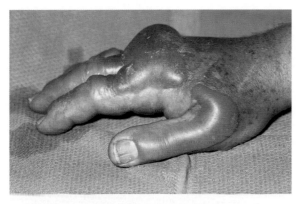

**Figure 20.24** Superficial and partial thickness burns to the dorsum of the hand.

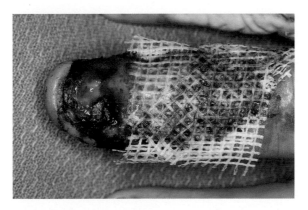

**Figure 20.25** Whitetail spider bite – necrosing due to toxins (required amputation).

## Spider bite

Figure 20.25 shows an inadequately managed whitetail spider bite injury. Due to cytotoxic reaction to the spider venom, the finger required amputation related to avascular necrosis.

## Bone injury

Fractures of the bones of the hand require immobilisation of the fracture site. The site of the fracture will determine the form of immobilisation applied. Several options are available. In the middle, proximal and carpal bones, the introduction of the use of titanium plates and screws has allowed early rehabilitation of the hand that was previously not available to the patient. Early mobilisation can minimise or prevent joint stiffness and the development of fibrous tissue that restricts full movement of the hand[3–6].

For some fractures, fine internal wiring may be utilised, or rigid straight wires may be inserted crossways through the middle phalanx or a single wire through the finger tip to stabilise the distal phalanx to maintain a stable position. Some of the steel wire pin will remain exposed so that when the fracture is healed it can easily be removed[3–6]. Pin site care is important and requires a protective cover to prevent injury to the patient, and others[8].

## Endoscopic hand procedures

Figure 20.4 displays the flexor retinaculum, a fibrous band responsible for securing the tendons, nerves, and blood vessels (that supply the hands) within the carpal tunnel (Figures 20.5 & 20.6).

Carpal tunnel syndrome is a painful disorder of the wrist and hand induced by compression of the median nerve. These symptoms may be worse at night than during the day. Following a range of examinations that include tests to nerves in both wrists, X-rays of the neck to exclude cervical nerve involvement, and hand therapy treatment modalities, surgery may be indicated.

Figure 20.26 (on the right of the picture), demonstrates an open procedure where the flexor retinaculum is divided by a scalpel. The left illustration demonstrates surgery undertaken with an endoscope. This latter form of surgery significantly reduces the surgical, inpatient, rehabilitation, and recovery time.

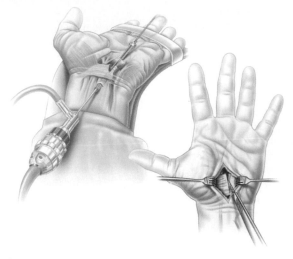

**Figure 20.26** Endoscopic and open surgical techniques for treating carpal tunnel syndrome.

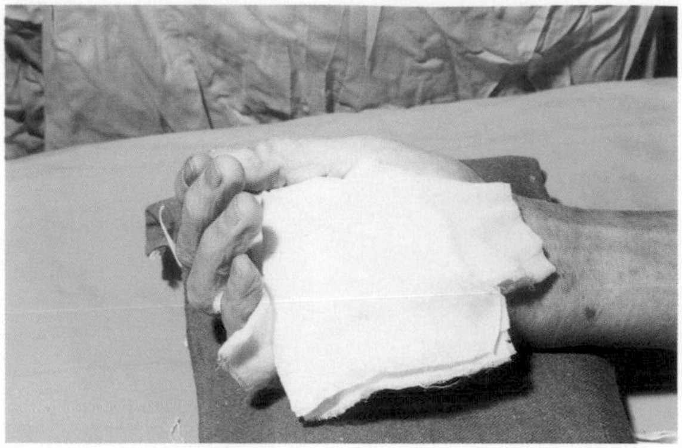

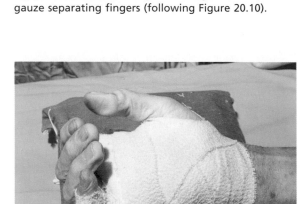

**Figure 20.27** Hand bandage 1 – filling in dead spaces – gauze separating fingers (following Figure 20.10).

## Wound bed management – securing the wound

Although most surgically managed, or injured hands, will be splinted, not all hand wounds will require compound dressings and splints (e.g. simple Dupuytren's contracture)[12–14]. Many surgeons may prefer to mobilise the hand early, and apply adhesive-backed silicone sheet/retention dressing material for suture line protection, stability, and flexibility of the hand. These dressings can also be applied over skin grafts to the hand.

Chapter 12 (Wound Bed Management) outlined the principles for the application of dressings and bandages including the hand. Figures 20.27–20.33 display the classic hand dressing, bandaging, external securing of the bandages, and the methods of elevation from operation to discharge[8].

Each repaired hand is splinted on the basis of:

- What position is most appropriate to achieve protection of underlying tissues
- Securing the desired position of function
- Position of least tension on the tendons, nerves, vessels and the skin[12–17].

Splints supporting internal dressings must stay securely in place for the period prior to the primary dressing. Failure to achieve this places the wound

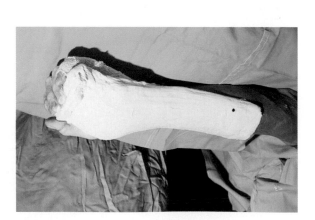

**Figure 20.28** Hand bandage 2 – fifth finger bandaged separately to rest of hand.

**Figure 20.29** Plaster of Paris slab splint for immobilisation of the hand.

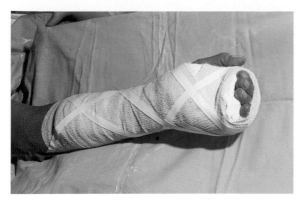

**Figure 20.30** Final taping to secure outer bandages – note hyperaemia following release of tourniquet.

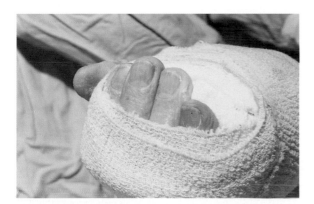

**Figure 20.31** Slight venous congestion of fifth finger postoperative surgery (compare with other fingers) – will normally resolve with elevation – may require bandage 'stretched'.

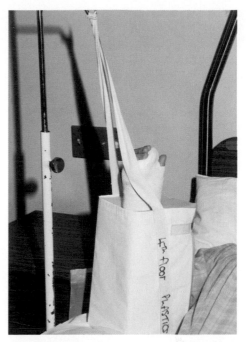

**Figure 20.32** Elevation in a box sling or orthopaedic sling.

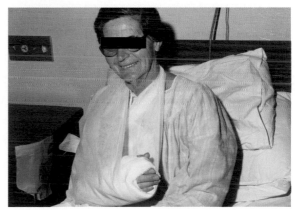

**Figure 20.33** Resting position in sling – elevate higher if any venous compromise.

and resultant hand function at risk. Figures 20.34 and 20.35 demonstrate the inadequate match of splint to the personality of the patient. When setting goals and outcomes these issues must be included.

## Postoperative nursing management

Neuro = the nerve; Vascular = the artery or vein.

When regional or local anaesthetic blocks have been utilised, sensory and motor functions are impaired. Until the block wears off, it is important to ensure that the patient is protected, by securing the arm appropriately. There is a potential for self-injury (e.g. fractured nose) due to loss of motor control of the limb. Neurological response will be absent in the presence of an active sensory and motor block and this must be considered when neurovascular observations are undertaken.

**Box 20.11** Postoperative risk management issues.

- Addressing the appropriate level of elevation to prevent arterial compromise or venous insufficiency/congestion
- The hand/limb must be elevated at the 'above the heart' level to ensure venous drainage – use one or two pillows, a normal or orthopaedic hand sling/support, or IV stand (Figures 20.31–20.32)
- Accuracy of neurovascular assessment and interpretation of data[15]
- Adequate pain management in the absence of a regional block or IV narcotic infusion[16]
- The protection of the wounds, and their dressings[17]
- Addressing a plan for discharge that focuses on the individual patient's needs
- The psychosocial issues related to a particular type of surgery, or injury that may be the result of partial or total loss of the hand or digits[18]
- The opposite hand should always be checked before assessing the injured hand (because coldness and blueness of the hands may be a normal feature for the particular patient)
- All digits, if practical, should be visible for individual assessment – this allows for each digit to be assessed separately
- Response to touch (neurological observation, sensory perception) will be absent if the nerve responsible for the zone of damage has also been injured or the zone has been blocked by local anaesthesia
- Vascular monitoring/observation can be approached using the five 'Ps' – pain, pulse, pallor, purple, pins and needles sensation[15]
- Pain must be well controlled to provide safety, comfort and co-operation[16]
- No movement of any digit must be allowed unless specifically instructed in writing by the plastic surgeon, as movement may cause rupture of, for example, a flexor tendon repair, repaired nerve, or anastomosed blood vessel(s)
- The patient should be well hydrated to provide good general circulation
- The patient must be physically warm to exclude hypothermia and avoid peripheral vascular shutdown.

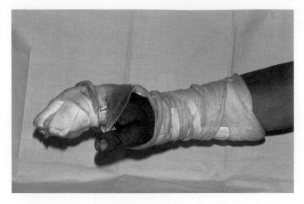

**Figure 20.34** Inadequately applied hand dressing and splint – 1.

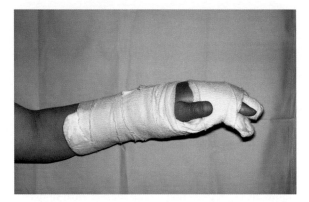

**Figure 20.35** Inadequately applied hand dressing and splint – 2.

**Review**

*Setting goals of care and preferred clinical and patient outcomes*, Chapter 2, Boxes 2.7–2.9.

**Table 20.3** Vascular observations of the hand – inadequate arterial flow.

| Observation | Response | Potential problem | Action |
|---|---|---|---|
| Finger/s pale/white<br><br>Pain intense and sharp, not relieved by narcotics<br><br>Capillary return greater than 3 seconds = arterial compromise<br><br>Patient pale, sweaty, restless and anxious<br><br>Patient may report 'pins and needles' feeling – this may indicate potential nerve involvement/injury | Lower the hand – does the colour move from pale/white to pink?<br>*No* – arterial flow is grossly impeded<br>*Yes* – arterial flow partially occluded<br><br>Does the patient have adequate general perfusion?<br><br>Check urinary output for signs of dehydration<br><br>Check for any wound drainage | *Intrinsic* = arterial clotting problems or problems of vessel wall spasm<br><br>*Extrinsic* = elevation of hand inappropriate – too high when arterial flow poor<br><br>? Tight bandages or dressings<br><br>?Tight plaster<br><br>?Haematoma causing pressure on vessels<br><br>?Wound edge sutures too tight<br><br>Pain causing peripheral vascular compromise<br><br>Inadequate general fluid perfusion | Notify the medical officer immediately and request immediate clinical response<br><br>'Stretch' release of bandages, or initiate cutting of bandages, (decompression management)<br><br>Give narcotic pain relief to relax muscle contraction<br><br>Document the adverse episode fully |

**Table 20.4** Vascular observations of the hand – inadequate venous flow.

| Observation | Response | Potential problem | Action |
|---|---|---|---|
| Finger/s blue/purple/mottled and swollen (*see Figure 20.30*)<br><br>Pain intense but dull and throbbing (briefly relieved by narcotics)<br><br>Capillary return less than 1 second, said to be 'brisk'<br><br>Patient may be pale, sweaty, restless and anxious | Elevate the hand higher than normal above the heart. Does the colour move from blue to pink?<br>*No* = venous outflow is grossly impeded<br>*Yes* = venous outflow partially occluded<br><br>Does the patient have adequate general perfusion?<br><br>Check urinary output for signs of dehydration<br><br>Check wound drainage output | *Intrinsic* = clotting problems – venous obstruction<br><br>*Extrinsic* = elevation of hand inappropriate<br><br>?Tight bandages/dressings<br><br>?Tight plaster or pressure at a particular point<br><br>?Haematoma causing pressure on vessels<br><br>? Wound edge sutures too tight<br><br>?Pain causing peripheral vascular compromise<br><br>?Inadequate general fluid perfusion | Notify the medical officer immediately and request immediate response<br><br>'Stretch' release of bandages or cutting of bandages (decompression management)<br><br>Give narcotic pain relief to relax muscle contraction<br><br>Document the adverse episode fully |

## Reactive hyperaemia

Figures 20.27 and 20.28 display the hand with tourniquet remaining on whilst placement of dressings is being undertaken. When the tourniquet is released, there is a red 'flushed' effect due to arterial inflow under pressure. This effect is referred to as reactive hyperaemia (Figures 20.29 and 20.30), and should not be confused with vascular compromise.

---

**Box 20.12** Decompression technique.

- Only the surgeon or an experienced nurse clinician should disturb the original dressings, as important tissues such as vessels, nerves, flexor tendons may be re-injured, and the entire surgical procedure deemed a failure
- Regardless of the original surgical procedure, or existing wound problem, the position of the fingers/hand should be maintained, with one person assisting, by holding the fingers in the original position whilst decompression is undertaken
- Failure to do this may result in spontaneous uncontrolled movement of the fingers, causing injury to the repaired vessels, nerves or tendons
- **Technique 1:** the crepe bandages and securing tapes (Figure 20.30) are left in place and may be artificially stretched with the point of a pair of heavy scissors or a metal spatula type instrument (only the surgeon or an experienced nurse clinician should do this)
- **Technique 2:** the bandages and dressings are cut through to the skin (Figures 20.33 & 20.34) on the opposite side to the wound site itself (protecting the wound) to relieve the overall pressure being exerted. Such is the fragility of some wounds/vessels in a swollen digit that a single strand of elastic crepe bandage may be responsible for compromising the arterial or venous circulation
- Should the circulatory problem remain unresolved, all dressing and bandages should be cut and the whole wound examined.

---

## Decompression of the wound bandages and dressings

Vascular compromise can be caused by either arterial or venous circulatory instability. The most common is venous. The common areas seen to be at risk in plastic surgery are the upper and lower limbs, the ears and the face. The most common cause of vascular compromise in the hand is excess compression (pressure) exerted upon the vessels that supply the fingers or overall limb.

When the wound or surrounding tissues are in danger from vascular compromise 'decompression' is the term given to the practice of releasing the compression exerted, by cutting the bandages and dressings down to the skin.

Figure 20.31 displays the blueness exhibited by venous compromise. By elevating the hand above the heart, this venous compromise may be resolved. Alternatively, decompression of the bandages will be required to release the external compressing effects of the bandages and allow circulatory flow to be restored.

---

**Box 20.13** Redressing the wound following decompression.

- Skin grafts or skin flaps of any type are best left undisturbed as much as possible, unless there is a problem with the flap
- The original cut/released bandages should be restored into their original position, and a loose crepe bandage applied over them, as the original dressings applied are always the best
- As normal or accepted perfusion observations are restored, or prior to discharge, any outside adhesive tape should be applied very gently, and reinforced with a loose but flexible elasticised tubular garment. This assists in reducing bandages from slipping, particularly in adolescents and children (Figures 20.36 & 20.37)
- Adolescent and poorly co-operative patients require additional measures to aid in the retention of the dressings and bandages
- In children, the application of cohesive bandages or a single outer layer of plaster of Paris can be useful in securing the bandages
- Figures 20.36 and 20.37 demonstrate a totally inadequate original application of a hand splint and bandage, totally weakening the desired function
- On patient discharge, the arm must be placed in a sling, or an orthopaedic collar and cuff, with a soft pad of foam at back of neck – this cushions the neck against the gravitational pull of the weight of the arm
- For children, safety pins can be used to secure both sides of the sling along the border of the immobilised hand and forearm, as this technique aids in preventing the hand being easily removed from the sling[8].

---

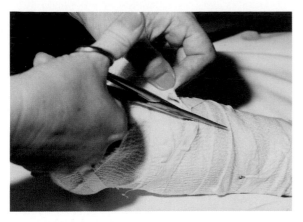

**Figure 20.36** First stage decompression of bandages.

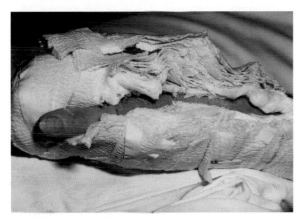

**Figure 20.37** Full decompression of bandages down to the skin.

> ### Box 20.14 Inpatient wound management by nurse clinicians.
>
> - Report any unusual or excessive fresh bleeding
> - Wound bed management – keep exposed wounds and surrounding skin as clean as possible
> - Ensure basic hygiene of, for example, fingernails
> - Ensure any exposed surgical pins are enclosed and not a source of potential injury to patients or other
> - Pin site care if required.

> ### Box 20.15 General nursing care.
>
> - Maintain fluid intake for adequate perfusion of the wound
> - Maintain arm and the patient in a comfortable position
> - Educate patient about pain assessment and reporting
> - Educate patient regarding prevention of shoulder discomfort and stiffness by demonstration of specific upper arm and shoulder exercises
> - Nutritional assistance if required
> - Psychological reassurance[1,9,18]
> - Social worker if necessary to arrange for assistance in the home.

> ### Box 20.16 Discharge education.
>
> - For other than major trauma, a large proportion of elective or uncomplicated hand surgery is done as day surgery or with an overnight stay. This means that all attending clinicians must be very vigilant for actual and potential problems prior to discharge and alert patients of observation protocols following discharge
> - Optimally, the patient should be phoned after 24 hours to check on comfort or any bleeding
> - Before the patient is discharged, the surgeon should be consulted to ascertain whether the patient is to be seen by the hand therapist prior to discharge or if appointments are to be made
> - Pain or discomfort must be controlled to ensure co-operation
> - With children, ensure primary carers are alerted to a disciplined need for elevation of limb and reporting of pain
> - The arm must be kept elevated above the level of the heart in a sling, or collar and cuff support, at all times during day and on one or two pillows at night or when sitting in a chair
> - The patient should report to the hospital emergency room or surgeon's rooms any excessive pain which is not relieved by instructed analgesic medication or limb elevation
>
> *Continued*

- The patient must request that the hand is fully assessed by a competent medical or nursing person, with hand surgery care experience, and the dressings should be decompressed to ensure any problems are minimised or prevented
- No secondary injury can be done to the wound by undertaking this, as long as no movement of the digits or hand occurs and the hand is bandaged as described in Figures 20.27–20.30.
- The hand dressings must not be removed completely unless ordered by the surgeon
- Leave dressings untouched – do not get dressings wet
- When showering, cover the hand and arm up to the elbow with a shower proof garment designed for this procedure for example (LIMBO™), or a clean plastic bag and secure with a rubber band(s) to exclude water (see: http://www.limbo.com.au)
- Report any offensive odour or wound discharge
- If given antibiotics, complete the course as instructed to avoid the potential for infection
- NO SMOKING
- Do not drive any motor vehicle, as it is illegal to drive one-handed unless licensed to do so
- Practise shoulder and elbow exercises as demonstrated. This is important in excluding joint stiffness in the shoulder and elbow due to inactivity and lack of normal use.

## Box 20.17  Patient discharge.

Patients must not be discharged unless:
- All safety and comfort risk management parameters and expected clinical outcomes are met
- The patient, or carer, understands the strict need to undertake all discharge instructions, in particular those instructions that deal with limb elevation and pain assessment/management
- The patient, or carer, understands the specific signs and symptoms that constitute actual or potential problems in the home environment
- The patient or carer has a pathway of reporting adverse events that provides a sense of safety and comfort.

# Primary dressing management – clinical application

## Box 20.18  Primary dressing management – preparing the patient.

- If nurses are not experienced in dressing management, discretionary judgement in attempting to undertake the task is required by the clinician when faced with varying degrees of complex hand wounds
- Many wounds have tie-over graft dressings, special flaps and complex Z-plasty repairs or combinations
- In plastic surgery, the rule is to seek advice and/or assistance, to learn from the experience, and do not injure or cause pain to the patient
- In some wounds, analgesia may be necessary prior to commencing the dressing as the hand is a sensitive organ, and the patient's fears of outcomes may be expressed through the dressing management
- Most patients have an intrinsic fear of pain or discomfort at the actual time of dressing removal, a sense of anticipation at the surgical outcome of the procedure, and how the wound will look
- When undertaking the primary dressing of any wound, physical and psychological preparation of the patient, and getting the proper equipment prior to undertaking the task, are important
- Place the patient on a recliner chair or a consulting room couch and ensure they are comfortable
- Many patients faint or feel nauseated when having hand dressings done. Have some sweets available for some extra sugar, and diversion
- Ensure the patient is warm – cover them with a light blanket
- Place the hand on an appropriate resting table, arm board, or flat pillow.

## Box 20.19  Primary dressing management – undertaking the dressing.

- Sit down on a chair and be comfortable, reassuring and talking to the patient during the procedure
- Gently remove the dressings, layer by layer, ensuring that the position of the hand does not alter
- Stop at any time if the patient expresses discomfort or distress
- Gently wash the hand in warm soapy water and softly dry all areas, including between the finger clefts

- Thoroughly clean away the old blood and crusts from the wound, and any desquamated skin
- Request that the surgeon inspect the wound
- Undertake the redressing of the wound as prescribed by the surgeon
- Because the thick skin of the hand is very likely to split open once rehabilitation begins, following primary dressing many surgeons will usually request nurse clinicians to apply conforming, flexible retention tapes to secure the suture lines and surrounding skin whilst early mobilisation is instituted
- Manufacturers provide detailed instructions with their products and these should be followed with attention to detail to ensure the desired effect is attained
- Sutures may not be removed from the hand for up to 10–14 days to ensure wound edge splitting does not occur as early rehabilitation is commenced
- Moisturise the areas surrounding the dressing with a skin moisturiser
- Plaster of Paris splints used immediately following surgery should not be reused, as all conforming qualities are lost with the removal of primary dressings and padding
- Hygiene cannot be guaranteed if bleeding, sweating, and moisture from showering has occurred
- Check with the surgeon as to any resplinting and further orders for care
- Additional splinting may be reinstated (by the hand therapist) through the use of lightweight thermoplastic conforming materials, with Velcro® to secure the splint and provide additional comfort and freedom
- Specialised dynamic splints for rehabilitating flexor tendons may be applied (Figure 12.1)
- For children, following complex reconstructive surgery, most primary dressings of the hand (e.g. skin grafts, major reconstruction) may require a short general anaesthesia, some appropriate sedation, or analgesia.

## Review

*Auditing preferred clinical and patient outcomes,* Chapter 2, Boxes 2.10–2.12.

## References

(1) Belcher D. A care plan for the patient having hand surgery. *Plastic Surgical Nursing*, 1989; **9**(3):126.
(2) *The electronic textbook of hand surgery* (e-hand .com). http://www.eatonhand.com/
(3) Aston S.J., Beasley R.W. & Thorne C.N.M. *Grabb and Smith's plastic surgery*, 5th edn. New York: Lippincott & Raven Publishers, 1997.
(4) McCarthy J.G. (ed.) *Plastic surgery, volumes 1–8.* Philadelphia: W.B. Saunders, Harcourt Brace, 1990.
(5) Ausher B.M., Erikson E. & Wilkins E.G. *Plastic surgery: indications, operations and outcomes.* St Louis: Mosby, 2000.
(6) Masson J.A. Hand 1: fingernails, infection, tumours, and soft tissue reconstruction. *Selected Readings in Plastic Surgery*, 1996; **8**(32):1–63.
(7) Mallett J. & Dougherty L. (eds) *The Royal Marsden Hospital manual of clinical nursing procedures*, 5th edn. Oxford, London: Blackwell Science, 2000.
(8) Storch J.E. *The hand: nursing management following injury or elective surgery.* Clinical teaching notes: post-graduate course in plastic surgery and wound management nursing, Australian Catholic University, 2000 (revised 2004).
(9) Grunert, B.K. & Maksud-Sagrillo, D.P. Psychological adjustment to hand injuries: nursing management (nursing care of trauma patients). *Plastic Surgical Nursing*, 1998; (Sept 22).
(10) Fortunato N. & McCullough S. *Plastic and reconstructive surgery. Mosby's Perioperative Series.* St. Louis: Mosby, 1998.
(11) Goodman T.A. (ed.) *Core curriculum for plastic and reconstructive surgical nursing*, 2nd edn. Pitman N.J.: ASPSN American Society of Plastic Surgery Nurses, 1996. http://www.aspsn.org
(12) Foss-Campbell B. Principles of splinting the hand. *Plastic Surgical Nursing*, 1998 (autumn); **18**(3):199–203.
(13) Kim D.C. Protecting hand splints. *Plastic Reconstructive Surgery*, 2000 (Oct); **106**(5):1220.
(14) Carlson M., Longaker M.T. & Thompson J.S. Wound splinting regulates granulation tissue survival. *Journal of Surgical Research*, 2003 (Mar); **110**(1):304–309.
(15) Kunkler C.E. Neurovascular assessment (Chapter 2). *Orthopaedic Nursing* 1999 (May/June); 63–71.
(16) *Therapeutic guidelines: analgesia*, 3rd edn. Department of Human Services, State Government of Victoria, Australia, March 1997/98.
(17) Terrill P.J. & Varughese G. A comparison of three primary non-adherent dressings applied to hand surgery wounds. *Journal of Wound Care*, 2000; (Sept); **9**(8):359–364.
(18) Clark C.C. Post traumatic stress disorder: how to support healing. *American Journal of Nursing*, 1997 (Aug); **97**(8):27–33. http://www.nursingcenter.com

## Recommended websites

**Demonstrating the complexity of the hand and its function**

http://www.1upinfo.com/encyclopedia/H/hand.html
http://www.methodisthealth.com/plassurg/anatomy.htm
http://catalog.nucleusinc.com/generateexhibit.php?ID=1997&A=2

http://www.eatonhand.com/hom/hom042.htm
http://www.nebraskamed.com/ortho/anhand.cfm#
http://www.newrenart.com/html/michelang.html
http://www.plasticsurgery.org/public_education/procedures/HandSurgery.cfm
http://www.plasticsurgery.com.au/index.html/
http://www.nlm.nih.gov/medlineplus/handinjuriesanddisorders.html

# Chapter 21

# Replant Surgery

**Replantation** is the term used to describe the re-attachment of a completely amputated body part by the restoration of the arterial inflow and venous outflow to the amputated part. The term differs from **revascularisation** where successful restoration of the circulation may occur, regardless of how small a remaining bridge of tissue is[1-6].

Digits on the hand are by far the most common body part presenting for replant or revascularisation surgery, but limbs, scalps, noses, male genitalia and ears have been replanted or revascularised, with varying primary success. Secondary or revision surgery is common[1 5].

Microsurgical repair techniques are required for blood vessels and nerves. Reattachment of other anatomical parts (e.g. tendons, bone and skin) is dependent on the region and degree/extent of injury[1-5].

---

**Review**

It is suggested this chapter is read in association with Chapters 18 and 19.

---

## Patient selection for replant surgery

Patients presenting for replantation of the upper or lower limb frequently have other associated major injuries that may require lifesaving management which preclude replantation of the amputated part(s).

Patients presenting with an amputated digit on the hand may not have other injuries but may have more than one digit amputated and decisions must be made on which finger(s) surgical salvage is to be attempted[1-5].

This is a critical time, and the patient must be honestly informed of the chance of the finger's survival, options, and in particular, the potential functional (usefulness) and aesthetic outcome. The distress of the injury can cloud the patient's and family's judgement and decision-making, and the clinical judgement of the surgeon may take precedence over the patient's wishes.

If there is any possibility of permanently retaining an important severed functional digit (particularly the thumb or index finger), most patients will generally request restoration of the finger regardless of the potential for stiffness, sensory deprivation and poor aesthetic outcomes.

Some patients who can see an immediate and future loss of income due to the extended time for surgery and rehabilitation will request amputation. This procedure will allow a patient to return to work within a couple of weeks, in most cases.

For many cultures, the loss of digits is a negative sign and any suggestion that amputation is the principal option of management can present a difficult ethical or religious problem for the surgeon when the chance of survival of the finger is zero.

---

**Box 21.1** Indications for replant surgery.

- Amputations at/below the level of the wrist (the higher the injury the longer the restoration of nerve recovery)
- Guillotine type injuries (clean sharp injury)
- Young fit persons, particularly children (healing potential parallels growth)
- Co-operative patients who can accept failure of surgery
- Non-smokers[1-7].

---

Patient selection must be rigorous and discussions must include the family, if resources are to be used appropriately and the success rate is worth the effort[1-5]. Patients should be informed of the contemporary research and availability of high quality prosthetic fingers for aesthetic purposes.

---

**Box 21.2** Contraindications to replant surgery.

- Patients who also present with life-threatening injuries
- Severe crush or avulsion injuries of the tissues
- Gross contamination
- Co-morbidity, for example, diabetes mellitus, heart disease, disease processes related to heavy smoking
- Prior surgery or trauma to the part
- Ischaemia time in excess of:
  - 6 hours for proximal to carpus (wrist), or 12 hours 'warm' ischaemic time
  - 12 hours for a digit

Successful cases have been reported at 24 hours+ for distal end of the digit, with 54 hours reported for a finger[1-7].

---

**Box 21.3** Surgical considerations.

- The success of replant surgery is determined by functional as well as cosmetic parameters and with the loss of these important attributes the patient may judge the surgery as a failure
- The principal aim is to save (prioritise) the best of the injured digits and specifically aim to save the thumb (considered 50% of the hand), index and middle fingers, for best functional result (e.g. pincer movement which allows the patient to undertake fine manipulative tasks – picking up small objects, doing up buttons)
- Surgeons will scavenge from non-replantable parts to replace those destroyed, for example, veins, arteries, nerves
- Cartilage may be 'banked' from amputated ears (e.g. can be temporarily stored in the subcutaneous layer of the abdomen)
- Replanted digits in children grow normally when bone is revascularised
- Following amputation of a body part, replantation surgery offers the possibility of a one-stage reconstruction for some patients

---

- The substantial cost of these procedures means that all efforts must be made to select patients who are able to meet specified criteria for potential retrieval success
- This includes an assessment of the patient's psychological health and capacity for compliance and co-operativeness in the complex postoperative and rehabilitation phase
- The immediate postoperative period can be fraught with problems of vascular compromise and later, infection, subsequently leading to amputation
- Long-term problems of minimal function, stiffness, cold sensitivity and pain often lead to amputation as a last resort[1-6].

---

**Box 21.4** Risk management to attain optimal outcomes.

- Efficient transport arrangements for patient and amputated part from injury site to hospital
- Amputated part is placed in a plastic bag, sealed and surrounded on the outside of the bag by ice
- Ice must not be placed in the with the amputated part as the lowered temperature will compromise the efficacy of the vessels
- The time of ischaemia is in parallel to the potential for survival
- Dedicated surgical team from presentation in the emergency room to the clinical ward areas
- Surgical team and operating theatre readily available to reduce avascular time
- Professional nurses proficient in vascular observations, documentation and reporting in the postoperative period
- Allied health professionals to support patient and family
- Psychologists
- Dedicated trained hand and upper arm rehabilitation therapists
- A sympathetic and objective approach by all to the possibility of failure[1-10].

## Box 21.5 Clinical risk management in vascular compromise.

- Venous compromise is the most common complication of microvascular surgery
- The risk of hypothermia and hypovolaemia must be addressed in the first instance
- Dedicated plastic surgical teams, who are committed to microvascular replant surgery, will have strict first-line monitoring protocols set in place
- The lowering of the haematocrit in the presence of normovolaemia and normothermia has been accepted as an important component for maintaining circulatory flow in micro vessels that are highly susceptible to thrombosis
- The decisions and timing for use of for example, therapeutic heparin, dextran, and/or medical leeches, are decisions that are based on the team's assessment of the risk potential and what is actually occurring
- Risk prevention is the most common clinical approach, but each patient must be treated on the specific patient's potential for replant success, existing morbidity and psychological attitude[1-7].

## Review

*Setting goals of care and preferred clinical and patient outcomes*, Chapter 2, Boxes 2.7–2.9.

## Box 21.6 Surgical approach.

- The tissue components, tendons, nerves, vessels, bones and skin are repaired in a specific order, with the vessels done last
- This provides the least degree of movement to the vessels protecting them from tension, shear and friction
- The microscopic size of arterial and venous vessels within the fingers may result in anastomosed vessels experiencing obstruction (venous the most common) during the first 72 hours
- This will often require subsequent surgery to release the obstruction

- In surviving digits, intermittent periods of ischaemia can finally lead to secondary procedures such as skin grafts and skin flaps to replace lost skin that is most vulnerable in these cases[10]
- Finally, if the replant of a thumb or index finger fails, depending on the level of digit loss, local tissue alternative reconstruction will be considered
- Complete loss requires a reappraisal and after the wound has healed, transplant of a big toe may be considered to replace the thumb[1-6].

# Postoperative nursing management

## Box 21.7 Safety.

- Due to the operative timeframe (may be up to 12 hours for multiple digits) and potential for vascular complications, specialist nursing care is essential
- Prevention of hypovolaemia and hypothermia is essential until patient and wound stability is assured
- Vascular complications may require a return to the operating theatre within the first 72 hours, escalating the overall seriousness of the patient's condition, requiring nursing care to be undertaken in the intensive care or high dependency unit[1-7].

## Box 21.8 Comfort.

- As with the seriously injured hand, continuous regional anaesthetic blocks (with a catheter inserted into the brachial plexus region) are commonly used in replant patients to provide continuous pain management and provide for easy access should secondary surgery be required
- Brachial plexus blocks are accepted to increase perfusion to the limbs, assisting circulatory integrity.

**Box 21.9** Vascular monitoring and wound management.

- Postoperative clinical patient management and vascular monitoring is identical to that for major flap procedures and major hand surgery, with the focus on risk management issues that may lead to vascular compromise[1–10] (see Chapter 20 – Tables 20.3 & 20.4)
- The vascular observation, analysis and reporting protocols of colour and other clinical indicators, provide the basics of clinical assessment and must be strictly adhered to (see Tables 20.3 & 20.4)
- Most vascular anastomosis or perfusion problems require immediate surgical attention if perfusion is to be restored and replant salvaged
- Other problems may be caused by development of haematoma, leading to increasing pressure and tension on the skin suture line exerting pressure on the anastomosis
- Removal of sutures and evacuation of the haematoma may resolve this problem
- Any signs of bandage or dressing tightness proximal to the wound should be constantly checked (as oedema may increase substantially) and the bandage decompressed quickly[10]
- Most replanted digits or parts will have only absorbing type wet normal saline dressings applied with immobility of the region using a resting splint or pillows for elevation
- It must be remembered that the fixed skin regions of upper or lower limbs will tolerate only a minimal increase in swelling.

**Box 21.10** Independence and general nursing management.

- In the postoperative phase, nurse clinicians must be critically conversant with both the physiological and psychological risk factors and nursing implications arising from long, complicated procedures, grief and loss issues, family concerns and the potential for failure[10]
- As with all long complex invasive surgery, on return to the clinical unit the patient may be seriously ill for the first 48–72 hours

- This requires the necessary preparation to be undertaken to address nursing risk management, for example[10]:
  - Prevention of hypovolaemia (a urinary catheter may be in place to measure fluid balance)
  - Prevention of hypothermia (ambient room warmth)
  - Addressing safety issues related to immobility, particularly deep vein thrombosis
  - Preventing pressure ulcers, particularly the heels (the patient may have been lying sedated, in a fixed position on the operating table, with little protection for many hours, increasing the risk of pressure to the skin)
  - Addressing increased pain from other wounds where, for example, skin or other tissue has been harvested.
- Ascertain the extent of additional surgical procedures being done prior to receiving the patient back postoperatively, for example, surgical flaps and/or skin grafts.

**Box 21.11** Summary.

- Replant surgery could be said to be one of the most complex and time-consuming, and often the least rewarding areas of reconstructive surgery[1–6]
- In the cases that go well, the rewards of retaining a functional and aesthetic body part are enormous for the patient
- Problems of cost, poor patient motivation, patient compliance, digital stiffness and sensory deprivation remain some of the main reasons for strict assessment criteria for the injury being used to gauge the potential for success
- Patients will frequently request amputation where poor surgical outcomes restrict adequate use of the finger or chronic pain is an issue[1–7]
- An extension of this surgery has been in the area of elective reconstructive transplant microsurgery. In the same patient, big toes have been transplanted to reconstruct thumbs with significant functional and aesthetic success[1–6]
- To date, the transplant of a limb from patient A to patient B has had limited success, mainly because of major tissue rejection problems and timing required for sensory and functional restoration.

### Discharge education

For discharge education, the education following hand surgery can be used, described in Chapter 20. For other replants, adjust as appropriate to the site.

### Case examples

#### Amputated thumb

Figures 21.1 and 21.2 demonstrate a hand with an amputated thumb where the patient requested a replant. The surgeon expressed some doubt about the success of the procedure as the amputation was not a guillotine injury (vessels were stretched and tortuous) which would have assisted the revascularisation. The thumb is 50% of the hand and this drove both the patient and surgical team to attempt to salvage the injured digit.

Figure 21.3 displays day 1 with an acceptable response to replant surgery – comparison with opposite non-injured thumb. Figures 21.4–21.7 demonstrate increasing venous compromise. Blistering and finally necrosis are shown. Figure 21.8 shows amputation and Figure 21.9 shows a neurovascular flap designed on the back of the index finger to be rotated to cover the amputated thumb. Split thickness skin graft was applied over the donor site.

#### Bitten ear

The patient presented following disagreement during a football match. An opposing team member had bitten a section of the right ear off. Replant microsurgery was undertaken based on previous studies of the blood vessels to the ear.

Leeches were attached immediately following anastomosis and maintained on site for three days, significantly minimising the anticipated venous insufficiency due to the small diameter of the vessels. Figure 21.10 demonstrates effective take and vascular proficiency maintained.

See recommended websites demonstrating the complexity of replant surgery at the end of this chapter.

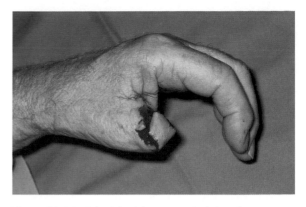

**Figure 21.1** Left hand with amputated thumb.

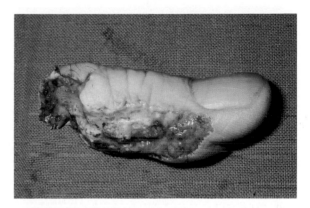

**Figure 21.2** Amputated thumb, left hand.

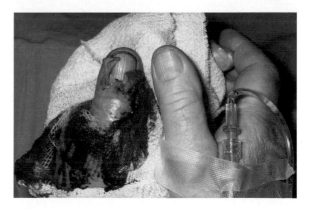

**Figure 21.3** Days 1–2 post replant – blisters beginning – venous congestion.

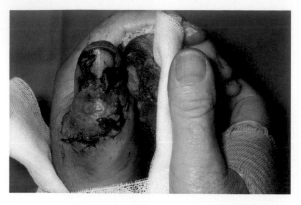

**Figure 21.4** Day 3 post re-plant – blisters increasing.

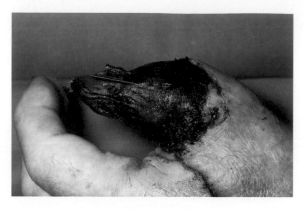

**Figure 21.7** Day 10 – totally avascular thumb.

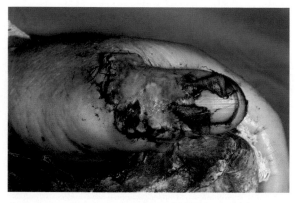

**Figure 21.5** Day 4 – post re-plant – thumb in demise.

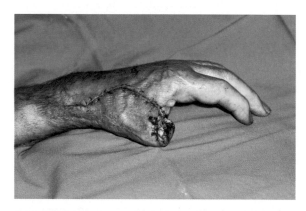

**Figure 21.8** Day 11 – amputation stump.

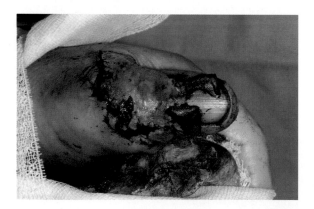

**Figure 21.6** Day 5 – thumb in demise.

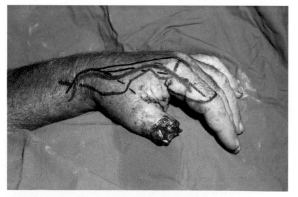

**Figure 21.9** Day 11 – neurovascular island flap designed to cover thumb – donor defect area will be covered with STSG.

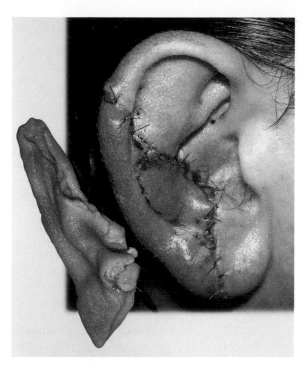

**Figure 21.10** Microvascular repair of amputated composite tissue from right ear based on modern understanding of vascular anatomy. With permission: Professor G.I. Taylor.

## References

(1) Aston S.J., Beasley R.W. & Thorne C.N.M. *Grabb and Smith's plastic surgery*, 5th edn. New York: Lippincott & Raven Publishers, 1997.

(2) Tittle B.J., English J.M. & Hodges P.L. Microsurgery: free tissue transfer and replantation. *Selected Readings in Plastic Surgery*, 1993 (Jan); **7**(11) 1–31.

(3) Kayser M.R. Surgical flaps. *Selected Readings in Plastic Surgery* 1999; **9**(2):1–63.

(4) McCarthy J.G. (ed.) *Plastic surgery, volumes 1–8*. Philadelphia: W.B. Saunders/Harcourt Brace, 1990.

(5) Ausher B.M., Erikson E. & Wilkins E.G. *Plastic surgery: indications, operations and outcomes*. St Louis: Mosby, 2000.

(6) Ruberg R.L. & Smith D.J. *Plastic surgery: a core curriculum*. St. Louis: Mosby, 1994.

(7) Morris A. McG. Stevenson J.H. & Watson A.C.H. *Complications of plastic surgery*. London: Baillière Tindall, 1989.

(8) Goodman T.A. (ed.) *Core curriculum for plastic and reconstructive surgical nursing*, 2nd edn. Pitman N.J.: ASPSN American Society of Plastic Surgery Nurses, 1996. http://www.aspsn.org

(9) Fortunato N. & McCullough S. *Plastic and reconstructive surgery*. Mosby's Perioperative Series. St. Louis: Mosby, 1998.

(10) Storch J.E. *Plastic surgery and wound management nursing*. Postgraduate curriculum guide, syllabus, and course notes for students. Melbourne, Australia: Australian Catholic University, and St Vincent's and Mercy Private Hospitals, 2000 (revised 2004).

## Recommended websites

**Demonstrating the complexity of replant surgery**
http://www.frps.org/rePlant.html
http://buncke.org/book/ch39/ch39_3.html
http://www.baps.co.uk/clinical_areas/trauma-hand.htm
http://www.orthop.washington.edu/hand_wrist/replantationsurgery/print
http://www.orthop.washington.edu/hand_wrist/replantationsurgery/03

# Chapter 22

# Tissue Expansion

## Background

Tissue expansion is a mechanical process that increases the surface area of local tissues available for reconstructive procedures. It is an integral component of the reconstructive ladder[1-11].

Although the selection of the site for expansion is critical, the increasing understanding of the blood supply to the skin has seen its application widened from the external skin to the oral and vaginal mucous membrane, for local reconstructive procedures[1,2]. This chapter will be confined to the skin.

---

### Box 22.1 Surgical stages.

- Assessment of the wound and surrounding tissue
- Selection of the site for insertion of the expander
- Inflation of the expander begins at time of insertion with incremental volumes at 3–7 day intervals until the desired expansion is achieved
- In the breast the total time of this phase may take 6–8 weeks to achieve
- Surgical procedure to reconstruct the defect.

---

## Surgical technique

The technique requires the insertion of a medically graded and approved Silastic® expander – a 'balloon' or 'bag' that may be placed under the superficial fascia of the skin, above the fascial layer, or under the muscular layer, according to the goal attempting to be achieved.

The expander has a one way or self/sealing valve/port (placed adjacently, under the skin) that allows the expander to be incrementally inflated (or deflated), expanding the muscle, fascia and the immediate, or surrounding, skin[1-11].

Inflating ports (most fitted with metal inserts) can be integrated into the expander and may be placed under the skin close to, or at a distance from, the prosthesis. Those with a metal component can be located from the outside by a magnet for the purposes of inflation or deflation. This ensures that the expander is not accidentally pierced.

The sizes and shapes of tissue expanders are varied to match the anatomical site of the body, contour required, skin available at the site, fill capacity, skin stretching capacity and amount of skin required[1-11]. Figure 22.1 demonstrates both a range of tissue expanders and permanent implants used in plastic surgery.

There are further examples on the websites provided at the end of this chapter.

---

### Box 22.2 Applications – common examples.

- Congenital malformations:
  - May be any part of the body
  - Reconstruct a congenital malformation for example, an absent breast (e.g. Poland syndrome, Figure 27.4)
- Breast for reconstruction – pre-expansion prior to myocutaneous free flaps
- Forehead, nose, ear, extremities:
  - Assist in reconstruction (following removal of a skin cancer or trauma) of the ear in association with soft tissue tube pedicle (Figure 19.10) or lower limb (Figure 17.11).
- Scalp
  - For replacement of hair-bearing skin, following burns to the scalp[10].

---

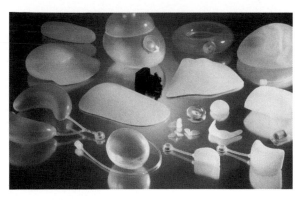

**Figure 22.1** Example of tissue expanders and permanent Silastic® implants.

**Box 22.4** Tissue expansion – the disadvantages.

- The length of time taken to expand the skin may be an issue for some patients
- The expander creates what can be an unsightly bulge when inserted for repair of the scalp or other visible areas of the body
- Following a one or two week interval of initial healing, after primary insertion, the procedure requires usually once or twice weekly visits to the surgeon for injection of normal saline that inflates the balloon
- The extent of expansion is dependent on the ability of the specific skin zone to expand, for example, in semi-fixed skin areas (e.g. lower limbs)
- For some people, the inconvenience and obvious appearance of an expander are significant deterrents for them to consider alternative options (e.g. camouflage prosthetics).

**Box 22.3** Tissue expansion – the advantages.

- Using the patient's own full thickness skin is the best choice where it is possible
- Using adjacent skin offers a near perfect match of colour, texture, and hair bearing qualities
- With the skin remaining connected to the donor area's blood and nerve supply, there is a smaller risk that it will fail
- Almost anyone in need of additional skin can benefit from tissue expansion, infants to elderly men and women
- Surgical tissue expansion is a relatively straightforward procedure that enables the body skin to progressively 'expand' existing skin, generating extra skin for use in reconstructing a defect. (It is a form of local skin flap)
- The use of tissue expansion as an option to reconstruct areas of deficient or defective tissue is now a common surgical option to provide missing or damaged skin, despite the need for 'staged' increases of the expander by:
  - The required injections of fluid over a period of weeks or months
  - Considerable potential complications
- Tissue expansion generally produces excellent results when reconstructing some areas of the face and neck, upper and lower limbs and buttocks.

**Box 22.5** Safety – clinical risk management.

- As with any operation, there are risks associated with surgery, and specific complications associated with those common to procedures where local circulation may be at risk
- The most common patient concern is that the Silastic® expander used in the procedure will crack/break or leak while it is in the body
- Whilst expanders are rigorously pre-tested and placed *in situ* with care, leaks may occur, but this is rare
- If the expander should leak, the solution (normal saline) used to fill the expander is harmlessly absorbed by the system and the expander can be replaced in a relatively minor surgical procedure
- Wound complications parallel those of skin flaps, for example, avascular necrosis, haematoma, seroma and infection related to the increased pressure exerted on the local vessels and nerves each time expansion is undertaken
- Unless these risks are appropriately managed, they may lead to muscle and skin necrosis, infection, expander extrusion, implant failure, constant pain, and underlying nerve injury
- Wound care and the maintenance of basic wound hygiene are important factors in preventing the entry of opportunistic bacteria

*Continued*

- A small percentage of patients develop an infection around or under the expander. While this may occur at any time, it is most often seen within a few weeks after the expander is inserted and is probably due to a small but unrecognised haematoma, or an area of avascular necrosis at the base of the expander
- It is important that the incremental expansion is not so overzealous that it causes avascular necrosis or tension on the suture line, so creating a site for infection
- In some cases, the expander may need to be removed for several months until the infection clears. A new expander can then be inserted should the patient wish
- Overall failure rates relate to the anatomy of particular tissue zones in which the expander is used (e.g. fixed skin areas) and attention to detail in dealing with actual and potential emerging vascular problems[1–8].

- If the pain becomes extreme and continuing, some fluid may need to be removed by the surgeon or the nursing clinician under medical supervision
- Following each expansion, patients must not be discharged from the clinic unless the safety of the overlying skin can be clearly demonstrated.

## Review

*Vascular observations of the hand*, Chapter 20, Tables 20.3 and 20.4.

*Setting goals of care and preferred clinical and patient outcomes*, Chapter 2, Boxes 2.7–2.9.

**Box 22.7** Wound bed maintenance – nursing care.

- Increasingly, the most common form of insertion is by endoscopy, minimising the length of the suture line
- Following the initial procedure of expander insertion, there should be no tension on the suture lines or the skin zone over the centre of the expander
- Tension is demonstrated by vascular changes (localised whiteness at and across the suture lines)
- It is important to ensure that any securing adhesive dressing tapes used, particularly across the suture lines, are not under any tension – this can result in skin blistering, and wound contamination, which may compromise the success of the entire procedure
- If a drainage tube has been inserted at the time of the initial procedure it should not be removed until the surgeon is satisfied that drainage is absolutely minimal, particularly observing for any primary leakage of the balloon
- Basic hygiene is important to prevent infection, particularly before and after each injection
- A small transparent film dressing can be applied over the injection site, for a few days, following each injection into the valve
- Moisturisation of the suture line/scar lines and expanding skin tissue (e.g. Vaseline®, Sorbolene or glycerin) is required to ensure softness, as the tenseness of dry skin may cause blistering or cracks in the thinner skin zones
- Moisturiser also restores pH of the skin, enabling it to provide barrier function.

**Box 22.6** Comfort – clinical risk management.

- Oral pre-emptive pain management should be considered prior to each increase in the volume of the tissue expander
- Regardless of the insertion site of the expander, each injection of normal saline that increases the volume of the prosthesis, challenges the integrity of the blood vessels and the peripheral nerves of the expanded tissue/skin and immediate surrounding tissues
- It is common for the balloon to be overinflated initially, causing ischaemic (arterial) pain and severe discomfort
- Assessing for neurovascular compromise related to compression/pressure exerted on the vessels and nerves, following each balloon filling, should be considered standard practice[12]
- Low level, sharp pain, with slow but increasing loss of sensation over the central region of the expander, is an important signal that subtle nerve and vessel pressure injury is occurring in the lower dermal/fascial layer
- Documentation by clinicians of neurovascular assessment, including pain scores, using numerical scales, is essential following each incremental inflation
- In a limb, elevation of the part is a key element of the resolution of pain as this reduces arterial blood inflow, and assists venous outflow

- The nurse clinician should reinforce the positive characteristics of the procedure without minimising any obvious difficulties – document the observations related to each visit or communication
- Any doubts and problems the patient may communicate should be listened to, and if necessary, reported to the surgeon, particularly those that relate to pain or loss of sensation over the expander site
- The patient should be educated that some degree of discomfort will be felt for a few days following further inflation
- Postoperative pre-emptive education regarding oral pain management and elevation of the part, where possible, provides comfort
- Patient education is important for the patient to be able to discriminate between normal short-term pain/discomfort, and ischaemic reportable pain
- Vascular assessment and reporting criteria education should be reinforced following each visit, with the patient observing for adverse events related to potential deflation or signs and symptoms of infection
- Extreme care must be taken to ensure avascular necrosis does not occur through inadequate communication of the pain threshold level and vascular observations required to be undertaken, and reporting parameters between patient, nurse and surgeon
- Directions regarding wound care should be provided in writing and reinforced verbally.

**Review**

*Auditing preferred clinical and patient outcomes,* Chapter 2, Boxes 2.10–2.12.

### Case example

An 18-year-old male was lying on top of a train ('train surfing') and suffered multiple injuries when the train went under a low underpass. Part of the multiple injuries sustained was a de-gloved sacral region, which was primarily skin grafted (Figure 22.2).

When all wounds were healed, the patient underwent the insertion of multiple tissue expanders to address the issues related to function and aesthetics (Figure 22.3). These were expanded and left in for 6–8 weeks.

### Post insertion and post removal of the tissue expanders – nursing care

The initial nursing care of this patient was complex as it required essentially remaining in the face down position with 30° side to side positioning for 72 hours to ensure there was no pressure on the skin flaps and drainage tubes.

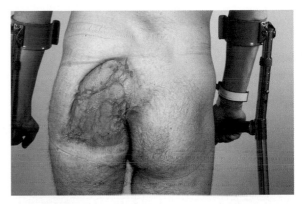

**Figure 22.2** Healed multiple split skin grafts following trauma management.

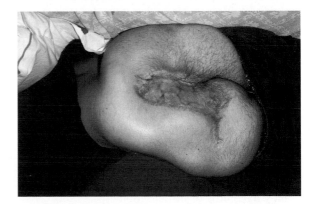

**Figure 22.3** Multiple insertion of tissue expanders (four) to replace scar tissue.

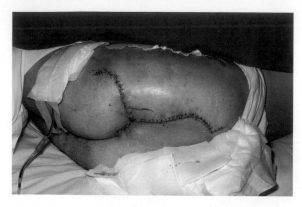

**Figure 22.4** Tissue expanders removed, scar tissue excised and reconstruction using expanded local skin (rear view) – internal negative suction drainage applied to exclude dead space and potential for development of haematoma.

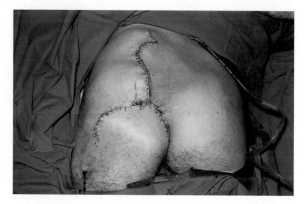

**Figure 22.5** Tissue expanders removed, scar tissue excised and reconstruction using expanded local skin (lateral view).

Each procedure required a nursing care plan that addressed the patient's safety, comfort, wound care and independence needs. Figures 22.4 and 22.5 demonstrate removed tissue expanders and reconstruction of normal tissue. The principal advantage of this will be:

- Significantly reduced risk of secondary injury (pressure ulcers) in the skin grafted tissue, which may have little or no sensation
- A more stable blood supply.

Following insertion and removal stages, physiotherapy assisted in early mobilisation. This allowed for independence that included hygiene (showering) and toilet privileges to be available to the patient. A soft, low residue diet was given for the first two weeks to ensure that there was no constipation and straining.

Tissue expansion, in this case, met the criteria of safety, comfort and independence, as well as protection, function and aesthetics.

See recommended websites following references for additional case examples.

## References

(1) Tissue expansion – emedicine – http://www.emedicine.com/plastic/topic406.htm
(2) Tissue expansion – emedicine – http://www.emedicine.com/ent/topic708.htm
(3) Radovan C. Tissue expansion in soft tissue reconstruction. *Plastic Reconstructive Surgery*, 1984 (Oct); **74**(4): 482–92.
(4) Kayser M.R. Surgical flaps. *Selected Readings in Plastic Surgery* 1999; **9**(2):1–63.
(5) Aston S.J., Beasley R.W. & Thorne C.N.M. *Grabb and Smith's plastic surgery*, 5th edn. New York: Lippincott & Raven Publishers, 1997.
(6) McCarthy J.G. (ed.) *Plastic surgery, volumes 1–8.* Philadelphia: W.B. Saunders, Harcourt Brace, 1990.
(7) Ausher B.M., Erikson E. & Wilkins E.G. *Plastic surgery: indications, operations and outcomes.* St Louis: Mosby, 2000.
(8) Goodman T.A. (ed.) *Core curriculum for plastic and reconstructive surgical nursing*, 2nd edn. Pitman, N.J.: ASPSN American Society of Plastic Surgery Nurses, 1996. http://www.aspsn.org
(9) Fortunato N. & McCullough S. *Plastic and reconstructive surgery.* Mosby's Perioperative Series. St. Louis: Mosby, 1998.
(10) Esposito C. & Dado D.V. The use of tissue expansion in the treatment of burn scar alopecia. *Plastic Surgical Nursing*, 1997; **17**(1):11–15.
(11) Hinojosa R.J. & Layman A.S. Breast reconstruction through tissue expansion. *Plastic Surgical Nursing*, 1996 (autumn); **16**(3):139–45, 176–8.
(12) Kunkler C.E. Neurovascular Assessment (Chapter 2). *Orthopaedic Nursing*, 1999 (May/June); 63–71.

## Recommended website

**Case demonstrations/examples**
http://www.plasticsurgery.org/surgery/recon.htm

- Tissue expansion – the leg
- Tissue expansion – arm and scalp
- Post mastectomy insertion of expander.

# Section V
## Applied Reconstructive Plastic Surgical Nursing 2

# Chapter 23

# Craniofacial Reconstruction

1. Congenital malformations
2. Craniofacial soft tissue and bony trauma
3. Craniofacial tumours
4. Craniofacial vascular anomalies

## Background

In the field of surgery, the establishment of normal anatomical landmarks is essential[1-4]. It is recognised that for optimal functional outcomes, the body's normal structure is designed to provide the best possible opportunities for the human organism to survive.

The craniofacial region contains some of the most fundamental structures required to do this, for example the brain, the facilities for hearing, seeing, digestion, taste, breathing and smell. Any threat to the integrity of the performance of these functions may pose a threat to life.

The term 'craniofacial' is now universally used to describe the anatomical region of the skull and face[1-11]. The span and variations of presenting congenital, post traumatic and disease-based conditions that occur in the craniofacial region, are vast and complex in their description, and beyond the scope of this text.

Sophisticated magnetic resonance radiological imaging (MRI) and 3-D bone structure imaging techniques are the result of state of the art digital imaging and these provide extraordinary anatomical views for accuracy in diagnosis and surgical reconstructive planning[1-4].

This chapter will aim to provide an outline of the common presenting conditions, an overview of the reconstructive procedures available, and the principles of nursing care.

## 1. CONGENITAL MALFORMATIONS

Despite the vast range of minor or major congenital aberrations and malformations that are seen in paediatric reconstructive plastic surgery, nature continues to demonstrate how extraordinary it is that the human organism so often gets it right. But when things go wrong, the consequences can be devastating for the child, the parents, and the extended family.

During pregnancy, some major and severe congenital conditions may be diagnosed at approximately 16 weeks following ultrasound or genetic testing[4]. This presents parents with fundamental decisions as to whether continuation of the pregnancy is to be an option.

Parents will be given every opportunity to make an informed choice with specific and objective unbiased information about the actual and potential positives and negatives of what is currently scientifically and psychologically known and documented.

Having a child born with congenital malformation(s) is a devastating and often an unexpected experience for many parents and surrounding family. This event frequently changes the whole dynamics of the relationships between all concerned. Parental despair and guilt will emerge and early counselling sessions with the surgeon and geneticists can assist the parents in a basic understanding of the origins of the conditions, and what can safely be achieved through treatment options.

Some major conditions observed in the child will present in a variety of patterns, and require appropriate age-related adjustments to professional patient care approaches. The primary needs of safety must be addressed and these include airway management and the initial and specific techniques for baby feeding, and ongoing nutritional needs.

Secondly, issues related to unrecognised or apparent growth dysfunction, intellectual changes or child behavioural problems can be addressed within the boundaries of overall management[1-4].

All of these areas must be handled in a seamless demonstration of professional skills, and undertaken in an attitude of compassion, and recognition of the immediate, and long-term physiological and psychosocial implications.

See recommended websites (craniofacial malformations) at the end of this chapter.

## Common presentations

It should be noted that in the presentation of congenital malformations, general classifications usually come under those conditions that are:

**Non-syndromic**   they essentially appear as a single entity; or

**Syndromic**   they present in association with other abnormal conditions[1-4].

The more common presentations are outlined.

## Craniosynostosis

One of the more common presentations observed at birth is a bony condition that relates to premature fusion of the bones of the cranium. This is called **craniosynostosis**[1-4]. Craniosynostosis is a birth defect of the brain characterised by the premature closure of one or more of the fibrous joints between the bones of the skull (called the 'cranial sutures'), before brain growth is complete. Closure of a single suture is most common.

The abnormally shaped skull that results is due to the brain not being able to grow into its natural shape because of the early closure of this single suture line. Instead, it compensates with growth in areas of the skull where the cranial sutures have not yet closed[1-4].

The condition can be gene-linked or caused by metabolic diseases such as rickets, or an overactive thyroid. Some cases are associated with other disorders such as 'microcephaly' (abnormally small head) and 'hydrocephalus' (excessive accumulation of cerebrospinal fluid in the brain)[1-4].

The first sign of craniosynostosis is an abnormally shaped skull. Other features can include signs of increased intracranial pressure and later developmental delays, or mental retardation, which are caused by constriction of the growing brain. Seizures and blindness may also occur.

Within this taxonomy exists a group of syndromic malformations of the facial bones that are further classified under particular terms, for example, Apert's syndrome, craniofacial microsomia, and Crouzon's syndrome[1-4]. The craniofacial syndromic bony malformation, Apert's syndrome, is associated with webbing malformations in the hands and feet (syndactyly, Figure 23.1) and not uncommonly, hydrocephalus.

Such is the complexity of this particular condition that in some presentations the patient may also present with cleft lip and/or palate (Figures 23.2 & 23.3), heart defects, and with varying degrees of neurological and intellectual impairments[1-4].

There are major and minor classifications of these very complex conditions and each case is managed according to the individual clinical medical presentation, assessment of mental status, and potential for improvement through surgery, medical, nursing, and allied health programmes[1-4].

## Craniofacial clefts

A second major group is classified under the term 'craniofacial clefts' where the vertical form of the face is malformed, creating the split in the bones and soft tissue, for example, bilateral cleft lip and palate[1-4].

The clinical adage is that if one malformation exists there is the real potential for additional abnormalities to be present. Primarily the child should be thoroughly investigated and assessed to exclude any conditions that may present physiological risks to the child's safety. Secondly, at a later stage, the immediate families may desire to be thoroughly investigated to exclude any gene-based aberrations or conditions existing within either parent groups.

## Common secondary syndromic conditions

- Soft tissue and bony malformations of the extremities, for example, finger and toe webbing called 'syndactyly' (Figure 23.1)
- Bony growth plate deficiencies
- Ear anomalies – partial or total absence of a single or both ears, various malformations
- Cleft lip and palate (Figures 23.2 and 23.3).

These may require, where possible, reconstructive surgery to restore important functions, and general aesthetics. Timing or staging of these procedures is usually related to physical growth development,

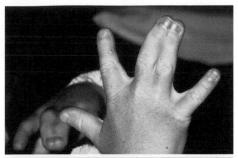

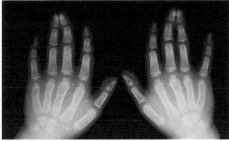

**Figure 23.1** Syndactyly – webbing of the fingers associated with Apert's syndrome.

important functional requirements, the parents desire to prepare the child for the outside world of other children, a wish for increasing independence, and the beginning of school life[1-4].

## Principal patient and medical risk issues

**Box 23.1** Principal and important functional deficits seen in major congenital craniofacial malformations.

- Increased intracranial pressure – requiring lifesaving/preserving surgery
- Hydrocephalus – requiring lifesaving/preserving surgery
- Visual abnormalities with underlying malformations – requiring lifesaving/preserving surgery which also relieves intraorbital pressure[1-4].

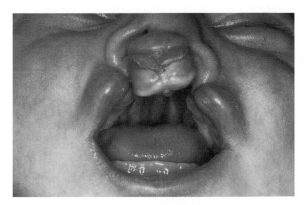

**Figure 23.2** Bilateral cleft lip and palate.

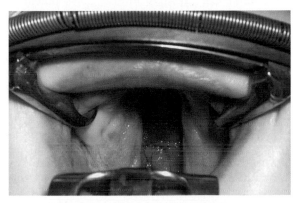

**Figure 23.3** Cleft palate (with intra-operative cleft palate mouth gag in place).

## History of craniofacial reconstructive surgery

In 1901, Dr Rene Le Fort, a French pathologist, published three consecutive papers on the now famous classification of facial fractures. Despite his controversial research methods (e.g. dropping various weighted balls on the faces of human cadavers provided by grave robbers), Le Fort accurately described the lines of weakness (e.g. based on the normal facial suture lines) in the face through which most fractures occurred following trauma.

These lines where the facial bones break following certain forms of trauma, have become known as the **Le Fort I, II,** and **III** fractures. Le Fort's original work has served as the foundation for the development of modern craniofacial and maxillofacial surgery. It has served as a guide for facial repair following trauma, correcting congenital facial anomalies, the rebuilding of the face following major tumour resections, and aesthetic reconstructive surgery (Figures 23.4 and 23.5).

For a range of reasons, Le Fort's work was put on hold. It would not make any profound impact on reconstructive surgical practices until the 1960s.

## Application of Le Fort's concept in the 1940s

The increased use of aeroplanes during World War II produced a large number of major facial deformities and stimulated attempts toward development of facial reconstructive surgery. Sir Harold Gillies, an English plastic surgeon, was a leading contributor in the reconstructive techniques of traumatic deformities. Gillies endeavoured to further advance this field by attempting to apply his trauma-based experience to the treatment of major congenital anomalies.

In 1949, Gillies performed the first elective Le Fort III osteotomy, a procedure which separates the facial bones from the skull with movement of the upper jaw forward. This was the first recorded attempt to radically correct congenital facial deformities with bony facial surgery. It is suggested that Gillies was unhappy with the result, due to a reversion of the bone movements, and never performed the procedure again[2].

## Modern craniofacial surgery

The pioneer and originator of modern reconstructive craniofacial surgery was Dr. Paul Tessier, a French plastic surgeon. Tessier reappraised Le Fort's studies, and renewed the interest of reconstructive plastic surgeons around the world with his research-based classifications of abnormal developments ranging from numbers 1–14. This allowed for innovative and selective operative procedures to be developed in the elective treatment for a broad range of congenital craniofacial malformations.

Tessier's approach was officially described at the 4th Congress of the International Confederation for Plastic and Reconstructive Surgery in Rome, in 1967, where he presented a successful case in which a facial advancement was surgically performed to treat a patient with Crouzon's syndrome. The Le Fort III osteotomy and bone advancement was designed to include a major portion of the orbits with the upper jaw. This generated great interest in the new and radical type of surgery. Tessier's procedures contravened the current surgical standards of the day. However, he proved that an assertive application of Le Fort's conceptual approach enabled correction of severe congenital deformities[2].

Tessier's technique included:

- A coronal incision (within the hairline – ear to ear) that included the dissecting/peeling down of the soft tissue from the facial bones, with simultaneous intracranial exposure
- Surgical fracturing of the skull and facial bones (with surgical saws) which permitted circumferential mobilisation of the orbits and enabled radical repositioning of the eyes and the skull
- The principle that the bones must be repositioned or reconstructed before the soft tissue can be repaired[1-4].

Subsequent growth of this specialty was very rapid. Surgeons from all over the world visited Tessier to learn these new operative procedures, and as a result of the surgeons he taught, craniofacial centres emerged across the world. Central to the success of this surgery was the adoption of a multidisciplinary team approach to provide safety and consistency with the most advanced treatments.

Historically, it could be said that the evolution of the knowledge from Le Fort's studies that defined the aetiology of trauma-based craniofacial conditions, has largely been responsible for:

- The understanding and expansion of emergency and elective reconstruction of craniofacial malformations
- The treatment of craniofacial injuries and reconstruction following major facial trauma
- The transference of the concepts and principles to aesthetic surgery developed to alter facial profiles by the redefining and repositioning of the facial bones[1-4].

## Surgical innovation

Surgical innovation and success have been paralleled by the modernisation and the availability of:

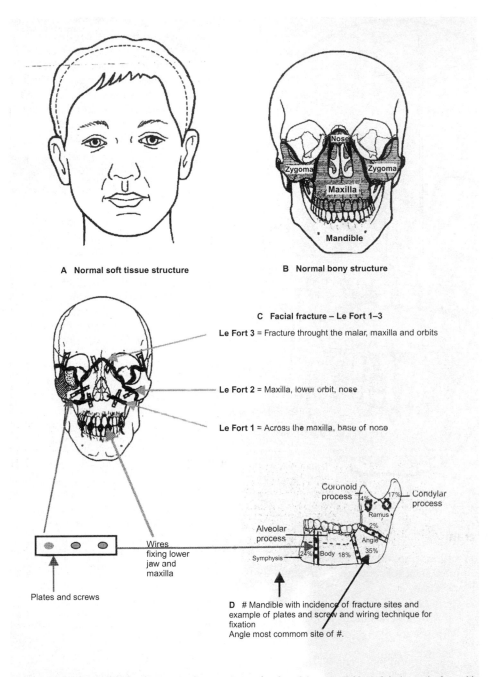

**A  Normal soft tissue structure**

**B  Normal bony structure**

Nose

Zygoma    Zygoma

Maxilla

**Mandible**

**C  Facial fracture – Le Fort 1–3**

**Le Fort 3** = Fracture throught the malar, maxilla and orbits

**Le Fort 2** = Maxilla, lower orbit, nose

**Le Fort 1** = Across the maxilla, base of nose

Coronoid process   4%   17%   Condylar process

Ramus   2%

Alveolar process

Angle   35%

Symphysis   24%   Body   18%

Wires fixing lower jaw and maxilla

Plates and screws

**D   # Mandible with incidence of fracture sites and example of plates and screw and wiring technique for fixation**
**Angle most commom site of #.**

*It is important to note that the above examples constitute only a few of the potential bony injuries to the face with or without associated soft tissue injuries.*

**Figure 23.4** Normal soft tissue and bony structure of the face with examples of typical fracture sites and methods of repair. Teaching notes, Jill E. Storch.

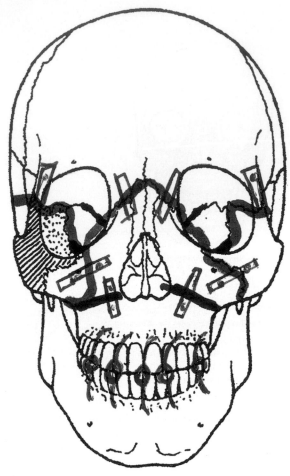

**Figure 23.5** Macro view of common repair of facial fractures – Le Fort I, II and III. Teaching notes, Jill E. Storch.

- Prevention and management of infection (particularly meningitis) by antibiotics that can penetrate the blood–brain barrier
- A multidisciplinary approach
- Increasing sophisticated radiological imaging
- A range of refined anaesthetic and safe operating room practices
- Specialised bone fixation materials (Figures 23.4 & 23.5)
- Specialist postoperative nursing care
- Psychosocial assessment, and the dedicated care by parents and significant others.

This specialty continues to grow rapidly due to contributions from craniofacial teams and increasing

technological innovations. This ensures that this leading edge surgery will continue to offer new hope and promise to patients, regardless of the aetiology, by appreciably improving the functional, and aesthetic, quality of life of many human beings who otherwise may have been condemned to a life being ostracised by much of society, hidden in the home, or confined to mental institutions[1–15].

## Craniofacial surgery – preferred outcomes of reconstruction

**Box 23.2** Preferred outcomes of craniofacial surgical procedures.

| | |
|---|---|
| **Protective** | Ensuring airway and neurological safety |
| **Corrective** | To correct malformations of the skull bones and/or face and that result from birth defects, trauma or tumours |
| **Restorative** | To restore optimal structural stability and functional outcomes |
| **Aesthetic** | To restore, or improve, the craniofacial aesthetics. |

### Essentials of the overall approaches to be undertaken

Craniofacial surgery requires a team approach with a multidisciplinary and case management approach that includes both the patient and significant carers, wherever possible[1–4].

The proposed order and type of interventions to be undertaken is based on:

- A needs assessments for patient safety
- Extent of the intervention(s) required to achieve the preferred outcomes
- Any morbid factors that may present risks to the preferred end outcomes.

A breakdown in any aspect of care may cause the significant carers or parents to lose faith in the process, and this may have long-term consequences should secondary procedures be required. The reconstructive surgeon(s) and nurse team leader must maintain a close observation on all aspects of the patient's management.

**Box 23.3** Range of the craniofacial multidisciplinary team participants.

- Clinical nurse specialist/co-ordinator
- Craniofacial surgeon
- Plastic surgeon
- Ear, nose and throat specialist (otolaryngologist)
- Geneticist
- Neonatologist
- Neurosurgeon
- Operating room nurses
- Surgical unit nurses including intensive care unit
- Nutritional specialist
- Oral surgeon
- Orthodontist
- Paediatric dentist
- Physical therapist
- Paediatrician
- Primary care physician
- Psychologist
- Speech therapist
- Social worker.

**Box 23.4** Primary management – assessment, risk assessment and planning.

- Following birth, specialist paediatric consultations for medical, neurological and opthamological status are undertaken to establish any need for emergency life-saving, or life-preserving interventions
- Following referral, computerised tomography, magnetic resonance imaging and 3-dimensional radiographic imaging/studies are undertaken to assess the degree of malformation, allowing senior team surgeons to determine the degree of bone malformation, and bone movements that may be necessary to bring about safe maximum structural and functional results
- Referrals on to other specialists are determined by prioritising the lifesaving/life-preserving needs of the infant
- In particular craniofacial malformations (e.g. craniosynostosis) early surgery/intervention is required to reconstruct/redefine the cranial vault to provide for the growth of the brain soon after birth
- In any surgery that exposes the brain, the primary life-threatening risk in the intraoperative phase is haemorrhage, and in the postoperative phase, meningitis[1–5]
- Early major reconstructive surgery is not undertaken unless both physical and functional results are identified to be in the patient's best interests with minimal risk to the patient's life
- Prior to undertaking any major craniofacial or bone reconstructive procedures, surgeons will examine 3-dimensional digital computer imaging, discuss it in multidisciplinary team meetings, rehearse the procedure on paper, use assembled plastic models, and if appropriate, make use of the autopsy room
- Timing of elective surgical intervention(s) is largely determined by the presenting status of the patient, parent's desire for change, and the perceived safety of the proposed procedure
- With children, parents must be included in all aspects of the decision-making process
- An integral part of any professionally planned procedure, surgical or nursing, is to 'walk' through the entire plan in the mind's eye, addressing potential risks/complications, and developing contingency plans to deal with potential adverse events or complications
- The need to primarily address or correct other associated conditions will be made before any decision is made for elective craniofacial reconstruction. These include:
  - Potential for respiratory compromise (e.g. Pierre Robin's syndrome – a complex congenital syndrome identified by a recession of the mandible)
  - Cardiovascular abnormalities (particularly heart valve anomalies)
  - Nutritional problems related to feeding difficulties.

## Paediatric craniofacial surgical approaches – examples

### Craniosynostosis – endoscopic approach

Based on current advancements of endoscopic surgical techniques, a recent important advancement described in the literature is the treatment of congenital craniosynostosis suitable for children five months of age and under.

This minimally invasive procedure utilises only incisions of 2 cm rather than full coronal incisions (ear to ear). Surgery is followed by the wearing of specially designed 'moulding' helmets (similar to safety helmets), which are mechanically adjusted weekly for up to 6–8 months[4–7].

See recommended websites (craniofacial malformations) at the end of this chapter.

---

**Box 23.5** Suggested advantages of the endoscopic approach.

- Minimises invasive anaesthetic procedures
- Does not require tracheostomy, wires, plates and screws
- Significantly reduced operating, and inpatient timeframes
- Minimises postoperative brain swelling, and the potential for haemorrhage and infection
- Significantly more cost effective, and less disruptive to the child.

---

- Modular Internal Distraction System (MID™) introduced by endoscopic technique utilising biodegradable devices:
  - Timing of surgery appears to be contentious and based on individual patient assessment
  - The utilisation of tracheostomy for airway management, and the postoperative placement in PICU, is determined by related abnormalities that may compromise the airway in the postoperative phase
  - Inpatient time is suggested to be approximately 2–4 days, depending on any related risk factors[4-7] (see also selected website references)
  - The significant advantages for the patient are similar to those outlined in Box 23.2.

## Craniofacial distraction osteogenesis

Based on original orthopaedic techniques of long bone lengthening which evolved from the work of Gavriel Ilizarov in Kurgan, Siberia, in the 1960s, advances have been made in the past 40 years, with the procedure now being applied to malformations of the craniofacial region.

These techniques have been further improved with external and internal distraction osteogenesis accepted as a surgical process for reconstruction of skeletal deformities. This involves gradual, controlled displacement of surgically created fractures resulting in simultaneous expansion of soft tissue, and bone volume.

---

**Box 23.6** Modular Internal Distraction System (MIDS™) techniques.

- Mid-face distraction using MIDS™:
  - A coronal incision is made and the surgeon divides the skull into two sections – the MIDS is applied, and special metal or biodegradable plates are implanted beneath the skin and the two sections are reattached
  - Over a period of approximately 4–8 weeks, with the use of an expansion screw, the plates are incrementally forced apart with new bone growing between the gap plates reshaping the skull.

---

## Open surgical procedure

As outlined in Tessier's technique[1-4].

## Adjunctive procedure for increasing amount to available soft tissue

Preoperative soft tissue expansion (see Chapter 22) has been described as a significant advantage where soft issue is minimal, or absent, prior to reconstruction utilising traditional osteotomy and bone grafting. Advantages that have been suggested include tension-free suture lines, use of like tissue and colour, and improved aesthetic results[10].

---

**Developments in treating congenital malformations of the mandible**

Some congenital bony malformations of the lower jaw (e.g. Pierre Robin's syndrome – a complex congenital syndrome identified by a recession of the mandible) are being primarily treated by the use of what are also referred to as 'distraction' techniques[5,8,9]. This is a similar concept to the Modular Internal Distraction System (MIDS™) described in Box 23.6.

The technique includes intra-osseous pins inserted into the cortex of the mandible. A frame is attached, and by a mechanical adjusting process, the bone is 'distracted' or 'stretched', and incrementally lengthened to a point where the lower jaw is essentially a 'normal' length for that individual patient.

This technique again reflects the methods used to lengthen the long bones of the limbs where congenital malformations or growth defects occur. Realignment of the teeth using intradental frames and wiring may be undertaken simultaneously to help achieve the desired aesthetic and functional outcomes.

## Fixation materials utilised in craniofacial surgery

Plates and screws used to fix facial and small bone 'fracture' sites are now more commonly made of:

**Titanium:** because of the strength of titanium, smaller plates and screws can be used in injured sites where access is difficult. In some cases of, for example, particular fracture regions of the jaw, this allows the patient to forgo the previous practice of locking/splinting of the upper and lower teeth in the postoperative healing phase. This modern approach enables the patient to eat and drink, within certain parameters, more normally, but with extreme care.

**Absorbable material:** plates and screws that have greater strength, integrate and dissolve within the bone over time are now becoming more readily available and used more frequently. As plates and screws are often required to be removed after the fracture or reconstruction is healed, these new materials have the potential to reduce hospital costs and require the patient to undergo only one procedure. At the time of writing, no long-term research was available to confirm or deny the efficacy of their use.

---

**Review**

*Setting goals of care and preferred clinical and patient outcomes*, Chapter 2, Boxes 2.7–2.9. Adapt as appropriate to the patient's clinical needs.
    *Perioperative management – children*, Chapter 16.

---

**Box 23.7** Discharge education.

- Ongoing wound safety management
- Nutritional management – as formulated with nutritional expert
- Comfort management – analgesia as prescribed
- Oral hygiene management
- Pin site care
- Suture line care as appropriate
- Parents reporting protocols if problems occur
- Reassurance that assistance is only a phone call away
- Referrals and appointments for ongoing management as directed by team leader.

---

## Congenital malformation of the upper lip and/or palate

The long history of reconstructive plastic surgery has always included the attempted non-surgical and surgical management of cleft lip and palate[1-4]. Figure 23.6 demonstrates one of the many medieval attempts at cleft lip repair.

See recommended websites (cleft lip and palate) at the end of this chapter.

Despite evolutionary advances in surgical reconstructive techniques, there are few conditions that require such prolonged detailed, disciplined and integrated management, and touch almost every facet of medical, nursing, and allied health sciences, than congenital malformation of the upper lip and/or palate.

Figure 23.3 exhibits a major cleft in the palate. Figures 23.2 and 23.7 exhibit the severity of a bilateral lip and cleft palate, with the lip repaired. Again, modern research into the blood supply to the skin is assisting in delivering better surgical results and Figure 23.8 shows contemporary cleft lip repair based on the research and knowledge of the micro blood supply within the upper lip and surrounding tissues.

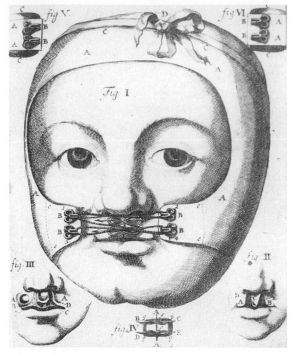

**Figure 23.6** Historical method of attempted repair of cleft lip based on use of head harness and lacing of edges together. Reprinted from: Wood-Smith D., 1967, with permission from Elsevier.

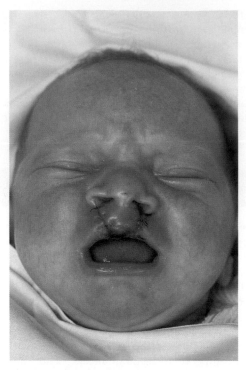

**Figure 23.7** Bilateral cleft lip repair – post repair.

**Box 23.8** Definition/classification/incidence.

- Cleft lip is the result of failure of fusion of the soft tissue of the upper lip during embryonic development
- Cleft palate is the result of inadequate fusion of the soft and/or hard palate during embryonic life
- Cleft lip or cleft palate may be incomplete, unilateral or bilateral
- Cleft lip is associated with cleft palate in 70% of unilateral cleft lip cases and 85% of bilateral cleft lips[1]
- Incidence – clefts: About 1:1000 births. Males are involved more frequently than females and the left side is involved more frequently than the right. Asians have a rate of 2:1000 births and Africans are reported as 0.5:1000. Figures vary in different races[1–4].

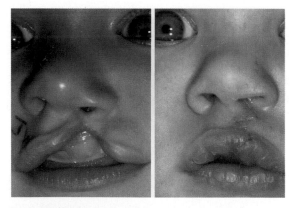

**Figure 23.8** Repair of cleft lip based on clinical research of the blood supply to the upper lip. With permission: Professor G.I. Taylor.

## Box 23.9 Aetiology.

- Most facial-based clefts (or bone/soft tissue divisions) are considered spontaneous and in only 30% of cases can an identifiable cause be found.

| | |
|---|---|
| **Familial** | 30% have positive family history, usually associated with multiple factors. |
| **Genetic** | syndromic or non-syndromic |
| **Environmental** | (suggested association) alcohol, smoking, anticonvulsants, retinoids, folate deficiency[1-4]. |

## Box 23.10 Multidisciplinary management pathways.

- Management begins immediately after birth and, for most children, will often continue until adulthood
- The long-term period of management is related to matching the required procedures for facial asymmetry, optimal dental and speech function, to overall growth development timeframes
- This congenital condition is a complexity of physiological and psychosocial patient needs, with patience and dedication required by all concerned, particularly the parents
- Clinicians will be mindful of the potential for associated congenital morbid factors, such as heart defects, vascular aberrations, and intellectual deficits, which may not be recognised until later stages as the child develops[1-4].

## Box 23.11 Clinical management of cleft lip and cleft palate.

- The surgeon will normally visit parent(s) and baby immediately after birth to provide reassurance, outline the primary treatment regime, and discuss the projected timeframe
- Parents are usually devastated and will frequently have strong feelings of guilt, failure and fear
- Continuing reassurance and reinforcement of assistance is essential
- As many of these babies are born premature, the staging of reconstruction is determined by appropriate management of any associated medical conditions, the nutritional status, and attainment of appropriate growth milestones[1-4]
- In both cleft lip and particularly cleft palate, safe and effective feeding is the initial, and often, enduring difficulty for parents but feeding methods are becoming increasingly more sophisticated in assisting the child and parents[1-4].

See recommended websites (cleft lip and palate) at the end of this chapter.

## Box 23.12 Clinical management of cleft lip – feeding.

- Each child will be individually assessed and a feeding regime planned to suit the degree of the malformation(s)[1-4,11-14]
- Breastfeeding for unilateral cleft lip is usually possible but in complex bilateral cleft lip which includes the anterior palate, the baby may have some difficulty in creating a sealed vacuum, leading to an inability to suck properly (i.e. proper oral closure cannot be undertaken to enable suction to be effective) or to get sufficient volume
- Frequent burping (expelling of stomach air swallowed during feeding) is very important for the baby's comfort
- Surgeons and specialist unit clinicians will usually have a preference for particular feeding implements and techniques to meet special needs, and the surgeon and specialist paediatric and lactation nurses will spend considerable time explaining this to the baby's carers (see Box 23.13 for feeding examples).

## Box 23.13 Clinical management of cleft palate – feeding.

- Infants with cleft palates cannot breastfeed as they cannot form a suction technique[1-4]
- Breast milk may be obtained by the use of a breast pump
- Clinicians specialising in cleft palate feeding, and lactation experts, will be consulted in the first in-

*Continued*

stance for guidance, and to provide the mother with confidence in the feeding process
- Special feeding teats, bottles, spoons, and individualised positions (e.g. sitting in a 30–40° position) for feeding techniques will be required to allow gradual flow, and prevent fluid regurgitation into the lungs
- Babies with cleft palate tend to swallow more air while feeding and may need more frequent burping than other babies
- Examples of feeders available include:

| | |
|---|---|
| **NUK nipple**® | this nipple can be placed on regular bottles or on bottles with disposable bags. The hole can be made larger by making a criss-cross cut in the middle |
| **Mead Johnson's Cleft Palate Nurser**® | this is a soft, plastic bottle that is easy to squeeze and has a large crosscut nipple. Any nipple that the infant prefers can be used with this system |
| **Medela's Haberman Feeder**® | a specially designed bottle system with a valve to help control the air the baby takes in, and to prevent milk from going back into the bottle |
| **Syringes** | these may be used in hospitals following cleft surgery and may also be used post surgery at home. Typically, a soft rubber tube is attached on the end of the syringe, which is then placed in the infant's mouth. |

- In some cases, supplements may be added to breast milk, or formula, to help the infant meet his/her calorie needs. Again, paediatric nurse lactation and nutrition experts can assist and should be consulted
- Close regular monitoring and charting of weight at all stages of primary infant care and developmental stages, prior to, and following surgery, is an essential component of ongoing management.

---

**Box 23.14** Clinical management – addressing feeding and nutritional difficulties.

- For some cleft palate babies, custom-designed space-occupying appliances called 'obturators' or 'feeding aid appliances'[5], may be designed to enable the baby to suck without fluid escaping through the nasal passages. These are similar to dental plates used to hold teeth[1–4]
- Custom appliances may also be designed to guide the alveolar (premaxillary) segments into place prior to surgery[1–4]

- With suitable cleft lip babies, some surgeons may create specifically designed 'lip adhesion' devices in an attempt to reduce the gap and assist in feeding[1–4]
- Babies should not be discharged from hospital unless parents are comfortable with the management of the baby's feeding and general care[1–4]
- Surgeons, paediatricians and nursing clinics must continue to ensure the parents are comfortable with feeding techniques, and weight charts must be checked at regular weekly intervals until discontinued by the surgeon or paediatrician
- For adults with an unrepaired cleft palate, obturators are custom designed to allow both feeding and speech to be enhanced. This technique is commonly practised in situations where continuing complications prevent complete closure of the palate, or in developing countries where surgery is unavailable, has failed, fistulas occur that cannot be repaired, or defects are so wide that surgery is not possible[1–4].

See recommended websites (cleft lip and palate) at the end of this chapter.

---

**Box 23.15** Cleft lip – decision-making for surgical intervention.

- The timing of surgical repair of a cleft lip is generally determined by the degree of impairment, the protocols of the particular surgeon, or specialist units, any associated morbidity and the overall health status of the child
- Modern paediatric anaesthetics and increasingly sophisticated techniques have allowed early timing of surgery[1–4]
- Some centres may do a Stage 1 procedure by 'suturing' the two edges of the lip together (called 'lip adhesion' – a modified cleft lip repair) prior to the baby's discharge from hospital to assist in feeding, and for aesthetic considerations[1–7]. This is principally dependant on the surgeon's judgement of each individual case, and the wishes and permission of the parents[1–4]
- Nutritional weight and overall growth may define timing of procedures and in cleft lip this usually seems to occur at between approximately 10–12 weeks[1–4]
- Simultaneous primary repair of the anterior (soft) palate may also be undertaken within some techniques[1–4]

- Pre-surgical orthodontics is becoming more common in babies to direct ongoing body/tissue growth, to enhance surgical correction, ultimate function, and aesthetics when surgery is undertaken[1-4] (see website references for examples at the end of this chapter)
- Bilateral cleft lip is an extremely difficult surgical repair procedure, and usually requires multiple procedures to correct the absent tissue and nasal deformities (e.g. secondary procedures such as Abbe flaps – using a tissue flap from the lower lip[1-4]
- Tissue expansion is now being discussed and used to assist in correction of tissue deficits and nasal deformities[10].

---

**Box 23.16** Cleft palate – decision-making in surgical intervention.

- Children with severe unilateral, or bilateral cleft lip, and/or cleft palate will usually require long-term and significant orthodontic treatment and speech therapy assistance
- Cleft palate (Figures 23.4 & 23.6) children are often prone to middle ear infections but there is differing opinion on what approaches should be medically taken
- Hearing may be affected because the muscles of the palate affect the ear, making the child more likely to develop 'glue ear', a condition where thick sticky fluid accumulates behind the eardrum as a result of an infection of the middle ear. Medically it is referred to as otitis media with effusion. It can cause temporary hearing loss but can be treated with antibiotics or, if it is an ongoing problem, with a minor operation to insert a tiny plastic tube (i.e. a grommet) into the eardrum through which the fluid can drain
- Primary surgery is usually undertaken at approximately 6–12 months of age depending on degree of deformity, nutritional status, and attainment of growth milestones
- Following complex cleft palate repair, palatal fistula may be a complication that is difficult to correct and may compromise speech quality
- Secondary and tertiary surgical procedures are a common feature of this condition
- For orthodontic integrity, a bone graft to the alveolus may be done at about 10 years of age to assist in growth of secondary front teeth. Orthodontic management dominates at this stage[1-5]
- The final plastic surgical operations are usually related to speech quality, quality of nasal airways, and cos-metic outcomes related to the shape of the nose, and this may continue until the patient is in adulthood[1-4]
- For some patients, as previously discussed, obturators may remain the only, or the preferred, alternatives to successive surgical procedures where closure is complex or constantly plagued with complications (e.g. palatal fistula)
- For nurse clinicians, patient education regarding obturator cleanliness, based on oral hygiene maintenance, is important for overall oral and dental management.

---

**Review**

*Setting goals of care and preferred clinical and patient outcomes*, Chapter 2, Boxes 2.7–2.9. Adapt as appropriate to the patient's clinical needs.

*Perioperative management* – children, Chapter 16.

---

**Box 23.17** Cleft lip – the primary surgery.

- Procedures may be prefaced by the application of custom designed orthodontic appliances/aids to guide the alveolar/premaxilla segments into place prior to surgery
- Primary surgical goal is to close the soft tissue gap
- Primary cleft lip surgical approaches are based on the degree of deformity
- Local anaesthetic (e.g. lignocaine) with adrenaline is commonly injected prior to the surgical procedure. This minimises bleeding during surgery and assists in reducing postoperative soreness
- Lip closure may leave the suture lines under significant tension
- Strengthening of the suture line may be required by the use of adhesive paper tapes for approximately 72 hours and following removal of sutures
- Postoperative haematoma or oedema may cause separation of the wound edges[1-4,13,14]
- Nasal and oral hygiene following feeding, and as required
- Suture line and surrounding skin may need basic moisturising – Vaseline® or antibiotic ointment
- Arms may need to be restrained at the elbow (as prescribed) to prevent access of the child's hand to the mouth and thus potential for secondary injury.

**Box 23.18** Cleft palate – the primary surgery.

- Local anaesthetic (e.g. lidocaine) with adrenaline is commonly injected prior to the surgical procedure. This minimises bleeding during surgery and assists in minimising postoperative soreness
- During surgery, palatal tissue flaps are raised based on their palatine arterial blood vessels to replace missing central palatal tissue. This is accomplished by dissecting the tissues from the lateral edges of the palate and joining the elevated tissues at the centre, thus closing the central gap
- This movement of tissue leaves raw exposed areas on each side of the palate which heal through granulation[1–4,13,14].

## Cleft lip/palate – postoperative nursing management

**Box 23.19** Safety.

- The use of a tongue stitch to maintain a patent and controlled airway has been largely abandoned but is extremely useful if postoperative bleeding occurs (Figure 23.9). If used, the stitch should be inserted at the mid level of the tongue transversely, not vertically, as any strain placed on the stitch will tear the tongue tissue
- In the immediate postoperative period, the primary risk potential is for airway compromise, or loss of airway control should the tongue stitch be removed prior to the child being fully awake
- Complications may occur (e.g. post cleft palate – postoperative haemorrhage) (see Box 23.20)
- Postoperative haemorrhage is uncommon following cleft lip repair but swelling should be observed, and some initial discomfort will be experienced by the child
- At no point should an artificial airway be placed in the mouth unless undertaken by the surgeon or anaesthetist, as this may cause a complete breakdown of the surgery due to external pressure, significantly increasing the risk of life-threatening bleeding
- Fluid imbalance (dehydration – hypovolaemia) may occur if the child has been fasting for long periods, blood loss is in excess of the child's capacity to compensate, or there has been inadequate fluid replacement – urinary output should be strictly monitored

- Physical distress may occur if pain/discomfort, and hypothermia is not addressed pre-emptively[16]
- Children must never be left unsighted or unobserved until fully awake
- Clinicians should never turn their backs on a child in the post anaesthetic phase, as the potential for falls/injury is high
- In the older child, or adolescents having secondary cleft palate procedures, postoperative haemorrhage is uncommon, but management may be based on post tonsillectomy regimes.

**Box 23.20** Emergency management following bleeding – cleft lip.

- If the parents are present, request they wait outside until the child's condition is settled
- If appropriate, give small dose of sedation by providing prescribed opioid if the child is restless and anxious
- Nurse the baby on their right side
- Do not introduce a plastic or metal suction device into the mouth – use a gauze swab placed over a gloved finger to mop up any blood in the cheek space
- Request someone call the surgeon and a resident medical officer immediately
- Strictly observe vital signs, especially patient oxygen saturation, colour, pulse rate and rate of breathing – call Code Blue if any doubt about airway problems
- Give oxygen as required
- Keep parents informed of what is happening as much as possible.

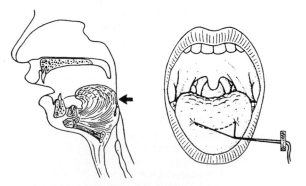

**Figure 23.9** Demonstrating the value of a correctly placed tongue stitch to assist in maintaining airway control post trauma and surgery.

**Box 23.21** Emergency management following bleeding – cleft palate.

- Seek immediate assistance
- Place the child on his/her right side to avoid regurgitation of blood and obstruction of airway
- Do not introduce a plastic or metal suction device into the mouth – use a gauze swab placed over a gloved finger to mop up blood in the cheek space
- If the parents are present, request they wait outside until the child's condition is settled/controlled
- Do not leave the child alone – call a Code Blue if there is no medical officer in the immediate vicinity or it is deemed necessary for patient safety
- If appropriate, give a small dose of sedation by providing IV morphine by infusion pump to reduce child's anxiety
- Strictly observe vital signs, especially patient oxygen saturation, colour, pulse rate and rate of breathing – give oxygen if possible
- If bleeding is constant or excessive, take a folded gauze swab, stand behind the head of the child, place the left hand on the back of the head for counter pressure and control of head movement
- With the right index and/or middle finger insert the folded gauze into the mouth, and gently exert pressure on the bleeding palate vessel until the doctor arrives (the risk of a bitten finger is better than an exsanguinated child)
- Save all blood soaked material for blood loss assessment
- Keep parents informed of what is happening as much as possible.

**Box 23.22** Comfort.

- Many anaesthetists will insert paediatric rectal analgesia (e.g. paracetamol) prior to commencement of the surgery, or immediately postoperatively to provide a therapeutic level of comfort as the anaesthetic analgesic drugs wear off
- Leading experts advocate the feeding of babies (glucose water or diluted normal feeds) within one hour of cleft palate and/or cleft lip repair, with excellent outcomes for comfort
- Continuing provision of oral pain/comfort management as prescribed (e.g. four-hourly for the first 72 hours), and to relieve additional discomfort by synchronising analgesia just prior to feeding times

- Distress raises the child's blood pressure, increasing the risk of small vessels oozing, clots dislodging and bleeding to commence
- Surgeons and lactation experts will prescribe a methodology with a progressive and timely regime for restoring normal fluid replacement and nutrition
- Return to normal feeding is related to the extent of the surgery and the child's early, medium and long-term nutritional and fluid needs
- The use of oral 'comforters' is not advocated and should only be used with permission of the surgeon
- Warmth, cuddling, soothing and satisfying dietary needs, are essential elements of a holistic approach to risk management.

**Box 23.23** Wound management and general nursing care.

For approximately one week after surgery, lip wounds are usually taped to protect against secondary injury and subsequent wound edge separation/breakdown

- Basic wound hygiene must be undertaken at regular intervals and as necessary
- Lip soreness and surrounding oral skin 'cracking' will occur if moisture is not maintained
- Vaseline® or antibiotic ointment should be applied before and after feeding, and after any toileting of the wound(s)
- Protocols for oral and nasal hygiene is essential following cleft lip and cleft palate procedures, particularly oral care following each feeding
- Suture (may be absorbable) removal following cleft lip is usually undertaken without the use of sedation or general anaesthetic – in some cases there may be the exception
- Sutures utilised in a cleft palate repair will be absorbed and do not require removal.

**Box 23.24** Independence.

- Some surgeons will request the use of arm splints/restraints to protect the wound from little hands scratching, etc., but the use of restraints is being seen less often, or has ceased[13,14]

*Continued*

- A specialist plastic surgery paediatric unit study has shown that there appears to be no evidence to support the standard use of child restraint, post cleft lip/palate[15]
- Use of restraints should be discussed with the individual surgeon prior to application
- Parent(s) may demonstrate anxiety in respect of surgical and wound outcomes relating to feeding practices and feeding routines
- Discharge parental education by specialist paediatric nurses competent in the feeding of children with feeding problems, in association with nutritional experts, and community nurses, needs to be ongoing
- Positive reinforcement helps the parents' confidence, and ability to manage is also essential, as many of these babies are very small and parents may feel inadequate, anxious, varying degrees of guilt, and fear of the unknown or unexpected.

## Psychosocial assistance

Parents may be alerted to support groups and encouraged to contact them for family support. Some surgeons have reservations about such groups, as they believe the children should be allowed to integrate into the normal community without feeling 'different'.

Groups such as these can be very reassuring to the parents, with additional counselling available. The difficulty arises when parents begin to compare treatment regimes, surgeons and overall care, and believe that they may be being disadvantaged in some way. Nurse clinicians should not suggest referral to these groups unless the surgeon's wishes are first ascertained.

Genetic counselling is an important part of the overall approach to care and this can alert patients to the potential of clefts in any further proposed offspring[1-4].

---

**Box 23.25** Discharge management.

- Ongoing wound safety management – restraint protocols
- Nutritional management – feeding, weighing
- Discomfort management – analgesia as prescribed
- Oral and nasal hygiene management
- Parents reporting protocols if problems occur
- Wound management as directed
- Reassurance
- Referrals and appointments as directed by team leader.

---

**Review**

*Auditing preferred clinical and patient outcomes,* Chapter 2, Boxes 2.10–2.12.

---

## 2. CRANIOFACIAL SOFT TISSUE AND BONY TRAUMA

**Box 23.26** Craniofacial trauma – adults.

- In adults, the most common presentation of craniofacial conditions in Western society is craniofacial trauma[1-4]
- Most presentations are associated with alcohol intoxication
- Of these, lacerations are the most common, caused mainly by glass, a knife, human or dog bite
- Fractures of the nose, zygoma/malar and mandible due to assaults and sporting accidents are also common
- The presentation of patients with facial fractures should alert clinicians to the potential risk of head/brain injury, cervical spine injury, vascular and nerve injuries of the soft tissue, lacerations to the tongue or palate (frequently missed), loss of teeth, and injury to the senses, particularly sight and hearing
- Fractures of the upper and lower face, with or without head or cervical spine injury may require life-saving interventions (e.g. tracheal intubation or tracheostomy) if the airway is compromised by bleeding
- Injuries that include the eye(s) may result in blindness in one or both eyes[1-4]. Critical clinical assessments must always take these into consideration.

See recommended websites (craniofacial soft tissue and bony trauma) at the end of this chapter.

## Box 23.27 Craniofacial trauma – children.

- Most injuries to the face seen in children are fractured nose (accidental or abuse), lacerations, and particularly dog bites, human bites (from other children), or cat scratches[1-4]
- Facial fractures in children occur in approximately 5% of all presenting facial injuries (e.g. fractured nose, play/sporting injuries, physical assault/abuse) and are treated in the same manner as adults[1-4]
- Some problems with dentition may result but this can be readily adjusted in the growing child
- Because of the fragility of a child's craniofacial bones and the brain, few children survive severe craniofacial injury[1-4]
- Those who do survive may be severely physically and intellectually compromised
- This is clearly demonstrated when accidents are reported that concern children, for example, horse riding, trail bike riding.

## Box 23.28 Principal life-threatening emergency treatment considerations in facial injuries.

- Maintenance of the airway (e.g. oral/tongue lacerations, fractured larynx, loss of consciousness) may require urgent tracheostomy[1-4]
- Identification of other injuries (e.g. brain, cervical spine, eyes, upper and lower limbs, pelvis or internal abdominal organ ruptures)
- Shock
- Identification of additional risk factors, and prevention of aspiration (alcohol, unknown/known presence of illicit drugs, lacerations in the oral cavity, loss of teeth)
- Prevention of additional haemorrhage (e.g. from tongue or palate lacerations, scalp lacerations, nasal fractures)
- Hypovolaemia.

## Box 23.29 Patient assessment 1.

- The patient's history (mechanism of injury) clinical assessment, physical examination
- Assessments of major facial injury presentations primarily include lateral spine X-rays to exclude vertebral fractures, while computed tomography (CT) and magnetic resonance imaging (MRI) are best to demonstrate brain damage[1-4]
- Where available, CT scans and 3-D bone studies are becoming the norm (in addition to the range of standard facial X-rays) to demonstrate extent of bone damage
- CT is useful in demonstrating the true extent of a bony injury and swelling in dead spaces, particularly around the eyes and maxillary region
- Bleeding from the ears should be observed for fractured base of skull
- Brachial plexus injury is often associated with, e.g. motorbike accidents, or horse falls, and may be missed in the flurry of care for other injuries, or if the patient is unconscious.

## Box 23.30 Patient assessment 2.

- In simple or compound wounds of the face, injury to the facial nerve must also be excluded, as facial paralysis is a severely debilitating functional and aesthetic condition[1-4]
- Nurse clinicians should be observant for nerve injury as varying degrees of motor deficiencies may not appear immediately obvious (e.g. due to anaesthesia, or if the patient is unconscious) until the patient is awake, and can co-operate in demonstrating specific facial movements such as a smile, or showing their teeth
- Any indications of motor or sensory deficits should be reported to the surgeon immediately
- If injured, the facial nerve or a significant branch may require immediate, or secondary multiple reconstructive procedures[1-4]
- There are varying degrees of functional recovery and aesthetic outcomes, even when nerve repair is performed at the original time of surgery to repair other injuries[1-4]

**Box 23.31** Patient assessment 3 – upper face – maxilla.

- The maxilla is the fixed/immobile structure, and the mandible is the mobile structure of the face (Figures 23.4 and 23.5)
- Any fracture of the face has the potential to compromise the function of adjacent zones
- Most fractures of the upper face (maxillary zones) are classified as Le Fort I, II or III, according to the position of the fractures that correlate with the suture lines that join the upper zones of the face as previously discussed (Figures 23.4 and 23.5)
- Although Le Fort III is considered the most serious, with craniofacial disjunction (skull separated from the face), the additional potential for life-threatening meningitis is high if the meninges are perforated (i.e. fracture of the cribiform plate), go undiagnosed, or antibiotics are not prescribed immediately
- Nurse clinicians should observe for any fluid arising from the nose (even bloodstained) and this should be carefully assessed (i.e. tested for glucose reaction – may require a specimen to be sent to pathology) to exclude leakage of cerebrospinal fluid
- In addition, the lachrymal process may be injured, resulting in permanent 'dry eye' syndrome if the initial diagnosis is not made, and reconstruction undertaken[1-4]
- Nurses should observe for this, notify any problems to the surgeon, and maintain eye care (ointment treatment as prescribed), as corneal abrasion may occur if pre- and postoperative care is not maintained
- Le Fort II–III fractures (Figures 23.4 and 23.5) are commonly seen following motor vehicle accidents where the individual is not using a seat belt, and the face hits the dashboard or the steering wheel, but may also be caused by cricket or baseball bats, severe physical assault, or the like
- Single facial fractures (e.g. caused by assault or sporting injury) may occur to the malar or zygoma and include severe injuries to the walls of the orbit[1-4]
- This may result in causing potential damage to the eye through a condition called a 'blow out' fracture – a common fracture seen in footballers and unsolicited assaults – mainly diagnosed on CT scanning[1-4]
- The conjunctiva, eye muscle and infra-orbital nerve may become caught in the fracture and cause damage to sight
- Concomitant injury may occur within the temporomandibular joint, causing dislocation fractures and pain on mastication.

**Box 23.32** Surgical management.

- Primary – lifesaving – identification and management of the airway, brain injury, cervical spine, eye injuries, ear injuries including aural cavity
- Secondary – life preserving – identification and management of additional injuries
- Bone realignment – precise reduction and fixation using titanium metal, intermaxillary wiring or biological plates and screws and/or metal frames
- Bone grafts may be required
- Concomitant dental repair may also be required
- Soft tissue repair – underlying structures including vessels, nerves, muscle and skin.

**Box 23.33** Post traumatic reconstruction – the upper face.

- Based on the surgical concepts and principles of major craniofacial surgery (Tessier's technique)
- For most major reconstructive surgery on the upper face an incision is made in the scalp and is called 'bicoronal' (both sides of the skull, extending from ear to ear)[1-4] (see the dotted line on the scalp in Figure 23.4)
- The skin is dissected (peeled) down to the maxillary region exposing the major regions of the bony structure allowing for a clear view of all bony landmarks and soft tissue attachments
- With the incision line in the hairline, wound closure following surgery will be sutures or staples leaving little or no visible scar
- In complex multiple facial fractures, external orthopaedic-type frames may also be placed, securing the upper and lower face by locking the maxilla and mandible firmly for healing purposes. Alternatively, the upper and lower teeth may be wired together, locking the maxilla and the mandible firmly in place
- Single incisions in the hairline above the ear (called a Gillies incision) may be appropriate to elevate simple malar fractures, alternatively, incisions in the line of the lower eyelid, to wire or plate orbital fractures are commonly used, and provide mostly acceptable aesthetic results[1-4].

**Box 23.34** Aetiology and outcomes of fractures of the mandible or lower face.

- After the nasal fractures, fractures of the mandible are the second most common facial bone injury (Nasal fractures will be discussed in Chapter 30 with rhinoplasty).
- Aetiology for both is biased toward sporting injuries and physical assaults
- Secondary dental complications, bilateral temporomandibular injury, dislocations, numbness (e.g. neuropraxia) related to mental nerve injury, trismus (inability to open the mouth) are a few not uncommon, but very important short term and long-term complications[1-4].

**Box 23.35** Mandible fixation techniques.

- Surgery on the mandible or lower face is undertaken mainly within the mouth as in dental surgery[1-4]
- Internal fixation requires incisions to be made into the oral mucous membrane inside the mouth (Figures 23.6 and Figure 23.7)
- Some internal bony fixations for difficult mandible fractures may require additional surgical access via a small incision in the skin of the face overlying the fracture site[1-4]
- 'External fixation' is a method of applying a specially designed orthopaedic type of frame placed on the outside of the face with pins inserted into the bone of the face via tiny skin incisions (pin holes) and bars attached (similar to long bone external fixation management)
- Though facial bone fixation frames are less commonly used, they remain an important option in cases of severe trauma where fixation of multiple facial fractures is necessary to maintain precise reduction and prevent movement
- Plates and screws (titanium or absorbable), wires alone, or in combination, will usually secure the fracture(s) in a stable and fixed position. This is the most common technical option
- In some instances the maxilla and mandible may be wired together for increased stability (Figures 23.6 & 23.7).

**Review**

*Risk management, setting goals of care and preferred clinical and patient outcomes, Chapter 2, Boxes 2.7–2.9.* Adapt as appropriate to the patient's clinical needs.

# Postoperative patient management following craniofacial reconstruction

**Box 23.36** Discharge management.

- Ongoing airway safety management – reinforce protocols
- Nutritional management – dietician referral for ongoing care
- Discomfort management – analgesia as prescribed
- Oral hygiene care as prescribed
- Wound care as directed
- Parents reporting protocols if problems occur
- Ongoing appointments and referrals as directed by team leader.

**Review**

*Auditing preferred clinical and patient outcomes,* Chapter 2, Boxes 2.10–2.12.

## 3. CRANIOFACIAL TUMOURS

**Review**

Common presenting skin lesions/tumours/neoplasms, Chapter 7.

## Facial and oral tumour presentation

### Box 23.37 Head and neck region.

- The skin – benign vascular lesions, benign (hyperkeratosis), basal cell carcinoma (BCC) squamous cell carcinoma (SCC), and malignant skin lesions (melanoma), mainly related to related solar exposure[1-4]
- The lower lip is a common site for squamous cell carcinoma as the mucous membrane is greatly exposed to the sun and other irritants
- Tumours of the upper lip, external nose and facial skin are commonly basal cell carcinoma
- Elderly patients may demonstrate a dark staining of the skin – a tumour referred to as Hutchinson's melanotic freckle – these may go on to become a true melanoma
- The ear in men is a common site for skin lesions, many of which are squamous cell carcinomas
- The oral cavity – squamous cell carcinoma, salivary gland-based tumours, melanoma (very rare) may be seen on the lower lip.
- Patients who are immune compromised demonstrate a high level in the incidence of skin cancer particularly squamous cell carcinoma, and late stage AIDS patients may have Kaposi sarcoma lesions on the face or within the oral cavity
- Combination of skin and bone – e.g. squamous cell carcinoma invading the jaw or naso-ethmoid region
- Tumours of the parotid gland (benign or malignant) present the potential for facial nerve injury leading to paralysis of the affected facial side[1-4]
- Oral, benign or malignant disease processes of the craniofacial (head and neck) region may present in any part of the anatomical structure and, being out of sight, are often late in presentation[1-4]
- Tumours of the mucous membrane of the lip are easily seen and identified, but oral cavity, maxilla, palate and naso-ethmoid regions are often aggressive in nature (grow quickly), and may remain hidden until they bleed, become functionally obstructive, or painful to the patient
- Many are identified at dental visits when patients present because of painful unhealed ulcers of the oral cavity, and/or bleeding[1-4]
- The aetiology may be mixed or unknown, but is suggested to be in response to constant and long-term irritation caused by cigarette and/or marijuana smoking, overingestion of alcohol, nutritional deficits or poor dental fitting/hygiene
- Work environments that allow for the inhalation of toxic fumes and materials such as dust and wood fibres, have also been implicated

- As the blood supply and flow to this region is very high, this provides a source of 'nutrition' to the tumour promoting its growth and early potential to invade the local lymph glands. This then increases the early potential for metastasis, and the extension of the tumour to other systems such as the lung and the bones[1-4]
- Oral tumours may differ according to the age of the patient and their anatomical position
- The most common malignant tumour in this area is called squamous cell carcinoma. In some anatomical areas, this tumour has a high incidence of metastatic spread to the adjacent lymph nodes and then particularly to the lungs, brain and bone[1-4]
- Although some malignant oral tumours may be less aggressive than others, the younger the patient, the more aggressively the tumour appears to act
- As with other malignant tumours that have metastatic properties, these tumours have been scientifically described and graded according to a disease stage that essentially relates to whether lymphatic and/or organ spread is present[1-4]
- Treatment decisions are made according to the overall presentation of each individual, for example, benign (a cyst) or malignant
- Tumour type, position in the craniofacial region and tumour grading will usually determine the treatment modality. This may include surgery, radiotherapy and chemotherapy collectively or individually, according to the type and extent of the disease, potential for survival, and the patient's wishes[1-4]
- In the area of the lips and oral cavity, significant impairment or loss of oral functions such as eating, chewing, drinking, and speech, may occur following extensive tumour excision and reconstruction
- Sight and hearing may also be affected, and patients may be left with a permanent tracheostomy and artificial feeding modalities, significantly altering their quality of life
- Some patients may choose palliative management rather than extensive surgery and this will be offered as a viable option if cure cannot be guaranteed
- Nurse clinicians should be highly conscious of the debilitating psychosocial effects of these life-threatening conditions and act to provide access to any professional assistance available to the patient and family
- For patients undergoing radiotherapy and chemotherapy, the attending oncology clinicians are particularly observant for any adverse physiological effects, presenting wound(s) or psychosocial problems, as often this may affect the patient's wishes to continue complex treatment programmes.

## Head and neck reconstructive surgery options

Options range from direct closure of small skin tumours, skin graft or skin flaps for larger tumours, to major flap surgery for oral tumours with combinations of surgical approaches selected to parallel the functional and aesthetic needs following excision of the tumour[1–4].

Reconstruction of the head and neck is particularly complex when surgeons undertake to remove an aggressive tumour, restore function and aesthetics in one procedure. As these are often older patients, with a myriad of morbid and co-morbid factors, they present significant medical, nursing and allied health challenges from the point of diagnosis to post surgery management, rehabilitation and return to community care[1–4].

Major flap reconstructive microsurgery is a common form of reconstruction, as the surgery required is often extensive, due to the spreading nature of the majority of tumours, and the complexity of the anatomy of the head and neck region.

A significant amount of new bone, muscle and skin (free vascular transfers and skin grafts) may be required. This creates multiple wounds and significantly increases the degree of patient morbidity and co-morbidity for medical and nursing clinicians to address.

---

**Review**

Flap reconstruction techniques, Chapter 18.

---

**Box 23.38** Important preoperative considerations for nurse clinicians.

- Preoperative preparation involves all applications of clinical risk management, and for major elective surgery this can be wide ranging depending on the extent and anatomical site of the surgery
- All embracing preoperative medical and nursing assessment is essential and referrals should include dieticians, physiotherapists, and social workers if family or economic disruption is anticipated
- Strict attention to the physical (particularly cardiorespiratory function) and psychological work ups is

important to establish a safe reconstructive surgery environment, and for the patient to have a sense of confidence in the procedure, and the desired outcomes
- For some head and neck cancer patients, percutaneous endoscopic gastrostomy (PEG) may be inserted up to two weeks prior to surgery to improve the patient's nutritional status, include vitamin supplements, and remain *in situ* for the period of proposed chemotherapy and radiotherapy significantly improving the nutritional status and quality of life of many of these patients
- During, or following, any treatment modality, patients must be observed and questioned regarding any difficulties experienced, particularly those regarding dietary/nutritional needs, weight loss/gain (measured regularly), oral hygiene, pain, wound care, general feelings, and psychosocial problems
- It is important to address the patient personally, if possible, and not to exclude him/her from the process of care and decision-making and where possible, the family or significant carers must be informed and included in all aspects of care and any changes in treatment programme for the patient's condition
- Family or carers may have different expectations and may be shocked at the extent of the reconstructive surgery required and the technology involved during the immediate postoperative period
- Preparation of the patient and relatives will reduce the visual impact and improve the acceptance of the methods required to secure the safest and best patient outcome[1–4].

---

**Review**

*Nutritional issues for reconstructive plastic surgical patients*, Chapter 9.

---

## Postoperative nursing management following craniofacial reconstruction

This section applies to:

- Facial fractures done as part of surgery to reconstruct/realign following congenital malformation
- Facial fractures due to injury
- Bony facial reconstruction following excision of tumours and local flap or free flap tissue reconstruction[1–4].

## Box 23.39 Safety 1.

- Before accepting patient from post anaesthesia care unit the clinician should ascertain if the upper and lower jaws have been locked together and what method has been used
- Patients with jaws locked together in the postoperative period (without tracheostomy) should be considered for admission to the high dependency unit for the first 24 hours for respiratory risk management
- For patients with tracheostomy, if returned to surgical unit, staffing must allow for appropriate close clinical one-to-one management for the first 72 hours, and limited to those who have the necessary clinical expertise in major flap reconstruction management
- Strict observance of the potential for cardiorespiratory compromise is required
- Immediate physical access to the patient is important if respiratory or cardiac compromise occurs, including equipment (wire cutters, etc.) that must be available at the patient's bedside
- The patient should be sitting upright and rest as much as possible until informed otherwise
- Suction equipment must be accessible at all times – this includes a large oral sucker and suction catheters
- When mobile, wire cutters, wire cutting scissors and dressing scissors pinned together must accompany the patient at all times
- Physiotherapy management to ensure cardiorespiratory integrity
- Primary postoperative oedema, both intra-orally and extra-orally will occur – corticosteroids may be prescribed to reduce swelling
- If a tracheostomy tube has been inserted prophylactically, one of the same size as in the patient's trachea and one of a smaller size must also be available in case oedema is excessive, and the tracheal hole and inner area size is reduced[12]
- An emergency tracheostomy tray with tracheal dilators must be easily accessible in the clinical area at all times in case of any adverse respiratory event.

## Box 23.40 Safety 2.

- Bleeding can also occur and swallowed blood may be a primary cause of vomiting. Have an emergency plan to deal with unexpected events such as vomiting or respiratory obstruction[12]
- Any intra-ocular pain must be reported immediately as the optic nerve or the optic canal may be injured or haematoma may have developed. This is a surgical emergency as irreversible blindness may occur[5–9,10–12]
- Head injury observations should be maintained where neurosurgery has been a part of the surgery or the patient has had a fracture of the middle third of the face
- Observe for cerebrospinal fluid dripping from the nose (which may indicate fracture of cribiform plate) or bleeding from the ears (which may indicate fracture of the base of the skull)
- Strict circulatory perfusion management and measurement of fluid balance
- Nutritional maintenance/support – dietician referral – vitaminised foods – education about dietary maintenance
- Nursing risk management – deep vein thrombosis, pressure ulcers.

## Box 23.41 Safety 3.

- Prior to discharge the patient must be instructed thoroughly on the appropriate method of maintaining airway patency
- The patient should **not** be discharged without wire cutters or scissors to cut rubber bands if these have been used to lock lower jaw to maxilla
- Use return demonstrations with a mirror provided by patient if wires and arch bars are used
- No bending or strenuous exercise, which may increase blood pressure levels in face
- No pressure should be exerted over any regions of the face and any bleeding should be reported immediately
- The patient must not smoke.

## Box 23.42 Comfort.

- Analgesia as prescribed and related to extent of surgery
- Craniofacial trauma – oral paracetamol 4–6-hourly preferred, as opiates may induce vomiting
- Diazepam may be required to relieve severe facial muscle or temporomandibular joint spasm, and patient anxiety.

**Box 23.43** General nursing and wound care.

- Wound care to repaired skin wounds must be attended to, with basic hygiene an important element to exclude infection
- Oral care – mouth toilet and hygiene (e.g. normal saline mouth washes) must be maintained and patient educated on management following discharge
- Use soft toothbrush, but this must be done with minimal lip and jaw movement until otherwise advised
- Moisturise the lips with Vaseline® or equivalent, to prevent cracking
- Eye care
- Nasal care
- Pin site care (if present).

**Box 23.44** Independence.

- Pen and paper for patient to communicate, if appropriate
- Physiotherapy for leg movement – assist in venous return and prevent deep vein thrombosis/pulmonary embolism
- Mobilisation as prescribed.

**Box 23.45** Discharge management.

- Ongoing airway safety management – reinforce protocols
- Nutritional management – dietician referral for ongoing care
- Discomfort management – analgesia as prescribed
- Oral hygiene care as prescribed
- Wound care as directed
- Should not drive unless wearing a alert tag regarding their respiratory risk if accidents occur
- Parents reporting protocols if problems occur
- Ongoing appointments and referrals as directed by team leader.

**Box 23.46** Summary.

- Whether the patient presents for management post trauma, or for elective surgery, the principles of pre- and postoperative nursing management are predicated on the concepts of risk management for all aspects of patient safety
- Some post trauma patients may require an emergency tracheostomy to secure the airway, as intubation is rarely possible due to oral obstructions, swelling, bleeding and floating teeth
- Because of the sheer urgency of the situation, tracheostomy is easier than intubation, is lifesaving, and is easily reversed at a later stage
- In some instances the adult patient who presents for elective major reconstructive oro/craniofacial surgery may require a temporary or a permanent tracheostomy for the management of the all-important airway
- The need for a permanent tracheostomy presents a new and challenging quality of life for the patient and he/she enters a whole different way of living
- This should be managed by specialist respiratory team clinicians
- Nutritional maintenance is a significant issue if wound healing, recovery and rehabilitation is to be initiated and sustained
- Intranasal feeding or insertion of a PEG preoperatively may be important options to be considered, particularly if immediate follow-up radiotherapy/chemotherapy is to be initiated for patients with malignant tumours.

**Review**

*Auditing preferred clinical and patient outcomes,* Chapter 2, Boxes 2.10–2.12.

## Postoperative risk issues

The patient's sense of safety is paramount and the patient should have access to the emergency alert system at all times. The patient should be initially housed close to the nurses' station until physiological safety is assured. It is best to use the biggest room on the surgical unit, as the amount of equipment required is very space-consuming, and relatively free access to the patient is important should an emergency occur[12].

## 4. CRANIOFACIAL VASCULAR ANOMALIES

Vascular malformations observed on the face and other regions of the body are classified under two headings – haemangioma and vascular malformations – which are totally biologically different. There appear to be groups in between that are bizarre and rare, but may give the appearance of a typical type[14].

See recommended websites (craniofacial vascular malformation) at the end of this chapter.

Primary assessment and diagnosis by a paediatric plastic surgeon are essential in the infant stage, to determine the true identification and classification of presenting lesions. This determines the appropriate primary and ongoing management, as many conditions are inoperable and, for a range of reasons, will require conservative management[14].

The pressure from the parents to operate for aesthetic purposes is often intense. Surgeons will resist and counsel the parents of the difficulties related to the vascularity of the face and a small loss of blood in a child can be life threatening. Notwithstanding, resolution will occur without loss of important aesthetic outcomes, for example, the upper lip.

True haemangioma grow quickly during infancy and regresses slowly during particular childhood stages (Figures 23.10 & 23.11).

Although capillary cavernous haemangioma may resolve slowly over time (at about age seven years), others may require surgery if adjacent physical functions are at risk, or ulceration, and life-threatening bleeding of the malformation seems imminent. The skin of resolved lesions may be suitable for resection for aesthetic reasons under controlled conditions.

The use of laser treatment for cutaneous haemangioma is controversial, and it is difficult for parents to believe nothing can be done to remove what appear to be superficial and aesthetically unsightly lesions. The aesthetic surgical outcomes may be disastrous if the lesions are thicker than previously thought and so the waiting time for resolution worth the wait[1-4].

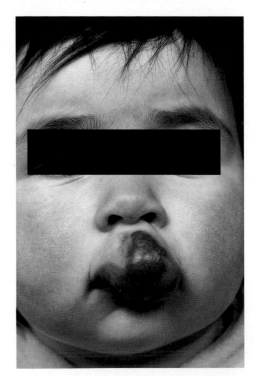

**Figure 23.10** Haemangioma, upper lip – anterior view.

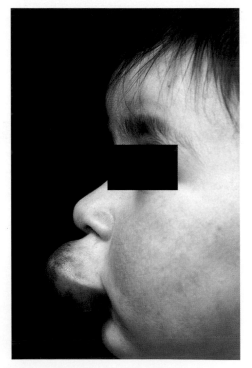

**Figure 23.11** Haemangioma, upper lip – lateral view.

## Special craniofacial vascular malformations – examples

Vascular malformations are developmental errors and may appear to be quite small during infancy[1-4]. These lesions never regress (with the exception of strawberry lesions) and frequently become quite large, often covering large areas of the face or body part. They are often externally recognised or described by their colours as 'strawberry', or resembling a 'port wine stain'. This simplicity of description may be misleading as their true nature may be disguised by accepting the colour as the diagnosis[1-4].

For example, Sturge-Weber syndrome (Figures 23.12 & 23.13) is a capillary malformation marked with a port-wine stain appearance (persistent throughout life) over a sensory dermatome of a branch of the trigeminal nerve of the face, and is commonly ipsilateral[1-4].

The markings may be seen in other parts of the body (Figure 23.13 – same patient as in Figure 23.12). The syndrome is frequently associated with complex

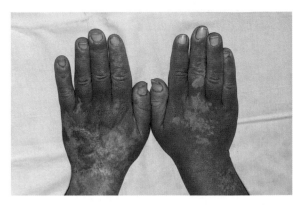

**Figure 23.13** Sturge-Weber syndrome – hand markings.

intracranial changes, intracranial calcification, cerebral cortex atrophy, and general or local seizures. Secondary glaucoma and optic atrophy may develop. The child may have hemiplegia and variable disabling cognitive and motor skills. The only known treatment is control of the seizures that are commonly associated with this syndrome.

Many clinical presentations may appear simple but in fact can be very complex, related to other vascular malformations in the brain, spine and/or general vascular system, and related to various syndromes. In addition, some superficial vascular malformations may be life-threatening if haemorrhage occurs due to swelling, dryness, ulceration or accidental trauma[1,5].

Surgery for any of these lesions is rare and only considered following sophisticated bone and complex vascular imaging, and assessment of the risk[1-4]. The complex nature of many of these presenting conditions requires the availability of a multidisciplinary team approach, a plastic surgeon, a neurosurgeon, a maxillofacial surgeon, dentists, specialist nursing staff, allied health professionals, psychologists and genetic counsellors, and other professionals co-opted as necessary.

With the extent of preoperative diagnostic investigations, extensive surgical planning and preparation, postoperative and rehabilitative management required, most patients (usually children) with these major congenital malformations, require management in a specialised paediatric surgical unit in major hospital where multidisciplinary care is available[1-4]. Added to this is the continuing reassurance and support parents can obtain from a team approach.

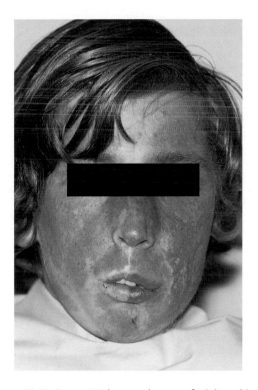

**Figure 23.12** Sturge-Weber syndrome – facial markings.

## References

(1) Aston S.J., Beasley R.W. & Thorne C.N.M. *Grabb and Smith's plastic surgery*, 5th edn. New York: Lippincott & Raven Publishers, 1997.

(2) McCarthy J.G. (ed.) *Plastic surgery, volumes 1–8.* Philadelphia: W.B. Saunders/Harcourt Brace, 1990.

(3) Ausher B.M., Erikson E. & Wilkins E.G. *Plastic surgery: indications, operations and outcomes.* St Louis: Mosby, 2000.

(4) Ruberg R.L. & Smith D.J. *Plastic surgery: a core curriculum.* St Louis: Mosby. 1994.

(5) Cohen S.R. Craniofacial distraction with a modular internal distraction system: evolution of design and surgical techniques. *Plastic Reconstructive Surgery*, 1999 (May); **103**(6):1592–607.

(6) Toth B.A., Kim J.W., Chin M. & Cedars M. Distraction osteogenesis and its application to the mid face and bony orbit in craniosynostosis syndromes. *Journal of Craniofacial Surgery*, 1998 (Mar); **9**(2):100–113, discussion 119–22.

(7) Burton R., *et al.* The miracle of growing bone: craniofacial distraction osteogenesis. *Currents*, 2002 (spring); **3**(2).

(8) McCarthy J.G., Schreiber J., Karp N., *et al.* Lengthening the human mandible by gradual distraction. *Plastic Reconstructive Surgery*, 1992 (Jan); **89**(1):1–8, discussion 9–10.

(9) Molina F., Ortiz Monasterio F. Mandibular elongation and remodelling by distraction: a farewell to major osteotomies. *Plastic Reconstructive Surgery*, 1995 (Sept); **96**(4):825–40, discussion 841–2.

(10) Menard R.M., Moore M.H. & David D.J. Tissue expansion in the reconstruction of Tessier craniofacial clefts: a series of 17 patients. *Plastic Reconstructive Surgery*, 1999 (Mar); **103**(3):779–86.

(11) Jackson I.T. & Beal B. Early feeding after cleft repair (Letter to the editor). *British Journal of Plastic Surgery*, 1997; **50**:217.

(12) Darzi M.A., Chowdri N.A. & Bhat A.N. Breastfeeding or spoon feeding after cleft lip repair: a prospective randomised study. *British Journal of Plastic Surgery*, 1996; **49**:24–6.

(13) Goodman T.A. (ed.) *Core curriculum for plastic and reconstructive surgical nursing*, 2nd edn. Pitman N.J.: ASPSN American Society of Plastic Surgery Nurses, 1996. http://www.aspsn.org

(14) Fortunato N. & McCullough S. *Plastic and reconstructive surgery.* Mosbys Perioperative Series. St. Louis: Mosby, 1998.

(15) Jigjinni V., Kangesu T. & Sommerlad B.C. Do babies require arm splints after cleft palate surgery? *British Journal of Plastic Surgery*, 1993; **46**:681–5.

## Recommended websites

**Craniofacial malformations**

http://www.childrensfaces.com/content/glossary/page2.htm (glossary of craniofacial terms)

http://www.chw.org/display/PPF/DocID/1823/router.asp (glossary of craniofacial terms)

http://www.erlanger.org/craniofacial/book/intro/history.htm

http://www.erlanger.org/craniofacial/book/intro/deformity.htm

http://www.craniosynostosis.net/ (craniosynostosis via endoscopic technique)

http://www.pedisurg.com/PtEduc/Craniosynostosis.htm (photographic examples provided – craniosynostosis)

http://www.kidsplastsurg.com/craniosynostosis.html (photographic examples provided – craniosynostosis)

http://www.stronghealth.com/services/surgical/plastic/craniofacial/hospitalcourse.cfm

http://www.emedicine.com/plastic/topic459.htm

http://www.baoms.org.uk/ce/ce_cranfac.html

http://www.erlanger.org/craniofacial/book/intro/deformity.htm

http://www.rch.org.au/plastic/units.cfm?doc_id=4833

http://www.centracare.com/sch/centers/pcw/child_cleft_cranio.html

**Craniofacial distraction osteogenesis**

http://www.uihealthcare.com/news/currents/vol3issue2/01distractions.html (distractions – photos – before and after)

http://www.chsd.org/1378.cfm (distraction osteogenesis – craniofacial reconstruction – photos before and after)

**Cleft lip and palate**

http://www.cleftadvocate.org/feeders.html (photos and examples excellent)

http://www.bfar.org/nipples.shtml (discussion on assisted nipple feeding – excellent)

http://www.aboutfaceusa.org/articles/feedingbabies.htm (excellent – feeding babies with cleft palate)

http://drstelnicki.com/2cleft.htm (excellent – feeding babies with cleft palate)

http://www.craniofacial.org/craniofacial_clefts.htm (photos and examples)

http://mercy.winningit.com/services/cleftLipSurgeryInformation.asp

http://www.plasticsurgery.org/public_education/procedures/CleftLipPalate.cfm (excellent)

http://www.umm.edu/plassurg/cleft.htm (excellent)

http://www.plasticsurgery.org/public_education/procedures/CleftLipPalate.cfm

**Craniofacial soft tissue and bony trauma**
Description and photos – excellent
http://www.erlanger.org/craniofacial/book/Trauma/Trauma_1.htm (excellent)
http://www.rad.washington.edu/mskbook/facialfx.html (excellent)
http://tristan.membrane.com/aona/case/max/max0202/ (excellent)
http://surgclerk.med.utoronto.ca/Phase2/Facial Fractures/FacialFractures_files/frame.htm (excellent)

**Craniofacial vascular malformations**
http://www.hopeforkids.com/body_hemangioma.html#images (excellent)
http://www.dermnetnz.org/index.html
http://hemangioma.com/hemangioma.html

# Chapter 24

# Ear Reconstruction

## Background

The ears are paired sensory organs comprising the auditory system, involved in the detection of sound, and the vestibular system, involved with maintaining body balance/equilibrium. The ear divides anatomically and functionally into three regions: the external ear (Figure 24.1), the middle ear, and the inner ear. All three regions are involved in hearing. Only the inner ear functions in the vestibular system.

The external ear (or pinna, the part that is visible), is composed of cartilage and skin, and has a relatively poor blood supply. The external ear serves to protect the tympanic membrane (the eardrum), and to collect and direct sound waves through the ear canal to the eardrum. About 2.7–3 cm long, the canal contains modified sweat glands that secrete cerumen, or earwax. Excess amounts of cerumen can block sound transmission.

The external size of the ear is 85% grown by the age of four years, and by year six the costal cartilage is suggested to be matured sufficiently to provide a reconstruction size and form similar to that of an adult.

The aetiology of ear abnormalities is considered under two headings – congenital and acquired. Boxes 24.1 and 24.2 provide examples of both.

---

**Box 24.1** Congenital malformations.

| | |
|---|---|
| Atresia | partial or complete absence may be seen as part of syndromic craniofacial malformations |
| Microtia | abnormally small – incidence about 1–7000, predominantly on the right side (may be seen as part of syndromic craniofacial malformations) |
| Macrotia | abnormally enlarged |
| Bat/shell ears | protruding ears or the absence of the antihelix fold (surgical procedure often referred to as an otoplasty)[1–9]. |

---

**Box 24.2** Acquired malformations – trauma and disease.

- Trauma – haematoma due to accident or assault, dog or human bite, burns, cauliflower ear (repeated damage, as in boxing, promoting thick fibrous tissue), motor vehicle accidents
- Benign cysts, benign tumours related to sun damage, keloid scars related to ear piercing
- Malignant skin tumours (70% due to sun damage, some pathology basal cell carcinoma but mainly squamous cell carcinoma with high metastatic spread, more common in males, occasionally melanoma[1–5]).

---

## Reconstructing the external ear

Such is the anatomical complexity of the ear and the nose, their recreation in order to appear normal and aesthetically acceptable to the patient, are stated to be two of the most difficult and challenging of all reconstructive procedures[1–9].

Ear reconstruction is a procedure to correct a malformation of the ear resulting from a congenital or acquired condition[1–9]. The operation may be a single procedure, or multistaged with a range of approaches. In using the patient's own tissues and/or adjuncts, multiple procedures may be required to reconstruct a single or matching set of ears.

Some reconstructive procedures in children (e.g. congenital conditions described, such as deformities of the helix or antihelix (Figure 24.2), 'bat', shell, or malformed ears (Figures 24.2–24.4), are planned to be fully completed prior to the child commencing school, corresponding to the child's growth, to prevent teasing from other children, and to minimise time away from school.

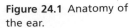

**Figure 24.1** Anatomy of the ear.

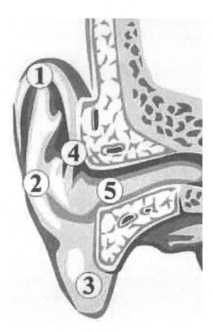

**Definitions of parts shown above**

1. **Helix** – the in-curve rim of the external ear
2. **Antihelix** – a landmark of the outer ear
3. **Lobule** – a landmark of the outer ear. The very bottom part of the outer ear
4. **Crest of helix** – a landmark of the outer ear
5. **External auditory meatus** – or external auditory canal. The auditory canal is the channel through which the sounds are led from the outside to the middle ear

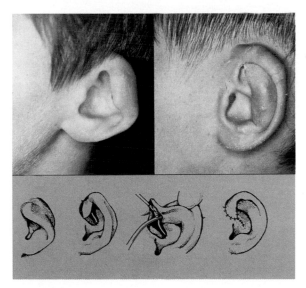

**Figure 24.2** Malformation of the upper rim of the ear.

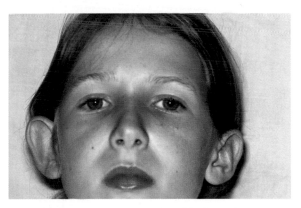

**Figure 24.3** Unilateral protruding (shell type) ear.

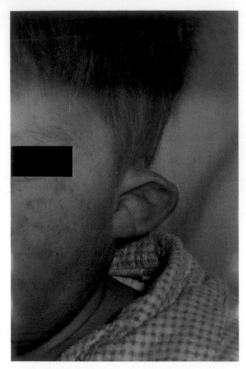

**Figure 24.4** Unilateral protruding (shell type) ear.

**Box 24.3** Elective ear reconstruction approaches – examples.

- Use of the patient's own local/regional tissue (e.g. skin, cartilage, bone) with or without the use of tissue expansion
- Costal cartilage from a rib is stated to continue to be the most reliable source of tissue for use as an underlying framework for skin cover
- Tissue expansion followed by insertion of a custom moulded Silastic® implant, placed under expanded skin
- Attaching a custom designed prosthetic ear by using clips/studs/magnets (Brånemark® technique), or surgical glue (see Chapter 25).

**Box 24.4** Reconstruction following trauma.

- Following animal or human bite, anti-tetanus and antibiotic cover is required
- Primary or secondary surgical repair by suturing
- Microvascular reconstruction following trauma (Figure 21.10)
- Elective reconstruction following the healing process.

Such is the anatomical complexity of the ear that its reconstruction, other than for a protruding ear(s) in the child or adult, may involve multistaged and/or microsurgical procedures or combinations[1–10].

**Box 24.5** Surgical options and risk management issues.

- Split to full thickness skin grafts – rarely used
- Local advancement skin flaps may be used for reconstruction following skin cancer[5]
- Tissue expansion (potential for over expansion with resultant avascular necrosis and prothesis extrusion) (see Chapter 22)
- Combined skin flaps and tissue expansion
- Tubed pedicles (potential for failure to vascularise, infection)
- Silastic prosthetic implants (potential for rejection, infection)
- Costal cartilage grafts (potential for pneumothorax during harvesting)
- Brånemark® reconstruction (potential for excess wound granulation at titanium implant sites) (see Chapter 25).

**Box 24.6** Preferred surgical outcomes of ear reconstruction.

| | |
|---|---|
| **Corrective** | to correct malformations of the ear that result from birth defects, trauma or tumours |
| **Restorative** | to restore optimal structural stability that assist in optimal function |
| **Aesthetic** | to restore, or improve, the visual aesthetics of the ear. |

**Review**

*Perioperative management – children*, Chapter 16.

---

**Box 24.7** Preoperative preparation.

- Nurse clinicians charged with the care of patients postoperatively should be clear regarding the extent of the surgery to be undertaken for children, as the parents may not have completely understood the extent of the donor sites required
- Clinicians should enquire from the surgeon the extent of the surgery and what potential clinical complications may occur postoperatively
- Enquiry should include any donor sites, drains, wound care, dressings, and potential complications that require a high level of postoperative monitoring/observation and discharge management[10]
- The absence or malformation of an ear can be emotionally traumatic at any age, and the risks of even minimal failure must be well understood by all concerned
- Pre-surgical preparation is extremely important with psychological considerations high on the list[11,12]
- Some procedures may be recognised as being more to appease the parents rather than the child. Children in their very early years may not appreciate the long-term implications that may occur in respect of their body image
- The patient's hair should be washed preoperatively and long hair should be tied back.

---

**Box 24.8** Intraoperative period – bat/shell ear reconstruction.

- Prior to surgery, surgical soap or Vaseline® may be applied to keep stray hairs away from the operation site. This makes early hair washing and the removal of old blood remaining postoperatively much easier
- In most instances local anaesthetic (lidocaine) and adrenaline is injected to reduce intra-operative bleeding, and provide postoperative comfort management
- This also separates the skin off the cartilage, assisting in the surgical dissection.

---

**Box 24.9** Wound dressings following surgery.

- Wound dressings will reflect the simplicity/complexity of the procedure undertaken
- Postoperative dressing application is undertaken to protect the avascular cartilage from excess compression and secondary injury (e.g. haematoma) (Figure 24.5)
- The potential complications related to dressing compression, requires special care to be taken when wound dressings are applied to the ear
- Vaseline® gauze, acriflavine impregnated wool, or normal soft wool is usually used to pack 'dead space' in the front of the ear and behind the ear, moulding the exact ear shape desired (Figure 24.5)
- Providing dressing uniformity in height, and contour, with the surrounding skull, assists in exerting equal compression as bandages are applied
- Any form of soft wool type dressing is preferable to gauze, as the roughness of the gauze is likely to cause skin irritation, causing children to attempt to prematurely remove the dressing
- The head may remain bandaged for up to two weeks postoperatively, or according to the surgeon's preference[6,7,9] (Figures 24.6 & 24.7)
- One research paper has shown that for the majority of patients having an aesthetic otoplasty, bandaging for two days may be sufficient[13]
- Hair washing and the application of 'branded' sports head bands, ski caps, knitted hats or elasticised, tubular, low compression bandages are becoming more commonly used for children and adult patients who are considered co-operative.

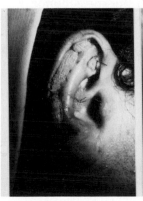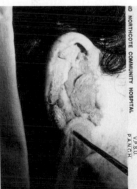

**Figure 24.5** Internal packing of ear contours (eliminating dead spaces) as part of dressing the ear post surgery.

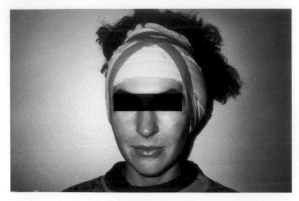

**Figure 24.6** External bandaging following surgery for protruding ears.

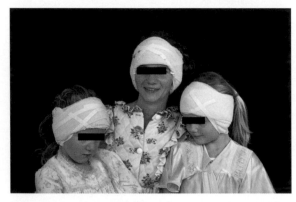

**Figure 24.7** Family of three children from same family, post surgery for protruding ears.

## Wound dressings – full thickness donor sites from behind the ear

Full thickness grafts are frequently harvested from behind the ear (Figure 24.8) for local defects following removal of tumours located in the antihelix.

Donor sites are commonly repaired with a continuous suture combined with a tie-over dressing on the suture line (Figure 24.9).

This fills the dead space, protects the suture line, and provides temporary compression. Bandages may or may not be applied if only one ear is operated upon. If bandaging is undertaken, both ears will usually be included. Wool should be placed in front of, and behind the ear to provide uniformity of height and to prevent irritation from the crepe bandage.

Post auricular full thickness donor site

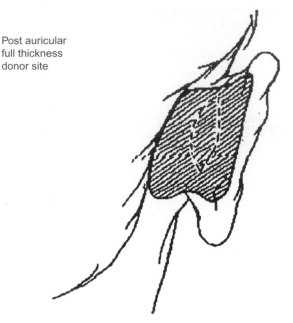

**Figure 24.8** Donor site full thickness graft from behind the ear.

# Postoperative nursing care – risk management issues

**Box 24.10** Clinical risk management – postoperative 1.

- The zone of the ear is a highly fixed skin region with a specialised circulatory system to the skin (cartilage has no discrete blood supply)
- Regardless of the reconstructive procedure undertaken, the actual or potential complications parallel those that exist for healing of any wounds[10]
- Complications may be accentuated by the adverse events peculiar to specific techniques used, particularly as the principal region for reconstruction may require more than one donor site[1–10]
- A potential complication post-harvesting of costal cartilage is pneumothorax[10]
- The incidence of haematoma, avascular necrosis of the skin/flaps, and infection, can be significant
- Scrupulous preoperative planning ensures the surgery is undertaken with high regard to the specifics of the local blood supply, and postoperative management is in the hands of experts at all levels of care[10].

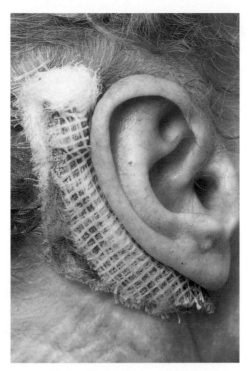

**Figure 24.9** Tie-over dressing to donor site to apply minimal compression and eliminate dead space and protect sensitive cartilage prior to traditional ear dressing (Figures 24.5 and 24.6).

## Clinical risk management – postoperative 2 – the ear wound(s)

---

**Box 24.11** Safety.

- Development of even a small haematoma (causing extreme pain and necrosis)[10]
- With the ear, two principal complications are seen, vascular compromise within the wound, indicated by pain, and unrelieved nausea and/or vomiting which in itself may be related to bandage compression and vascular compromise[1–10]
- Following a 'perfect' operation, the undue pressure of wound dressings and bandages may cause:
  - Avascular 'spotting' with ulceration developing
  - Tension on skin edges that may cause wound breakdown
  - Any single or combination of complications may compromise the entire reconstruction.

---

- Vascular compromise/pain/wound monitoring is based on the potential for circulatory compromise mainly to the cartilage and a strict record of any pain and/or blood loss should be maintained and reported immediately
- Vascular compromise is an urgent complication, which should be reported immediately, and relieved by bandage decompression to prevent avascular necrosis of the cartilage and draped over skin[6–12]
- Excessive compression of head bandages may result in air pressure changes within the inner ear (the labyrinth), affecting balance and inducing vomiting
- Primarily, an antiemetic should be given, but continuous vomiting will cause distress and a raised intracranial pressure. This may generate wound bleeding, haematoma etc.
- If vomiting or nausea is not relieved, bandage decompression must be considered
- Decompression of the bandages must be with permission from the surgeon, and bandages should be cut down to the skin in a vertical line at the forehead site
- This action allows for pressure to be released immediately and, as vomiting, pain or severe discomfort is relieved, a new securing bandage can be applied over the existing bandages without disturbing the inner dressings
- Failure of either or both of these complications to be relieved by decompression will require the entire wound dressing(s) to be taken down and the wound fully inspected. This should be anticipated by the clinician and redressing components pre-emptively made available to save time
- Pain management and sedation may be required to settle the patient
- Pain may be related to 'tie-over' dressings (e.g. skin grafts) compressing fragile tissues, particularly cartilage
- Complex redressing should not be undertaken in an uncooperative patient or in a patient who is distressed.

---

**Box 24.12** Comfort.

- In the postoperative phase, the declining efficacy of local anaesthesia and vasoconstrictors may see the precipitation of pain and wound bleeding
- Whilst regional blocks that provide long-term analgesia are state of the art, they may mask the

*Continued*

development of a haematoma or any bleeding – any strikethrough bleeding should be reported immediately

- The nurse clinician should review analgesia given in the post anaesthesia care unit and provide for analgesia to be given orally (or rectally, if appropriate, in children) as ordered strictly four-hourly for the first 72 hours[14,15]
- Pain not relieved by analgesia should be reported immediately
- This pain may be accompanied by nausea and vomiting (see above under *Safety*)
- Children need to be free of pain and nausea, warm and comforted with a sense of safety, as crying and irritability can raise the blood pressure and increase the tension on the wound(s) and potential for bleeding[14,15]
- In both children and adults, additional wounds may be present
- Pain may be quite significant from donor sites such as the hip (movement) or chest wound sites (breathing), and provision for comfort measures should be made for these or other wounds
- Following complex multisited procedures, narcotic analgesia may be required initially for one to two doses, and, for some patients, a short term narcotic infusion may be useful[14,15]
- Pain may result from blood that has leaked into the ear labyrinth
- The ear should be checked with an auriscope and carefully cleaned with saline soaked cotton buds
- Temporomandibular joint pain may result from children or adults clenching or grinding their teeth – oral analgesia and/or low dose diazepam may be required to relieve the spasm and resultant pain.

## Review

*Setting goals of care and preferred clinical and patient outcomes*, Chapter 2, Boxes 2.7–2.9. Adapt as appropriate to the patient's clinical needs.

---

**Box 24.13** Wound management – general nursing care.

- Assess for the presence of other wounds including, for example, wound drainage sites if skin, cartilage, costal cartilage or bone is used, and that additional drainage bottles are present
- If costal cartilage has been harvested the potential for pneumothorax is significant and the patient may have a chest tube inserted to assist in ventilation of the lung
- For procedures that include insertion of tissue expander(s), see Chapter 22
- Following aesthetic otoplasty or other similar procedures, dressings may be changed on day one postoperatively to assess for haematoma or malpositioning, which is easier to correct in the early stages[6–9]
- Nurse clinicians removing the primary and secondary dressings should be extremely careful at all stages to ensure that bleeding or pain and that dislodgement of dressings does not occur
- For congenital malformations, and skin tumours of the ear, skin grafts or flaps may be used, and primary dressings may also be undertaken on day 1 postoperatively[1]
- Some procedures may be left open without dressings, particularly tubed pedicles, which require vascular monitoring
- For dressings left intact for a longer period, it is important to observe for bleeding through the bandages, or poorly-filled drainage tubes or collecting bottles, as children cannot support excessive blood loss
- The removal of dressings postoperatively requires the patient to be in a reclining position and the bandages cut as for decompression (middle of the forehead down to the skin)
- Each layer is removed individually and gently. If no further dressings are required, the patient may go home and gently shower and wash the hair under warm (not hot) water
- Hair drying should be undertaken by gentle towelling – not rubbing – or using hair dryer on cool – not hot
- Emphasis is put on the need for protection and safety of the ears(s), as cartilage is slow to heal and the procedure may fail
- Headbands should remain on overnight to protect against secondary injury to the ear
- A soft diet is required for the first 7–10 days as excessive or hard chewing will cause discomfort to ears, as the temporomandibular joints are very close[11].

## Box 24.14 Independence

- Most procedures are undertaken as day or short stay procedures
- Early mobilisation is usually possible but this is dependant on the extent of donor sites that may compromise full mobility for a few days
- Decisions will be based on an overall assessment of the safety of the wounds and the patient
- Children will require diversionary activities and should be persuaded towards quietness and protection of the wounds – structured play, not rough and tumble games.

## Box 24.15 Discharge management.

**The patient should be given the following verbal and written advice:**

- Do not remove dressings unless otherwise instructed
- The ears must remain free from any undue pressure at all times
- Do not consciously lie on the ear(s)
- Quiet activity – resting as much as possible for the first few days or until instructed
- Wear knitted ski hat or beanie over dressings in bed at night to secure the bandages
- Soft diet – no straining
- Report any excessive pain, unusual odour or bleeding to your surgeon or nearest emergency room
- Do not get bandages wet, and if this does occur return to the surgeon's rooms for changing
- When dressings are removed, wear a favourite tennis headband, knitted ski hat or beanie at night for about four weeks to ensure ears do not accidentally fold forward – cartilage heals slowly and is easily fractured.

## Review

*Auditing preferred clinical and patient outcomes,* Chapter 2, Boxes 2.10–2.12.

## References

(1) Atlantic Coast Ear Specialists. *Anatomical tour of the ear.* http://www.earaces.com/anatomy.htm
(2) Biavati M.J. & Leach J.L. *Ear reconstruction.* http://www.emedicine.com/ent/topic79.htm
(3) Davison S., Thomassen J. & Cohen M. *Ear reconstruction and salvage.* http://www.emedicine.com/plastic/topic213.htm
(4) Tennessee Craniofacial Centre. *Microtia reconstruction.* http://www.erlanger.org/craniofacial/book/Ear/Ear_2.htm (excellent – photos – surgery)
(5) Kavanagh, K.T. *Scalp advancement flap for ear reconstruction in a patient skin cancer.* http://www.entusa.com/ear_reconstruction.htm (excellent)
(6) Aston S.J., Beasley R.W. & Thorne C.N.M. *Grabb and Smith's plastic surgery,* 5th edn. New York: Lippincott & Raven Publishers, 1997.
(7) McCarthy J.G. (ed.) *Plastic surgery, volumes 1–8.* Philadelphia: W.B. Saunders, Harcourt Brace, 1990.
(8) Ausher B.M., Erikson E. & Wilkins E.G. *Plastic surgery: indications, operations and outcomes.* St Louis: Mosby, 2000.
(9) Ruberg R.L. & Smith D.J. *Plastic surgery: a core curriculum.* St. Louis: Mosby, 1994.
(10) Morris A. McG., Stevenson J.H. & Watson A.C.H. *Complications of plastic surgery.* Baillière Tindall: London, 1989.
(11) Goodman T.A. (ed.) *Core curriculum for plastic and reconstructive surgical nursing,* 2nd edn. Pitman, N.J.: ASPSN American Society of Plastic Surgery Nurses, 1996.
(12) Fortunato N. & McCullough S. *Plastic and reconstructive surgery. Mosby's Perioperative Series.* St. Louis: Mosby, 1998.
(13) Barltey K.V. How long should ears be bandaged after otoplasty? *Journal of Laryngology and Otolaryngology,* 1998 (June); **112**(6):531–2.
(14) Keuren K.V. & Eland J.A. Perioperative pain management in children. *Nursing Clinics of North America,* 1997 (March); **32**(1):31–44.
(15) Mooney K.M. Perioperative management of the paediatric patient. *Plastic Surgical Nursing,* 1997(summer); **17**(2):69–75.

## Recommended websites

**Photo galleries of pre-operative, surgical procedure and post surgery outcomes**
http://www.plasticsurgery.org/index.cfm
http://www.earreconstruction.com/surgical-technique.html
http://www.plasticsurgerydoctors.com/procedures/plasticsurgeryprocedureindex.html
http://www.plasticsurgery.com.au/index.shtml

# Chapter 25

# Camouflage Prostheses

## 1. CAMOUFLAGE PROSTHESES – ANAPLASTOLOGY

### Background

Camouflage prosthesis is also called **anaplastology**, which comes from the Greek *ana*, again, plus *plastos*, formed. It is defined as a synergy of art, science and technology restoring the human anatomy, by the use of artificial materials[1,2]. It is also the term applied to custom designed appliances made for the purpose of obscuring or disguising missing or malformed anatomical parts. The name given to these professional and sculptural masters, worldwide, is anaplastologists. This is to distinguish them from those who make prosthetic limbs. Anaplastology differs from prosthetics and orthotics in that the emphasis is on the aesthetics or the appearance of the devices created, rather than functional priority.

Traditionally, when anatomical parts have been missing as a result of congenital malformation, trauma, or disease, man has attempted to disguise the difference to appear what may be considered 'normal'. History records masks, artificial glass eyes, wooden and metal noses, wooden legs, and a range of disguises used for both good, and evil purposes[3–5]. It is stated that over 400 years ago Ambrose Pare pioneered the attachment of an artificially constructed ear, for aesthetic purposes[5]. The loss of ears or noses was a common occurrence in, for example, sword fighting, or as the mark of an adulterer.

During World War I and World War II, despite the large human sacrifice, numerous men and women survived. Of those who survived, many experienced significant losses of body parts, and particularly facial anatomy. This was predominantly seen in airmen due to burns acquired following aircraft crashes. In addition, with the increasing salvage of patients after successful removal of some malignant tumours, patients began requesting camouflage techniques that would allow them to return into normal society. The art and science of reconstructing artificial craniofacial parts, by sculpturing missing parts for the individual, gained increasing momentum.

Following World War II, with the advent of new synthetic materials (e.g. firm and soft plastic materials), and improved cosmetic paint colours, this meant these could be mixed and manipulated to closely match the individual's own skin colour and markings. All of these advances resulted in the firm establishment of the place of camouflage techniques and artificial devices.

### Anaplastology in the 21st Century

When replacing missing tissue, the use of the patient's own skin has always been the optimal choice for reconstruction, and despite the leaps made in reconstructive surgery such as free flap transfer and tissue expansion, for various reasons, alternatives may need to be sought. For example, some tissues are unsuitable or insufficient for local reconstruction, lacking an adequate regional or local blood supply due to radiotherapy, post burns, or where the local area is surrounded by solar damaged tissue. Tissues that develop hypertrophic or keloid scars also present difficulties when attempting to locally reconstruct missing parts.

> **Box 25.1** Role and function of camouflage devices and anatomical prosthesis.
>
> - The desired goal of any camouflage device or prosthesis is to assist in restoring optimal function and aesthetics
> - The prosthesis helps to protect exposed delicate tissues, covers exposed cavities, can provide, for example, artificial fingers, hands, feet, breasts, ears to support eyeglasses, or hearing aids, and restore appearance

- Techniques developing prosthesis as permanent attachments are the state of the art
- A well-made prosthesis can facilitate the return of an individual to most of their normal activities and eliminate the need for bandages and eye patches
- Because the prosthesis is not living tissue, there are some obvious limitations – the prosthesis may not restore normal movement, does not blush or tan and must be removed for cleaning
- Even a well-made prosthesis may be detectable under close observation
- Cosmetic make-up has also significantly improved in helping to disguise scars and lines that mark the meeting point of the prosthesis and normal skin
- The prosthesis can address physical rehabilitation, but some patients may also require psychological counselling or spiritual direction.

## Issues in use of camouflage devices and anatomical prostheses

Two complex problems have prevented a greater acceptance of prostheses:

- The lack of availability of non-irritating adhesives that could allow the prosthesis to be worn for long periods of time without skin damage
- Translucence of the prosthesis that occurred in certain forms of light, which could clearly distinguish (demarcate) between normal skin and artificially constructed materials[1-3].

Until the research and introduction of osseointegration, beginning in the 1950s, prosthetic body parts were attached to the body in a variety of ways, most of which:

- Were often uncomfortable and painful to wear
- Inadequately matched the original body part
- Could not be worn for long periods of time
- Had problems with patients' experiences of allergies to adhesives
- Required to be attached to, for example, spectacles.

The definition of success of the aesthetic outcome of any prosthesis is evaluated by:

- The manner in which it incorporated into the adjacent structural features as to be concealed and appear as 'normal' for that person
- The patient's acceptance[1-3].

Despite difficulties experienced, for many people, these appliances served important functional and aesthetic purposes, allowing them to move freely in the community, and for some patients this remains so. Patients will always be given choices, and many older patients may still prefer to use simple alternatives such as a custom designed nasal prosthesis, attached to their spectacles.

### Case examples

**Patient one** (Figures 25.1–25.5). Although these pictures may seem extreme, they demonstrate the challenges that anaplastologists face when inoperable lesions (e.g. infiltrating basal cell carcinomas) present, and patients desire some degree of normal structural view of themselves.

Inoperable, the patient's wound was dressed daily with calcium alginate in an attempt to limit any bleeding and this was covered with layers of non-adherent plastic coated dry dressings.

As previously described in Chapter 6, basal cell carcinomas are infiltrating lesions, and are rarely

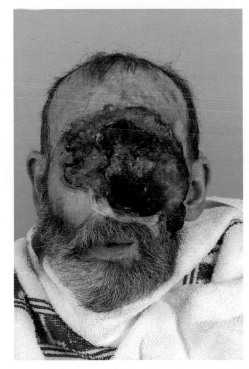

**Figure 25.1** Infiltrating basal cell carcinoma of the face tissue and bone structure.

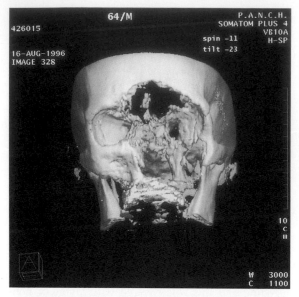

**Figure 25.2** Anterior view CT scan of facial bone destruction.

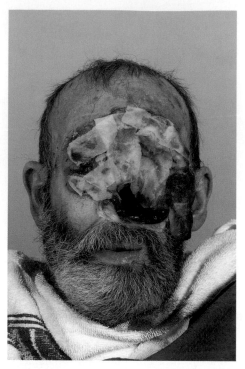

**Figure 25.4** Calcium alginate dressings used in an attempt to minimise facial bleeding.

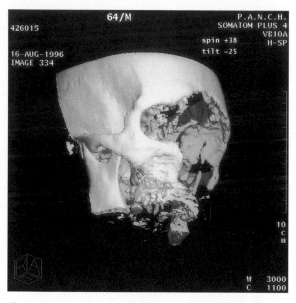

**Figure 25.3** Lateral view CT scan of facial bone destruction.

metastatic. Computed tomography (CT) scans shown in Figures 25.2 and 25.3 demonstrate the potential destructive nature of these infiltrating malignancies on the face. These patients will usually die from haemorrhage due to the tumours penetrating major arterial vessels.

**Patient two** (Figures 25.6 and 25.7) had a full thickness skin removal of a melanoma of the lower right leg, and the defect was skin grafted. A contoured silicone prosthesis was constructed and this could be worn under tights to disguise the anatomical defect, visible when trousers were not worn.

**Patients three and four** (Figures 25.8–25.11) demonstrates the use of a prosthesis attached to eyeglasses for ease of use, and to suit the defect.

See recommended websites (camouflage prosthesis – anaplastology) at the end of this chapter.

## 2. OSSEOINTEGRATION AS A RECONSTRUCTIVE PROCESS

**Osseointegration** is the term applied to the implantation, fixation, integration, or fusion of the metal,

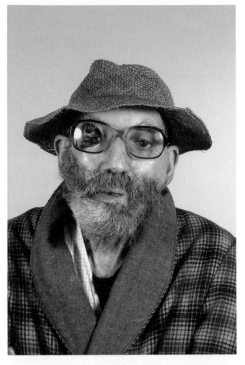

**Figure 25.5** Masterful facial sculpture designed to provide camouflage and aesthetics.

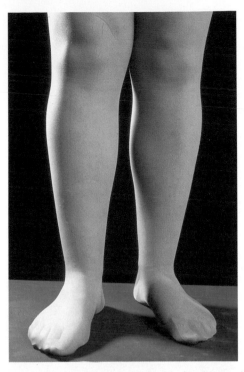

**Figure 25.7** Sculptured silicone mould glued into place to provide camouflage.

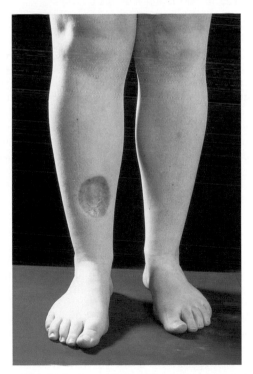

**Figure 25.6** Right lower limb with contour defect due to excision of melanoma.

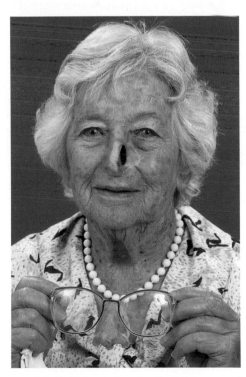

**Figure 25.8** Full thickness basal cell carcinoma excised left side of nose.

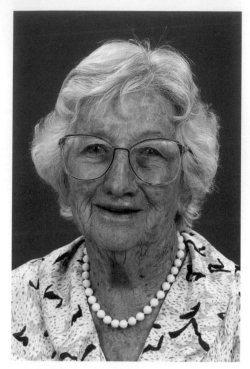

**Figure 25.9** Camouflaged by contoured prosthesis attached to glasses.

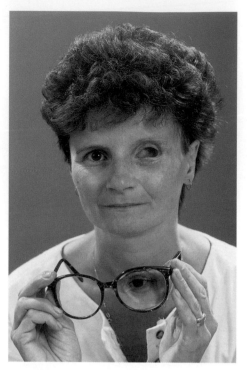

**Figure 25.10** Post removal of eye tumour.

titanium, designed as studs or screw appliances, into bone, free from any relative movement[3,4,6,7]. Customised replications of missing body parts are then clipped on, or attached through a magnetised format. This is one the most innovative procedures of the 20th and 21st Centuries to tissue-based reconstructive procedures, and non-tissue integrated anaplastology prosthetic alternatives.

## The concept of osseointegration

During the 1950s, Brånemark demonstrated the efficacy of pure titanium (e.g. purity is graded on a scale of 1–4), in its ability to become permanently incorporated, or fused, into living bone. He showed that this could be attained without fracturing or interfering with the local blood supply of the surrounding fragile periosteum and bone[3–7].

There is an important difference between integrated pure titanium and bone and other materials. Titanium can co-exist with none of the complications commonly seen from other inserted metal materials

(i.e. stainless steel) or internal/external Silastic® or plastic prostheses (i.e. infection, rejection, extrusion, allergies to adhesives, ability to be worn for only short periods), and in all but a minimum of patients can be left in place permanently.

Brånemark introduced the technical/biological term 'osseointegration' and this term continues to describe the concept and principles of the technique, and range of available applications[6]. Following years of research, in 1965, the practical application of the concept was demonstrated through the 'integration' of a tooth into the mandibular or maxillary bone, utilising titanium as a stabilising base. This technique allowed for the restoration of missing teeth free from the use of frames, plates, etc. In 1979 it was reported that the technique had been applied to the attachment of an ear to the mastoid region thus opening a new field of application[6].

Clinical risks and potential complications of osseointegration are suggested to relate to:

• Lack of application to the strict criteria related to patient selection

- Inadequate understanding of the surgical techniques required in application
- Failure to recognise and prepare actual and potential 'at risk' patients with preoperative hyperbaric oxygen regimes[1-3]
- Inadequate patient hygiene practices during and following the procedural process.

## The surgical application process

The inserted titanium appliances inserted into the bone are referred to as **abutments**[1-5]. The device is also referred to as a load bearing appliance. In some instances, abutments may be jointed together by a solid gold bar to strengthen the static appliance to withstand the load bearing required by the application of the external prosthesis. These implants (abutments and load bearing devices) are capable of sustaining absent load bearing structures in almost any body region, and their construction is paralleled to functional and stabilising requirements.

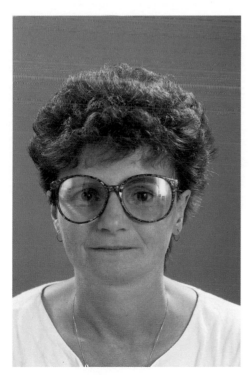

**Figure 25.11** Eye prosthesis attached to glasses.

The external prosthetic structures for ears, nose or eyes are artificially sculptured and attached by clips or magnets to reproduce the normal anatomical and aesthetic form. The technique may be used as a single entity, or in association with soft tissue/bony reconstructive surgery[1-5]. Case example 2, later in this chapter, provides an excellent example of the aesthetic contrast of earlier camouflage methods (attached to the patient's glasses) and modern osseointegration of a nasal implant.

> **Box 25.2** Indications for application of osseointegration in the craniofacial region.
>
> - Patients who are a poor surgical risk for complex/multiple reconstructive procedures
> - Patients who do not wish to have major reconstructive surgery
> - Patients who have been received radiotherapy in the surrounding areas adjacent to that selected for the osseointegration procedure
> - Poor local tissue due to, for example, multiple excisions for skin tumours
> - Patient wish for prosthetic replacement of the nose, the eye, fingers
> - Absence of lower half of the ear
> - Some congenital malformations (e.g. absence of anatomical structures) such as those seen in the ear(s)
> - In combination with major/complex soft tissue and bone reconstructive procedures to the craniofacial region.

> **Box 25.3** Preoperative surgical/nursing preparation.
>
> - The patented criterion applied to the surgical application of this technique is that specific surgical educational courses must be undertaken in order that the exclusive instrumentation and appliances can be purchased and used
> - This ensures an excellent level of quality control in application, patient selection, guidelines for nursing care, and a very high level of success rate and preferred clinical outcomes
> - Awareness of strict patient selection, surgical timing, and the timeframe of this procedure, is important
>
> *Continued*

- Initial and continuing patient education, with patient commitment to the process
- In relation to craniofacial osseointegration, preoperative skin, hair, oral and general hygiene is extremely important and assists in the initial success of the procedure
- As the timeframe for the entire procedure to be completed may be between three to six months, depending on the site, there is considerable time for nursing staff to ensure that patients are disciplined in the continuing ritual of hygiene maintenance[8]
- Preoperative hyperbaric oxygen treatment regimes are reported to be responsible for the success of the procedure in patients who are deemed 'at risk', for example, due to previous irradiation, previous surgery, previous infection, scarred tissue, or generally poor skin and soft tissue regions due to long-term UVB exposure.
- As the timeframe for the entire procedure to be completed may be between three to six months, depending on the site, there is considerable time to ensure that patients are disciplined in the continuing ritual of hygiene maintenance.

Osseointegration is a form of reconstruction but is not a solution for all patients. It is a procedure that has a specific application in selected patient circumstances, particularly those who are committed to ongoing disciplined hygiene practices[7].

## Recent research innovations

One of the interesting aspects of contemporary research has been what is termed 'osseoperception'. This is the ability of some patients to 'perceive' or recognise a stimulus that parallels a normal vibratory feedback, related to movement. This continuing research has important implications for osseointegrated prostheses, in anatomical regions (e.g. the finger tips) where neural feedback for safety is important[6].

---

**Box 25.4** Surgery and construction of the prosthesis.

- As in all complex reconstructive surgery, planning of the sites of the abutments is important as it is fundamental that they have the ability to withstand the proposed prosthetic load to be placed upon them
- The planning and timeframe of the preparation for surgery, and insertion of the abutments before the prosthesis is finally attached, allows the prosthetic scientist to design, sculpture and colour with exactness
- This provides a prosthesis that matches the appropriate size, colour and aesthetics and is appropriately designed to the particular patient.

---

**Box 25.5** Postoperative nursing care.

| | |
|---|---|
| Safety | as an elective procedure, safety is determined by the age of the patient, any associated clinical medical or psychological morbidity, and general responses to recovery from the anaesthesia |
| Comfort | can usually be managed with a strong oral analgesia four-hourly (strictly) for the first 72 hours if necessary, reducing in dosage as required |
| Independence | the procedure is relatively straightforward in the hands of specialists but education and patient co-operation in independent care and early reporting of any adverse events is important[8]. |

### Box 25.6 Wound management.

- Primary wound care protocols are according to each surgeon's preferences, and it is important to clinically observe for any adverse events such as inflammation and oedema
- Initially, 4–6-hourly wound and pin site care is required for five days, or until the incision has integrated with the abutment
- This can subsequently be incorporated into daily wound hygiene (daily shower)
- The application of Vaseline® ointment is usually prescribed as a prophylactic measure
- With the titanium so inert and integrating into the tissues and bone with little or no inflammatory response, little more than daily normal skin hygiene is required.
- The efficacy of topical antibiotic ointments has not been scientifically substantiated so Vaseline® is perhaps a much cheaper and adequate substitute, if necessary
- Complications can occur if disciplined and basic hygiene is not practised
- Early in the postoperative phase, following the placement of abutments, some small areas of hypergranulation tissue may be observed close to the insertion sites
- Compression, hypertonic saline dressings (that shrink and destroy the cells), followed by moist wound healing dressings, and regular hygiene practices, have been used with excellent results[6]
- As stated above, wound bed preparation is essential and this must be sustained with a disciplined lifetime of wound bed management and pin site care (see Chapter 12)
- Continuing problems may eventually require the removal of the abutment, as a last resort.

### Review

*Setting goals of care and preferred clinical and patient outcomes, Chapter 2, Boxes 2.7–2.9. Adapt as appropriate to the patient's clinical needs.*

### Case examples

**Patient 1:** Figure 25.12 shows a young man who was born without a right ear, and was selected as suitable for osseointegration. Figure 25.13–25.15 exhibit the process, and Figure 25.16 the outcome.

**Patient 2:** is an elderly male patient who underwent amputation of the nose for a basal cell carcinoma which had infiltrated into the columella and nasal structure. Figure 25.17 shows the use of a nasal camouflage prosthesis attached to the patient's glasses and Figure 25.18 the inserted abutments and load bearing appliance. Figure 25.19 shows the significantly improved aesthetics by the use of osseointegration.

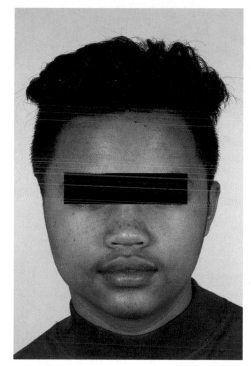

**Figure 25.12** Young man with congenital absence of the right ear.

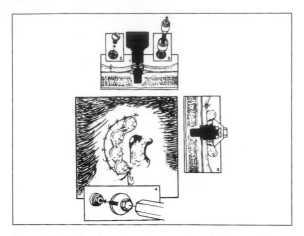

**Figure 25.13** Setting osseointegration abutments into the bone.

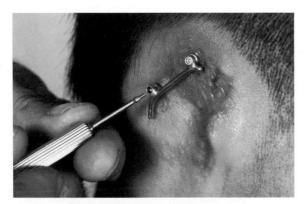

**Figure 25.14** Adding a gold bar for additional load bearing strength.

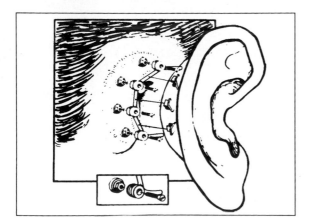

**Figure 25.15** Magnetised points on bone and prosthesis abutments.

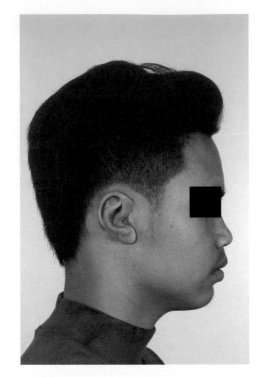

**Figure 25.16** Osseointegrated prosthesis in place.

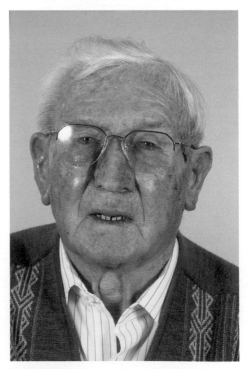

**Figure 25.17** Elderly man with nasal prosthesis attached to glasses.

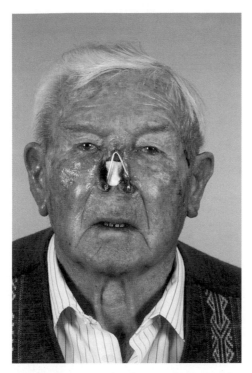

**Figure 25.18** Abutments in place ready for nasal osseointegrated prosthetic attachment.

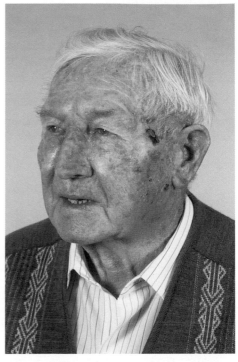

**Figure 25.19** Osseointegrated prosthetic sculptured attachment with marked aesthetic improvement.

See recommended websites (osseointegration) at the end of this chapter.

---

**Box 25.7** Discharge management.

- Although some patients may be youthful, many patients who have this procedure are elderly, may have problems remembering treatment regimes and will require assistance with their care
- This situation must be individually addressed and the education for general and wound site hygiene focused on written instructions, prescribed times and frequent check-ups by the surgeon, and nurse clinicians, to ensure co-operation and the integrity of the prosthesis
- In addition, the co-opting of significant carers can ensure minimal surrounding skin complications

---

- In the author's experience, continuation of pin site care was often a difficulty at the site of the ear, as the patient experienced problems in viewing the 'wound' or external prosthetic abutments[6] – educating significant carers will aid in this instance
- Surrounding skin-care, including removal of dry encrusted skin, dry scabs, etc., should be preceded by replacement of moisture in the dry skin, to allow ease of removal
- An effective and inexpensive method of keeping the pins clean from any exudate is to use warm, pH-balanced soap alternative and water, drying with a soft towel or using cotton buds, and giving a final clean with a medical alcohol substance[6]
- Observing for any over granulation at the pin sites must be ongoing as this may precede critical colonisation and infection
- Any wound problems should be reported to the surgeon immediately to prevent/minimise any risk to the continuing success of the procedure[6].

## Review

*Auditing preferred clinical and patient outcomes,*
Chapter 2, Boxes 2.10–2.12.

## References

(1) American Anaplastology Association. *Definitions.* http://www.anaplastology.org/AAAindex.php.

(2) Medicine Net. *Anaplastology definition.* http://www.medterms.com/script/main/art.asp?articlekey=24556

(3) Aston S.J., Beasley R.W. & Thorne C.N.M. *Grabb and Smith's plastic surgery,* 5th edn. New York: Lippincott & Raven Publishers, 1997.

(4) Ausher B.M., Erikson E. & Wilkins E.G. *Plastic surgery: indications, operations and outcomes.* St Louis: Mosby, 2000.

(5) McCarthy J.G. (ed.) *Plastic surgery, Vol. 1–8.* Philadelphia: W.B. Saunders, Harcourt Brace, 1990.

(6) Brånemark R., Brånemark P-I., Rydevik B. & Meyers R.R. Osseointegration in skeletal reconstruction and rehabilitation. *Journal of Rehabilitation Research & Development,* 2001 (March/April); **38**(2):1–8. http://www.vard.org/jour/01/38/2/brane382.htm

(7) Wilkes G.H. & Wolfaardt J.F. Osseointegtation: alloplastic versus autogenous ear reconstruction: criteria for treatment selection. *Plastic Reconstructive Surgery,* 1994 (Apr); **93**(5):967–79.

(8) Storch J.E. *Plastic surgery and wound management nursing.* Postgraduate curriculum guide, syllabus, and course notes for students. Melbourne, Australia: Australian Catholic University, and St Vincent's and Mercy Private Hospitals, 2000 (reviewed 2004).

## Recommended websites

**Camouflage prosthesis – anaplastology**
http://www.facialprosthesis.com/cv.htm (facial)
http://www.cpmart.com/ (breast prosthesis)
http://www.gesichtsepithetik.de/eng/
http://dukehealth1.org/plastic_surgery/prosthetic/svcs.asp
http://www.hopkinsmedicine.org/medart/production/prosthetics/sld050.htm

**Osseointegration**
http://www.rehabtech.eng.monash.edu.au/OPRA
http://www.entific.com/osseointegration.asp
http://www.vard.org/jour/01/38/2/brane382.htm

# Chapter 26

# Urogenital Reconstruction (Hypospadias)

## Background

**Hypospadias** is a congenital malformation in which the male urethral opening is on the under surface of the penis. The malformed urethral opening may be close (distal) to where it is normally situated (90%), mid shaft, or proximal (closer to the testes) (10%).

The malformation may be associated with one or more abnormalities (e.g. suggested to be approximately 17%)[1]. The degree and extent of any associated malformations will determine which functionally need to be corrected first.

**Chordee** is the term used in association with hypospadias where there is a curvature of the penis that inhibits the normal ability of the patient to straighten the penis (Figure 26.1). The degree of curvature determines the necessity for phasing of the surgical process, and this may require more than a one-stage procedure. In small/limited curvatures this is usually corrected at the time of initial surgery, and in some instances may require a small secondary procedure at a later stage[1-11].

The incidence in the USA is stated to be approximately 1:350 live male births, and the rate is suggested to be higher in different regions of the world[1-11]. This condition is of extreme psychosocial concern to both the child as he grows, and the parents who may believe that the sexual potential of the male adult may not be realised.

## The surgical pathway

Although reconstructive procedures are usually undertaken by paediatric urology surgeons, many reconstructive plastic surgeons in different regions of the world still undertake the surgery. As in other con-genital malformations, it is important from a psychological perspective that, if possible, surgery is undertaken before the child mixes socially with others, and particularly before entering the school environment.

The child's pathway in life should be as free as possible from taunting and bullying because of perceived or real difference(s). It is customary that the malformation of hypospadias is repaired early in the child's life (preferably prior to one year of age if the child is grown sufficiently) to assist in normal growth, and avoid recall regarding the procedure. If the condition of hypospadias goes unrepaired as a child (Figure 26.1) problems of sexuality, difficulty with intercourse, and major psychological problems will emerge as adulthood approaches. Fortunately, the condition is usually recognised as a baby and the condition corrected as appropriate to the deformity.

Such is the anatomical understanding and technical expertise of surgeons, the reconstruction of distal hypospadias has evolved from a multistaged to a single stage procedure, conducted principally as day surgery or overnight stay[1].

In children with more proximal conditions, the complexity of the repair (e.g. catheter/stents, drain, grafts, tissue flaps) requires an inpatient stay that may be up to four days, in the absence of any complications[1-3]. Surgical complications (e.g. haematoma, graft, flap failure, urinary retention) may extend the inpatient stay beyond this.

The preferred outcome of surgical interventions is to provide a penis that is functionally and aesthetically normal. The principal factors that may prevent this are:

- The degree of the original deformity
- The tissue available for reconstruction
- Postoperative complications
- The overall success of the procedure.

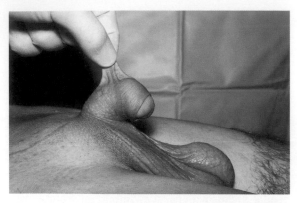

**Figure 26.1** Young male with unrepaired hypospadias (minimal chordee deformity).

---

### Box 26.1  Preoperative preparation.

- During the surgical consultation, the degree of deformity is determined and a decision made as to the most appropriate surgical approach
- A penis with a severe curvature (chordee) that requires grafting will usually require staged procedures
- Parents will be questioned regarding the presence of hypospadias or urinary tract conditions within the existing family circle and counselled as appropriate
- The surgical procedure will be outlined and, with the operative consent obtained, preparatory management put into place
- Prior to the main procedure, the child will be investigated for the presence of other congenital malformations which are not uncommon in children with hypospadias (e.g. undescended testes, kidney abnormalities, or hernias)
- In addition, there will be checking of the patency and efficacy of the upper urinary tract by ultrasonography for the presence of any structural abnormalities, blood examination, and urine tests to exclude any existing infections that may potentially compromise the procedure
- Nurse clinicians participating in the preparation of the child must be aware of the anxiety, fear and guilt that may be felt by the parents – as commonly experienced for any congenital malformation[12–14]
- Reassurance during investigations and information regarding the child's safety, comfort, wound care, and postoperative management, may require constant reinforcement
- The discovery of additional malformations will increase the degree of anxiety parents feel
- Some surgeons may prescribe a rectal suppository the

day prior to the procedure to ensure evacuation of the bowel and reduce any postoperative straining that may bring on bleeding[10]
- The child is bathed and admitted on the morning of the procedure
- Premedication may be administered but, with the child at only 12 months old, or younger, this may be omitted in some cases
- Prophylactic antibiotics are usually administered to prevent potential urinary infection and these may be given IV, prophylactically, prior to commencement of, or during, the surgical procedure.

---

### Box 26.2  Surgical reconstruction.

- Choice of anaesthesia is determined by the extent of the surgery itself, postoperative analgesia needs, and length of the child's hospital stay[1–10]
- General anaesthesia augmented with a caudal regional anaesthetic block may be administered pre-surgery, or at the completion of the procedure (suggested to be associated with reduced bladder spasm postoperatively), in association with a choice of narcotic, rectal analgesia, and sedation[14–17]
- Penile anaesthetic blocks are also useful for comfort measures
- Prior to the surgical reconstruction, urethroscopy/cystoscopy is undertaken to ensure the normal patency of the urethra (e.g. urethral strictures, incompetent urethral valves)
- In specific cases (e.g. some proximal conditions) a percutaneous suprapubic catheter may be inserted for temporary urinary diversion. Children accept this technique more readily that urethral catheters
- The degree and extent of the surgery is matched to the position and degree of deformity and available skin. Z-plasty, local flaps, or full thickness skin grafts from local skin may be required
- With severe hypospadias, absence of sufficient local penile skin may require harvesting of buccal mucosa (the oral cavity), abdominal wall or inner arm skin for grafting
- A Mini-Vac® drain may be left in for 24 hours, or a No. 8 French gauge Silastic® tubing catheter (referred to as a 'stent' or 'splint'), may be left in the urethra for 3–14 days
- Urine drainage will be allowed to flow into a soft nappy, or free flow into a bag for accurate measurement of output
- Absorbable sutures will be used for the repair process to exclude formal suture removal.

**Box 26.3** Safety 1 – risk management and postoperative nursing care.

- Each surgeon will select the dressing to parallel the extent of the surgery, and the need for temporary 'splinting' of the penis with a catheter, if skin grafts or skin flaps have been used
- Compression type dressings (dressings and mini bandaging) may cause tissue ischaemia and loss of flaps, grafts or any fragile zones of tissue[1]
- The penis wound may be dressed with a Bioclusive™ dressing to provide minimal compression, and to ensure that any adverse events can be readily observed[5]
- Donor sites will be dressed according to the site and wound thickness – usually primary suture
- Buccal donor sites will be sutured with absorbable sutures, and the mouth will require oral hygiene care
- The decision on the use of restraints in the first 7–10 days postoperatively is based on individual surgical decisions[7]
- No arbitrary advice can be provided other than to say that some experienced surgeons base the decision on the extent of the surgery, the age of the child, and the level of co-operation from the child
- The ability to interfere with the dressings and remove catheters increases with age, degree of discomfort and existing behavioural difficulties, and these are often the determining factors
- A significant study completed on 117 children (reported in 2001) with an average age of 2.2 years, who underwent a one-stage procedure, concluded that postoperative dressings were unnecessary on discharge, that children fared better overall when dressings were not applied and soft nappies were used, pain was significantly reduced, neomycin antibiotic ointment was applied, and patient and parent anxiety lessened[11]
- These studies are very valuable and can provide a basis for change of rituals to evidence-based development of protocols for improved quality of care for particular patients
- The high level of vascularity in the penis is both an asset (sexually) and a disadvantage (surgically) as the potential for haematoma where surgery is complex can cause major postoperative complications[1–11]
- Haematoma requires evacuation as an urgent procedure to prevent loss of grafts or flaps
- Early evacuation of the haematoma is important to ensure that zero areas of tissue are lost and early return to the operating theatre is essential to reduce the risk of continuing complicating factors

Wound dehiscence – usually caused by haematoma, swelling/oedema, leading to avascular necrosis of the flaps is a potential risk factor.

**Box 26.4** Safety 2 – risk management and postoperative nursing care.

- Bladder spasm – (extremely painful, and suggested to be caused by the presence of a catheter as a foreign body) may be relieved by narcotic analgesia by suppository, anticholinergic or antispasmodic medications, diazepam (used as a muscle relaxant), a warm bath, or a repositioning the catheter[1–5,7,10]
- Experienced nurses will identify and report the early onset of the condition[12,13]
- Surgeons will usually have a standard reporting protocol, and attempt to take pre-emptive measures to provide relief before spasm becomes too severe
- Fluid maintenance is essential to prevent dehydration, maintain renal function, prevent urinary retention and encourage regular urine output
- Avoidance of urine retention and bladder spasm is essential for patient safety and comfort
- Urinary tract infection – the risk of urinary tract infection is managed by prophylactic antibiotics and may be commenced prior to, or via, IV and following during surgery
- The ability to void sufficient urine is the primary prerequisite to discharge, and an adequate fluid intake is required for this to occur[1–13]

**Review**

*Setting goals of care and preferred clinical and patient outcomes*, Chapter 2, Boxes 2.7–2.9. Adapt as appropriate to the patient's clinical needs.

## Box 26.5 Postoperative (late) complications.

- Fistula
- Diverticulum
- Strictures of the meatus
- A range of flow difficulties (e.g. spraying whilst urinating)
- Surgical correction for any late complications is usually undertaken after about six months when all healing has taken place and the exact nature of the problem(s) can be accurately assessed[1–11].

## Box 26.6 Comfort – pain management, vascular status and wound protection.

- Evidence-based pain management is an essential clinical nursing goal of postoperative management[14–17]
- If caudal regional blocks or penile blocks have been used for patient comfort, wound/vascular complications may be developing without the sensation of pain being present[14–17]
- The colour (vascular integrity) of the end of the penis should be strictly monitored, and signs of arterial compromise (white) or venous compromise (dark blue) reported to the surgeon immediately
- The type, specific location, and description of any pain or vascular changes outside the expected parameters of basic discomfort must be reported immediately as time is of the essence if major complications are to be avoided
- Metal/plastic 'tents' or frames should be placed over the pelvic region to prevent the weight of sheets/blankets on the wound, prevent pain, and for easy wound inspection
- Minor types of procedures, at the distal end of the penis rarely cause difficulties when regular pain regimes, warm baths, hygiene, feeding, physical comforting, and favourite toys are provided
- Soft disposable nappies will usually keep little hands away from the wound, in the absence of discomfort
- The more proximal the malformation the more complex the surgery may need to be, and the incidence of pain due to haematoma, or avascular necrosis, has a higher index of concern
- Surgeons/units should have evidence-based pain/discomfort management protocols, wound observation/monitoring, recording and reporting procedures, and these should be followed explicitly[14–17]
- Antibiotics to prevent local wound and urinary infections are usually given prophylactically particularly in complex reconstructive procedures.

## Box 26.7 Clinical wound management.

- Topical antibiotic ointments, non-adhesive-type dressings and/or a bandage may be applied for only 24 to 48 hours and removed in a warm bath, and then topical ointments applied regularly, to maintain softness and reduce scabbing and cracking of the skin
- The application of Vaseline® impregnated gauze should be avoided as it will stick to the wound and cause severe pain on removal
- The use of talcum powder must also be avoided to prevent contamination of the wound
- Catheter hygiene and maintenance is extremely important
- The catheter tubing needs to be doubly secured and placed where the child cannot access it (difficult!), as reinsertion of the catheter under anaesthesia may be required if it is 'accidentally' removed.

## Box 26.8 Independence.

- Parents will be anxious, and every effort must be made to allay their fears regardless of the extent of the surgery.
- The level of co-operation from the child is generally related to his age, pain, discomfort and individual development and general behaviour (see Chapter 16)
- The overall management of children prior to, or following, these procedures is not always as easy as is described in textbooks
- The degree of surgical and nursing skills required in the child's care is matched by the extent of psychological counselling required for the parents even in what has been a simple, uncomplicated, and successful clinical outcome
- Complex, complication-ridden surgical experiences, can be devastating encounters for the parents and the child
- The success or failure of the procedure of hypospadia repair largely determines the patient's sense of personal body image, sexual potential of the individual, and the ability to function in society with independence and self assurance.

**Box 26.9** Discharge management.

- Primary discharge education depends on the procedure, but is focused on:
  - Maintaining fluid balance
  - Complications or problems in urinating, including volume and frequency
  - Preventing pain/discomfort[14-17]
  - Maintaining general hygiene
  - Wound care as prescribed and observing the colour of the tissues
  - Observing for any signs and symptoms of swelling, inflammation, or infection.
- Many parents may fear touching dressings/wounds or attending to stent/catheter care. This can be overcome by parent education and return demonstrations of care processes prior to the child's discharge
- Written and oral instructions, and names and phone numbers for emergency or continuing routine care, must be provided to reduce the anxiety of the parents should problems occur
- For the first few days, parents should be contacted by phone to assess if they are coping, to answer their questions, and to reassure that help is readily available if required.

## Review

*Auditing preferred clinical and patient outcomes,* Chapter 2, Boxes 2.10–2.12.

## References

(1) Santanelli F. & Grippaudo F.R. *Urogenital reconstruction, penile hypospadias.* http://www.emedicine.com/plastic/topic495.htm#target1

(2) Gatti. J.M. *Hypospadias.* http://www.emedicine.com/ped/topic1136.htm

(3) Badger J.A. *Hypospadias repair.* http://www.circlist.com/anatterms/hypospadias.html

(4) University of Pittsburgh Treatment Center. *Hypospadias treatment options.* http://pediatricurology.upmc.com/Hypospadias/Treatment.htm

(5) Aston S.J., Beasley R.W. & Thorne C.N.M. *Grabb and Smith's plastic surgery,* 5th edn. New York: Lippincott & Raven Publishers, 1997.

(6) McCarthy J.G (ed.) *Plastic surgery, volumes 1–8.* Philadelphia: W.B. Saunders, Harcourt Brace, 1990.

(7) Ausher B.M., Erikson E. & Wilkins E.G, *Plastic surgery: indications, operations and outcomes.* St Louis: Mosby, 2000.

(8) Ruberg R.L. & Smith D.J. *Plastic surgery: a core curriculum.* St. Louis: Mosby, 1994.

(9) Stone C., *Plastic surgery facts.* London: Greenwich Medical Media Limited, Alden Press, 2001.

(10) Morris A. McG., Stevenson J.H. & Watson A.C.H. Complications of plastic surgery. London: Baillière Tindall, 1989.

(11) McLorie G., Joyner B., Herz D., McCallum J., Bagli D., Merguerian P. & Khoury A. A prospective randomised clinical trial to evaluate methods of postoperative care of hypospadias. *Journal of Urology,* 2001 (May); **165**(5):6669–72.

(12) Goodman T.A. (ed.) *Core curriculum for plastic and reconstructive surgical nursing,* 2nd edn. Pitman, N.J.: ASPSN American Society of Plastic Surgery Nurses, 1996. http://www.aspsn.org

(13) Storch J.E. *Plastic surgery and wound management nursing.* Postgraduate curriculum guide, syllabus, and course notes for students. Melbourne Australia: Australian Catholic University, and St Vincent's and Mercy Private Hospitals, 2000 (reviewed 2004).

(14) Keuren K.V. & Eland J.A. Perioperative pain management in children. *Nursing Clinics of North America,* 1997 (March); **32**(1):31–44.

(15) Prince J. *Acute pain management.* http://www.medicineau.net.au/clinical/anaesthetics/AcutePain.html

(16) Chalkiadis G. *Pain management in children.* http://www.rch.org.au/paed_handbook/proc/index.cfm?doc_id=1752

(17) Lloyd-Thomas A. Paediatric pain management – the next step? Paediatric Anaesthesia, 1997; **7**(6): 487. http://www.blackwell-synergy.com/links/doi/10.1046/j.1460-9592.1997.d01-131.x/abs/

# Section VI
## Applied Reconstructive Plastic Surgical Nursing 3

# Chapter 27

# Breast Surgery

1. Augmentation mammoplasty
2. Reduction mammoplasty
3. Mastopexy
4. Subcutaneous mastectomy (female)
5. Gynaecomastia (male)
6. Breast reconstruction postmastectomy

---

**Box 27.1** Definitions 1.

| | |
|---|---|
| **Breast atrophy** | reduction of breast size usually post breastfeeding |
| **Breast hyperplasia** | an increase in the *number* of the breast cells |
| **Breast hypertrophy** | an increase in the *size* of the breast cells |
| **Breast agenesis/aplasia** | congenital absence of breast tissue |
| **Breast hypoplasia** | congenital small or absence of breast tissue |
| **Breast ptosis** | drooping of breast tissue usually due to, for example, breastfeeding |
| **Gynaecomastia** | enlargement of breast tissue in the male aetiology may be physiological, pathological, or pharmacological[1-7]. |

---

**Box 27.2** Definitions 2.

- Simple mastectomy or breast conserving procedures = removal of varying amounts of breast tissue for benign or malignant conditions – sentinel node biopsy may determine extent of lymph node removal
- Breast augmentation = artificial breast enlargement
- Breast reduction (or reduction mammoplasty) = removal of excessive breast tissue[1-7]
- Subcutaneous mastectomy = removal of breast tissue for example, in women who have a fear of familial-based cancer
- Subcutaneous mastectomy removes the entire breast tissue but leaves the nipple and areola (the pigmented circle around the nipple) in place

- Subcutaneous mastectomy is not a satisfactory prophylactic operation because of the danger of residual small amounts of breast tissue in the skin and nipple
- Subcutaneous mastectomy is also undertaken for women who wish to create a masculine appearance (trans-sexual, or gender reassignment)
- Mastopexy = tightening and uplifting of existing breast skin without removal of breast tissue – prosthesis may also be inserted to increase volume
- Breast reconstruction = rebuilding of the breast following removal of breast tissue (principally related to malignancy – may be related to cystic disease of the breast) by a range of surgically designed axial pattern flaps, or free vascular transfer using the patient's own tissue
- May be reconstructed with or without tissue expander or breast prosthesis[1-7].

## Blood and nerve supply to the breast

The arterial blood supply to the breast is rich and its principal sources are the perforating branches of the intercostal (10%), internal thoracic (60%), lateral thoracic (30%) and thoracoacromial arterial trunks. Terminal branches of these primary vessels are, in addition to other smaller vessels, responsible for the nipple–areolar zone (Figure 27.1).

The breast has two principal venous drainage systems: one deep and one superficial. The main portion of the deep drainage is via the perforating branches of the internal mammary vein and the remaining is via perforators into the intercostal veins and is carried posteriorly to the vertebral veins.

Lymphatic drainage principally follows the venous system, and although most of the lymph is drained through the axillary region, the thoracic

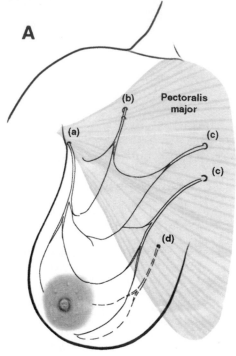

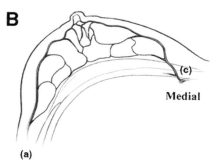

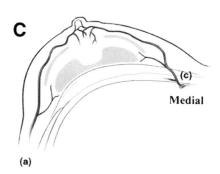

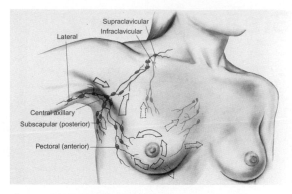

**Figure 27.2** Lymphatic drainage of the breast – important implications following diagnosis of breast cancer.

channels may carry 3–20% (Figure 27.2). Sensory nerve supply to the nipple region is discrete and vulnerable, provided chiefly by the lateral cutaneous branch of the T4 intercostal nerve[1-5].

> **Box 27.3** Generic background information.
>
> Abnormalities of the breast may result from complex congenital malformation, for example:
>
> - Poland syndrome, first described in 1841 by the eminent surgeon, Poland. Complex aetiology, principally associated with chest wall defects (e.g. malformation/absence of pectoral muscles, breast hypoplasia or aplasia), limb abnormalities. 1:25,000 live births; male: female ratio = 3 : 1; involves 75% of the right side of the upper body (Figure 27.3, female; Figure 27.4, male)
> - Accessory nipple(s) with or without breast tissue (Figure 27.5)
> - Single causes (e.g. injury – post burns), disease (benign or malignant tumours), or alterations in size or form mainly resulting from cell number, or cell size, breastfeeding, or gravity
> - Reconstructive surgery of the breast(s) is very common and covers a wide range of procedures that

**Figure 27.1** Schematic diagrams showing the dominant blood supply to the breast in A and B from: (a) the lateral thoracic; (b) acromiothoracic; (c) perforators of the internal thoracic; and (d) perforators of the anterior costal arteries. Figure 27.1C shows the annulus (circular breast ligament) and plane separating this from the blood supply to the skin. With permission: Professor G.I. Taylor.

aim to achieve symmetrical breasts in size, cleavage, and aesthetic outcomes for the patient whilst retaining, where possible, the normal breast and particularly nipple function

- Techniques are constantly aiming towards 'scar-less' surgery using, for example, endoscopy and liposuction procedures
- In selected patients, research into the blood supply to the breast is enabling previous procedures to be advanced by less intrusive surgical interventions
- Even in expert plastic surgical hands, these procedures can be technically difficult, and matching the patient's preferred requirements with the available options can be very challenging to achieve the exactness demanded by the patient
- Regardless of the reason the patient gives for requesting surgery, the patient who arrives with a photo from the latest fashion magazine requesting to 'look like this' is likely to present surgical and psychological challenges
- The malpositioning and/or inversion of the nipples, wound dehiscence and adverse scarring following any breast procedure versus acceptable outcomes, is a significant sphere of concern for all patients, and frequently an area of patient/surgeon conflict
- In all areas of plastic surgery, the use of pre- and postoperative photographs is an integral part of the discipline for the patient records, teaching purposes, and photographic evidence, if required, in cases of litigation[1–8].

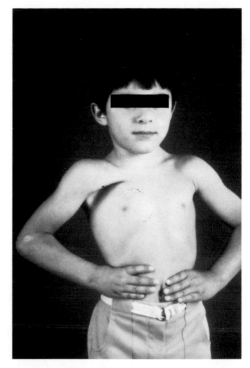

**Figure 27.4** Poland syndrome (male) – more severe case.

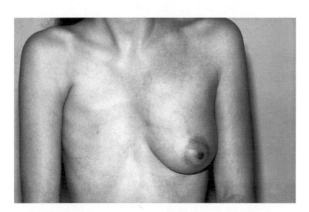

**Figure 27.3** Poland syndrome (female) – absence of breast, hand anomaly, malformation of arm and chest muscles (pectoralis major and pectoralis minor).

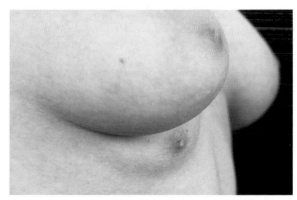

**Figure 27.5** Congenital malformation – right sided accessory breast/nipple.

# 1. AUGMENTATION MAMMOPLASTY

## Background

Breast augmentation was first recorded in 1895 when a German surgeon transplanted a giant lipoma (encapsulated fat tissue) from the back of a woman into her breasts. The outcome of the procedure is not recorded[1-5].

Contemporary breast augmentation involves a surgical procedure designed to augment (enlarge) the size of a breast(s) by devices described as 'prostheses'. This may be achieved by:

- The introduction of a silicone envelope inflated by injected saline
- A double envelope which contains an inner silicone gel sachet, contained within an outer wrapping inflated by injected saline
- Tissue expanding devices (see Chapter 22)
- The combined use of tissue flaps alone, or with breast prosthesis, or tissue expanding devices.

It is suggested that between one and two million American women have undertaken the procedure, and whilst some individuals have experienced minimal problems, for other women the postoperative, and after period, has been plagued with problems including asymmetry, capsular contraction, infection and ulceration, causing extrusion of the prosthesis. Most studies demonstrate an initial 86% satisfaction rate with problems that do occur appearing to be in the longer term[1-3].

It is important that prior to any undertaking to proceed with surgery the patient is fully cognisant of the implications of implanted material on breast screening procedures for malignant tumours. Some women may wish to undergo a breast screen prior to surgery and this option should be offered.

See recommended websites (augmentation mammoplasty – pre and post surgery photographic outcomes) at the end of this chapter.

## Box 27.4 Breast prostheses.

- Breast prostheses are designed in varying sizes, styles and textures that aim to enlarge or replicate missing contour, volume and form of the individual person
- The prosthesis may be designed to represent a spe-

cific form or a fixed size, or as an expander type where the volume can be increased or decreased, as the patient desires
- The latter may be used for expanding the skin following a mastectomy prior to reconstructive surgery using the patient's own tissue and may be included within the total reconstructive process[1-8]:
  - Cosmetic enlargement (and left in place with the filler removed) and incrementally filled until the preferred size is reached. This also allows for fluid to be removed should the patient request a lesser size, or the skin exhibits signs of tension and vascular problems (e.g. skin, post burns – post irradiation)
  - Expanding the skin prior to breast reconstruction using the patient's own tissue (e.g. TRAM flap), or used in combination with tissue (e.g. latissimus dorsi muscle) to attain the preferred volume, form and aesthetic outcome.
- Surgeons will have preferences for specific manufacturers, style and texture of prosthesis (e.g. round, teardrop), and precise patient needs, principally based on research product efficacy, and company policy of accredited service.

## Box 27.5 Risk management issues – issues related to silicone gel.

- Prosthesis that contain only silicone, have been suggested to be associated with 'leeching' of the silicone into the tissues
- Conditions related to disturbances within the immune system, and a potential association with the development of cancer of the breast and other vague disease processes, have been suggested, but there remains no definitive evidence to support these propositions[1-9]
- With the controversial nature of the research/evidence, in 1992 – restated 1995, the Federal Drug Administration in the USA removed silicone breast prostheses from the market place, except for specified clinical trials conducted under strict ethical research-based guidelines[2]
- The use of silicone prostheses is banned in many other countries[2]
- Individual cases of litigation and class actions, related to a range of complications suggested to be as a result of the effects of silicone on the immune system, are not uncommon[3].

**Box 27.6** Risk management issues and potential adverse outcomes.

- Primary wound complication may relate to existing morbidity, such as diabetes mellitus, previous irradiation, previous surgical procedures, infection, or heavy smoking
- As many patients may be taking the contraceptive pill or hormone replacement therapy (HRT), the risk of, for example, deep vein thrombosis should not be overlooked, and risk prevention strategies instituted according to the perceived risk of all existing and potential morbidity[1–10]
- Surgical and wound complications related to the implant include:
  - Haematoma          <6%
  - Seroma              <3%
  - Infection           <4%
  - Deflation           <6%
  - Extrusion, capsular contraction <38%–50% (dependent on grading system)
  - Hypertrophic scars >5%
  - Aesthetic (prosthesis malposition or unfavourable shape problems – nipple asymmetry) or any patient dissatisfaction related to the operative and aesthetic outcome[2].
- One case of toxic shock syndrome was reported in 1995 (*Staphylococcus aureus*)[2]
- There is no scientific evidence to prove that the prosthesis interferes with lactation.

## Risk management issues – summary

Breast augmentation remains one of the most commonly sought-after plastic surgery procedures, and equally one of the most controversial. Nonetheless, despite the worldwide debate and range of complications that may occur following the procedure (principally related to the normal response/rejection of foreign material), it continues to be undertaken by large numbers of women under less than optimal safe conditions and in non-accredited agencies.

Following even planned, safe procedures, many patients may register unhappiness at the prosthetic size/positioning, nipple position, or have a range of grievances, including real or perceived loss of nipple sensation, and any such concerns or issues must be referred to the surgeon for a consultation, with a relative degree of urgency[1–7,9,10].

In a Swedish research paper published in 2003[11], it was suggested that women who undergo breast augmentation as cosmetic surgery, are more likely to commit suicide than women from the general population. Breast malignancy and lung cancer due to heavy smoking were linked to the high incidence.

**Review**

*Setting goals of care and preferred clinical and patient outcomes*, Chapter 2, Boxes 2.7–2.9. Adapt according to risk management issues and clinical patient needs.

**Box 27.7** Preoperative preparation – primary considerations.

- Purely cosmetic procedures undertaken to enlarge a woman's breasts (or a man's during gender reassignment) require stringent and disciplined physiological and psychological assessments, patient preparation and fully informed consent[1–8]
- The cessation of smoking must be considered a criterion for proceeding with the surgery
- The patient taking aspirin, or similar pharmacological agents for cardiovascular conditions, may not be considered appropriate for surgery (i.e. postoperative bleeding) unless specialist medical management is instituted
- Because of the distribution of the sensory nerve, patients must be alerted to the potential postoperative partial, temporary or random loss of innervation in particular nipple zones
- For periareolar incisions the site may be anatomically determined by the risk of loss of innervation in a particular breast/nipple zone
- Preoperatively, many surgeons use digital imaging to demonstrate and document the patient's preference for size and shape, and in some cases, to demonstrate the unrealistic nature of the patient's expectations[12]
- Following patient assessment, psychiatric or psychological opinions may be sought should it be considered that the patient expectations are unrealistic
- Because of the sensitive and litigious nature of this procedure, the surgeon will have more than

*Continued*

one consultation with the patient and every potential risk/complication communicated orally, and in writing

- In addition to written documentation in the patient's notes, some surgeons will make an audio recording of consultations to ensure there has been no misunderstanding about any aspect of the procedure, potential complications, and realistic expectations
- Explicit written consent that confirms an understanding of the procedure, potential complications and long-term effects must be provided to the patient
- Practice nurses must be cautious in their discussions with the patient, and confine remarks and advice to their professional role of assistance[6–8]
- Patients will be instructed on the brassière (bra) type (without underwire), appropriate size, and number they should bring with them
- More than one bra is required in case of slight wound edge bleeding, and for hygiene purposes
- Many surgeons/practice nurses recommend patients use specific sports type bras for their overall firmness
- Preoperatively, methods of applying and removing the bra should be demonstrated to patients to ensure that the arms are not moved inappropriately in the early stages after the surgery.

## Review

*Intraoperative patient management*, Chapter 16.

## Box 27.8 Perioperative phase – supplementary information.

- Choice of anaesthesia (general anaesthesia, or local anaesthesia and sedation) is based on any existing patient morbidity, the site and size of the incision, muscle manipulation, patient preference of site, prosthesis size, and proposed length of inpatient stay[1–8]
- Anaesthesia may also be related to any proposition to undertake any additional procedures
- Local anaesthesia (lidocaine or bupivacaine) and epinephrine, may be injected prior to surgery as the anaesthetic of choice and/or, providing pain management and reduction of bleeding from small vessels[6–8]
- Strict sterile conditions in the intraoperative care of the prosthesis is important in order that inadvertent

contamination, by for example, glove powder, does not occur. Powderless gloves should be used

- The prosthesis may be inserted via a surgical incision, or endoscopic technique
- Insertion points are predetermined through prior discussion with the patient:

| | |
|---|---|
| **Axillary** | via the axilla – suggested to present the least complications[6] |
| **Periareolar** | via the nipple |
| **Inframammary** | groove under the breast |
| **Umbilical** | via an incision at the umbilicus |

- Prosthesis may be inserted in front, or behind, the pectoral muscle, the latter is usually preferred to minimise risk of capsular contraction
- A prosthesis inserted under the pectoral muscle appears to bleed more, as the muscle is dissected from the chest wall leaving an oozing wound bed
- Surgical diathermy heat probes are used to seal off any obvious and potential postoperative bleeder vessels
- Pneumothorax is a potential complication when dissecting the pectoralis minor muscle off the chest wall in very thin patients and patients following previous breast surgery[2]
- Following insertion of the implant through an incision, the appropriate volume is inserted, the inner wound tissue layers are closed, and the skin wound is sealed with a continuous suture to attain the optimal scar
- Wound drains are rarely used, to prevent potential contamination and infection
- Suture lines may be reinforced with medical grade (adhesive) paper dressing strips
- Simple external occlusive waterproof (polyurethane film) wound dressings are applied over the incision site, and usually a predetermined volume size bra is applied immediately
- The prophylactic use of antibiotics has been demonstrated to have no effect on the incidence of postoperative infection, consequently it is suggested that they should not be prescribed[2].

# Postoperative nursing management – special issues

## Box 27.9 Safety.

- Principal complication in the immediate postoperative phase is haematoma that includes pain, exponential to the degree of bleeding/swelling[1–10]
- Observation/monitoring is by gently gliding the hands across the upper surface of the breast for any abnormal or compact swelling greater than the existing firmness of the prosthesis itself[8]
- If the procedure is bilateral, both sides should be checked and compared for any increasing swelling
- Internal vacuum pressure therapy drainage systems are rarely used (potential for infection) but, if inserted, are commonly removed within 24 hours in the absence of any excess drainage
- Any attempt by the patient to recommence smoking to relieve apprehension should be counselled against, documented by the attending nurse clinician and reported to the surgeon
- Patients must be strongly encouraged to practice prescribed physical movement of the lower limbs to aid in the prevention of deep vein thrombosis and cardio-respiratory compromise
- Patients who have been on, or continue to take, contraceptive medication should be advised to maintain the wearing of venous support stockings
- Suture line, or incision wound care, is usually minimal (i.e. basic wound hygiene) – if intradermal sutures are used, aim at minimising scars
- Scar closure and scar outcomes may be further improved with the applications of skin closure strips, changed daily, for up to four months[6].

## Box 27.10 Comfort.

- Pain or severe discomfort related to chest wounds and injury to intercostal muscles, has the potential to limit the patient's required respiratory function
- Narcotics may be necessary, initially, and the strength of the oral discharge analgesia prescribed appropriate to providing comfort for full respiratory function, is required
- Analgesia should be prescribed to be taken preemptively, particularly for the first 72 hours, when the inflammatory phase is expected to begin abating

- Pain not controlled by normal or strong analgesic management, beyond expected parameters, must be assessed in relation to the development of a haematoma, or the patient's individual threshold
- Analgesic medication that includes aspirin should be avoided to reduce risk of bleeding, and the patient should be informed of this.

## Box 27.11 Independence.

- For most patients who undergo solely aesthetic augmentation mammoplasties, the procedure is undertaken in day, or 23-hour surgery units allowing mobility to be early, and a return to activities of daily living recommenced in stages, over two to three weeks[6,7]
- Particular restraints on excessive arm movements, heavy lifting, level of sexual activity, and overall general exertion should be discussed and reinforced
- Although this information will be provided preoperatively, it is essential that the patient has a high level of understanding of the risks of not following the guidelines (in writing) following discharge.

### Review

*Auditing preferred clinical and patient outcomes,* Chapter 2, Boxes 2.10–2.12.

## 2. REDUCTION MAMMOPLASTY

### Background

Breast reduction is a surgical procedure to reduce the size/volume of breast tissue[1–7]. This may be undertaken as a unilateral procedure to correct breast size imbalance (e.g. congenital malformation, a unilateral mastectomy for benign or malignant tumours) or as bilateral procedure.

Patients are usually women in the older age group, undergoing reduction procedures having often lived a life of discomfort and embarrassment due to large, heavy, or pendulous breasts.

The breast reduction surgical procedure chosen is based on the size of the breasts, current medical morbidity, the amount desired by the patient for removal and the potential morbidity related to specific surgical approaches. Surgeons will discuss with the patient the desired breast size in relation to height and weight, surgical options, potential risks and complications, and postoperative management Again, digital imaging[12] is useful in demonstrating what is possible and for assisting the patient to select a preference.

Preoperative breast screening for malignancy is advisable for patient and surgical risk management. In tissue zones with significant depths of fat, problems of fat necrosis can occur[13,14] but modern research into the blood supply to the breast is assisting to reducing the incidence (Figure 27.1 and 27.10).

Following a successful procedure, patients will often express extreme satisfaction.

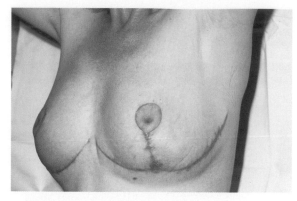

**Figure 27.7** Breast reduction – inferior pedicle technique – excellent sizing outcome – complicated by nipple inversion and scar hypertrophy.

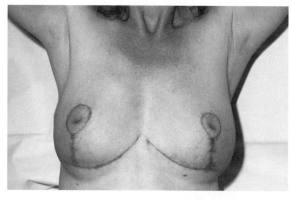

**Figure 27.8** Breast reduction – inferior pedicle technique – scarring, uneven nipples, nipple inversion.

---

**Box 27.12** Common surgical techniques for breast reduction.

- Various pedicle-based procedures
- Free nipple graft technique (FNGT)[1-7] (Figure 27.9)
- Open surgical approaches utilising $CO_2$ lasers for specific 'tissue tightening/uplifting' techniques
- Liposuction techniques
- Endoscopic approaches
- Modifications of existing techniques related to specific blood and nerve supply territories (Figures 27.1, 27.9 & 27.10).

---

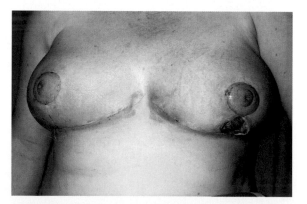

**Figure 27.9** Wound breakdown at inverted 'T' junction (meeting point of flaps) following major breast reduction utilising free nipple grafting technique.

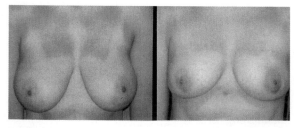

**Figure 27.6** Breast reduction – inferior pedicle technique – optimal aesthetic outcome.

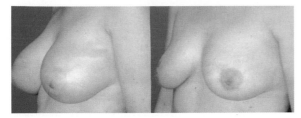

**Figure 27.10** Sub-glandular breast reduction outcome: before, and after one year – an advanced technique for removal of fatty tissue. The incision line is disguised in the peri-areolar zone – based on anatomical research (see Figure 27.1). With permission: Professor G.I. Taylor.

See recommended website list (breast reduction and mastopexy – pre and post surgery photographic outcomes) at the end of this chapter.

## Indications for breast reduction

### Box 27.13 Physical and psychosocial indications for breast reduction.

- To correct congenital asymmetry of the breasts
- Desire to reduce the size of the breasts
- Neck and back pain – pins and needles in the hands due to neck strain
- Irritation, skin grooving, and chafing of the shoulders because of breast weight on the bra straps
- Maceration and dermatosis in the inframammary groove
- Painful breast tissue
- Morbidity associated with disturbances in mobility
- Potential loss of breast and nipple sensation
- Issues of body image in all age groups
- Difficulty in buying clothes with matching size top and bottom[1–7].

### Box 27.14 Clinical risk management – 1.

- Failure to fully inform the patient of approach options and potential complications of whichever procedure is surgically advocated

- Errors of surgical/operative planning, surgical approaches, surgical technique, are suggested to precipitate the principal postoperative risks/complications
- Inappropriate patient selection and inadequate patient preparation – usually related to medical morbidity
- Breast reduction surgery is often undertaken in the mature aged woman who may potentially be at medical risk, particularly of silent or overt deep vein thrombosis
- Risk management that takes into consideration known morbid factors and issues peculiar to varying degrees of immobility, obesity, smoking and other lifestyle dynamics must be addressed[1–8,13,14]
- In obese patients some surgeons will request some loss of weight to address potential complications related to the medical morbidity normally associated with obesity, such as mobility, deep vein thrombosis, chest infections, and wound breakdown due to the poor blood supply to fatty tissue[13,14]
- As for any major elective surgical procedure, exercise and preoperative physiotherapy education in posture, stomach breathing, controlled soft coughing, and practising active leg movement are important preparatory measures[15,16]
- On admission, the use of prophylactic subcutaneous low molecular weight heparin to reduce the potential for deep vein thrombosis is a medical decision, and is commonly prescribed for patients over 25 years of age – newer generation alternatives are coming on the market,[1–9] (see Chapter 15).

### Box 27.15 Clinical risk management – 2.

- Breast haematoma, seroma, fat necrosis and/or infection, are the principal postoperative surgical risks
- In most cases, the inferior pedicle design is the technique of choice and delivers an excellent aesthetic result with the least complications
- In specific patients, the inferior pedicle procedures may avoid many of the complications of the other procedures
- In large pendulous breasts, the inferior pedicle technique can place the vascularity of the nipples at risk if the pedicle becomes kinked or is under excessive tension
- Wound problems related to avascular necrosis of the skin may be caused by devascularisation of the skin

*Continued*

through poor technique, excessive skin tension (flap necrosis) or smoking
- For patients who require the removal of 1000–2500 g of breast tissue or greater, per breast, breast reduction (by breast amputation) with the nipples repositioned by free nipple grafting, may be the preferred surgical technique[2]
- Greater amounts have been removed using the inferior pedicle based procedure, with procedural safety
- Secondary complications of inverted or loss of nipple(s) may result from the weight of long inferior pedicles (e.g. kinking of vascular pedicle leading to avascular necrosis of the nipples – inverted nipples).

### Review

*Setting goals of care and preferred clinical and patient outcomes*, Chapter 2, Boxes 2.7–2.9. Adapt according to risk management issues and clinical patient needs.

## Postoperative nursing management

### Box 27.17 Safety.

- Many of these procedures are increasingly undertaken as day or 23-hour surgery in operating rooms attached to the surgeon's consulting suites, or surgical centres
- Patient assessment, medical and psychological preparation, patient and appropriate procedure selection, is critical to avoid adverse events
- For highly motivated, co-operative and normally fit individuals requesting breast reduction surgery, short stay periods may be suitable
- Following surgery on patients with existing or potential morbid factors, the management of significant and continuing pain, or potential complications related to compromised mobility and wound care, may require a minimum of 48 hours of expert observation
- Home, or a local non-hospital environment is inappropriate unless there is a professional nurse on call, and immediately available, should complications arise
- Physiological and psychological care of the patient is consistent with that for any person who has undergone significant surgery
- As has previously been discussed, the issues of maintaining cardiorespiratory integrity, adequate perfusion, thermoregulation, and prevention of deep vein thrombosis, are paramount[8]
- All excised tissue should be referred to the pathologists for examination (e.g. for malignancy).

### Box 27.16 Clinical risk management – 3.

- Principal complications related to the FNGT:
  - Continuing excess weight placed on injured tissues, and micro vessels surrounding/at the inframammary groove and 'T' junction, can be considerable causing primary vascular compromise
  - Inverted 'T' junction wound breakdown (e.g. suture line dehiscence) (Figure 27.9)[1–4]
  - Requirement for nipples to be separated from blood supply, and repositioned as a free nipple graft – vascular risks issues related to full thickness skin graft 'take'. This may result in avascular necrosis of the nipples.
- Avoidance of wound tension may be assisted by accurate selection of the bra to be worn postoperatively, transferring and spreading the breast weight more equally, exerted by posture and gravity
- The use of vacuum pressure therapy internal drainage systems is a surgical decision and based on each individual case
- Any drainage systems inserted require monitoring as to amount and type of exudate
- Drains are usually removed if the serous exudate is less than 20 ml over a 24 hour period, and this generally occurs at the 48 hour timeframe with the inflammatory response reducing
- Greater than this amount and/or abnormal type of fluid exudate requires a surgical assessment to determine the clinical reasons (e.g. development of fat necrosis or seroma).

## Box 27.18 Comfort.

- Comfort, co-operation and reduced co-morbidity can be significantly assisted with a short-term patient-controlled narcotic analgesic pump/syringe, or strict four-hourly high strength oral analgesia, reducing according to need after 72–96 hours
- This allows not only for comfort, but also co-operation in maintaining cardiorespiratory integrity, and early increasing degrees of essential mobility to prevent physiological complications
- As many patients are overweight or obese, early mobility is extremely important.

## Box 27.19 Wound and general nursing care.

- Normal swelling and discomfort will occur in relation to the inflammatory process
- Gentle sliding of the hands across the top of the breast line and along the side of the chest areas is the best method (other than the presence of increasing severe pain) in assessing for the clinical development of a haematoma or abnormal fluid collections
- External signs of bleeding should be noted and reported
- With the patient placed in a firm fitting bra post surgery, any adverse fluid collections are usually obvious quite early, and parallel the degree of pain experienced
- In procedures where the nipples have been temporarily separated (excised) from the breast tissue, they are repositioned by the full thickness grafting technique and this normally includes tie-over dressings – this aids close adherence of the donor to the recipient site – failure of nipple grafts to take can be a significant and devastating complication when this procedure is undertaken
- Specific monitoring of the suture lines (colour, swelling, tension), and around the regions of the nipples and 'T-junction' is important to pre-empt vascular complications of the skin and subcutaneous tissues[1–4]
- Regardless of the technique used, choice of supportive bra type and size is important to firmly support the uplift, and reduce the drooping effect of gravity on the base of the wound, and tension on the repositioned nipples
- Bras with underwire are contraindicated to protect the suture lines, particularly following the FNGT
- Supportive bras are encouraged to be worn 24 hours per day for approximately 6–8 weeks
- Open management of nipples requires regular monitoring for the integrity of their blood supply, and maintaining continuity of moisture levels by application of Vaseline®
- Non-adherent padded dressings or soft nipple protectors may be required over the moisturised nipples to prevent shear and friction when patient is mobile, and to prevent soiling the bra[8]
- Post healing: patients will often comment that the most common late 'complication' is the spreading of scars experienced after healing has taken place (Figure 27.8)
- The postoperative application of polyacrylate tape daily, for several weeks/months in the hope of reducing scar hypertrophy, may be useful in some patients (for examples, see: http://shop.store.yahoo.com/ehms1/mefix.html)
- Stretching of the scars may be unavoidable in older patients due to the increasing loss of normal dermal elastic memory/recoil.

**Box 27.20** Independence and discharge management.

- At day one post surgery, the patient at medium to high risk may require assistance to mobilise and go for short walks, increasing according to wellness
- If previously applied, thrombo-embolitic devices (TEDs®) stockings should be removed, and anti-embolic stockings suitable for mobile patients (e.g. medically prescribed) should be measured to fit the individual patient and applied pre-discharge
- Patients must be instructed to continue to wear these as prescribed, for at least for one month and up to four months as risk for deep vein thrombosis and pulmonary embolism is suggested to be higher in older patients following major surgery (although not supported by evidence this is suggested to be potentially prophylactic)
- Maintenance of any prophylactic antiembolic therapeutic regimes
- Following discharge, and in the absence of complicating factors, surgeons and practice nurses must provide the patient with written guidelines for the limiting of early strenuous activities, lifting, driving, etc., and the timeframes for commencing any activity that may compromise the procedure. They must provide for increasing the patient's return to activities of daily living, which can be expected in approximately four weeks
- Written and verbal guidelines should be provided for pain/discomfort management, hygiene, wound care on discharge with specific reporting mechanism should any adverse event occur.

**Review**

*Auditing preferred clinical and patient outcomes*, Chapter 2, Boxes 2.10–2.12.

## 3. MASTOPEXY

**Box 27.21** Background.

- Breast ptosis or flaccid (drooping) breast tissue is commonly caused by breastfeeding, age, atrophy or rapid weight loss

- The degree of ptosis is categorised within three levels according to the level of the nipple, in relation to lower contour of the breast[1-7] (Figure 27.6 shows an example of ptosis associated with excess breast tissue)
- Mastopexy is a surgical procedure performed to correct or provide a preferred aesthetic outcome by tightening the breast skin with similar surgical approaches to that of breast reduction but without the removal of breast tissue
- In order to achieve breast symmetry, mastopexy may be a component of breast reduction, breast augmentation or breast reconstruction
- Principal complications are related to wound problems associated with avascular necrosis of the skin, which may be caused by devascularisation through poor technique, excessive skin tension (flap necrosis), or continued smoking[1-7,9].

**Box 27.22** Clinical risk management issues.

- Preoperative medical and nursing morbidity
- Risks associated with general major surgical procedures
- Haematoma
- Tissue flap necrosis due to wound tension, wound infection
- Malpositioning of the nipples
- Scars
- Patient dissatisfaction.

**Review**

*Setting goals of care and preferred clinical and patient outcomes*, Chapter 2, Boxes 2.7–2.9. Adapt according to risk management issues and clinical patient needs.

*Perioperative nursing management*, Chapter 15.

*Postoperative clinical nursing management*, see risk management, safety, comfort and independence for breast reduction, earlier in this chapter

*Auditing preferred clinical and patient outcomes*, Chapter 2, Boxes 2.10–2.12.

## 4. SUBCUTANEOUS MASTECTOMY (FEMALE)

### Box 27.23 Background.

- Subcutaneous mastectomy is the removal of breast tissue that may be undertaken if there is a major fear of familial cancer or for painful multiple cystic conditions of the breast[15]
- It is not common for any of the lymph nodes to be removed
- Subcutaneous mastectomy may be unilateral or bilateral
- Simultaneous augmentation mammoplasty, or the use of external breast prosthesis may be utilised to restore breast form
- The procedure may also be undertaken in younger women with a desire to appear more masculine in their appearance
- All tissue removed requires pathological examination
- An internal vacuum pressure therapy drainage system may be inserted for up to 48 hours to prevent/minimise development of haematoma in dead space left by tissue removal.

See recommended websites (simple or subcutaneous mastectomy including photographs of pre and post surgery outcomes) at the end of this chapter.

### Box 27.24 Clinical risk management issues.

- Preoperative medical and nursing morbidity
- Risk associated with major general surgical procedures
- Haematoma, tissue flap necrosis, wound infection
- Scars.

### Review

*Setting goals of care and preferred clinical and patient outcomes*, Chapter 2, Boxes 2.7–2.9. Adapt according to risk management issues and clinical patient needs.

*Auditing preferred clinical and patient outcomes*, Chapter 2, Boxes 2.10–2.12.

*Perioperative nursing management*, Chapter 15.

*Risk management, safety, comfort and independence for surgical mastectomy* earlier in this chapter[6,7,15,16].

## 5. GYNAECOMASTIA (MALE)

### Box 27.25 Background.

- Gynaecomastia is a benign breast condition, with enlargement of ductal and connective tissue in the male.
- It occurs in 75% of males at puberty, with 75% disappearing within several years[1–7,17]
- Before surgery can be considered the patient must be fully assessed for any abnormal conditions, for example: hormonal changes, local breast tissue cancer, systemic cancerous conditions, familial, some drug use (including marijuana, heroin), or as part of a congenital syndrome, e.g. Klinefelter's syndrome)[1,7,17]
- The procedure is mainly aesthetically based, especially in the younger male, with a preference to wear fashionable T-shirts or other close fitting upper body clothing
- A basic understanding of the pathology is important as it can provide an indication of potential postoperative complications, such as haematoma[1–7,17]
- Three types are described:

  | | |
  |---|---|
  | **Florid** | less than four months in duration, hypervascular and highly likely to bleed postoperatively |
  | **Fibrous** | more than 12 months in duration |
  | **Intermediate** | 4–12 months in duration. |

- The condition is usually graded on a 1–2–3 scale (with grade 1 the least growth)
- Final decisions for a surgical procedure are determined largely by the grade and the potential for optimal medical and aesthetic outcomes.

---

**Box 27.26** Gynaecomastia – the surgery.

- Existing and potential medical and nursing morbidity determine preoperative preparation
- The surgical procedure has been commonly referred to as a **subcutaneous mastectomy**
- The most common methods of surgical tissue removal is by:
  - Open incision (for severe growth deformities) via a periareolar incision
  - Ultrasound assisted liposuction (becoming a more common approach)
  - Endoscopic removal (via an incision in the axilla)
- Local anaesthesia and a vasoconstrictor (for example, lidocaine or bupivacaine and adrenaline) are injected following general anaesthesia for pain control, and attempts to control any postoperative bleeding
- Although gynaecomastia is considered a benign condition, all available tissue should be examined by a pathologist, to exclude malignancy (uncommon, about 1%, but aggressive).

---

**Box 27.27** Clinical risk management issues – postoperative.

- Haematoma remains the most common immediate post surgical complication[17]
- Haematoma frequently requires a return to the operating room for surgical evacuation
- The insertion of vacuum pressure therapy drainage systems and attempts at wound compression do not appear to alter the incidence of haematoma
- Attempts at compression by application of chest binders or 'tight' circular chest bandaging does not stop bleeding of larger microvessels, rather blood is dispersed into the surrounding available dead space or dissected tissues
- Compression has the effect of significantly increasing the risk of compromising cardiorespiratory function, if pain is not controlled, and particularly in those males who smoke, or in the older age group with accompanying morbid factors[8]
- Tissue flap necrosis, wound infection would be the other significant complications
- Risk management for deep vein thrombosis is required, particularly in the older male, those who smoke, sit for long periods in cars, or at desks, and have sedentary lifestyles

---

- The same clinical risk management practices should be implemented for males as for females
- Secondary complications include a dish-like appearance of the breast, nipple retraction, visible scars in open surgery, and patient dissatisfaction, particularly in the younger males
- Safety, comfort and independence with discharge management are as previously described for breast reduction.

See recommended websites (gynaecomastia – including photographs of pre and post surgery outcomes) at the end of this chapter.

---

**Review**

*Setting goals of care and preferred clinical and patient outcomes*, Chapter 2, Boxes 2.7–2.9. Adapt according to risk management issues and clinical patient needs.

*Perioperative nursing management*, Chapter 15.

*Postoperative clinical nursing management*, risk management, safety, comfort and independence for surgical mastectomy, earlier in this chapter[6,7,15,16].

*Auditing preferred clinical and patient outcomes*, Chapter 2, Boxes 2.10–2.12.

---

## 6. BREAST RECONSTRUCTION POSTMASTECTOMY

### Background

The incidence of breast cancer in women who reach 70 years of age is approximately 10%, and higher (one in five women) in some societies and communities. Global breast screening systems are highlighting the early age (under 40 years of age) in particular demographic groups of the incidence of breast cancer[1–5].

Some malignant breast tumours are aggressive in nature and others less so, but for the patient the diagnosis of breast cancer is one that is frightening and distressing. From whatever direction it is observed or experienced, the procedure of mastectomy for breast cancer is one of the most profound psychological and physical experiences in any woman's life.

The removal of a breast(s) for benign or malignant tumour(s) is associated with significant psychosocial morbidity and, for some patients, the potential or actual diagnosis of 'cancer' is/may be life-threatening in the short, medium or long-term.

The past 25 years have seen alterations in the approaches to breast surgery for cancer from major mutilating surgery attempting to eradicate the disease, to sophisticated science-based tumour removal that conserves breast tissue, using sentinel node biopsy to conserve important axillary lymph glands as much as possible, without compromising the necessity for a tumour-free breast[1-4].

Approaches to reconstructive surgery have paralleled these changes with research-based approaches to reconstruction (e.g. Figures 27.11–27.13), and this has allowed restoration of breast form to become a common procedure rather than one that is rarely or successfully performed[1-7].

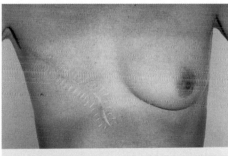
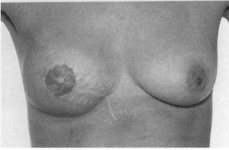

**Figure 27.11** Breast reconstruction using latissimus dorsi flap and insertion of prosthesis for volume and contour – nipple reconstruction undertaken as a secondary procedure – donor sites selected to match opposite nipple colour.

The high incidence of breast tumours, benign and malignant, paralleled with the desire of many women to avail them of appropriate reconstructive surgery, regardless of the prognosis, reinforces the continuing and fundamental importance of female body image to individuals and society as a whole.

See recommended websites (breast reconstruction following mastectomy including photographs of pre and post surgery outcomes) at the end of this chapter.

---

**Box 27.28** Surgery for breast cancer.

- A simple or total mastectomy is the removal of breast tissue, but does not include the axillary lymph glands
- Breast conserving procedures also referred to as partial or segmental mastectomy, or lumpectomy (*en bloc* of tumour), where minimal tissue is removed ensuring clear tumour margins
- A modified radical mastectomy removes the breast tissue and the axillary lymph nodes – the pectoralis major and minor muscles remain intact
- A radical mastectomy is a surgical procedure undertaken for the total removal of breast tissue, which also includes all of the axillary lymph glands, and the pectoralis major and minor muscles.

---

## Approaches to reconstructive surgery of the breast

Breast reconstruction is a procedure with the goal of rebuilding the breast through a range of surgically designed procedures that may include, for example:

- Insertion of a prosthesis
- Muscle/skin axial or free flaps
- Tissue expansion
- Combination of techniques which may be a single procedure or require multiple stages.

The choice of reconstructive procedure for the individual patient is dependent on a range of factors but principally reflects the amount of tissue to be replaced that can provide an acceptable aesthetic form, matching the opposite breast. In some

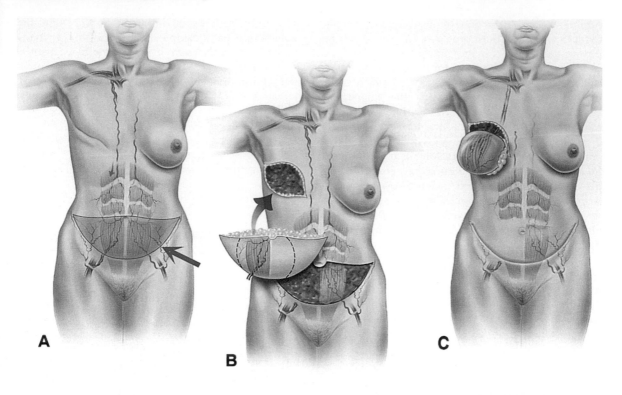

**Figure 27.12** Illustrative demonstration of TRAM flap technique based on blood supply to the skin research. With permission: Professor G.I. Taylor.

instances, this may also necessitate a procedure on the normal breast for the purpose of symmetry.

The procedure may be undertaken immediately post mastectomy, as a secondary procedure when the mastectomy wound(s) has healed, or when chemotherapy and/or radiotherapy is complete.

Immediate reconstruction, where appropriate, can have positive psychological outcomes for the patient, as the need for immediate adjunctive chemotherapy may delay the reconstruction, add to the patient's distress and general feelings regarding the entire condition and perceived outcome.

Overall support and a positive sense of self-survival are essential elements of the whole unsettling and potentially life-threatening episode. The desire for restoration of the breast form (aesthetics) is high and the challenge for reconstructive surgeons has been to find a range of procedures that can match the needs of the individual patients. This is reflected in the current range of available surgical options/procedures undertaken to restore breast form.

As stated, breast reconstruction may be a single or staged set of procedures, or a combination of methods undertaken simultaneously, for example nipple reconstruction (often required), may be undertaken at the time of the primary operation, or secondary to the procedure at a later date. Use of part of the opposite nipple, labial or groin tissue, and surgical tattooing are some of the approaches used. The aim is to match the opposite nipple in size, colour and texture[1-7].

## Alternatives to surgical reconstruction

It is important to point out that not all women may choose to have reconstructive surgery and will elect to use external custom-made prostheses that fit into a bra size suited to the physical proportions of the

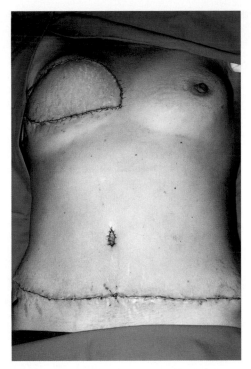

**Figure 27.13** Clinical example of excellent post surgical result following TRAM flap – nipple replacement undertaken as a secondary procedure.

- Augmentation mammoplasty – may be used as immediate or secondary reconstruction where minimal tissue is removed
- Tissue expansion (the most common procedure used for immediate reconstruction where loss of breast tissue and skin is not extensive), followed by nipple reconstruction if required
- Mastectomy – tissue expansion followed by latissimus dorsi muscle reconstruction rotated from the patient's back with skin attachment to the breast region – tissue expander relocated behind muscle – secondary nipple reconstruction
- Latissimus dorsi muscle reconstruction rotated from the patient's back (with or without skin attachment) to the breast region (a prosthesis may be inserted) may be used as an immediate reconstructive procedure
- Transverse rectus abdominis musculocutaneous flap (TRAM flap). Muscle may remain attached to its vascular pedicle, or relocated by free transfer and microsurgery. May be used as immediate or secondary reconstruction – (Figures 27.12a and 27.13 – example of surgical tissue transfer) – nipple reconstruction undertaken as a secondary procedure
- Free flaps based on the gluteus maximus muscle or from the lateral thigh are infrequently used because of donor defect and postoperative complications[1–6,10,18,19].

person. Some patients will make this choice initially and then, as their survival appears to be more likely, may choose to have surgery. Alternatively, if primary reconstruction fails, external prostheses may be the only option available to the patient.

Making choices and decisions in the presence of a potentially life-threatening condition is not simple, particularly when adjunctive treatment modalities are required and significant others and family are involved. Each patient must be treated as an individual – options and potential risks must be explained, and psychosocial support that focuses on, for example, grief, loss, anger, and fear, provided as an integral part of the entire complex physiological and psychological experience.

The range of reconstructive procedures is governed by the type of tumour, the amount of tissue removed, and an agreement between the surgeon and the patient on what is considered safest and most appropriate.

## Transverse rectus abdominis muscle flap breast reconstruction

Because of the inherent and perceived problems associated with foreign materials, for example silicone, inserted into the body with the potential for rejection, infection and a range of undesirable morbid factors, there is a constant search for natural alternatives.

One of the 'Holy Grails' of reconstructive surgery has been:

- The use of the patient's own skin/tissues that can be moved *en bloc* from one site to another without compromising the quality of the tissue and its blood supply
- Tissue that provides the qualities of preferred function and aesthetic form

• Leaving an inconspicuous scar at both the donor and recipient sites.

For many patients requesting breast reconstruction, the application of the free vascularised TRAM flap procedure is now considered to be moving closer to the achievement of that goal.

---

**Box 27.30** General considerations that are important in the selection of the TRAM flap.

- The blood supply to the transverse rectus abdominis muscle is the superior epigastric (non-dominant artery), and inferior epigastric (the dominant artery)
- The integrity of the flap outcome is at significant risk in patients who smoke, are obese or have physiological morbidity (e.g. diabetes mellitus, vascular disease)
- Previous abdominal surgery (e.g. caesarean section, hysterectomy) may have the capacity to compromise the integrity of the original donor vascular territory
- Conventional TRAM flaps remain connected to their own blood supply, e.g. use the superior epigastric blood supply and this may lead to a partial loss of skin (15–20%)
- Free vascular transfer of the TRAM using the inferior epigastric artery significantly improves the rate of success (between 1 and 5% in skin loss)[1]
- Flap delay techniques (see Chapter 19) are improving skin loss to zero in some cases
- The incidence of hernia in the abdominal wall, with the loss of the inferior anterior rectus sheath is approximately 6% for conventional and free vascular transfer of the muscle
- Hernia prevention techniques are undertaken utilising repair of the abdominal wall with a strong synthetic mesh material – this is usually undertaken following the harvest of the donor flap prior to closure of the abdominal wound[1-4] (see Chapter 28, major abdominoplasty)
- The relevance of this latter information is significant in that understanding the type of reconstruction that has been undertaken and heightens the awareness of the risks and potential complications that can be expected can be related to the importance of staging postoperative rehabilitation, for example, exercise, heavy lifting, etc.

---

**Box 27.31** Nursing risk management issues – TRAM flaps.

- Nursing management must be approached as a multisited major surgery with compounded clinical/physiological risks, and psychosocial implications if/when complications occur – see Chapters 15 and 19
- Free vascularised TRAM flap transfer may be up to five major surgical procedures in one undertaking:
  - Varying degrees of mastectomy, or reopening of previous breast wound(s)
  - Harvesting of the donor flap and its vascular pedicle
  - Abdominal wall reconstructive surgery
  - Microsurgery for attaching the flap to its recipient site, according to the availability of recipient vessels (may have been injured during the mastectomy procedure)[1-4]
- The undertaking of bilateral free vascular TRAM flap transfer exponentially compounds the potential physiological risks, and flap survival risk.

See recommended websites (breast reconstruction including pre and post surgery photographic outcomes, and overview of timeframes and rehabilitation programmes, at the end of this chapter.

---

**Review**

*Setting goals of care and preferred clinical and patient outcomes*, Chapter 2, Boxes 2.7–2.9. Adapt as appropriate to the patient's clinical needs.

*Safety, comfort and independence*, Chapters 15 and 19.

*Perioperative clinical management*, Chapters 15 and 19.

*Reconstructive flap management*, Chapters 18, 19 and 22

*Postoperative management following major abdominoplasty*, Chapter 28.

## Clinical vascular monitoring/observation and documentation

The nurse clinician's ability to translate vascular observations from early warning systems to adverse events may be the difference between success (Figure 27.12 & 27.13) and degrees of potential flap failure (Figures 27.14–27.16).

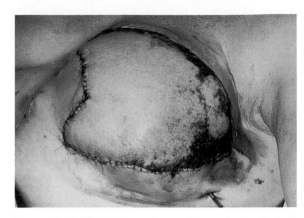

**Figure 27.16** TRAM flap outcome demonstrates that all but small areas of the black zone (distal portion) slowly recovering. Only this zone will require excision and split skin graft or be allowed to granulate.

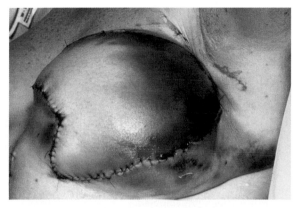

**Figure 27.14** TRAM flap demonstrates early importance of identifying differences in colour zones of bruising versus vascular compromise at various levels, and specifically indicated at right hand corner (*colour blue/black at 3 o'clock*), avascular necrosis.

Figures 27.14–27.16 show increasing bruising and potential avascular necrosis. This increased bruising is marked out in Figure 27.15 and distal flap end clearly demonstrates differences in vascular perfusion levels. Figure 27.16 clearly shows the need to be able to distinguish between bruising and vascular compromise. Only a small distal portion of the total flap was lost.

### Review

*Auditing preferred clinical and patient outcomes,* Chapter 2, Boxes 2.10–2.12.

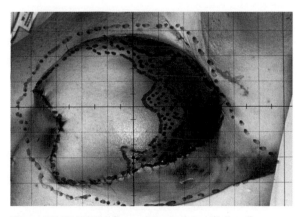

**Figure 27.15** TRAM flap, objectively outlining the zones of potential recovery using colour tracing. Some recovery at right hand zone but colour black at 3 o'clock indicates definite avascular necrosis.

## References

(1) Ausher B.M., Erikson E. & Wilkins E.G. *Plastic surgery: indications, operations and outcomes.* St Louis: Mosby, 2000.
(2) Aston S.J. Beasley R.W. & Thorne C.N.M. *Grabb and Smith's plastic surgery*, 5th edn. New York: Lippincott & Raven Publishers, 1997.
(3) Stone C. *Plastic surgery facts.* London: Greenwich Medical Media Limited, 2001.
(4) McCarthy J.G. (ed.) *Plastic surgery, volumes 1–8.* Philadelphia: W.B. Saunders, Harcourt Brace, 1990.

(5) Ruberg R.L. & Smith D.J. *Plastic surgery: a core curriculum*. St. Louis: Mosby, 1994.

(6) Fortunato N. & McCullough S. *Plastic and reconstructive surgery*. Mosby's Perioperative Series. St. Louis: Mosby, 1998.

(7) Goodman T.A. (ed.) *Core curriculum for plastic and reconstructive surgical nursing*, 2nd edn. Pitman, N.J.: ASPSN American Society of Plastic Surgery Nurses, 1996. http://www.aspsn.org

(8) Storch J.E. *Plastic surgery and wound management nursing*. Postgraduate curriculum guide, syllabus, and course notes for students. Melbourne, Australia: Australian Catholic University, and St Vincent's and Mercy Private Hospitals, 2001 (revised 2004).

(9) Morris A. McG., Stevenson J.H. & Watson A.C.H. *Complications of plastic surgery*. London: Baillière Tindall, 1989.

(10) Codner M.A., Cohen A.T. & Hester T.R. Complications in breast augmentation: prevention and correction. *Clinical Plastic Surgery*, 2001 (July); **28**(3):587–95, discussion 596.

(11) Koot V.C., Peeters P.H., Granath F., *et al*. Total and cause specific mortality among Swedish women with cosmetic breast implants: Prospective study. *British Medical Journal*, 2003; **326**:527–28.

(12) VanderKam V.M. & Achauer B.M. Digital imaging for plastic and reconstructive surgery. *Plastic Surgical Nursing*, 1997 (spring); **17**(1):37–8.

(13) Armstrong M. Obesity as an intrinsic factor affecting wound healing. *Journal of Wound Care*, 1998 (May); **7**(5):220–21.

(14) Soper D., Bump R.C. & Hurt W.G. Wound infection after abdominal hysterectomy: effect of the depth of subcutaneous tissue. *American Journal of Obstetrics and Gynecology*, 1995; **173**:465–71.

(15) Smeltzer S.C. & Bare B.G. *Brunner and Suddarth's textbook of medical-surgical nursing*, 9th edn. New York: Lippincott, Williams & Wilkins, 2000.

(16) Mallett J. & Dougherty L. (eds). *The Royal Marsden Hospital manual of clinical nursing procedures*, 5th edn. Oxford, UK: Blackwell Science, 2000.

(17) Rohrich R.J., Ha R.Y., Kenkel J.M. & Adams W.P. Classification and management of gynecomastia: defining the role of ultrasound assisted liposuction. *Plastic Reconstructive Surgery*, 2003 (Feb); **111**(2):909–23, discussion 924–25.

(18) Koutz C.A. & Quarnstrom M.A. Breast reconstruction after mastectomy. *Clinical Reviews*, 2000; **10**(11):95–107.

(19) Hultman C.S. & Daiza S. Skin sparing mastectomy flap complications after breast reconstruction: review of incidence, management, and outcome. *Annals of Plastic Surgery*, 2003 (Mar); **50**(3):249–55, discussion 255.

## Recommended websites

**Augmentation mammoplasty, including pre- and post-surgery photographic outcomes**

http://www.aesthetic.yourmd.com/ypol/user/userMain.asp?siteid=221060 (breast conditions – highly recommended)

http://rejuven8u.com/plasticsurgery/secondarybreast.html (managing complications following prosthesis insertion)

http://www.nationalsurgery.com/FCSC/procedures-cosmetic-reastaugmentation.php (breast augmentation)

http://www.plasticsurgery.org/public_education/procedures/AugmentationMammoplasty.cfm (breast augmentation)

http://www.fda.gov/cdrh/breastimplants/biintro.html (breast augmentation)

http://www.fda.gov/cdrh/breastimplants/birisk.htm (breast augmentation)

http://www.plasticsurgery.org/index.cfm (breast augmentation)

http://www.plasticsurgery.org/public_education/procedures/TissueExpansion.cfm (breast augmentation)

http://www.plasticsurgerydoctors.com/procedures/plasticsurgeryprocedureindex.htm (breast procedures)

http://www.plasticsurgery.com.au/index.shtml (breast procedures)

http://www.plasticsurgerydoctors.com/procedures/plasticsurgeryprocedureindex.html (breast procedures)

**Breast reduction and mastopexy breast reduction and mastopexy including pre- and post-surgery photographic outcomes**

http://www.locateadoc.com/gallery.cfm/Action/List/ProcedureID/89 (breast reduction photos – before and after surgery)

http://www.laserbra.com/ (breast reduction describing technique using $CO_2$ laser)

http://www.plasticsurgery.com/gallery/list.asp?spid=1&procid=31 (breast reduction photos – before and after surgery)

http://www.plasticsurgery.org/public_education/procedures/Mastopexy.cfm (mastopexy photos – before and after surgery)

http://www.plasticsurgery.co.za/breduction.html (breast reduction photos – before and after surgery)

http://www.plasticsurgery.org/index.cfm (breast reduction photos – before and after surgery)

http://www.plasticsurgery.com.au/index.html (breast reduction photos – before and after surgery)

**Simple or subcutaneous mastectomy including pre- and post-surgery photographic outcomes**
http://www.breastcancer.org/simple_mastectomy.html
http://www.breastcancer.org/tre_surg_mastectomy.html

**Gynaecomastia, including pre- and post-surgery photographic outcomes**
http://www.plasticsurgery.org/index.cfm
http://www.plasticsurgery.org/public_education/
    procedures/Gynecomastia.cfm

http://www.plasticsurgerydoctors.com/procedures/gyne
    comastia.html

**Pre- and post-surgery photographs and outcomes on breast reconstruction, including an overview of timeframes and rehabilitation programmes**
http://www.plasticsurgery.org/index.cfm

# Chapter 28

# Body Contouring

1. Abdominoplasty
2. Thigh lift
3. Liposuction

## Background

The removal of adipose tissue from the abdomen was initially reported towards the end of the 19th Century[1]. These procedures gained momentum in the 1950s when surgical techniques were refined to parallel an increasing understanding of the blood supply to the regions and significantly minimise the common complications of fat/skin necrosis.

The 1970s saw the introduction of liposuction, a revolutionary concept that has changed surgical approaches to the removal of fat tissue from a single modality to one of choices, according to the anatomical region, and the desire for scar minimisation.

Adipose or fatty tissue may now be safely removed from almost any region of the body where it exists, as long as the risks/complications related to known adverse events during and after surgery are addressed.

Combined procedures of open surgery and liposuction are common, as the selection of the most appropriate procedure can be tailored to meet the patient's requests. For many patients the previous need for open surgery has been minimised or, in some cases, eliminated, with planned multiple liposuction procedures[1-8].

## Physiology of fat formation

Subcutaneous fat forms an important insulating layer of varying thickness for the body, situated between the skin and the muscle fascia. Under normal conditions, fat is deposited at a superficial and a deep layer, proportional to the anatomical part.

Following weight gain, the fat is deposited with the deeper layer and this is sex specific, with women experiencing enlargement in the regions of the lower anterior abdomen, the iliac area, and the sub-trochanteric zones. These zones present the significant areas of concern and constitute the major female patient presentation for surgical removal/contouring.

## Selecting the procedure to suit the preferred patient outcomes

When patients present for the removal of unwanted adipose or fatty tissue, or lax skin, most surgeons select a surgical approach based on anatomic findings aligned to clinical guidelines or classification systems, for example, Category I (CI) = liposuction alone, to Category VI (CVI) = complete circumferential abdominoplasty[1-3].

The most common are Category 1 and Category IV[1-4]. Other classifications may include combined excision of tissue and liposuction on a scale where Category 1 = minimal procedure and Category IV = major procedure(s) [1-4].

These are not arbitrary, but provide flexibility in providing discretionary judgement guidelines of what is safe for the patient, and what meets the preferred aesthetic outcomes. Some patients may require staged, or repeated procedures, when multiple and/or substantial areas of the body are to be considered for adipose tissue removal.

## 1. ABDOMINOPLASTY

## Background

The aetiology of excess adipose (fatty) tissue and/or excess skin alone, may be related to age, morbidity, past pregnancy, dietary and lifestyle habits, lack of reasonable exercise and familial, syndromic, or genetic causes. The common presenting age group for surgery is approximately 35–40+ years of age[1-4].

Skin laxity following pregnancy, or loss of weight, are common reasons for presentation for removal of skin alone, without the removal of deep levels of adipose tissue, but the procedure may continue to be referred to as a **lipectomy** or **mini-abdominoplasty**, Category II or III[1–4].

---

### BOX 28.1 Principal definitions.

| | |
|---|---|
| **Lipo** | from the Greek prefix *lipo-* meaning 'fat' |
| **Adipose tissue** | pertaining to tissue composed of fat cells |
| **Cellulite** | the fibrous septae (retinacula cutis), that anchors the skin, distorting laterally as fat cells increase in size and number – skin continues to loose elasticity with age |
| **Abdominoplasty** | major surgical removal of deep and superficial fat layers and/or skin by excision from the abdominal region, repair of the abdominal muscle wall, and relocation of the umbilicus |
| **Mini-abdominoplasty** | removal of skin and hypodermal layer, which usually contains minimal levels of adipose (superficial) tissue (mainly loose skin and hypodermal attachment) without the repositioning of the umbilicus |
| **Surgical thigh lifting** | benefits hips, buttocks, inner and outer thighs – anterior and posterior thighs – more commonly undertake by surgical liposuction |
| **Liposuction** | the surgical removal of subcutaneous fat through multiple small incisions in the skin, by a mechanical vacuum aspiration (suction) technique or by ultrasonic suction-aspiration[1–8]. |

---

## Principal surgical techniques

### *Endoscopy*

An endoscope is a tubular instrument that provides illumination and visualisation of the operative area through minimal incisions. It contains a side arm, which allows for the insertion of instruments that can be manipulated to carry out a range of surgical techniques at a significant distance from the site of surgical incision. Internal images can also be viewed on a monitor, with significant magnification, allowing for, for example, microvascular anastomosis[1,3].

An important benefit of this technique in plastic surgery is the ability to undertake certain procedures leaving only a small scar. Its greatest drawback is in its inability to address skin excess. An endoscopic abdominoplasty is ideal for patients who have weakened muscles of the lower abdomen, but still have relatively tight abdominal skin.

Endoscopic abdominoplasty will help tighten the abdominal muscles and can be combined with liposuction to remove excess fat, but endoscopic abdominoplasty is unable to tighten loose/excess skin in the abdominal region. As stated, this is its greatest limitation.

In some studies, research indicated that an endoscopic abdominoplasty was more beneficial to male patients than to females in addressing the muscle laxity when skin elasticity still existed, but there is no doubt that an endoscopic abdominoplasty can make a big difference for patients of both sexes, as long as the skin has retained a certain amount of elasticity[1,3].

See recommended websites (endoscopy and abdominoplasty, including pre and post surgery photographic outcomes and overview of timeframes and rehabilitation programmes) at the end of this chapter.

## Surgical abdominoplasty

**Abdominoplasty** (Figure 28.1) is referred to as the surgical removal of skin, and varying levels/depth of fat layers at the site of the abdomen. The procedure includes the plication of the abdominal wall muscles and the suturing, or application of Marlex mesh, to strengthen the wall, with the umbilicus repositioned/transposed (approximately 10 cm above the pubis) to recreate the correct aesthetic positioning[1–4] (Figure 28.2).

A 'mini' abdominoplasty is often undertaken in conjunction with liposuction (liposuction limited to above the umbilicus and possibly over the iliac

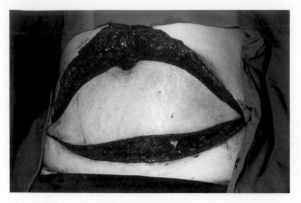

**Figure 28.1** Incision for open abdominoplasty and resiting of umbilicus.

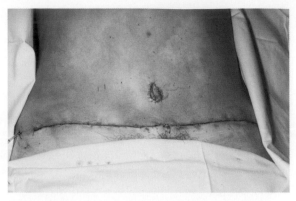

**Figure 28.2** Wound repair following abdominoplasty – excellent result – resiting of umbilicus.

crests). Open 'mini' abdominoplasty surgery is confined to below the umbilicus with skin and minimal fat removed relative to the safe degree of skin tension. Translocation of the umbilicus is not required and in patients with minimal skin laxity, some techniques may utilise endoscopic tightening of the abdominal muscle bands[1-4].

### The obese patient

**Panniculectomy** (in obese patients) is a major surgical procedure for removal of the large abdominal apron of fat. Panniculectomy may be performed in conjunction with other scheduled surgery, such as hysterectomy.

Panniculectomy in obese patients is usually performed in a hospital, due to the medical and nursing morbid status of these patients and the extensive nature of the surgery. Patients may be hospitalised for one or two weeks or more, and complete wound healing may take several months[1,3].

Major abdominoplasty procedures, where moderate to large volumes of fat and skin are removed, constitute major surgery with the potential for all the accompanying life-threatening and postoperative wound complications[1-4,8-10].

When liposuction is also undertaken at other anatomical sites, this further increases the risks for medical and nursing morbidity, and the potential for additional major complications. With critical patient selection and preoperative planning, risks and complications can be prevented or minimised by hospi-

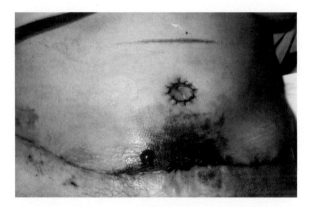

**Figure 28.3** Post open abdominoplasty for excess adipose tissue – early avascular fat and skin necrosis – observe blisters associated with venous compromise at zone of greatest tension and least blood supply.

talisation for several days for monitoring, and observation for any early signals of medical or wound problems.

Figures 28.3–28.5 show avascular necrosis of skin where the flaps meet as points of high wound tension with subsequent wound breakdown requiring surgical debridement, skin grafting and specialist wound management.

What can be clearly demonstrated is that the greater depth of adipose tissue, the greater the risk potential for fat necrosis, subsequent skin necrosis, and development of sinuses and potentially a chronic wound status[9,10].

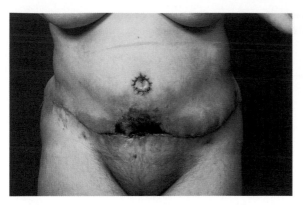

**Figure 28.4** Resolved surrounding zones of avascular fat/skin tissue compromise leaving central zone of necrosis – requires surgical excision.

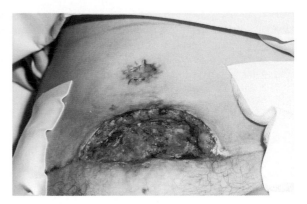

**Figure 28.5** Post excision of avascular necrosis – split thickness skin graft was applied to accelerate wound closure, VAC System® applied to stabilise graft from movement, seal wound, to assist in 'take', and to reduce wound size.

**BOX 28.2** Principal risk management issues – complications 1.

- Extensive abdominoplasty procedures that severely restrict the patient's mobility in the early postoperative phase have a higher overall general complication rate than liposuction alone in the abdominal region
- Immobility and obesity are significant predisposing factors for thromboembolism (1%), vascular deep vein thrombosis/pulmonary embolism (PE), or fat embolism (monitor for chest pain and petechia – tiny purple or red spots on the chest wall)
- Deep vein thrombosis › PE → death
- Deep vein thrombosis leading to PE has a mortality rate of approximately 1:1000 cases
- Whilst the mortality rate may appear low, the continuing morbidity following episodes of silent, or demonstrated and treated, deep vein thrombosis, and/or PE, are significant, lifelong and potentially life-threatening
- Whilst the patient is in hospital, TEDs®, or advanced sequential calf pumping devices, and prescribed specific movement of the legs that activate the calf muscles, is important to increase the reduction of venous stasis that comes with immobility
- It is essential that risk assessment and medical decisions regarding risk management for pre-emptive antiembolic therapy, and discharge treatment modalities (e.g. appropriate graduated compression stockings), are maintained therapeutically for up to four months post surgery
- A urinary catheter may have been inserted prior to surgery to review perfusion status due to major fluid shifts in the first 48–72 hours. This is a medical decision and will relate to the extent of the surgery
- For the patient in the postoperative phase, the catheter reduces the effort of using urinals, but the down side may be the potential for urinary retention on removal, or urinary tract infections. A balance is required in making decisions regarding the patient's overall safety, and sometimes tradeoffs may need to be made
- Major adverse episodes may occur, for example wound breakdowns, systemic infection or deep vein thrombosis, necessitating bed rest and/or additional surgery (Figures 28.3–28.5). This may require the patient to remain in hospital for longer periods or return to hospital following discharge
- Patients who are required to be bedbound, or have limited mobility, for a short timeframe require risk management assessments (e.g. for pressure ulcers, fat necrosis due to weight, falls, psychological issues) as elements of their wound bed management, and these should be undertaken to ensure the patient's ongoing safety
- Prior to discharge, a complete wound bed assessment and educational programme for wound bed management are important to ensure that a holistic approach continues
- This may also include the assistance of allied health professionals who are experts in rehabilitation towards normal staged remobilisation, and a return to the activities of daily living and a preferred quality of life[1–4,8].

## BOX 28.3 Principal risk management issues – complications 2.

- Haematoma – may not be obvious immediately, due to normal postoperative swelling – may require surgical evacuation[1-4]
- Infection (approximately 5% – mainly avascular fat) – requires antibiotics, bed rest and, potentially, surgical intervention[1-4]
- Avascular necrosis of the skin, umbilicus, with or without dehiscence (1–5%)[1]. This may be caused by previous or continued smoking, wound tension at the sites at risk (point of flap joins) (Figures 28.3–28.5), patient falls, or accidental events, previous operations reducing local blood supply, or undrained haematomas
- In most cases can these be treated with conservative moist wound healing dressing management (avascular skin or eschar can be easily debrided with surgical scissors or scalpel, as it is insensate) and healing can be expected within six to eight weeks
- Surgical debridement in the operating room may be necessary for large areas, with skin grafts applied to granulating regions, and to accelerate the healing process
- Seromas occur frequently and are generally attributed to the early resumption of overvigorous activity[1-4]
- Aspiration may be required but because of the recurrence rate and the fact that most will resolve over time, surgeons will not aspirate more than once
- Patients should be reassured and requested to observe and report any adverse changes
- Patients should be provided with individual rehabilitation programmes that match the level of surgery
- Aesthetically poor/unacceptable wound outcomes may occur with malpositioning of incision lines or the umbilicus
- Secondary procedures to revise scars may need to be considered[1-4]
- Medical decisions regarding further surgery are not usually considered until full healing has taken place and original scars have resolved or demonstrate any undesirable hypertrophy.
- Late:
  - Scarring
  - Altered sensation
  - 'Dog' ears, requiring surgical revision[1-4,8].

## BOX 28.4 Preoperative preparation.

- Regardless of the extent of the procedure, preoperative assessment, patient selection, choice of the most appropriate surgical approach for the individual patient, and preoperative planning that is based on physiological risk management and the patient's existing morbidity, are critical to the clinical outcomes (see Chapters 9 & 15)
- Liposurgery should not be seen as a complete surgical programme of weight reduction, and preoperative preparation may require patients to lose weight as a sign of their commitment to an ongoing lifestyle change to avoid repetitive surgery and medical morbidity
- A suggested programme of good diet and exercise preoperatively should be instituted as a positive incentive for a commitment to rehabilitation
- Full medical assessments (particularly of those patients with congenital syndromes), reviews of existing medications, patient discussions, and referrals to allied health professionals (e.g. dieticians, physiotherapists) to improve cardiovascular function by minimising the potential for further morbidity and postoperative co-morbidity (e.g. chest infections, deep vein thrombosis/PE) may be included as part of the preoperative work up
- Patients with pre-existing morbid factors, including a history of diabetes mellitus, smoking or cardiovascular dysfunction, should be assessed for pulmonary function, and undergo a programme of preparatory respiratory exercises provided by a physiotherapist
- Previous operation scars (e.g. caesarean section, hysterectomy) may compromise the circulation of the remaining tissue and this is considered when surgeons are planning for the safest approach
- Specialised contour compression garments, measured to suit the individual patient and anatomical sites, should accompany the patient into hospital or day surgery centres and be applied immediately postsurgery[1-4].

---

**BOX 28.5** Perioperative phase – supplementary information to Chapter 15.

- A urinary catheter may be inserted to establish adequate/accurate fluid balance
- Therapeutic venous thrombosis prevention strategies are initiated
- Several choices of anaesthesia are available and vary according to the extent of the procedure
- Procedures that include reconstruction/repair of the abdominal wall will usually require a general anaesthesia that includes muscle relaxants, to relax the abdominal muscle wall
- General anaesthesia with infiltration of local anaesthesia (lidocaine) mixed with a vasoconstrictor (adrenaline). Patient controlled analgesia is required postoperatively
- Epidural regional block with sedation is the anaesthesia of choice. The epidural catheter may be left *in situ* and analgesia maintained by regular 'top-ups' for the first 48–72 hours allowing early mobility
- Spinal anaesthesia with sedation (not used very often, but remains an option)
- Local anaesthesia (lidocaine or bupivacaine with adrenaline) and sedation
- Systemic antibiotic therapy is usually instituted intra-operatively and continued postoperatively where the depth of fat tissue presents a risk of avascular necrosis[1–4].

---

# Postoperative clinical nursing management

---

**BOX 28.6** Safety.

- Compression 'girdles' with adjustable Velcro® should be applied that initially deliver gentle compression and retention of dressings. Firmer adjustments to suit the mobilising patient can be made as this occurs[1–4]
- The initial application of 'rigid' abdominal binders should be avoided to prevent fat necrosis, pressure on internal drainage tubes and compromise respiratory function, particularly at the level of the diaphragm (see recommended websites at the end of this chapter)
- The patient should be positioned in a semi-Fowler's (flexed) posture with three to four pillows under the legs to relieve stress and tension on the repaired

abdominal muscles, and wound suture lines, to assist in venous return, and prevention of venous stasis[1–6]

- Pain that is not adequately and continuously controlled following any major abdominal surgery (particularly if the abdominal wall is tightened) can result in substantial alteration in cardiorespiratory function with reduced movement of the diaphragm, significantly reducing respiratory reserves
- Clinicians should assess lung and diaphragm expansion with a stethoscope to ensure full respiratory integrity is present
- As alterations to the integrity of the cardiorespiratory and perfusion systems pose a significant risk to overall homeostasis (e.g. venous return) and wound repair, pain management must be pre-emptively arranged, managed with diligence, particularly in the first 72 hours, or until comfortable mobilisation can be undertaken
- In patients at high risk, a respiratory physiotherapist may be required to be in attendance as soon as possible after the patient's return to the surgical unit, to ensure respiratory integrity, and to ensure continuity in the strict regime/programme of breathing and coughing exercises
- Patients should be given a soft pillow to be held against their abdomen when asked to gently cough or take deep breaths, as a counter to overexertion on the wound, and to provide a level of psychological security
- Patients who have had major abdominal surgery that includes the abdominal wall (including TRAM flaps), should be checked postoperatively for bowel sounds and flatus to ensure that paralytic ileus (a complication that may manifests itself by a decrease or absence of intestinal peristalsis following abdominal surgery) has not occurred[1–4].

---

**BOX 28.7** Comfort.

- Following major procedures, particularly when the abdominal wall has been repaired, in the first 24–48 hours a continuous epidural, or IV patient controlled analgesic (PCA), provides the optimal medical/nursing environment for delivering comfort and enabling the patient to co-operate in the range of risk prevention strategies required for patient safety
- Effective oral analgesics should be commenced as soon as possible, allowing a therapeutic level to be

*Continued*

established as the PCA or epidural analgesic is slowly reduced down prior to removal (see Chapter 11)
- Less major procedures will require strong oral analgesic management, decreasing as the patient recovers and mobilises (see Chapter 11)
- Patients should be educated regarding the potential for constipation when using analgesic medications containing codeine and appropriate measures taken to ensure that there is absolutely no straining when going to the toilet as this may result in wound breakdown/dehiscence
- Patients should also be encouraged to drink adequate amounts of water to aid fluid balance, circulatory integrity and in gastrointestinal activity[1-4].

## BOX 28.8 Wound bed maintenance – general nursing care 1.

- An overall wound bed assessment should be undertaken to enable a global understanding of the surgery has been undertaken, general physiological and psychological status of the patient, drainage systems, suture lines and wound dressings
- Because of the significant area of dead space remaining after most major abdominoplasty procedures, the patient may return to the surgical unit with internal negative pressure drainage systems (e.g. RediVac®) in place for approximately the first 48–72 hours
- The goal is to reduce the incidence of haematoma development and assist in the interface of tissues to assist healing
- Because of the need for early mobilisation, a specific plan for each patient is essential:
  - Constant uncontrolled upper body movement may cause shear and friction within the wound
  - Control of wound tension is essential as the patient attempts to become totally vertical
  - Temporary loss of negative pressure losing the interface of the tissues may result in microvascular vessels in fat tissue being slow to establish a viable blood supply, leading to avascular fat necrosis
- These issues present major conflicting tensions in avoiding the risk of deep vein thrombosis, cardiorespiratory complications and other medical-based morbid factors associated with immobility
- The need for timely immobility allowing the wound to heal and gain strength must be balanced against the need to prevent physiological complications[1-4].

## BOX 28.9 Wound bed maintenance – suture lines – general nursing care 2.

- Being able to shower helps the patient's psychological sense of recovery, and wounds that are non-exudating can be dressed with surgical film materials
- Self-care encourages movement and distractions from any negative feelings
- Continuous intradermal sutures (dissolving type or non-dissolving type) are commonly used to provide the least scar deformity and these are reinforced with skin coloured medical adhesive paper tapes applied to support the skin wound edges
- Tapes should not be applied to 'hold the wound together' (as discussed previously in Chapters 11–13), as tension, shear and friction will quickly cause skin blisters and local inflammation (Figure 28.6)
- Sutures that require removal may be taken out at about 10–14 days (may be up to 21 days), depending on the tension within the wound and the degree of activity prescribed for the patient
- Skin-coloured medical adhesive paper tape is then applied to assist in reducing spreading or hypertrophic scar development
- The timeframe for wearing an abdominal binder is determined by the surgeon in relation to the healing soft tissue wound
- This may further be determined by perceived strength of the abdominal wall as this tissue is slow to heal with the constant movement of breathing, moving, etc[1-4].

## BOX 28.10 Independence.

- Initially, the patient is highly dependent on the nursing staff and gradually gains a degree of shared dependency (interdependent – co-dependency) and finally recovers a greater degree of independence as pain and discomfort resolve, and self-care and mobility increase
- Mobility is largely dependent on the patient's age and extent of the surgery, with minor abdominoplasty allowing the patient to be discharged, in care, within 24–36 hours
- A return to activities of daily living according to the surgeon's instructions and in some cases, assistance from allied health professionals and the wearing of compression garments during the day provides the

patient with comfort and a feeling of physical security [1–7]

- Major abdominoplasty procedures may necessitate a two to three night stay with gradual removal of drainage tubes, PCA, urinary catheter, and restoration of mobility
- No excess tension should be allowed on the wound and as the patient mobilises, particular degrees of body flexion (bending) is prescribed until wound strength is sufficient to withstand the normal range of movements
- Restoration to normal mobility is related to age and the extent of the procedure, but is generally completed in about six weeks
- Mobility commences with a week of assisted home rest post discharge, and a return to sedentary activities, wearing of graduated compression antiembolic stockings (up to four months), and prescribed walking distances to prevent deep vein thrombosis (high risk patients), and very gradual level of manual lifting type work at two to three weeks [1–4].

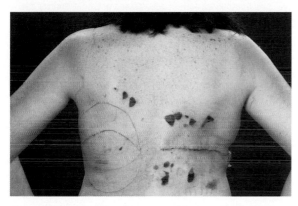

**Figure 28.6** Skin blistering caused by surgical adhesive wound tapes applied under tension with constant shear and friction related to constant movement (e.g. breathing, upper body movement).

**Review**

*Setting goals of care and preferred clinical and patient outcomes*, Chapter 2, Boxes 2.7–2.9. Adapt according to risk management issues and clinical patient needs.

*Auditing preferred clinical and patient outcomes*, Chapter 2, Boxes 2.10–2.12.

## 2. THIGH LIFT

> **BOX 28.11** Background and principles of management.
>
> - Indications for thigh lift include excess fat, but more particularly excess skin related to skin laxity following repeated weight gained and lost
> - Most common zones of concern are:
>   - Hips
>   - Outer, inner, anterior or posterior thighs.
> - Liposuction combined with abdominoplasty can assist in attaining the required aesthetic result
> - Major abdominoplasty can benefit the upper anterior and medial thighs
> - Risk management and complications as for abdominoplasty and major liposuction procedures (Boxes 28.3–28.4)
> - Preoperative preparation, perioperative, including anaesthesia, and postoperative nursing management as for abdominoplasty, including supportive thigh garment therapy
> - As this is major surgery, hospital care is usually for two or three days post surgery
> - With the significant wounding, wound bed management and monitoring for haematoma, suture line tension, avascular fat or skin, or fluid collections, are extremely important
> - Foley catheter removed on day 1 or 2
> - May be some postural difficulty in voiding and bowel movements
> - Mobility is gradual and staged
> - Sedentary activities at about two weeks, full mobility at approximately 6–8 weeks [1–4].

**Review**

*Setting goals of care and preferred clinical and patient outcomes*, Chapter 2, Boxes 2.7–2.9. Adapt according to risk management issues and clinical patient needs.

*Auditing preferred clinical and patient outcomes*, Chapter 2, Boxes 2.10–2.12.

## 3. LIPOSUCTION

### Background

### BOX 28.12 Liposuction.

- Fashionable obsession with thinner bodies has bought younger patients requesting adipose tissue reduction with minimal open surgical intervention
- Liposuction is a surgical process of body contouring by the suction or aspiration of subcutaneous and deep adipose (fatty) tissue through small incisions, utilising various sized cannulae appropriate to the size of fat tissue and anatomical region (e.g. abdomen, thighs, upper and lower limbs)[1-4]
- The method can be employed as a single technique or in conjunction with conventional surgery in any area of the body, and is used in both males and females
- It has additional applications in the temporary reduction of lymphoedema, and for gynaecomastia (excess adipose tissue in male breasts)[1-8]
- As a technique, it is now the most common plastic surgical procedure in the Western world
- Traditional tumescent liposuction, or more recently, ultrasonic techniques are the two most commonly described
- Rather than attempt to achieve authentic weight loss, many patients may present quite frequently for minimal adipose tissue liposuction removal for contouring purposes
- This is achieved by selective liposuction with small incisions for maximum corrective effects, in the hands of expert plastic surgeons[1-8]
- Both described techniques have advantages and disadvantages, and the efficacy of one over the other has yet to be scientifically proven.

### Conventional liposuction – tumescent technique

For ease of cannula movement and assisting postoperative pain management this technique requires significant amounts of lidocaine, or Marcain® with adrenaline, pre-injected into the sites selected for liposuction. Three main types and sizes of cannula are available, blunt, bullet and spatula, but many surgeons may have custom designed cannulae[1-4,8].

### Ultrasonic assisted liposuction (UAL)

Ultrasonic energy is transmitted to a transducer, which transforms the sound waves into mechanical vibrations. These are further transmitted to a titanium probe or cannula that has been inserted into an area of fat. With vibrations of approximately 20 000 cycles per second the fat is melted and can be evacuated away by a vacuum pump. This leaves the collagen network intact, significantly minimising the bleeding[1-8].

See recommended websites (liposuction and compression garments including pre and post surgery photographic outcomes, and overview of timeframes and rehabilitation programmes) at the end of this chapter.

### Box 28.13 Patient selection.

- Anatomical patient assessment and selection for the procedure to match the aesthetic outcomes desired by the patient, are based on the surgeon's preferred criteria and patient classification (see '*Selecting the procedure to suit the preferred patient outcomes*' later in this chapter)
- Objective assessment profiles provide guidelines as to the most appropriate procedure(s) required to achieve the preferred aesthetic outcomes, free from complications[1-4]
- Patients may require multistaged procedures if the whole body is to undergo a major contouring change[1-8].

### Box 28.14 Risk management and potential complications.

- The overall complication rate following major liposuction procedures is suggested to be about 10%[1-5]
- Deaths have been reported from liposuction alone, sepsis secondary to necrotising fasciitis, hypovolaemic shock, and fat embolism[1-5]
- Major physiological complications include major blood loss, hypovolaemia, deep vein thrombosis, PE, and fat emboli

- Strict risk management in relation to each specific patient and threshold volumes to be aspirated (e.g. 1500 cc) is suggested to avoid postoperative problems[1-5]
- Major wound complications include haematoma, seromas and infection
- Skin necrosis where aspiration has been too close to the skin and pitting may occur
- Varying degrees of decreased skin sensation are common but it is expected that sensation will return within 3–6 months. Patients should be alerted to this pre- and postoperatively to avoid accidental injury[1-5].

- Fluid replacement must be accurately calculated and this is based on the amount of fluid injected, absorbed, removed and demonstrated renal function
- Autologous blood may be obtained up to three weeks prior to surgery if deemed necessary and preoperative iron supplements or diet rich in beetroot and green vegetables provided
- Full blood examinations for haemoglobin, hematocrit levels, clotting anomalies should be obtained preoperatively
- A postoperative haemoglobin and hematocrit may be assessed where extensive liposuction has been undertaken[1-5].

## Review

*Setting goals of care and preferred clinical and patient outcomes*, Chapter 2, Boxes 2.7–2.9. Adapt according to risk management issues and clinical patient needs.

### Box 28.15 Anaesthesia.

- Choice of anaesthesia is based on the extent of the procedure and range from local anaesthesia and sedation, to general anaesthesia and full monitoring strategies as for a major surgical intervention
- Liposuction procedures over small to moderate regions and small volumes of fat can be undertaken as simple outpatient or day surgery procedures[1-8]
- For large areas of liposuction an anaesthetist or nurse anaesthetist must be present for all procedures due to the cardiovascular effects of large volumes of local anaesthesia and vasoconstrictors that may be used
- In addition, significant fluid loss, for example, when full body contouring is undertaken, can also cause significant cardiovascular compromise[1-5]
- The procedure should be categorised as 'major' with all the risks associated with major fluid shifts and alterations in general circulatory homeostasis
- Full monitoring facilities should be used, with IV lines available for fluid and blood replacement if/as required
- A urinary catheter may be inserted preoperatively for the first 24–48 hours to assess third space fluid shifts, and volume replacement needs

### Box 28.16 The surgery.

- Surgery can be time (up to 3–4 hours) and energy consuming where large regions are to be embarked upon, and multiple approaches are utilised, each having specific application and advantages for use in different body regions[1-8]
- **Ultrasound assisted liposuction**: ultrasonic energy is used to break up the fat globules and allows the material to be aspirated. Suggested to be less energy consuming as the fat melts and breaks down into a more fluid consistency[1]
- **Tumescent infiltration**: extensive body areas are infiltrated with large volumes of local anaesthetic and vasoconstriction mixtures. Suggested to significantly reduce blood and fluid loss, limiting the need for fluid replacement, and to provide long-term postoperative pain management[1]
- **Endoscopic liposuction** may be undertaken in regions that are small, for example lower eyelids, and is generally confined to the facial zones where specific encapsulated fat globules are evident and close to important structures
- **Endoscopic tightening** of the abdominal wall may be undertaken as part of the overall liposuction procedure
- In some procedures aspirated fat may be reinjected into other regions for restoration of lost contour such as facial regions (e.g. lip, glabella) or depressed scars following trauma[1-4]
- The required effects often only last for about six months, mainly as the fat is readily absorbed or may cause fat necrosis as a complication.

## Box 28.17 Postoperative nursing and wound bed management.

- General principles of care are as for abdominoplasty, modified to address the age of the patient, existing medical morbidity and the extent of the surgery
- Compression garments, producing a form of external negative pressure are applied to the areas of surgery immediately postsurgery to assist in reducing haematoma and seroma by eliminating dead space previously occupied by the adipose tissue
- Pain management is usually controlled by strong oral analgesia given strictly four hourly for the first 72–96 hours, and slowly decreased as oedema subsides
- Night sedation is usually appropriate for the first two to three days where generalised soreness related to the inflammatory and oedema phase is experienced
- Continuing tiredness may be related to blood loss (haemoglobin should be checked) but early mobility is encouraged with a return to activites of daily living as soon as possible[1–5]
- Patient education is provided, including written instructions for rehabilitation and monitoring and reporting of adverse events[1–8].

## Summary

Plastic surgery, particularly the purely aesthetic component, presents many challenges for the nurse practitioner, regardless of the practice site. Expectations for optimal outcomes are high and the patient rarely expects less than what he/she requests.

Physiologically, understanding the blood supply to the skin, risk management, and medical and nursing complications that can occur regardless of the procedure require eternal vigilance and a commitment to attention to detail.

Psychosocially, the final result, how the patient feels about themselves, and their place in society, cannot be separated from the body, and in the ultimate analysis it is this that will determine the patient's level of satisfaction.

## Review

*Auditing preferred clinical and patient outcomes,* Chapter 2, Boxes 2.10–2.12.

## References

(1) Aston S.J., Beasley R.W. & Thorne C.N.M. *Grabb and Smith's plastic surgery*, 5th edn. New York: Lippincott & Raven Publishers, 1997.

(2) Stone C. *Plastic surgery facts*. London: Greenwich Medical Media Limited, 2001.

(3) Ausher B.M., Erikson E. & Wilkins E.G. *Plastic surgery: indications, operations and outcomes*. St Louis: Mosby, 2000.

(4) Fortunato N. & McCullough S. *Plastic and reconstructive surgery. Mosby's Perioperative Series*. St. Louis: Mosby, 1998.

(5) Pravecek E.L. & Worland R.G. Tumescent abdominoplasty under local anaesthesia with IV sedation in an ambulatory surgical facility. *Plastic Surgery Nursing*, 1998 (spring); **18**(1):3843.

(6) Ablasa V., Jones M.R., Gingrass M.K., Fisher J. & Maxwell G.P. Ultrasound assisted lipoplasty – part 1: an overview for nurses. *Plastic Surgical Nursing*, 1998 (spring); **18**(1):13–15.

(7) Ablasa V., Jones M.R., Gingrass M.K., Fisher J. & Maxwell G.P. Ultrasound assisted lipoplasty – part 1: Clinical management. *Plastic Surgical Nursing*, 1998 (spring); **18**(1):16–25.

(8) Goodman T.A. (ed.) *Core curriculum for plastic and reconstructive surgical nursing*, 2nd edn. Pitman, N.J.: ASPSN American Society of Plastic Surgery Nurses, 1996. http://www.aspsn.org

(9) Soper D., Bump R.C. & Hurt W.G. Wound infection after abdominal hysterectomy: effect of the depth of subcutaneous tissue. *American Journal of Obstetrics and Gynecology*, 1995; **173**:465–471.

(10) Armstrong M. Obesity as an intrinsic factor affecting wound healing. *Journal of Wound Care*, 1998 (May); **7**(5):220–221.

## Recommended websites

**Endoscopy, including photo gallery of pre- and post-surgery**

http://www.plasticsurgery.org/public_education/procedures/Endoscopy.cfm

**Abdominoplasty, including photo gallery of pre- and post-surgery**

http://www.plasticsurgery.org/public_education/procedures/Abdominoplasty.cfm

http://www.plasticsurgery.com.au/procedures/tummytuck.shtml

**Liposuction, including photo gallery of pre-surgery and post-surgery outcomes**

http://www.plasticsurgery.org/public_education/procedures/Lipoplasty.cfm

http://www.plasticsurgery.org/public_education/procedures/LiposuctionTumescent Technique.cfm

http://www.plasticsurgery.com.au/procedures/liposuction.shtml http://www.centerforderm.com/brochures/liposuction.html

**Compression garments**

http://www.c-d-i.com (examples of postoperative compression garments)

http://www.homerecovery.com (custom-made compression garments and range of aesthetic surgical recovery products)

http://www.dalemed.com (custom-made compression garments and range of aesthetic surgical recovery products)

# Chapter 29

# Aesthetic/Reconstructive Surgery of the Face

## Background

It is often said that 'beauty is in the eye of the beholder' and it is this view and perception that individuals may have of themselves, and believe that others may have of them, that largely drives aesthetic surgery.

It is the dominant reason that many people desire surgery to restore, or create, what is accepted within society as a normal appearance, or to identify with modern images[1-6].

---

**Box 29.1** Application of aesthetic/reconstructive surgery of the face – examples.

- Functional deficits such as congenital soft tissue malformations
- Congenital syndromes causing laxity of the skin
- Post trauma effects (e.g. post traumatic burns and soft tissue incorporating bone injury, congenital facial nerve palsy, amputated parts)
- Disease processes such as benign or malignant tumours
- Facial nerve palsy related to removal of an acoustic neuroma
- To aesthetically improve the ageing face
- In an attempt to redefine the total concept of the individual's identity.

---

Because of the complexity of what the patient desires and the range of approaches and interventions available, there is rarely one single surgical approach that addresses the total wishes of the patient, or relieves the anxiety they may be experiencing. Digital imaging is an important adjunct in demonstrating what is reasonably possible and in addressing a patient's unrealistic expectations[7].

## Facial rejuvenation

Figure 29.1 provides a flow chart of options available for superficial and deep tissue facial rejuvenation.

Facial rejuvenation may be considered within two principal headings:

### Superficial changes

- Skin maintenance
- Chemical peels
- Laser application
- Dermabrasion.

### Deep changes

Corrected by open surgery (Figure 29.2) – procedure aimed at addressing the effects of ageing and gravity.

### Aetiology and nursing management principles

Ageing is a normal biological progression and a range of medical and surgical procedures have been designed to improve, or camouflage, the process for those who desire to retain a youthful appearance for as long as possible. By far the most common patient presentation is seeking facial rejuvenation due to photo ageing, or the normal ageing process[1-6].

---

**Review**

*Physiology of the ageing of the skin*, Chapter 7.

---

With the reducing age of individuals seeking interventions, a large number of people who would previously seek open surgery at a later age, will now use

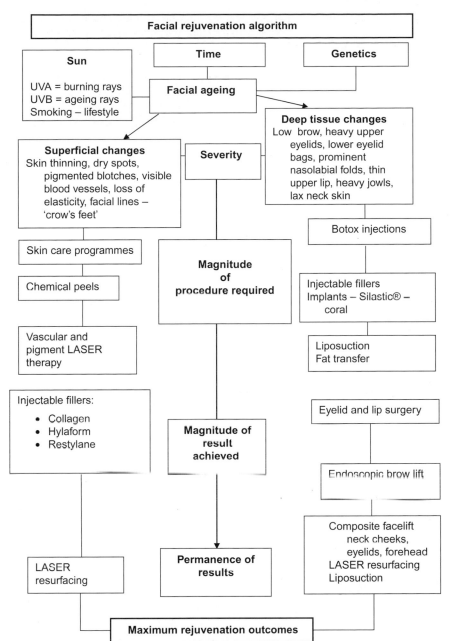

**Figure 29.1** Decision-making in facial rejuvenation.

modern skincare programmes, and/or facial resurfacing as a lifetime method of skin management (e.g. skin creams, local skin care programmes, microdermabrasion or laser resurfacing). Others will seek traditional open aesthetic surgery when these procedures no longer deliver the aesthetic look desired, for a range of psychosocial reasons.

Regardless of the surgery or treatment requested, and the decisions made in relation to any proposed procedures, pre- and postoperative photographic evidence including any digital imaging records must be documented.

Photographic and written documentation is also useful should the surgeon determine that the individual is not suitable for any form of intervention due to medical morbid factors, psychiatric reasons, or potential for major complications.

Such is the plethora of procedures offered, and variation in the information available regarding the entire range of aesthetic procedures, this chapter will deal only briefly with the more common procedural options generally considered, or offered to the patient.

Before any treatments are proposed, the following must be ascertained:

- Existing or past morbidity
- Smoking levels/habits
- Lifestyle habits – lack of exercise
- Alcohol consumption
- Recreational drug taking
- Current medications.

There is some discussion regarding the discontinuation of medications prior to surgery that have the potential to cause bleeding postoperatively. Medications that, for example, are physiological necessary and maintain cardiovascular homeostasis should not be altered or ceased without consultation with the patient's treating physician.

Previous elective facial surgery or facial injuries are also considered as potential complicating factors in wound healing. Patients seeking facial rejuvenation surgery are highly discriminating in describing their needs and in displaying their displeasure at clinical and aesthetic outcomes which do not achieve these needs.

## Superficial facial rejuvenation – facial resurfacing

In many people over the age of 30 years, photo ageing (exposure to the elements, particularly constant exposure to harsh sun, or the effects of the cold weather), lifestyle, smoking, and the normal stages of reforming collagen begin to decline (loss of type III collagen and elastin), and start to become evident.

The continuing exposure to these rudiments are the major causes of ageing that will show the exter-

nal physical signs of facial lines, and many younger people will seek advice on uncomplicated treatments to slow down, or reverse the process.

**Box 29.2** Facial resurfacing – general principles utilised by surgeons to guide their advice to presenting patients.

- The deeper the skin problem is, the deeper the treatment required to achieve the desired result
- The deeper the treatment required, the greater the risks, side effects, trade-offs and downtime for the patient
- Superficial treatments involve minimal down time, rapid healing, minimal postoperative redness, and little or no depigmentation
- The deeper the treatment, the longer it takes to heal and the greater the potential for prolonged redness and/or hyperpigmentation
- In deep treatment, there is a higher risk of greater long-term reduced pigmentation and demarcation lines
- Advantages include the greater chance of smoothing deeper lines and/or scars
- Skin care maintenance, chemical peeling, laser treatment, or varying degrees of dermabrasion, are procedures undertaken without surgical excisions
- They may be used as a single treatment modality and in certain circumstances in conjunction with surgery to address major ageing conditions
- Facial resurfacing techniques may also be used in the selective treatment of benign or malignant lesions (laser), scars, or conditions such as acne
- In the USA these procedures may be undertaken by accredited practice nurses under the supervision of specialist plastic surgeons.

## Skin maintenance

**Box 29.3** Skin care maintenance – the clinical principles.

**Level 1**

- Tretinoin-based programmes. Tretinoin skin preparations are a family of drugs all similar to vitamin A. These products are generally prescribed for acne but have been shown to reverse some of the effects of photo-ageing by increasing cell turnover, vascularity and skin thickness. They may be used alone, pre-operatively, and postoperatively following surgical resurfacing treatment[1-4].

### Level 2

- Glycolic acid is an alpha-hydroxy acid based on normally occurring organic acids obtained from various fruits, and synthesised in the laboratory
- Glycolic acid is made in concentrations greater than that found in basic skin care maintenance products, and is used in a range of low level 'peels'. GlyDerm® is an example of this
- The procedure involves a series of treatments about six weeks apart and provides a total skin care regime from treatment to recovery
- Glycolic acid products do not truly peel the skin or treat fine lines, but give the skin a highly refreshed appearance
- There is no down time and thus it may be undertaken during a normal working day and repeated every four to six weeks[1-4]
- Specialist trained skin care practitioners conduct specific clinics providing this service. (Lower grade products, not requiring medical prescription, are available over the counter of department stores and chemists/drug stores).

### Level 3

- An alternative skin care maintenance product (e.g. MicroPeel plus®, a BioMedic® product which contains salicylic acid) may produce a higher level removal of superficial dead skin cells and stimulates new living cells to reactivate the renewal process[1-4]
- This may require to be undertaken on a day off from work but involves no down time, as such
- Only specialist practitioners should be consulted and plastic surgical practice nurses can advise on this.

that traumatise the skin, removing deep lines and restoring smoothness of the skin by the healing response to injured epidermis and the upper dermal layer creating a contracting – resurfacing effect – average penetration 0.3–0.6 mm[5]
- Chemical peeling is a technique dependent procedure. That is, there should be a full understanding of the pharmacological products, formulas, and the potential positive/adverse outcomes that may result from using varying degrees of potency
- Formulas are available that produce specific injury at levels from the stratum corneum to reticular dermis
- This requires a very accurate assessment of the patient's skin and a decision on the preferred outcome prior to undertaking the procedure
- Phenol is the most common of the true chemical peeling agents. It is highly toxic and produces a deep peel[5]
- Phenol is absorbed systemically, detoxified in the liver, and is excreted in the urine. It should only be used in the hands of experts as cardiac arrhythmias, mainly atrial, have been recorded in 39% of patients, so ECG monitoring and facilities to address cardiac arrest are essential[5]
- Occlusive, semipermeable membrane moist wound healing dressing or similar, are applied as a mask, according to the depth of the injury
- A large number of surgeons prefer to use only Vaseline® (petroleum jelly) and non-adherent dressings with a tubular elastic type dressing for retention of the dressings. This allows for easy dressing change over the first 48–72 hours with the excess exudate
- Trichloroacetic acid (TCA) is less toxic and is not absorbed systemically, thus is suitable for patients with cardiovascular, renal or hepatic disorders
- TCA produces a milder peel and is suitable for treating mild sun damage through to superficial lines.

See recommended websites (skin maintenance) at the end of this chapter.

## Chemical peels

**Box 29.4** Skin resurfacing – clinical principles.

- The purpose of chemical peels is to create an 'injury' to the skin by a controlled process of applying agents

**Box 29.5** Chemical peels – principal contraindications – risk management issues.

- Oily skin
- Scleroderma
- Post radiated tissue
- Active herpes simplex 1
- Severe skin damage by the sun
- Individuals with dark skin tones[5].

---

**Box 29.6** Chemical peels – post-peel risk management issues.

---

- Major complications include full thickness skin loss, hypertrophic scarring and infection
- Lesser wound complications vary from mild skin bleaching or hypertrophic scarring to severe hyperpigmentation and prolonged erythema
- Patients must be appropriately educated pre treatment, regarding the risks, discomfort, need for complexity of wound care during recovery, down time associated with the varying degrees of peel depth, and potential adverse clinical outcomes
- Patient dissatisfaction at results.

---

**Box 29.7** Chemical peels – wound bed repair and management.

---

- A considerable degree of burning sensation and significant oedema is experienced for the first 24–48 hours depending on the depth of the peel
- Pre-emptive and regular four to six-hourly oral analgesics (rapid working and extended effects) and cold compresses can provide some initial comfort in the first 24–48 hours
- Alternatively an occlusive semipermeable membrane moist wound healing dressing or similar may be applied and this may provide a relative degree of pain relief
- Some surgeons prefer the wounds left open and Vaseline® or neomycin ointment applied
- Dressings are usually removed after 24–48 hours and the wound will resemble a superficial partial thickness burn
- The skin is then dusted with antimicrobial thymol to encourage crusting
- Moist wound healing occlusive dressings may be re-instated but most surgeons prefer to leave the wound open (with ointments of choice applied, e.g. Vaseline®, antibiotic ointment or topical sunblocking agents with moisturisers)
- Regimes of eschar care/removal must be strictly followed according to the individual surgeon's instruction for the best results (i.e. NO premature picking or removal of eschar)[1–8]
- Many companies (e.g. GlyDerm® or SkinCeuticals®) now provide pre-peel preparation product regimes, and similar for post-peel recovery skin care, in a total 'start to finish' kit form

- Working with a selected accredited company, the practice nurse can encourage and supervise a disciplined daily regime that the anxious patient can follow with minimal effort and anxiety
- The practice nurse can also provide regular patient monitoring and can report any adverse events/feedback to the surgeon
- Downtime is dependent on the depth level of peel and patients must be aware of this.

See recommended websites (post-peel skin care) at the end of this chapter.

---

## Laser application

**Laser** is an acronym for **L**ight **A**mplification by **S**timulated **E**mission of **R**adiation[1–7]. The properties of laser light allow for the transmission of a high-energy beam over a significant distance without diminution of its potential energy or other properties at the point of absorption[1–10].

The various types of lasers are named according to the specific 'medium' in which the light is generated, for example, argon, erbium, carbon dioxide ($CO_2$) and Nd:YAG (short for neodymium-doped yttrium aluminium garnet). Each medium has its own specific wavelength, and consequently absorption characteristics, with each type being more suitable for some procedures than others. More sophisticated machines are being developed that combine a range of features in one machine, allowing for greater treatment choices at single sittings according to the patient's specific pathological needs in different facial or body zones[1–10].

### Ablation

A basic understanding of physics and the technical application of each 'medium' that is necessary to achieve the specific desired level of ablation, without destroying deep dermal cells can be useful.

Lasers used for skin resurfacing are mainly $CO_2$, Erbium, or Nd:YAG and the wavelengths of each are within an invisible spectrum. The energy generated is rapidly converted to heat on absorption in water

(water in cells within the skin). Controlled laser beams discharge their heat, burning the skin on contact, with minimal penetration. This 'burning' is referred to as 'ablation' and in order to attain the desired level of penetration for ablation to occur, more than one 'pass' of the beam may be required to be undertaken.

Ablation can be paralleled to burn depths that occur when skin is exposed to various levels of heat. Superficial and partial thickness burning/ablation, retains the residing hair follicles and sweat glands, allowing healing by normal contracting and resurfacing forces to occur.

The depth of the ablation selected is related to the condition being treated. For example, localised ablation is for superficial treatments for benign lesions, local scar revisions, resurfacing for zones of acne scarring, or specific ageing lines around the mouth or forehead.

Full face resurfacing is undertaken at varying levels within particular zones of superficial and deep facial lines, and this may be combined with surgical facelift procedures[1-10].

Regardless of the type of surgical laser machine being used, specific safety precautions and risk criteria for laser used are based on the American National Standards Institute[1-10]. All staff working within, or adjacent to the zone of use, must be educated and certified regarding the use and protection afforded by these standards. The potential for fire and patient/staff injury is high where these standards are disregarded.

---

**Box 29.8** Risk management issues 1 – contraindications for laser resurfacing of the skin.

- Active herpetic lesions
- Accutane therapy 6–12 months prior to proposed surgery
- Unbleached, dark skin
- Skin conditions (e.g. scleroderma)
- Previous radiation therapy
- Poor patient co-operation with preoperative preparation of skin.

---

**Box 29.9** Risk management issues 2 – preoperative management.

- Medical assessments may be required if the patient has morbid conditions that may compromise recovery, for example, diabetes mellitus, coagulopathies, or congenital syndromes that affect normal dermal/epidermal skin layer repair
- Specific/disciplined skin maintenance/preparation begins three to six weeks prior to procedure (see Box 29.4)
- Laser resurfacing is a powerful stimulator for the herpes simplex virus and preoperative anti-viral aciclovir prophylaxis (e.g. Zovirax®) is recommended for all facial resurfacing[1-7]
- Prior to some procedures, antibiotic prophylaxis may also be appropriate where recent low grade infections have been present (e.g. 'pimples' or active acne).
- Patient education regarding postoperative treatment regime.

---

**Box 29.10** Clinical risk management issues – special considerations.

- Patients who may be at greater risk of adverse reactions following resurfacing procedures are those with active herpes simplex or other viral infection, collagen diseases or autoimmune disorders, or those who have undergone recent treatment with Roaccutane® for acne (see: http://www.roaccutane.com.au), or recent irradiation, etc.[1-5].
- Special precautions are necessary for patients with skin sensitivity, allergies, atopic skin reactions, seborrheic dermatitis and eczema
- Dark skinned persons have a greater tendency to develop pigment changes
- Extreme caution is required with those who have a previous history of scar hypertrophy and/or keloid formation[1-7]
- Some controversy exists regarding the safety of performing laser resurfacing at the same time as open surgery facelifting procedures because of the risk of necrosis in the region of the distal pre-auricular skin
- For eyelid surgery, and/or endoscopic brow lift, laser resurfacing is often an integral part of the procedure
- These are individual surgical decisions which will be based on many of the above considerations, and professional discretionary judgement as to the efficacy and safety for the individual patient[1-8].

**Review**

*Setting goals of care and preferred clinical and patient outcomes*, Chapter 2, Boxes 2.7–2.9. Adapt according to risk management issues and clinical patient needs.

---

**Box 29.11** Perioperative management.

- Emla®, a skin absorbing local anaesthetic cream is frequently used for small regions, and for wider areas local anaesthesia without vasoconstrictors (these limit tissue absorption of laser light)
- For large areas and full facial laser ablation, regional or general anaesthesia is administered
- Intravenous corticosteroid medication, followed by pharmacological defined reducing doses, is often used for full face resurfacing to assist in the reduction of swelling.

---

**Box 29.12** Postoperative management – wound bed repair and maintenance.

- Erbium laser applies a low level resurfacing technique thus producing less thermal injury. But because it is in the germinative skin layer (which holds the skin's water) there is a significant amount of wound exudate. Less exudate is observed with $CO_2$ ablation which goes deeper, absorbing water and coagulating micro vessels as laser passes are made
- Following $CO_2$ resurfacing, or ablation where the depth is greater, the wound/s are usually dressed with occlusive semi-permeable membrane moist wound healing dressings or a similar non-adherent dressing for 24–48 hours, depending on the degree of exudate
- Many surgeons prefer to manage the wounds open with frequently changed cooled normal saline gauze, until ooze and warmth related to the major inflammatory response have ceased or declined significantly after about 48 hours
- Initial stage is followed by frequent facial bathing, and the application of Vaseline®, neomycin or 1% hydrocortisone ointment, to prevent or limit desiccation
- The use of a child's bib with plastic backing can reduce the staining of clothes

---

- Following dressing removal, Vaseline® or neomycin ointment is applied or, again, the staged application of products provided in the 'kit' form are used
- Newly healed skin is extremely sensitive, so only recommended skin care products should be applied so as not to precipitate additional reactions
- Surgeons and practice nurses can advise on the most appropriate for individual cases, used in their practices (e.g. the use of the skincare 'kits', which are directed to specific levels of ablation, can be useful guidelines)
- Regular four to six-hourly oral analgesia, and night sedation (e.g. low dose lorazepam) assists in comfort for the first 48–72+ hours
- Healing takes about three to five days for superficial resurfacing, and seven to ten days for deep ablation
- At about one to three months post laser resurfacing, more advanced skin care maintenance programmes may be slowly and gently introduced, but this will only be advised in the absence of any post-healing problems (e.g. itchiness or increased pigmentation).

---

**Box 29.13** Late postoperative results and complications.

- Laser resurfacing can deliver very dramatic positive changes but, as in all surgery, complications can occur
- Of significant concern are complications such as herpes simplex or bacterial infections
- Depending on the depth of treatment, skin type and the region treated, prolonged erythema and itching may continue for six months or longer
- Ongoing cool compresses, steroid creams and/or antihistamine medications may be required[1–4]
- Hypertrophic scarring is a major complication[1–4]. This may be avoided by the surgeon undertaking a test patch prior to deciding on substantial surgery
- Some patients (e.g. with olive or dark skin) are prone to blotchy pigmentation. Tretinoin and hydroquinone can help to reduce this
- In the long term (up to two years) some reduced pigmentation and lines of treatment zone demarcation can be of concern to the patient
- The application of high quality medical grade camouflage make-up products, which include the highest levels of sunscreen protection, and are long acting, are usually suggested by the surgeon or practice nurse
- These can greatly reduce anxiety of patients undergoing this form of skin treatment who wish to return to work as soon as possible[10]
- Laser treatment may also be an adjunct to facelift procedures to remove circumoral and glabella wrinkles.

See recommended websites (laser resurfacing, herpes simplex treatment options, camouflage make-up) at the end of this chapter.

## Dermabrasion

### Box 29.14 Dermabrasion.

- Dermabrasion is a resurfacing technique utilising a motor driven hand piece (12 000–15 000 rpm) that drives/rotates various sized diamond tipped burrs[1–4]
- The technique aims to 'abrade' the epidermis and superficial layer of the dermis, resulting in dermal contraction and epidermal resurfacing
- It is usual to undertake a test patch behind the ear before engaging in a full procedure, allowing healing to take place and judging the efficacy of the outcome, particularly in relation to altered pigmentation
- It may also be an adjunct to facelift procedures to remove circumoral and glabella wrinkles
- Wound management and postdermabrasion complications are similar to TCA peels
- Frequent micro dermabrasion techniques are becoming more popular in skin care centres, reducing down time related to peels.

## Botox treatment

**Botox**® is a formulation of *botulinum* toxin type 'a'. It is derived from the bacterium *Clostridium botulinum*. This bacterium produces a protein that blocks the release of acetylcholine and relaxes muscles. Type 'a' is just one of seven different types of botulinum toxin (a, b, c1, d, e, f, and g), and each has different properties and actions. No two of these botulinum toxins are alike.

Botox® may be injected 2–3 weeks prior to laser surgery in the glabella (e.g. frown lines) and lateral eye skin (e.g. 'crow's feet' wrinkling). When applied, purpose-made preoperative skin preparation management products have demonstrated that results are better and healing is accelerated.

See recommended websites (Botox® treatment) at the end of this chapter.

**Review**

*Auditing preferred clinical and patient outcomes,* Chapter 2, Boxes 2.10–2.12.

## Facelift (rhytidectomy)

Despite the extensive promotion of the benefits of a lifetime of protecting the skin, many patients will continue to request/require facial rejuvenation by closed or open surgical methods to address increased skin wrinkling and gravitational changes.

Also known as rhytidectomy, facelift is a major surgical procedure undertaken to camouflage the signs of ageing by the undermining of the facial skin, tightening facial muscles, and excising excess skin (Figure 29.2). It may or may not be accompanied by adjunctive procedures that enhance the overall result/outcome of the surgery.

For example, the endoscopic approach is becoming an increasing feature of brow and facelift surgery. The choice of which of single or combined procedures is most appropriate is a surgical decision determined by the age of the patient and degree of restoration seen as necessary. Superficial liposuction, laser resurfacing, dermabrasion and/or chemical peels may be undertaken at the same sitting, prior to or following deep tissue surgical intervention.

Prior to committing to an open facelift the surgeon will examine the patient's skin, facial features and neck, to ascertain the degree of intervention appropriate to attain what the patient requests. As with almost all plastic surgery, an objective selection criterion is used in order that the choice of the procedure meets the needs of the patient, age and existing morbidity.

It also requires a commitment by the patient to co-operate in all aspects of skin preparation, medical care, time required for aftercare, down time (no smoking) and ongoing skin maintenance programmes[1].

For patients who are undergoing medical treatment for, for example, hypertension and/or psychological conditions, previous deep vein thrombosis or previous anaesthetic problems, medical consultation must be undertaken with the treating physicians to ensure risks to the patient are avoided. Clarification

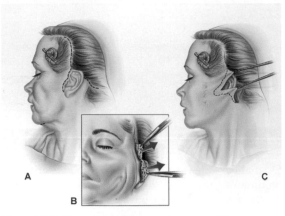

**Figure 29.2** Open face lift procedures – incisions and undermining of skin related to knowledge of vascular anatomy. With permission: Professor G.I. Taylor.

of continuation or changes to treatment requirements should be obtained in writing.

---

**Box 29.15** Summary of management principles and approaches.

- The procedure of facelift is not suitable for most rare congenial conditions that affect the normal dermal contraction of the skin
- The overall procedural aims of facelift are to remove loose skin, excise excess fat, tighten facial muscles, and firmly redrape the skin over the facial bony structure
- Facelift procedures aim to achieve what laser or chemical peel cannot completely achieve
- Deep tissue plastic surgery encompasses a process that exposes the tissues beneath the dermis (Figure 29.2)
- Facelifts may be at a superficial level (e.g. for young persons – under 40 years – often endoscopic, or minimal incisions around the ears) or at a deep level (e.g. older persons – over 40 years – open with adjunctive resurfacing procedures) and may be undertaken on both females and males
- Where severe facial lines are an issue, staged laser or chemical peels may precede facelift in selected patients
- Facelift may be undertaken in association with other adjunctive surgical procedures such as blepharoplasty, and varying degrees of facial rejuvenation procedures
- Although the use of endoscopic surgery is becoming

increasingly common, for some outcomes open surgery may be the preferred option
- Blepharoplasty, and circumoral laser therapy or dermabrasion, are often used in association with facelifting procedures, and endoscopic adjuncts and liposuction may be included simultaneously.

---

**Box 29.16** Clinical risk management 1.

- Haematoma is the most common surgical postoperative complication (2–5%)[1] and with the age of the patient being older than persons usually presenting for open aesthetic facial surgery (patients are usually over 40 years of age), a full medical examination, list of medications, and a medical workup are essential
- Because of the higher level of blood supply in the male face, the complication of haematoma is greater than in females[1]
- In both sexes, problems of hypertension, recurring particularly during and after the surgical procedure, risk of deep vein thrombosis/PE, potential coagulation anomalies, smoking, lifestyle, etc., require to be addressed to prevent or minimise complications that may compromise the surgery, or place the patient in a life-threatening situation for a major elective cosmetic procedure
- This technique should be considered a major surgical procedure and all the preparatory protocols should parallel this
- Following examination and return of all tests required, a second or third consultation with the patient will confirm or deny the appropriateness of the procedure for the individual patient
- With high patient expectations of the potential result, and for patients at medical risk, lesser invasive procedures may be suggested
- Patients must be fully informed of the risks, side effects and potential long-term complications verbally, and in writing. The consent for operation should reflect any information provided.

---

**Box 29.17** Clinical risk management 2 – postoperative potential risks and complications.

- Injury to the nerves that control the facial muscles, regions of numbness, bleeding, infection, poor healing, hypertrophic scarring and asymmetrical results

- Avascular necrosis of the skin zones around or behind the ears can occur, significantly delaying healing, and compromising the aesthetic results
- It is reported that the potential for skin necrosis is 12 times the average (1–3%) in patients with a current history of smoking[4]
- Early side effects include temporary bruising, swelling, skin tenderness and sense of tightness
- Following surgery males will need to shave behind the ears, as the hair bearing skin will have been repositioned higher than previously.

See recommended websites (facelifts) at the end of this chapter.

## Review

*Setting goals of care and preferred clinical and patient outcomes*, Chapter 2, Boxes 2.7–2.9. Adapt according to risk management issues and clinical patient needs.

### Box 29.18 Perioperative management.

- A sedative (e.g. lorezepam) is generally prescribed for the patient the night prior to the procedure, to provide a good night's sleep, and general relaxation
- General anaesthesia with local anaesthetic and vasoconstrictors
- Local anaesthetic and vasoconstrictor (combined with IV sedation). This has an active duration for the procedure of up to four hours but may be supplemented if the procedure is extended
- Patients should have adequate fluid balance management and continuous cardiorespiratory monitoring
- Long procedures present risks of physical pressure point compromise and physical discomfort, and special attention should be paid to this
- If the patient has a full bladder this will cause discomfort and may be misinterpreted as the local anaesthesia losing its effect
- Immobility poses risk of deep vein thrombosis and provision for this (TED stockings and heparin therapy) should be considered as an integral element of pre-, intra- and postoperative care
- Surgical procedures undertaken under general anaesthesia require the use of mechanical calf stimulation to sustain venous return.

### Box 29.19 The surgery.

- The surgical dissection includes loosening of the skin off the fascia and then the redraping of the loose skin over the facial skeleton
- This results in excess skin, in the form of skin flaps, in front of and behind the ears – excess skin is excised
- Overzealous excision of the excess skin in these wound zones is the principal area of tension, resulting in avascular necrosis, particularly as a result of postoperative oedema and facial movement
- It is interesting to note (see Chapter 7, mobility of the skin and implications in wound repair) that in most facelift procedures the tightening of the platysma muscle, a component of the superficial musculoaponeurotic system (SMAS) has become an integral part of the modern facelift procedure
- This element of the procedure has significantly increased the effectiveness and longevity of the procedure
- The medial borders of the platysma muscle are suggested to become ineffective in assisting to retain firmness of the skin under the chin as the individual ages
- Risks/complications may be associated with tension at the distal end as the skin is tightened towards the ear incision. This can result in avascular necrosis, the major complication of the procedure (Figure 29.2, tissue flaps)
- It must be appreciated that the older the patient, the thinner the skin, and any additional excess tension (e.g. caused by haematoma and oedema) combined with the fragility of the blood supply, places greater stress on the wounds, and thus increases the potential for wound complications associated with skin vascularity
- These wounds usually recover by specialist wound care assisting the granulation process
- Depending on the extent of the surgery, facelift and adjunctive procedures may be undertaken as day, or overnight stay
- Internal negative pressure drains are usually removed after 24 hours
- Patients are usually required to remain for two hours after drain removal to ensure no bleeding occurs from micro vessels trapped in the drain tubing holes.

## Postoperative nursing management

### Box 29.20 Safety.

- Conforming primary head dressings and firm (not tight) compression bandages may be applied for 24–48 hours
- Alternatively, the primary application of conforming adjustable head/facial compression garments, which aim to distribute compression more evenly, is becoming more popular
- Regardless of what dressing is chosen, the aim is to prevent/minimise bleeding postoperatively, as with the vasoconstricting agent used in the local anaesthesia beginning to lose its efficacy, blood pressure increasing, and general patient movement, the potential for bleeding increases
- Haematoma may be diagnosed by gently gliding the hands across the upper and lower surface of the face for any abnormal or firm swelling greater than the existing firmness of the skin itself
- Both sides must be checked, and compared for any increasing or 'firm' swelling zones particularly in regions of least resistance, and where gravity, for example, the lower cheek or neck area, allows a haematoma to collect
- Should a significant haematoma develop, the surgeon may remove sutures and allow the collected blood to be removed. In some cases the patient may require to be returned to the operating theatre for haematoma evacuation and checked for any arterial bleeders, under optimal surgical conditions
- The author has seen two cases where haematoma developed so quickly in the neck, compressing the trachea, that emergency tracheostomy was required to restore the airway due to failed tracheal intubation
- As previously indicated, internal negative pressure drainage tubes may be inserted, and if used, are usually removed within 24 hours
- Any attempt to recommence smoking or ingest alcohol (raises blood pressure) to relieve apprehension, should be counselled against, documented by the attending nurse clinician, and reported to the surgeon
- Small regular doses of oral diazepam are useful in apprehensive patients for short periods of time
- Risk management for the prevention of deep vein thrombosis/pulmonary embolism is paramount, and regular mobility/exercises encouraged
- Patients discharged as same day surgery must be given strict instruction to regularly undertake short walks at regular intervals and pillows under the legs at rest, to aid venous return.

### Box 29.21 Comfort.

- Pain or severe discomfort has the potential to restrain the patient from adequate respiratory and body movements and early, regular mobility
- With the extensive use of local anaesthesia, pain can usually be controlled with oral analgesia
- Pain not controlled by normal oral analgesic management, and expressed beyond expected parameters, must be assessed in relation to the development of a haematoma, or the patient's individual threshold
- Patients must be strongly encouraged to engage in physical movement appropriate to the prevention of deep vein thrombosis and cardiorespiratory compromise
- Self regulation is difficult if the patient feels uncomfortable in the initial important hours postoperatively when the risk of complications can be high in medium to high risk patients
- Night sedation (e.g. lorazepam or similar) may be appropriate for two to five days for comfort and to relieve anxiety[11].

### Box 29.22 Wound bed repair and management.

- Haematoma and/or necrosis of the skin flaps can compromise the healing down time and require moist wound healing dressings to reduce scarring as much as is possible
- Head dressings and conforming elastic bandages or appliances are often removed between 48 and 72 hours or earlier, depending on the surgeon's guidelines, and sutures may be removed at approximately five to seven days
- Depending on the degree of surgery, the application of conforming elasticised skull and facial support garments may be recommended for several days and/or at night only
- Vaseline® or neomycin ointment is applied regularly on the suture line to maintain softness of the skin and prevent cracking
- Reduced potential for scars may be improved with the applications of skin coloured adhesive surgical paper tape as often, and for as long as possible, up to four months
- High quality medically recommended camouflage make-up, with sunblock included, is suggested as an ongoing protection from the effects of photo ageing
- This allows the patient to return to the community early and with confidence.

**Review**

*Guidelines for wound care* of additional procedures such as laser treatments, discussed earlier in this chapter.

---

**Box 29.23** Independence and discharge management.

- With the majority of patients undergoing solely aesthetic facial surgery earlier than previously, most are conducted as day or 23-hour surgery, and mobility is expected to be early, with return to activities of daily living recommenced in stages, over several weeks
- Bruising will remain for up to three weeks and if other procedures have been included an increased complexity of wound care is required
- Although this information will be provided preoperatively, it is essential that patients have a high level of understanding of the risk of not following the guidelines, in writing, following discharge
- Many patients may express unhappiness with the result or have a range of grievances, including facial numbness, scarring or excessive bruising, and any such concerns or issues reported to the practice nurse must be referred to the surgeon for a consultation as soon as possible
- Patients who remain in hospital following major facelift surgery should be assisted to mobilise from day one after surgery, moving onto a chair, and going for short walks, increasing according to wellness, before being discharged after 48 hours into assisted care[1-4]
- On discharge, previously applied TED stockings should be removed and antiembolic stockings suitable for mobile patients should be measured to fit the individual patient and applied pre-discharge
- Patients must be instructed to continue to wear them and exercise as prescribed, for up to four months, particularly patients considered at high risk
- Following discharge, and in the absence of complicating factors, surgeons and practice nurses must provide written guidelines for increasing activities and timeframes, and full return to normal can be expected in approximately 10–14 days (but with some bruising unresolved) with application of medical grade camouflage make-up
- Full activities can commence in approximately three weeks and limited exposure to the sun maintained for up to nine months, but only with 15+ moisturising sun block cream applied every two hours
- A successful procedure can be expected to last for up to five years but is dependent on lifestyle (e.g. smoking and alcohol ingestion), limited exposure to the elements and disciplined overall skin care management as an integral part of sustaining a long-term and successful outcome.

---

**Review**

*Auditing preferred clinical and patient outcomes*, Chapter 2, Boxes 2.10–2.12.

---

## Reconstructive surgery to the eyelids

---

**Box 29.24** Aesthetic eyelid surgery – blepharoplasty.

- Blepharoplasty is a procedure to correct the excess of skin in the upper lids, and may be combined with removal of excess skin and fat (prolapse of orbital fat) in the lower lids
- In selected cases only the upper lids may be corrected when visual field defects occur (congenital or acquired ptosis or drooping eyelid)
- Similar forms of eyelid surgery may be performed to alter, for example, the oriental appearance to the western appearance
- Blepharoplasty is commonly undertaken at the same time as a facelift and/or brow lift
- A contraindication to undertaking the surgery is a condition called 'dry eye' syndrome (keratoconjunctival sicca)
- Tests for lacrimation can confirm the degree of the condition, which can also be a complication of surgery
- The operative procedure can take up to two or more hours depending on the severity of the condition and corrective procedure undertaken
- It is usually undertaken using local anaesthesia and sedation as a day surgery or outpatient.

See recommended website (blepharoplasty) at the end of this chapter.

---

**Box 29.25** Clinical risk management issues and potential complications.

- The principal major complication is haematoma and increasingly severe pain in the eye, and patients should be monitored for increasing swelling and level of pain
- Increasing pain and swelling can be a sign of emerging retrobulbar (behind the eyeball) haematoma and should be reported immediately to the surgeon
- Immediate measures should be undertaken (e.g. remove any sutures or incision line tapes) to prevent pressure on the eye globe and retina, which may result in potential blindness[1-7]
- A second important complication is the mechanical injury to the tear duct and iatrogenic 'dry eye' syndrome. As stated above, it should be established preoperatively that this did not exist before the decision to operate was made, to avoid litigation
- Dry eye syndrome requires the instillation of artificial tears and may be necessary for the rest of the patient's life
- Most problems are temporary, for example, discomfort, swelling, bruising, itching, sensitivity to light and excessive tear production, which may occur for about three weeks
- Any rubbing and use of harsh paper tissues should be discouraged.

---

**Box 29.26** Clinical nursing management – wound bed repair and maintenance.

- Bandaging of the eyes should be avoided and no external or occlusive compression applied
- The patient is required to have the head elevated at 30° for at least the first 24–48 hours
- At the completion of the procedure the eyelids will be separated by about 2–3 mm but full closure will be restored when local anaesthetic and postoperative swelling resolves
- Eye toileting and instilling of eye ointment is undertaken regularly, this protects the cornea from any injury – pharmacological eye drops may be prescribed

---

- Use of contact lenses for the first few days should be avoided to minimise/prevent irritation and subsequent desire to rub the eyes
- A container containing normal saline and some ice cubes is most appropriate with continuous cool (not ice cold) saline soaked gauze applied for comfort, and to reduce swelling for the first 24–48 hours
- Oral analgesia taken four to six-hourly at regular intervals for the first 72 hours will assist in comfort measures, and low dose night sedation may also be of assistance.

---

**Box 29.27** Ectropion of the lower eyelid.

- Ectropion is a condition which may be caused by sagging of the facial skin as a result of the ageing process accentuated by gravity where there is an inability of the upper and lower eyelids to close, protecting the cornea
- Secondary problems are conjunctivitis, eye irritation and excessive tear production in an effort to protect the cornea
- The corrective procedure is both functional and aesthetic and full thickness skin grafts (usually harvested from the upper eyelids or from behind the ears) are inserted into the skin of the lower eyelid releasing the tension and allowing the lower lid to close normally
- Tie-over dressings are used to secure the grafts at the recipient site (Figures 17.35 & 17.36)
- This procedure may also be undertaken following burns of the face to restore normal eyelid closure.

---

**Review**

*Setting goals of care and preferred clinical and patient outcomes*, Chapter 2, Boxes 2.7–2.9. Adapt according to risk management issues and clinical patient needs.

**Box 29.28** Discharge management – general issues related to facial surgery.

- Discharge education should explain to the patient the need for monitoring and reporting swelling and pain
- Wound bed management, eye toileting, administration of ointment, and the necessity of sitting up at least 30° to assist in venous drainage, and reduction of swelling by gravity is reinforced
- All instructions regarding avoidance of deep vein thrombosis should be followed with due diligence as the general age group seeking facelift are usually high risk patients, often with a past history of smoking and lifestyle risks
- Gradual resumption of normal activities is usually within 10–14 days as bruising resolves and exposure to the elements, particularly the sun, should be avoided as much as possible
- If this cannot be totally avoided, the patient should wear a hat and use prescription sunscreen eyeglasses for protection in highly lit areas and the outdoors[1–7]
- Makeup should be avoided until allowed by the surgeon and then only high quality medically recommended camouflage make-up (non-irritating) may be applied until bruising, etc., resolves. This allows the patient to return to the community early, and with confidence[1–7].

**Review**

*Auditing preferred clinical and patient outcomes,* Chapter 2, Boxes 2.10–2.12.

## References

(1) Aston S.J., Beasley R.W. & Thorne C.N.M. *Grabb and Smith's plastic surgery*, 5th edn. New York: Lippincott & Raven Publishers, 1997.

(2) McCarthy J.G. (ed.) *Plastic surgery, volumes 1–8* Philadelphia: W.B. Saunders, Harcourt Brace, 1990.

(3) Ausher B.M., Erikson E. & Wilkins E.G. *Plastic surgery: indications, operations and outcomes.* St Louis: Mosby, 2000.

(4) Stone C. *Plastic surgery facts.* London: Greenwich Medical Media Limited, 2001.

(5) Fortunato N. & McCullough S. *Plastic and reconstructive surgery.* Mosby's Perioperative Series. St. Louis: Mosby, 1998.

(6) Goodman T.A. (ed.) *Core curriculum for plastic and reconstructive surgical nursing,* 2nd edn. Pitman, N.J.: ASPSN American Society of Plastic Surgery Nurses, 1996. http://www.aspsn.org

(7) American Society of Plastic and Reconstructive Surgical Nurses. Lasers in plastic surgery. *Plastic Surgical Nursing,* 1997 (autumn); 17(3):123–79.

(8) Anderson S.V. Laser resurfacing: a survey of pre and post procedural care. *Plastic Surgical Nursing,* 1998 (winter); 18(4):229–34.

(9) Weinstein C., Ramirez O. & Pozner J.N. Postoperative care following laser resurfacing: avoiding pitfalls. *Plastic Reconstructive Surgery,* 1997 (Dec); 100:1855–66.

(10) VanderKam V.M. & Achauer B.M. Digital imaging for plastic and reconstructive surgery. *Plastic Surgical Nursing,* 1997 (spring); 17(1):37–8.

(11) Valente S.M. Anxiety among clients for plastic surgery. *Plastic Surgical Nursing,* 2002 (summer); 22(2):55–62.

## Recommended websites

**General aesthetic surgery – includes photo gallery of pre- and post-surgery**

http://www.plasticsurgery.org/index.cfm

http://www.plasticsurgerydoctors.com/procedures/plasticsurgeryprocedureindex.html

http://www.plasticsurgery.com.au/index.shtml

http://www.plasticsurgery.org/public_education/procedures/endoscopy.cfm

**Resurfacing – skin maintenance**

**Level 1** http://www.tretinoin.com/

http://www.nlm.nih.gov/medlineplus/druginfo/medmaster/a682437.html

**Level 2** http://www.icnglyderm.com

**Level 3** http://www.micropeel.com

**Chemical peels**

http://pubs.ama-assn.org/cgi/collection/dermabrasion_chemical_peels

**Post peel care**

http://www.skinceuticals.com

**Example of facial compression binders suitable for securing dressings in place**

http://www.fstubbs.com/noflash/lipo/facial.htm

**Facial laser resurfacing**

http://www.plasticsurgery.org/public_education/procedures/SkinResurfacing.cfm

http://www.infoplasticsurgery.com/laserresurface.html

**Herpes simplex and treatment options**
http://www.aad.org/pamphlets/herpes.html

**Camouflage make-up**
http://www.dermablend.com
http://www.skin-care-style.com/dermablend.asp
http://www.colortration.com
http://www.sachacosmetics.com/camouflage.htm

**Botox®**
http://www.botox.com(s)ite/professionals/faq/home.asp

**Aesthetic facial surgery including photog allery of pre-surgery and post-surgery outcomes**
http://www.plasticsurgery.com.au/procedures/facelift.shtml

http://www.plasticsurgery.org/public_education/
procedures/rhytidectomy.cfm
http://www.plasticsurgery.org/public_education/
procedures/facialimplants.cfm
http://www.plasticsurgery.org/public_education/
procedures/endoscopy.cfm

**Blepharoplasty**
http://www.plasticsurgery.org/public_education/
procedures/blepharoplasty.cfm

# Chapter 30

# Nasal Surgery

1. Rhinoplasty – septo-rhinoplasty
2. Post traumatic reconstruction – forehead rhinoplasty
3. Post tumour excision reconstruction

## Background

Nasal surgery aims to redefine the shape, and improve the **function** and **aesthetics** of the nose in the following circumstances:

- Congenital craniofacial malformations (e.g. cleft lip/palate) (see Chapter 23)
- Trauma:
  - Accidental – nasal fractures, sporting, motor vehicle accident, soft tissue included
  - Assault/abuse
  - Animal or human bites.
- Burns – scarring, loss of function and form
- Reconstructive surgery following removal of tumours
- Septal perforations due to cocaine sniffing.

## 1. Rhinoplasty – septo-rhinoplasty

### Box 30.1 Rhinoplasty.

- The desire to surgically redefine the size, and/or shape of the nose as a whole, or in part for aesthetic purposes (Figures 30.1 and 30.2)
- This surgery is referred to as a **rhinoplasty**
- Surgery may be undertaken as an open, closed, or combined procedure, and may include minor skin reduction at the alar bases
- Surgery may require bone (hip – skull, outer table) or cartilage grafts (rib)
- Silastic® implants may be used – initial good results but may be rejected and migrate out
- Cheek and/or chin implant may be inserted to correct overall facial asymmetry
- Chin surgery (bony reduction) may be undertaken to correct overall facial asymmetry

- More than one procedure may be necessary to satisfy the patient's requirement
- Surgical decisions are based on the degree of surgery to be undertaken and/or the surgeon's preference for specific surgical approaches.

### Box 30.2 Congenital malformations – trauma – septal perforations.

- Reconstructive procedures for post trauma (e.g. major assault, motor car accidents, gunshot wounds) and congenital malformations, associated with for example, cleft lip and/or palate, present significant surgical challenges
- Reconstruction may require adjunctive rib or hip bone grafts to replace missing or malformed structures to assist in form, function and aesthetics
- For children with cleft lip or cleft palate, surgery begins in the first 12 months of life and will often require primary and secondary procedures related to function and aesthetics of the middle third of the face
- Additional surgery to correct the position and function of the jaw may be required
- Trauma (accidental, sporting injury, or assault), may fracture the nasal bones and the septal cartilage, resulting in a distortion referred to as septal deformity or a 'crooked nose'
- This usually results in an alteration to nasal breathing and often leads to allergic conditions developing, due to the fragility and constant inflammation of the nasal mucous membrane
- In sportspersons (usually footballers or basketball players), full corrective surgery is not usually undertaken until the individual retires from active partici-

*Continued*

449

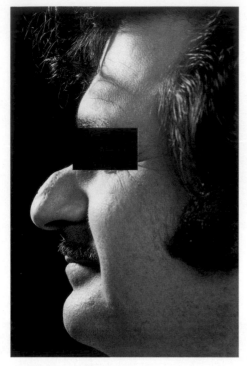

**Figure 30.1** Nasal deformity.

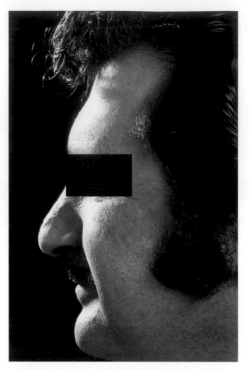

**Figure 30.2** Post-rhinoplasty.

pation in the sport as further injury intensifies the degree of the injury and corrective requirements
- The procedure will be designated septo-rhinoplasty on the admission and operating schedules
- The procedure may or may not require bone/cartilage grafts
- Habitual use/sniffing of cocaine powder (inhaled via the nose) may result in avascular necrosis of an area of the septum, leaving a perforation or hole that may require reconstructive surgery
- In addition to its considered euphoric effects, pharmacologically, cocaine acts as a local anaesthetic with vasoconstricting properties on the septal mucus membrane – cocaine soaked (4%) gauze packs or cotton buds are commonly used as preoperative nasal packs prior to intranasal surgery, and sinus washouts conducted in outpatient settings.

**Box 30.3** Preoperative risk management issues 1.

- Rhinoplasty or reconstruction of the nose is often suggested to be one of the most difficult surgical procedures where the patient's expectations of the aesthetic outcome, regardless of the aetiology, are for perfection rather than mere improvement
- Many patients requesting aesthetic rhinoplasty will present with a picture cut from a magazine and request surgery to accomplish the almost impossible
- The use of digital imaging that clearly depicts the whole of the patient's face, and demonstrates the likely improvement that nasal surgery would make to the overall profile, is an essential tool in aesthetic surgical practice
- More than one consultation may be required with some patients and records of all discussions, photographs and written agreements for potential improvement, should be maintained
- The patient must understand that the operation does not instantly produce their preferred outcome, as

oedema, and contracting healing tissues, may alter what is observed immediately post surgery, and several months later

- As previously stated, if patients believe that they have been promised the perfect outcome, they are very unforgiving and will seek redress through litigation
- 10% of patients are recorded to express dissatisfaction post surgery, with the most common complaint being that of nasal tip definition, such as too bulbous, too pointy, or upturned
- A secondary procedure to revise the nasal tip is a commonly requested procedure
- The most challenging cases that present are suggested to be those who have undergone previous aesthetic nasal surgery and are expressing varying degrees of dissatisfaction
- Secondary procedures to correct perceived or real anomalies can be technically more difficult than primary procedures, and may require cartilage and/or bone grafts
- Some surgeons may refuse to operate on patients who appear to have unrealistic expectations, as they can foretell a litany of continuing displeasure, dissatisfaction and, ultimately, litigation
- Practice nurses must be extremely discreet, and refrain from criticism of any kind regarding prior procedures or the patient's expectations
- Surgeons may seek peer review of the surgery, and psychiatric consultations to ascertain if there is any underlying pathology, particularly in patients who spend a lifetime undergoing aesthetic surgery with varying levels of dissatisfaction
- Because patient outcome expectations are very high, and the patient is usually very anxious, continuing patient support is important, and, regardless of the perceived insignificance of a patient's complaint, it must be taken seriously, recorded and reported to the surgeon, and resolved as soon as possible.

---

**Box 30.4** Clinical risk management issues – preoperative preparation 2.

- If the patient is an adult or adolescent, the nurse clinician should explain the importance of not smoking (smoking aggravates the nasal passages and airway, impairs blood flow to wound, and will potentially compromise the outcome) prior to and after the operation
- The patient history should be reviewed in relation to any morbid conditions, specific medications

which may instigate bleeding, or compromise wound healing

- Comprehensive patient education should be provided as to what to expect postoperatively (e.g. in particular, if nasal packs are to be used, rib cartilage or bone graft are required and drainage tubes are to be inserted)
- Instructions should be provided regarding mouth breathing, as the nose may be blocked temporarily and at different degrees for up to two to three weeks, due to oedema
- Patients should be encouraged to practise this preoperatively to be accustomed to the change
- Nasal sprays may be routinely prescribed pre- and postsurgery (e.g. oral corticosteroids, or corticosteroid-based spray preparations, to assist in preventing irritation, sneezing and swelling of the mucous membrane
- Irritated/sensitive mucous membrane is common in patients who have previously fractured their septum, or suffer from allergies and bleed readily
- In patients with a history of herpes simplex, a prescribed prophylactic treatment of aciclovir (Zovirax®) may be considered
- The anaesthetic should be discussed as most procedures are undertaken under local anaesthesia and sedation as day surgery patients
- Patients may be apprehensive about being 'awake'
- Following some specific cases, a 23-hour stay may be required, as post trauma or repeat nasal surgery has the potential to bleed more postoperatively, because it may be necessary to refracture the bones, realign the septum, and clear the turbinates
- The choice to insert postoperative nasal packing or special splints is made on the basis of the procedure and potential for bleeding
- Men should be requested to shave on the day of surgery to assist in securing the nasal dressings.

See recommended websites (general aesthetic surgery, rhinoplasty – includes photo gallery of pre and post surgery) at the end of this chapter.

---

**Review**

*Setting goals of care and preferred clinical and patient outcomes*, Chapter 2, Boxes 2.7–2.9. Adapt according to risk management issues and clinical patient needs.

## Anaesthesia

---
**Box 30.5** Anaesthetic choices.
---

- General anaesthesia – including cocaine (4%) nasal packs pre-operatively, and injected local anaesthesia with a vasoconstrictor for reduction of intraoperative and postoperative bleeding, and to provide postoperative analgesia
- General anaesthesia with induced hypotension may also instituted by the anaesthetist to reduce intraoperative bleeding
- Local anaesthesia and sedation – cocaine (4%) nasal packs pre-operatively, and injected local anaesthesia with vasoconstrictor for reduction of intra-operative and postoperative bleeding and analgesia
- The IV sedation commonly administered, midazolam, has an action that prevents the patient from remembering the event – this is referred to as 'retrograde amnesia'
- IV fluid replacement is given to maintain fluid balance normally taken in over the 24-hour period, and to prevent dehydration
- Total physiological monitoring for continual assessment of the patient's safety status.

## Surgery

---
**Box 30.6** Surgical options.
---

- The open technique (incision across the columella exposing the whole of the anatomy of the nose)
- Closed, with incisions made in the inside alar region
- Combined closed/opened.

---
**Box 30.7** Postoperative clinical risk management 1.
---

- Postoperative nasal packing and/or nasal splints may be required for 24–48 hours
- Spontaneous major uncontrolled bleeding (epistaxis) may originate from the removed turbinates but usually the nasal septum, when the nasal mucosa overlying a dilated blood vessel is injured

- This often occurs following discharge and must be reported to the surgeon immediately and the patient advised to go to the nearest medical centre
- Nose picking by the patient is stated to be a common cause but the patient should be questioned regarding any recent secondary injury or medications taken for discomfort such as aspirin or anti-inflammatory drugs
- Initially, bed rest, sitting the patient up in Fowler's position, applying icepacks on the back of the neck, and compressing the base of the nose for 10–15 minutes will usually stop the bleeding
- Secondary procedures may require insertion of cocaine nasal packs, IV morphine, fluid replacement, insertion of a specially designed or Foley catheter and further use of ice packs
- Failure of the bleeding to stop may require more radical surgical interventions similar to those used for uncontrollable nasal bleeding due to other medical causes.

---
**Box 30.8** Postoperative clinical risk management 2.
---

- Some patients may require a rib graft for reconstructing the nasal form
- Perforation of the pleura may occur and this will require chest drain inserted (under water seal) for a few days to maintain intrathoracic pressure
- This is not life-threatening but may shock the patient if they awake to find a chest tube *in situ*
- Adequate pain management (e.g. narcotics initially), respiratory observation and chest physiotherapy management are important, to minimise any respiratory compromise
- Clinicians should reassure the patient and provide support to restore confidence in the outcome of the overall procedure
- Bone grafts required to be harvested from the hip can be extremely painful postoperatively and negative pressure suction drains inserted for approximately 48 hours
- Adequate pain management (e.g. narcotics initially) is extremely important in order that the patient can be mobilised early and with the least degree of discomfort
- During the operative procedure a rare, accidental perforation of the cribiform bone plate that protects the brain dura may occur
- The dura may accidentally be perforated, exposing the brain to external bacteria (e.g. similar as to that

described in trauma or accidental surgical reconstructive fractures of the middle third of the face, discussed in Chapter 23)
- When changing the nasal bolsters the presence of clear/serous fluid may be a clinical indicator of this serious problem
- A test for glucose, both with a glucose stick and a pathology specimen must be undertaken to exclude the potential for the presence of this condition (brain fluid is high in glucose content)
- This can be an extremely dangerous (life-threatening) complication as meningitis may result from the exposure of the brain to the external environment
- Urgent treatment with IV antibiotics is required, and failure of the dura to spontaneously repair/seal off unassisted may require surgical intervention by major neurosurgery, and a fascia lata graft taken from the leg used to repair the hole/defect.

## Postoperative nursing risk management issues – 3

### Box 30.9 Safety.

- Initial monitoring should be half-hourly, for blood pressure, pulse and oxygen saturation
- Respiration should be counted as $CO_2$ retention may be occurring if the respirations are slow and shallow, as breathing changes from nasal to mouth
- Encouraging regular deep breathing and gentle coughing (throat clearing) if possible, is important in the previously sedated patient who is slowly recovering respiratory independence and to prevent potential for respiratory compromise (e.g. long anaesthesia and general lethargy postoperatively)
- The clinician should monitor for excessive swallowing as this can be as sign of potential silent bleeding down the back of the throat
- Swallowed blood precipitates gut irritation and vomiting (altered pH), so IV fluid should be maintained until the patient is drinking normally and any nausea/vomiting has ceased, to prevent dehydration
- Antiemetics should be given to control nausea and vomiting, or anxiety, and sucking of ice chips can be helpful in providing small amounts of fluid replacement and reducing a 'dry mouth' feeling.

### Box 30.10 Comfort.

- In the absence of other adjunctive procedures as outlined above, patients will initially have general feeling of facial discomfort and will often complain of headache and anxiety[1–8, 10]
- This may be due to dehydration and/or a combination of facial discomfort related to inflammation and swelling/tension in this fixed skin region
- Oral analgesia (non-aspirin based), explanation of the potential cause, sucking of ice chips, cold packs to the eyes, and reassurance, is usually adequate to control this
- Unresolved headache and a rising body temperature (fever) may be an indication of more serious complications for example, septal haematomas, or other serious problems such as meningitis.

### Box 30.11 Wound bed repair and maintenance.

- Prescribed timing of nasal toileting, with normal saline and cotton buds, and care of any incisions are essential to maintain hygiene and prevent infection
- The presence of bruising, 'black' eyes and swelling are relatively normal postoperative events
- Normal saline soaked gauze dipped in a container with ice cubes used as cold compresses can provide comfort and be very soothing
- Oedema is usually present for about two to three weeks and complete swelling resolved between three and 12 months post surgery
- The timeframe for swelling resolution is essentially related to the extent of the procedure and the patient should be informed of this[1–7]
- The nasal structure will usually have some form of skin protecting and conforming splinting technique (e.g. adhesive surgical tape) applied across the nose and around the nasal tip, to secure the nasal tip in position
- This tape also provides a base for an overlying splint and may remain or be changed (as a retention splint) after the original plaster of Paris or metal overlying splint is changed
- A plaster of Paris moulded plastic (Figure 30.3) or metal splint (see example of range of plaster of Paris splints, Figure 30.4) may then be applied to protect from secondary injury, and immobilise the nasal bony structure in position

*Continued*

- Splints can also diminish swelling acting as a gentle, counteracting compressing support
- All splints should be applied with the degree of post-operative oedema in mind, for example, rigid metal or plastic splints have a high incidence of wound necrosis and tissue sloughing if tightly applied and post-operative oedema is significant[1]
- Clinicians must inform the patient to report any sharp pain, which would signify local skin ischaemia
- The length of time the splint remains in place depends on the surgeon's protocols and the extent of the surgery
- Plaster of Paris splints can become messy with the use of wet packs to the eyes and some surgeons may use these initially, remove them after 48 hours, clean and redress the region, and then apply a skin coloured plastic or metal splint which is more socially acceptable and easier to provide regional hygiene
- The patient will often have a dry mouth from continuous oral breathing, and frequent oral care and gentle mouthwashes should be advocated for comfort and retention of moisture of the mucous membrane
- Frequent application of Vaseline® or lip moisturiser is maintained to prevent the mucous membrane cracking and bleeding.

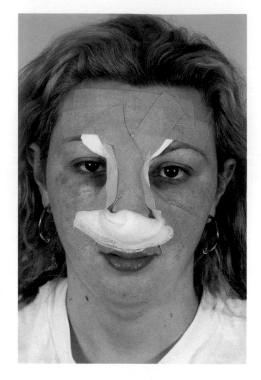

**Figure 30.3** Example of plaster of Paris nasal splint – and simple nasal drip collector.

**Box 30.12** Wound care – change of nasal bolsters.

- The nurse clinician should change the nasal bolster as required and record the colour of any exudate, and volume of any blood loss
- The bolster should be gently removed to prevent bleeding from any wounds around the alar base
- Nasal wounds should be kept clean by using swab sticks or cotton buds dipped in normal saline to remove crusts
- This is followed by the applications of Vaseline® or neomycin ointment or as prescribed by surgeon
- Custom-made nasal bolsters are useful as some patients may experience skin irritation from frequent removal and replacement of retention tapes. They are easy to change and are more aesthetic
- Renew the dressing tray by bedside, educating the patient in self-care and, as previously stated, request a return demonstration prior to discharge.

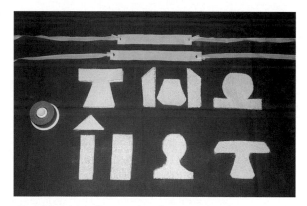

**Figure 30.4** Small example of range of plaster of Paris nasal splints – metal and moulded plastic also available.

See recommended website (latex-free nasal bolsters) at the end of this chapter.

---

### Review

*Setting goals of care and preferred clinical and patient outcomes,* Chapter 2, Boxes 2.7–2.9. Adapt according to risk management issues and clinical patient needs.

---

### Box 30.13 Independence.

- Patients will require physical and psychological support to return to activities of daily living
- Educating the patient to restore independence in self-care, wound hygiene and wound protective practices that do not compromise the procedure, allows greater acceptance of the outcome
- Many self-care procedures in nasal hygiene make the patient feel uncomfortable. This requires patience on the part of the clinician – it is useful to show the patient how to do this in front of a mirror and then ask them to demonstrate that they have mastered this.
- Patients will be interdependent for a day or so as they recover from the anaesthetic, and the return of the general feeling of the sensitivity of the nose
- Contact with the practice nurse 12–24 four hours post discharge and reinforcement of instructions regarding nasal care, discomfort, diet and maintenance of fluid intake, slowly increase the patient's ability to return to independence
- Patients should be encouraged to keep appointments for surgical follow-up and any comments made by the patient to the practice nurse or the surgeon, recorded in the patient's notes
- In the absence of any complications the patient can expect to be back to work in one to two weeks and increasing degrees of activities in two to four weeks according to the surgeons instructions
- Accidental trauma to the nose or sunburn for at least eight weeks must be avoided
- The final appearance following a relatively major rhinoplasty can be expected within one year or slightly longer.

---

### Box 30.14 Wound management – nasal packs.

- Nasal packs may be inserted in the nose postoperatively following fractured nose, rhinoplasty, nasal reconstruction, forehead flaps to the nose or any nasal procedure that requires packing to reduce postoperative bleeding, secure a graft or simply to retain a normal nasoseptal cartilage position
- Many nasal procedures include surgery to the nasal turbinates demonstrate a high propensity to cause bleeding postoperatively and this is a common cause for nasal packing, for compression, in the first 24–48 hours
- Example of nasal packs used:
  - Bismuth and Iodoform impregnated gauze
  - Glove fingers
  - Vaseline® impregnated gauze
  - Gelfoam® gelatin sponge
  - Sorbsan™
  - Kaltostat®
  - RhinoRocket® nasal tampons.
- Septal splints made from X-ray sheeting or similar, should be removed under supervision of the surgeon if the nurse is inexperienced as they can be difficult to remove in an anxious patient, and result in secondary injury[8]
- For many patients the insertion and removal of nasal packs appears to instil a greater fear than the entire surgical procedure
- Clinicians should be conscious of this and approach the removal of nasal packs with confidence, professionalism and concern for the patient's sensitivity regarding the procedure.

---

### Box 30.15 Removal of nasal packs – equipment and procedure.

- Plastic surgery nasal dressing pack, special plastic instruments, extra gauze, two kidney dishes, cotton buds, plastic backed absorbent pads, normal saline, gloves, ice pack and ice for patient to suck[8].

**Procedure:**

- The clinician should check the patient's notes for confirmation of time for pack removal, as packs should not be removed until ooze has ceased 24–48 hours postoperatively

*Continued*

- Patients should not be discharged until two to four hours after the packs are removed, in case bleeding occurs. This allows the patient to settle, and be observed for any problems of new ooze of blood
- Explaining the procedure in detail to the patient and encouraging questions is important as the patient is usually very anxious, and may have low pain threshold
- Giving pre-emptive oral analgesia 30–45 minutes prior to pack removal can assist in relaxing the patient and provides pain/discomfort relief, as this is often the most anxiety-provoking episode for the patient of the whole inpatient or return to surgery time
- Sit the patient in high Fowler's position, as this is an easier position for the procedure and allows the patient to bend forward as the packs are removed and fall into the dish, with minimal discomfort
- Instruct patient to breathe slowly and comfortably through the mouth as this helps to prevent the patient from retching from taste of any old blood whilst packs are removed
- Apply ice packs to the back of the neck as this aids in restricting blood vessels to the face, preventing further haemorrhage
- Encourage the patient to suck chips of ice – this helps to reduce anxiety further, and is a form of distraction
- Give the patient a kidney dish to hold under the nose as this allows packs to fall directly into a receptacle
- If the packs are sutured in place or together to prevent them falling back and being swallowed, cut the suture and discard
- Commence removal of packs separately, slowly and with even energy using forceps, disposing each pack into the kidney dish
- An even tension will minimise discomfort for the patient
- Packs may be a single piece of Vaseline® gauze packed into each nose
- Cover the packs immediately with a paper towel as some patients often have a feeling of revulsion at the sight and smell of the packs
- Once the pack are removed, clean the outer alar with normal saline soaked cotton buds
- Gently insert the cotton buds into the nares and clean in a rotating fashion
- This action will remove any blood clots present, allows easier breathing and prevents an environment for infection
- Apply a nasal bolster and monitor blood loss as removal of packs may cause raw areas to bleed. Instruct patient to rest quietly in bed for two hours, head elevated, continuing to suck on chips of ice

- Give the patient the call buzzer, as restricted movement allows ooze or bleeding to slow/stop and prevents the patient rising from the bed quickly, and from possibly fainting (postural hypotension).

**Box 30.16** Discharge management.

- Leave plaster/splint untouched – do not remove unless instructed
- Gently cleanse the eyes as necessary with water and cotton buds, and cleanse nose gently with water and cotton buds as instructed. Only clean the areas which can be seen by looking in the mirror
- Do not blow your nose, and refrain from bending or strenuous exercise as this may cause any small clots to dislodge and encourage bleeding to commence
- Numbness of the nasal tip may continue for some time, so strict adherence to the use of a moisturiser that includes UV blocking agents should be reinforced as sunburn will occur, creating a wound. Do not go out in the sun without a protective hat, use sun lamps or have hot showers or saunas until the surgeon permits
- Normal saline or sterile water nasal sprays may be prescribed if the nasal mucosa remains dry and irritating, and Vaseline® or similar should be applied as a moisturiser to prevent cracking and the discomfort of dry skin
- If sudden or abnormal bleeding (epistaxis) occurs at home:
  - Sit down
  - Place ice on back of the neck
  - Suck a piece of ice
  - Try to relax
  - Ask someone to contact the surgeon, or arrange to go to the nearest hospital emergency department.

See recommended websites (modern treatment for epistaxis) at the end of this chapter.

## Home monitoring following discharge

Patients should be called by phone within 12 hours of discharge to ascertain the colour of any exudate, level of bleeding, pain, nausea, vomiting, unresolved headache, and any general wound problems the patient may be experiencing. These should be referred to the surgeon and resolved as soon as possible according to the level of need.

---

**Review**

*Auditing preferred clinical and patient outcomes,* Chapter 2, Boxes 2.10–2.12.

---

## 2. Post traumatic reconstruction – forehead rhinoplasty

### Box 30.17 Wound bed management.

- The flap pedicle remains intact until vascular uptake is assured at approximately 2–3 weeks (Figure 30.5)
- Vascular monitoring is required, and any signs of vascular compromise (arterial or venous) will require particular sutures to be removed to relieve the tension
- Compromise is usually related to the vascular pedicle being kinked and this may be exacerbated by wound oedema and venous obstruction
- Four to six-hourly wound care with Vaseline® impregnated gauze, or gauze and antibiotic ointment is inserted under the pedicle to collect exudate, exclude blood collecting in the eye(s) and maintain wound hygiene
- Extreme care must be taken in order that the dressing or oedema does not place stretch/tension on the pedicle
- Suture line care is required 4–6 hourly with neomycin ointment applied to prevent dryness and breaks in the skin
- A nasal pack is usually inserted at the time of surgery to stabilise the flap and reduce movement of the pedicle – this may be removed after 48 hours
- Eye and nasal toilets are required 4–6-hourly and as necessary
- Pedicle is severed with the nasal component set into the nasal defect and any remaining tissue excised or replaced in the donor site to minimise the donor defect.

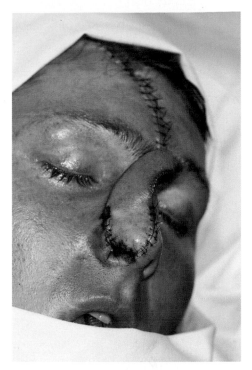

**Figure 30.5** Forehead rhinoplasty reconstruction post trauma.

## 3. Post tumour excision reconstruction

### Box 30.18 Wound bed management.

- Skin tumours are common on and around the nose and reconstructive procedures are based on the type of tumour, areas to be excised, site and tissue available for reconstructive purposes
- Tumours may also include cartilage and bone
- Skin tumours (often basal cell carcinomas) are relatively common on the face
- Small lesions are usually excised sutured primarily
- Larger tumours may require local flaps (Figures 30.6–30.8) or skin grafts for function and aesthetics (see Chapters 17 and 19)
- Wound management – according to repair type; see also Box 30.17.

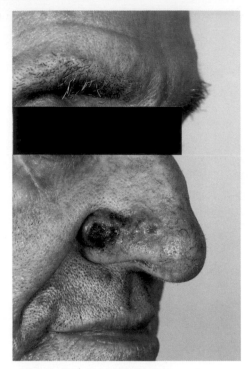

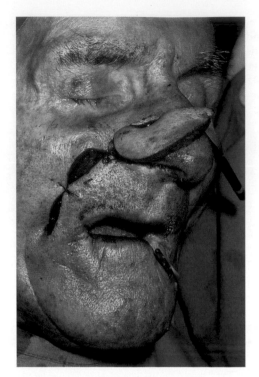

**Figure 30.6** Removal of small malignant skin tumour at the alar base.

**Figure 30.7** Defect repaired with local flap.

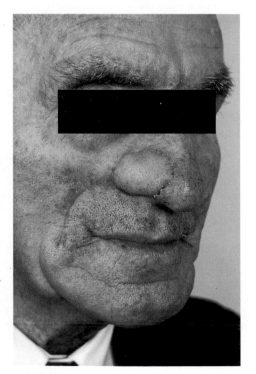

**Figure 30.8** Reconstruction by major local flap reconstruction.

## Review

*Setting goals of care and preferred clinical and patient outcomes*, Chapter 2, Boxes 2.7–2.9. Adapt according to risk management issues and clinical patient needs.

*Auditing preferred clinical and patient outcomes*, Chapter 2, Boxes 2.10–2.12.

# References

(1) Aston S.J., Beasley R.W. & Thorne C.N.M. *Grabb and Smith's plastic surgery*, 5th edn. New York: Lippincott & Raven Publishers, 1997.

(2) McCarthy J.G. (ed.) *Plastic surgery, volumes 1–8*. Philadelphia: W.B. Saunders, Harcourt Brace: 1990.

(3) Ausher B.M., Erikson E. & Wilkins E.G. *Plastic surgery: indications, operations and outcomes*. St Louis: Mosby, 2000.

(4) Stone C. *Plastic surgery facts*. London: Greenwich Medical Media Limited, 2001.

(5) Ruberg R.L. & Smith D.J. *Plastic surgery: a core curriculum*. St. Louis: Mosby, 1994.

(6) Fortunato N. & McCullough S. *Plastic and reconstructive surgery*. Mosby's Perioperative Series. St. Louis: Mosby, 1998.

(7) Morris A. McG., Stevenson J.H. & Watson A.C.H. *Complications of plastic surgery*. London: Baillière Tindall, 1989.

(8) Goodman T.A. (ed.) *Core curriculum for plastic and reconstructive surgical nursing*, 2nd edn. Pitman, N.J.: ASPSN American Society of Plastic Surgery Nurses, 1996. http://www.aspsn.org/

(9) Storch J.E. *Plastic surgery and wound management nursing*: postgraduate curriculum guide, syllabus, and course notes for students. Melbourne, Australia: Australian Catholic University, and St Vincent's and Mercy Private Hospitals, 2000 (revised 2004).

(10) VanderKam V.M. & Achauer B.M. Digital imaging for plastic and reconstructive surgery. *Plastic Surgical Nursing*, 1997 (spring); **17**(1):37–8.

(11) Valente S.M. Anxiety among clients for plastic surgery. *Plastic Surgical Nursing*, 2002 (summer); **22**(2):55–62.

# Recommended websites

**General aesthetic surgery, rhinoplasty – includes photo gallery of pre- and post-surgery**

http://www.plasticsurgery.org/public_education/procedures/CosmeticPlasticSurgery.cfm#15

http://www.plasticsurgery.com.au/procedures/nose.shtml

http://www.facialsurgery.com/ClkoffTPgt7_3016_12mh.html

http://www.nynose.com/

**Modern treatment for epistaxis**

http://wwwpatientcarenp.com/pcnp/articleDetail.jsp?id=110648

http://www.emedicine.com/ped/topic1618.htm

http://ehealthforum.com/health/subject79_211328_treat.html

http://www.physsportsmed.com/issues/1996/08_96/davidson.htm

**Latex-free nasal bolsters**

http://www.dalemed.com

# Index

Page entries for tables shown in **bold** type.
Page entries under main headings refer to general or introductory aspects of the topic.